Please return to: **WITHDRAWN**

PHARMA
R & D LIBRARY

ORAL MUCOSA IN HEALTH AND DISEASE

ORAL MUCOSA IN HEALTH AND DISEASE

EDITED BY

A. E. DOLBY

MD, BCh, FDS RCS Eng

Professor of Periodontology
The Welsh National School of Medicine
University of Wales, Cardiff

BLACKWELL SCIENTIFIC PUBLICATIONS
OXFORD LONDON EDINBURGH MELBOURNE

© 1975 Blackwell Scientific Publications
Osney Mead, Oxford
85 Marylebone High Street, London W1
9 Forrest Road, Edinburgh
P.O. Box 9, North Balwyn, Victoria, Australia

All rights reserved. No part of this publication
may be reproduced, stored in a retrieval system,
or transmitted, in any form or by any means,
electronic, mechanical, photocopying, recording
or otherwise without the prior permission of
the copyright owner.

ISBN 0 632 00101 1

First published 1975

Distributed in the United States of America by
J.B. Lippincott Company, Philadelphia,
and in Canada by
J.B. Lippincott Company of Canada Ltd, Toronto

Printed and bound in Great Britain by
Butler & Tanner Ltd
Frome and London

CONTENTS

Contributors   xiii

Editor's Preface   xv

1   Structure and Function of Normal Human Oral Mucosa   1
C.A. SQUIER, N.W. JOHNSON AND MARGARETE HACKEMANN

1:0	Introduction	1
1:1	The Functions of Skin and Oral Mucosa	1
1:1:1	Barrier function	2
1:1:2	Thermal regulation	3
1:1:3	Sensitivity	3
1:1:4	Secretion and excretion	3
1:2	The Organization of Skin and Oral Mucosa	4
1:2:1	Component tissues of skin and oral mucosa	4
1:2:2	Appendages of skin and glands in oral mucosa	5
1:2:3	Stratification of epidermis and oral epithelium	9
1:2:4	Components of the dermis and lamina propria	11
1:2:5	Regions showing specialized functions	13
1:3	The Epithelium: Keratin-producing Cells	18
1:3:1	Cell division and tissue turnover	18
1:3:2	Cell differentiation and keratin synthesis	27
1:3:3	Barrier function: the structural basis of permeability	40
1:4	The Epithelium: Non-keratinocytes	44
1:4:1	Types of non-keratinocytes	44
1:4:2	The melanocyte and epithelial pigmentation	51
1:5	The Boundary between Epithelium and Connective Tissue	55
1:5:1	The structure of the basement membrane	56
1:5:2	The origin of the basement membrane	58
1:5:3	Functions of the basement membrane	59
1:5:4	Epithelial–mesenchymal interaction	60
1:6	The Connective Tissue	64
1:6:1	Cells of the connective tissue	64
1:6:2	Fibre types and ground substance	77
1:6:3	Blood vessels and lymphatics	84
1:6:4	Nerves	86

Contents

1:7	Age Changes in Oral Mucosa and Skin	88
1:7:1	Changes in epithelial structure	88
1:7:2	Changes in epithelial turnover	90
1:7:3	Changes in connective tissue	90
1:7:4	Changes in appendages and glands	92
1:8	Further Reading	92
1:8:1	Skin	92
1:8:2	Oral mucosa	94
1:9	References	95

2 The Physiological Responsiveness of the Oral Mucosa: The Role of Saliva — 113
T.W. MACFARLANE AND D.K. MASON

2:0	Introduction	113
2:1	Secretion and composition	114
2:1:1	Secretion	114
2:1:2	Factors affecting composition	116
2:2	The Physiology of Saliva in Relation to the Oral Mucosa	118
2:2:1	Mucosubstances	118
2:2:2	Antibacterial factors	120
2:2:3	Permeability	122
2:2:4	Taste	124
2:2:5	Blood coagulation	126
2:2:6	Comparison with skin	126
2:3	Reduced Secretion	127
2:3:1	Clinical implications	127
2:3:2	Tests for functional activity	129
2:4	References	130

3 Immunoglobulin Systems of Oral Mucosa and Saliva — 137
PER BRANDTZAEG

3:0	Introduction	137
3:1	T and B Cells	139
3:2	Immunoglobulins: Classes and Characteristics	144
3:3	Immunoglobulins of Oral Fluids	151
3:3:1	Quantitation of Ig	151
3:3:2	Salivary secretions	152
3:3:3	Gingival crevicular fluid	159
3:3:4	Jaw cyst fluid	161
3:4	Immunoglobulins of Oral Tissues	163
3:4:1	Methods of detection	163
3:4:2	Major salivary glands	168

3:4:3	Buccal and labial mucosa—comparison with skin	176
3:4:4	Palatine and pharyngeal tonsils	183
3:4:5	Gingiva	185
3:4:6	Dental pulp	193
3:5	The Role of Immunoglobulins in the Physiology and Pathology of the Oral Cavity—concluding remarks	193
3:6	References	200

4 Oral Mucous Membrane Markers of Internal Disease: Part I 215
J. HAROLD JONES

4:0	Introduction	215
4:1	Diseases of the Gastrointestinal Tract	215
4:1:1	The Peutz–Jegher's syndrome	216
4:1:2	Oesophageal reflux	216
4:1:3	Peptic ulceration	216
4:1:4	Malabsorption	217
4:1:5	Acrodermatitis enteropathica	217
4:1:6	Crohn's disease and ulcerative colitis	217
4:2	Internal Malignancy	218
4:2:1	Metastases	218
4:2:2	Non-metastatic markers	218
4:2:3	Herpes zoster	218
4:2:4	Multiple mucosal neuromas	219
4:2:5	Mycosis fungoides	219
4:3	Diseases of the Connective Tissue	219
4:3:1	Systemic lupus erythematosus	219
4:3:2	Progressive systemic sclerosis (scleroderma)	220
4:3:3	Dermatomyositis	221
4:3:4	Polyarteritis nodosa; variants and similar diseases	221
	(a) Classical polyarteritis	221
	(b) Cutaneous polyarteritis nodosa	221
	(c) Wegener's granulomatosis	221
	(d) Giant cell arteritis	222
4:4	Granulomatous Diseases of Unknown Aetiology	222
4:4:1	Boeck's sarcoid (sarcoidosis)	222
4:4:2	Melkersson–Rosenthal syndrome	223
4:5	Oral Manifestations of the Accumulation of Metabolic Products	223
4:5:1	Amyloidosis	223
4:5:2	Cystinosis	225
4:5:3	Haemochromatosis	225
4:5:4	Hurler's syndrome	226
4:5:5	Lipoid proteinosis (hyalinosis cutis et mucosae)	226
4:5:6	Porphyria	226

4:5:7	Xanthomatosis	227
4:5:8	Miscellaneous deposits	227
4:6	Oral Manifestations of Systemic Reticulohistiocytic Proliferation	228
4:6:1	Histiocytosis X	228
4:7	Conclusions	228
4:8	References	229

5 Oral Mucous Membrane Markers of Internal Disease: Part II 233
M. M. FERGUSON

5:0	Introduction	233
5:1	Endocrine Glands	233
5:1:1	Pituitary gland	233
	(a) Growth hormone	234
	(b) Gonadotrophic hormones	235
	(c) Non-specific action from anterior pituitary	236
5:1:2	Adrenal cortex	236
	(a) Hypoadrenocorticalism	236
	(b) Hyperadrenocorticalism	238
5:1:3	Thyroid gland	239
	(a) Hypothyroidism	239
	(b) Hyperthyroidism	240
5:1:4	Parathyroid glands	240
5:1:5	Pancreatic islets	240
5:1:6	Gonads	241
	(a) Puberty	243
	(b) Menstrual cycle and oral contraceptives	243
	(c) Pregnancy	244
	(d) Menopause and post-menopause	244
	(e) Oestrogen-sensitive aphthae	245
5:2	Diseases of the Blood and Haematopoietic System	246
5:2:1	Defective haemostasis	246
5:2:2	Anaemia	247
5:2:3	Polycythaemia	248
5:2:4	Leukopaenia and agranulocytosis	248
5:2:5	Leukaemia	249
5:3	Nutrition and Oral Mucosa	250
5:3:1	Proteins and amino acids	252
5:3:2	Fatty acids	253
5:3:3	Vitamins	254
	(a) Vitamin A	254
	(b) Vitamin B_1 (thiamine)	255
	(c) Vitamin B_2 (riboflavin)	256
	(d) Nicotinic acid	258
	(e) Vitamin B_6	260

		(f) Pantothenic acid	261
		(g) Biotin	262
		(h) Vitamin B_{12}	262
		(i) Folic acid	267
		(j) Vitamin C	270
		(k) Vitamin D	271
		(l) Vitamin E	272
		(m) Vitamin K	272
	5:3:4	Minerals and trace elements	272
		(a) Iron	272
		(b) Zinc	276
		(c) Magnesium	277
		(d) Copper	277
		(e) Other trace elements	278
	5:4	References	278

6 Oral Cancer 301
W.H. BINNIE

6:0	Introduction	301
6:1	Clinical Features	302
6:1:1	Carcinoma of the lip	302
6:1:2	Intraoral carcinoma	303
6:1:3	Verrucous carcinoma	306
6:2	Incidence and Mortality	306
6:3	Survival	314
6:4	Aetiological Factors	319
6:4:1	Smoking	321
6:4:2	Tobacco chewing habits	323
6:4:3	Alcohol	324
6:4:4	Syphilis	326
6:4:5	Iron deficiency	327
6:4:6	Dental factors	328
6:5	References	330

7 Premalignant Lesions of Oral Epithelium 335
D. GORDON MACDONALD

7:0	Introduction—The Concept of Premalignancy	336
7:1	Lesions of Oral Epithelium which may be Premalignant	337
7:1:1	Leukoplakia	337
7:1:2	Candidal leukoplakia	340
7:1:3	Nicotine stomatitis	341
7:1:4	Erythroplakia	342
7:1:5	Lichen planus	343

Contents

7:1:6	Squamous cell papilloma	344
7:1:7	Chronic ulceration and mechanical irritation	345
7:1:8	Oral epithelial atrophy	345
	(a) Syphilis and leukoplakia	345
	(b) Oral submucous fibrosis	346
	(c) Kelly–Paterson syndrome	347
	(d) Atrophy in iron deficiency and vitamin B deficiency	348
7:2	Further Factors of Relevance to Premalignant Lesions and Malignant Transformation	348
7:2:1	Site	348
7:2:2	Age	350
7:2:3	Sex	350
7:2:4	Size of lesion	351
7:2:5	Natural history	351
7:3	Aetiology of Premalignant Lesions	352
7:4	Diagnosis of Premalignant Lesions	356
7:4:1	Epithelial atypia	356
7:4:2	Epithelial atypia as an indicator of premalignancy	358
7:4:3	Evaluation of epithelial atypia	359
7:4:4	Carcinoma in situ	361
7:4:5	Other possible aids to diagnosis of premalignant lesions	362
7:5	References	364

8 Bacterial and Viral Diseases and the Oral Mucosa 371
J.C. SOUTHAM

8:1	Bacteria	371
8:1:1	Introduction—bacterial ecology of the oral mucosa	371
8:1:2	Mutation and infective transfer	371
8:1:3	Antibiotic stomatitis	373
8:1:4	Acute ulcerative gingivitis	374
8:1:5	Actinomycosis	377
8:1:6	Tuberculosis	378
8:1:7	Leprosy	380
8:1:8	Syphilis	381
8:1:9	Infective endocarditis—the role of oral bacteria	384
8:2	Viruses	387
8:2:1	Mechanisms of viral disease	387
8:2:2	Diagnosis of viral infections	388
8:2:3	Antiviral agents	390
8:2:4	Classification of viruses	392
8:2:5	Smallpox virus	392
8:2:6	Molluscum virus	392
8:2:7	Measles virus	392
8:2:8	Mumps virus	393
8:2:9	Herpes simplex virus	393
8:2:10	Varicella–zoster virus	397

Contents xi

    8:2:11 Epstein–Barr virus 398
    8:2:12 Cytomegalovirus 400
    8:2:13 Papilloma virus of man 400
    8:2:14 Polyoma virus 400
    8:2:15 Coxsackie virus 400
    8:2:16 Australia antigen 401
    8:2:17 Diseases with a possible viral aetiology 404
  8:3 References 405

9 Oral Ulceration: Immunological Aspects 415
A.E. DOLBY

  9:0 Introduction 415
  9:1 Mechanisms of Immunological Injury 415
  9:1:1 The type I reaction 415
  9:1:2 The type II reaction 418
  9:1:3 The type III reaction 419
  9:1:4 The type IV reaction 421
  9:1:5 Autoimmune disease; peripheral and central origin 425
  9:2 Recurrent Oral Ulceration 427
  9:2:1 Mikulicz's recurrent oral aphthae 427
  9:2:2 Immunological findings in Mikulicz's recurrent oral aphthae 427
  9:2:3 Herpetiform ulceration 430
  9:2:4 Behçet's syndrome 431
  9:3 Pemphigus, Bullous Pemphigoid, Benign Mucous Membrane Pemphigoid 432
  9:4 Periodontal Disease 436
  9:5 Lichen Planus 437
  9:6 Antigens of Oral Mucosa and Skin 439
  9:7 HLA Antigens and Oral Mucosal Disease 440
  9:8 References 441

10 Disturbance of Salivary Gland Secretion: Sjögren's Syndrome 447
D.M. CHISHOLM AND D.K. MASON

  10:0 Introduction 447
  10:1 General Features of Sjögren's Syndrome 447
  10:1:1 Clinical features 448
  10:2 Oral Manifestations 450
  10:3 Diagnostic Techniques 451
  10:4 Laboratory Investigations 457
  10:4:1 Histopathology and lymphoreticular neoplasia 459
  10:4:2 Pathogenetic considerations 460
  10:5 Treatment and Management 461
  10:6 References 462

11 Candidal Infection of the Oral Mucosa 467
D.M. WALKER

11:0	Taxonomy, Culture, Identification	467
11:1	Candida as a Commensal Organism on Mucosa and Skin	467
11:2	Predisposing Factors	470
11:3	Non-specific Defence Mechanisms	475
	Salivary factors	475
	Epithelial barrier	476
	Iron deficiency	477
	Non-specific cellular defence	479
	Serum factors	480
	Candidal fungaemia	482
	Disseminated candidosis	483
11:4	Immune Response to Candida	483
11:4:1	Humoral immunity	483
	Antigenic structure of candida	483
	Diagnostic usefulness of candidal antibody estimations	484
	Protective or destructive role of humoral immunity in oral candidosis	485
11:4:2	Specific cellular immunity in candidosis	486
	Defects of cellular immunity	487
	Macrophage function in candidosis	489
	Immunological rehabilitation	489
11:5	Mechanisms of Pathogenesis	490
11:6	Classification of Oral Candidosis	491, 492–94
11:7	Pathogenesis of Oral Mucosal Candidosis—chronic hyperplastic candidosis (candidal leukoplakia—aetiology)	491
11:7:1	Defect in surface defence mechanisms	491
11:7:2	Defect in immune system—chronic hyperplastic candidosis (candidal leukoplakia)	495
11:8	References	499

CONTRIBUTORS

W.H. BINNIE FDS RCS Glasg, DDS McGill, *Department of Oral Medicine and Pathology, Guy's Hospital, London*

PER BRANDTZAEG Cand.odont, MS, PhD, *Immunohistochemical Laboratory, Institute of Pathology, University of Oslo, Rikshospitalet, Oslo 1, Norway*

D.M. CHISHOLM BDS, PhD, *Lecturer, Department of Oral Medicine and Pathology, Dental Hospital and School, University of Glasgow, Glasgow*

A.E. DOLBY MD, BCh, FDS RCS Eng, *Professor of Periodontology, Welsh National School of Medicine, Dental School, Cardiff*

M.M. FERGUSON BSc, MB, ChB, BDS, *Nuffield Dental Research Fellow, Department of Oral Medicine and Pathology, Dental Hospital and School, University of Glasgow*

MARGARETE HACKEMANN BSc, PhD, *Junior Scientist, Clinical Research Centre, Medical Research Council, Northwick Park, Middlesex*

N.W. JOHNSON MDSc, FDS, FRACDS, PhD, *Reader, Department of Oral Pathology, The London Hospital Medical College, London E1*

J. HAROLD JONES LDS RCS Eng, MB, BCh, MD, MRCPath, *Professor of Oral Medicine, Turner Dental School, University of Manchester, Manchester*

D.K. MASON, BDS, MD, FDS RCS (Ed & Glasg), MRCPath, *Professor of Oral Medicine and Pathology, Dental Hospital and School, University of Glasgow, Glasgow*

D.G. MACDONALD BDS, MRCPath, *Senior Lecturer in Oral medicine and Honary Consultant in Oral Pathology, Department of Oral Medicine and Pathology, Dental Hospital and School, University of Glasgow, Glasgow*

T.W. MACFARLANE BDS, MRCPath, *Lecturer, Department of Oral Medicine and Pathology, Dental Hospital and School, University of Glasgow, Glasgow*

J.C. SOUTHAM MA, MB, BChir, BChD, MRCPath, *Senior Lecturer in Dental Surgery, University of Edinburgh*

C.A. SQUIER MA, PhD, *Lecturer, Department of Oral Pathology, The London Hospital Medical College, London E1*

D.M. WALKER, BDS, FDS RCS Eng, MB, BCh, *Lecturer in Oral Medicine and Oral Pathology, Welsh National School of Medicine, Dental School, Cardiff*

EDITOR'S PREFACE

This book represents a critical presentation of modern scientific knowledge relating to oral mucosa and is intended primarily for graduates with a clinical or biological interest in the oral mucosa. It is intended also to serve as selective reading for undergraduate students.

The knowledge relating to the structure, function and disease of the oral mucosa has increased considerably during the past decade. Equally, the necessity for the interpretation of this basic knowledge has become of great importance to the clinician who seeks to base his practice on scientific principles. The contributors to this book have endeavoured to fulfil such an interpretative role. In addition to a reappraisal of the knowledge relating to the structure and physiology of oral mucosa comparison has been made with these features in the skin. The relationship of oral mucosal disease to systemic disease has been re-examined. Particular attention has been paid to those oral mucosal diseases in which a greater understanding of the disease process has arisen.

I would like to thank the authors for endeavouring to maintain, successfully, a coherent theme throughout the text. I would like also to thank the publishers, Blackwell Scientific Publications Limited, Osney Mead, Oxford, for their full co-operation, in particular Mr Per Saugman who has given generous support during the preparation of the book. Lastly, I would like to thank Mrs V. Davis for invaluable secretarial assistance.

CHAPTER 1
STRUCTURE AND FUNCTION OF NORMAL HUMAN ORAL MUCOSA

C.A. SQUIER, N.W. JOHNSON
AND MARGARETE HACKEMANN

1.0 Introduction

In writing this chapter we have attempted to provide an account of the structure of oral mucosa which will serve as a framework both for the physiological features described in subsequent chapters and for the pathological changes described in the second half of the book.

As the title suggests we have deliberately set out to relate the histology and ultrastructure of oral mucosa to its function as the lining tissue of the oral cavity, while at the same time considering some of the similarities and differences between this tissue and that covering the rest of the human body, the skin.

The account therefore begins with a survey of the major functions of oral mucosa and skin, followed by a general account of their organization. Sections 1:3 to 1:6, which follow, deal in more detail with the various components. Finally the way in which these tissues age is discussed.

References to recent original work are given throughout the text and a list of more general references is included at the end of the chapter which provide more comprehensive accounts of many aspects.

1:1 The Functions of Skin and Oral Mucosa

In discussing the functions of human skin it is easy to become preoccupied with details of the functional adaptations shown by this tissue and to forget what is perhaps its most significant role—its aesthetic qualities. To a great extent we describe (and judge) people by their skin—by its colour and texture, its hairiness, its dryness or its oiliness. Of course these aesthetic qualities are only the superficial manifestations of more basic properties that enable the skin to function as an efficient covering tissue, and thus

enable the organism to survive in its environment. These properties may be considered under the following headings:
Barrier function,
Thermal regulation,
Sensation,
Secretion and excretion.
In the following section these will be described and discussed in relation to the functions of oral mucosa. Other roles that are sometimes suggested for the skin include highly specific metabolic functions, such as the synthesis of vitamin D and cholesterol (Kandutsch 1964), and storage. There is little information about these processes in the oral mucosa, and they will not be discussed further in this chapter.

1:1:1 Barrier function

The skin is the barrier between the organism and the potentially hostile world around it. As well as protecting the deeper tissues from mechanical damage and solar radiation and preventing the entry of micro-organisms and toxic substances, the skin has in terrestrial animals to prevent dehydration of the body. This protective barrier function resides primarily within the epidermis, although both the dermis and the skin appendages, the hairs and glands, contribute to the effectiveness of the system, and it is worth remembering that should the primary epidermal barrier be breached, there are available in the dermis the protection provided by the inflammatory and immunological defence reactions.

The oral mucosa, while having the same embryological origins as the skin and showing in many ways a similar morphology, has less of a role to play as a barrier layer. There is mechanical insult, such as the trauma of mastication, but the lining of the oral cavity is rarely exposed to solar radiation. Information regarding the permeability of the oral mucosa is confusing, for despite the suggestions that the mucosa shows a permeability far greater than any region of the skin, salivary flow creates a perpetually moist mucosal surface without, apparently, causing waterlogging of the tissues. In the opposite direction a loss of interstitial fluid to the exterior is less likely to occur because of the humidity of the oral cavity, although a barrier to outward movement does seem to exist within the epithelium. Thus the oral mucosa is not simply a highly permeable lining membrane but has barrier functions similar to those of skin, the weakest link possibly occurring at the gingivo-dental junctions where the continuity of the epithelial surface is interrupted by the penetration of teeth.

1:1:2 Thermal regulation

The large surface area presented by the skin to the external environment makes it the most important factor in maintaining thermal homeostasis in mammals and this function is largely subserved by the connective tissue. Surface features such as creases and grooves increase the area while the presence of hair and subcutaneous fat provides insulation. The dermis is provided with an extensive vascular system and the blood flow to the skin is greatly in excess of the metabolic demands of the tissue. The presence of arterio-venous anastomoses enables the flow through the dermis to be regulated; increasing the blood flow leads to increased heat loss when the external temperature is lower than body temperature. When the external temperature is higher, heat loss is dependent on evaporation of water secreted by the sweat glands.

To what extent the human oral mucosa participates in thermal regulation is unclear because of a lack of detailed information on the organization and behaviour of blood vessels in this region. In the much-quoted example of the dog, it is known that during panting there is considerable heat loss from the tongue in which well-developed arterio-venous connections are present (Liebow 1963). Their existence in human mucosa does not appear to have been established (Hellekant 1972; see section 1:6:3).

1:1:3 Sensitivity

Much of the information reaching the nervous system from the outside is collected and transmitted by an extensive cutaneous nerve plexus. Sensory nerves terminate in both the epidermis and dermis over the entire body but are particularly concentrated, and show specialized receptor endings, in such regions as the palms and soles.

The oral mucosa has an equally extensive sensory innervation, terminating in both simple and organized nerve endings. The discrimination of certain sensations such as touch and temperature has been shown to be greater in certain oral regions, such as the lip, than in the skin; in mammals taste buds are located in the oral epithelium.

1:1:4 Secretion and excretion

The skin participates to a certain extent in both these processes although it is difficult, and perhaps meaningless, to try to separate these functions. Thus, although the sweat produced by the sweat glands contains water and small quantities of urea and salts, the prime function is the reduction of body temperature as a result of evaporation at the surface. The sebaceous glands produce a lipid-rich material that coats the skin while the secretion of apocrine glands probably represents a reduced expression of scent glands present in other animals.

In the oral cavity there are no sweat glands or apocrine glands and few sebaceous glands; the major secretion of the oral mucosa is provided by the salivary glands, whose activity maintains the moist surface of the mucosa and assists the mastication and passage of food. Saliva also has slight digestive functions and its secretory immunoglobulin system is an important component of the bodies defences (see Chapters 2 and 3).

1:2 The Organization of Skin and Oral Mucosa

Although skin and oral mucosa have the same basic structural components there are obvious differences between them. Compared to skin, oral mucosa is relatively moist, smooth and transmits the colour of the underlying vasculature more readily. Hairs, sweat glands and to a large extent sebaceous glands, are absent.

Skin shows a unique surface pattern of grooves and ridges on the palms, soles and digits, and everywhere there are extensive creases which probably serve as an adaptation to movement; with ageing there is an increase in surface creasing and wrinkling as a consequence of decreasing elasticity of the dermis (see section 1:7). The mucosal surface does not have such an intricate surface pattern and, possibly because of the more flexible nature of the tissue, rarely shows creases in areas where movement occurs. There are, however, characteristic surface features in certain regions: the clinical stippling seen in healthy gingiva represents small epithelial indentations which do not seem to involve the connective tissue (Rosenberg & Massler 1967; Owings 1969), the palatine ridges and the various papillae of the dorsal surface of the tongue are projections which include connective tissue as well as epithelium.

1:2:1 Component tissues of skin and oral mucosa

Skin is most simply divided into an outer epithelial component, the *epidermis*, and an underlying connective tissue, the *dermis* or *corium* (Figs. 1:1 and 1:2). The junction between the two tissues, the *dermo-epidermal junction*, is the site of the basement membrane and is distinct in histological sections, frequently showing an undulating boundary produced by the interdigitation of epidermal ridges, the *'rete ridges'* (or 'rete pegs'), with the *papillae* of the dermis. Two layers are usually recognized within the dermis, a superficial zone of loose connective tissue adjacent to the epidermis and surrounding the epidermal ridges—the *papillary layer*—and a deeper zone of denser connective tissue called, because of the net-like appearance of the fibre bundles, the *reticular layer*. The junction between these layers is not distinct. Beneath the skin is the *hypodermis*, a layer of connective tissue containing varying amounts of fat together with nerves and blood vessels and parts of various appendages and glands. There is no clear demarcation between the dermis and subcutaneous tissues.

The oral mucosa differs from skin in being a moist lining tissue, although in many other ways it shows similar morphological features and can be divided into equivalent regions. However, the terms epidermis and dermis are usually reserved for skin, the corresponding regions in oral mucosa being the *oral epithelium* and *lamina propria* (Figs. 1.1 and 1.2). The mucous membrane lining the gastrointestinal tract contains a third layer, the muscularis mucosa, consisting of smooth muscle and elastic tissue which separates the lamina propria from the underlying connective tissue of the submucosa. The absence of this layer from the oral cavity except in the region of the soft palate is another point of resemblance to skin and makes the recognition of a true submucosa more difficult and according to some authors, unjustified (Provenza 1964).

1:2:2 Appendages of skin and glands in oral mucosa

Present in the skin and derived largely from the ectodermal component are various appendages such as the hairs and hair follicles, sebaceous glands, apocrine glands, eccrine sweat glands and nails.

Developmentally, sebaceous and apocrine glands both form as outgrowths from hair follicles, which extend into the reticular layer of the dermis and sometimes deeper. Follicles are distributed over the whole body surface except for the palms, soles and muco-cutaneous junctions at densities of 40–1000 per cm^2 (Scheuplein & Blank 1971). In man, hairs probably serve mainly a sensory function and have a limited protective and insulative role. Opening into the neck of the follicles in most areas are the ducts of sebaceous glands. These are found in the skin at densities of 100–900 per cm^2 (Montagna 1963). Although these glands usually form part of the hair follicle complex (or pilo-sebaceous unit) they are present at muco-cutaneous junctions, where follicles are absent, and open directly on to the skin surface. Sebum, consisting mainly of lipid, is produced by holocrine secretion, which involves the complete breakdown of the secretory epithelial cells; while this secretion can emulsify with sweat and may spread over the skin to reduce water loss, its function is uncertain.

Apocrine glands are situated in the subcutaneous tissue and open into the hair follicles in the regions of the axilla, mammary glands, pubis, eyelids

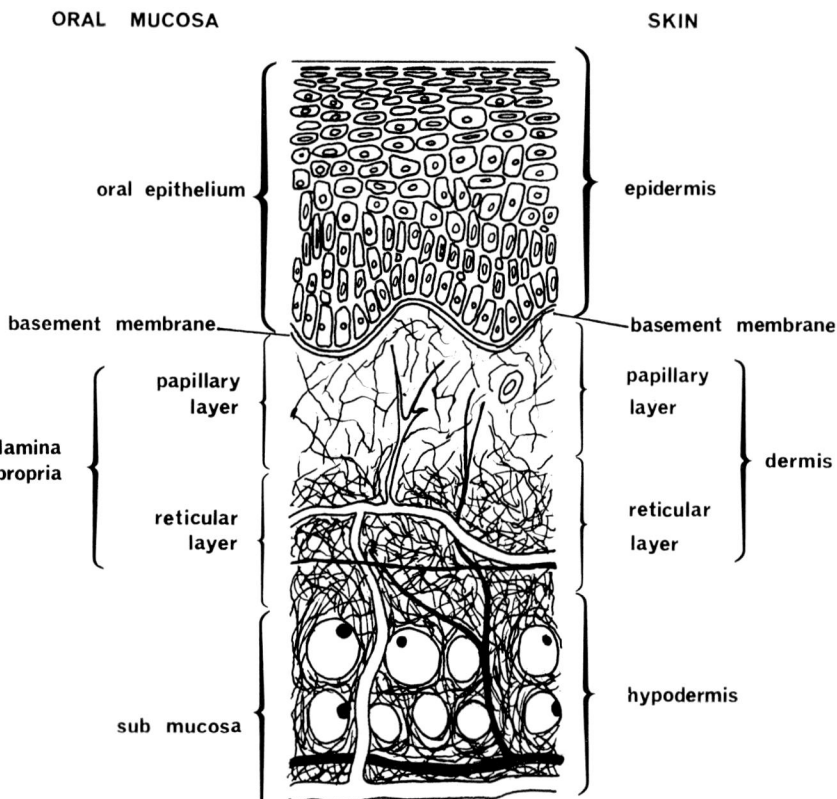

Fig. 1.1. Diagram of the organization of the major tissue components of skin and oral mucosa.

and auditory meatus. The secretion is produced in small quantities as an oily viscous fluid quite unlike sweat. It probably has no useful function in man although it is responsible for body odour on bacterial decomposition.

The eccrine sweat glands are derived from the epithelium independently of the hair follicles and are distributed over the surface of the skin in numbers varying from 200–800 per cm^2 (Scheuplein & Blank 1971). The coiled secretory portion of the gland is situated in the dermis and secretes a copious watery fluid which is modified in the duct carrying it to the surface so that the secretion becomes hypotonic. These glands serve the important function of temperature regulation as well as keeping the surface of the skin moist.

Apart from their individual functions, the appendages and glands described above all contribute to the permeability characteristics of the skin

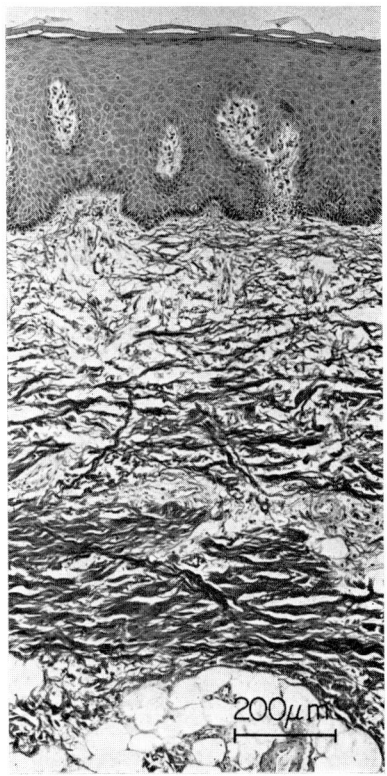

Fig. 1.2. Light micrograph showing a section of keratinized human palatal mucosa which illustrates the components referred to in Fig. 1.1. Bar represents 200 μm; stained Van Gieson.

for, by penetrating the epidermis, and particularly the barrier region of the horny layer, they provide parallel diffusion pathways through the skin. Such pathways may provide a significant means of passage for substances which penetrate only slowly through the stratum corneum (Scheuplein & Blank 1971).

None of the structures described above, with the exception of the sebaceous glands, are encountered in the oral mucosa although there is a single report of a hair follicle in buccal mucosa (Miles 1960). It is of interest to note that the filiform papillae of the tongue have a pattern of keratinization not unlike that seen in the hair cortex (Farbman 1970). The occurrence of pale yellow spots in the upper lip and buccal mucosa originally known as Fordyce's spots have been shown by Miles (1963) to represent sebaceous glands, similar to those usually associated with hair follicles in the skin. They are present in all parts of the cheek mucosa, particularly the middle zone, in 60–75% of adults and have also been reported in alveolar mucosa and dorsum of tongue (Knapp 1971). This distribution has led to suggestions that they arise during development when ectoderm possessing some of the potential of skin migrates into the oral cavity. Their function in this site is in some doubt; it is conceivable that they could provide lubrication, but as Miles (1963) points out, their universal absence from the lower lip weighs against such a suggestion.

Neither the skin nor the oral mucosa possess the intra-epithelial secretory cells found in the intestinal lining but the oral mucosa differs markedly from skin in containing salivary glands as the major glandular element. The secretion of these glands is responsible for maintaining the moist surface characteristic of the mucous membrane, acts as a lubricant and provides for some digestion of food in the oral cavity. Salivary glands may be classified in various ways according to their function, their size or their position. Most commonly they are divided on size into major and minor glands. The major salivary glands, the parotid, submandibular (sometimes also called submaxillary) and sublingual are large glands situated some way from the oral cavity and opening into it by long ducts. Minor salivary glands, situated in the deeper layers of the mucosa and in the submucosa, are grouped in several areas of the oral cavity. The role of the salivary glands will be considered in detail in Chapter 2.

Associated with the connective tissue surrounding the salivary glands are lymphocytes, and aggregates of these cells may be scattered throughout the glands; small lymph nodes are sometimes enclosed within the parotid gland. Small nodules of lymphoepithelial tissue resembling histologically the large tonsils of Waldeyers ring may occur variously in the soft palate, ventral surface of tongue and floor of mouth (Knapp 1970). In the posterior part of the oral cavity are the largest accumulations of lymphoid tissue, the lingual, palatine and pharyngeal tonsils, which are collectively referred to as Waldeyers ring. Here the overlying epithelium invaginates to form deep crypts within the lamina propria which is extensively infiltrated with lymphocytes, neutrophil leucocytes and plasma cells.

1:2:3 Stratification of epidermis and oral epithelium

Some of the greatest differences between skin and oral mucosa are evident in the surface layers of their epithelia. Everywhere the epidermis differentiates to produce a superficial keratin layer which serves as a tough,

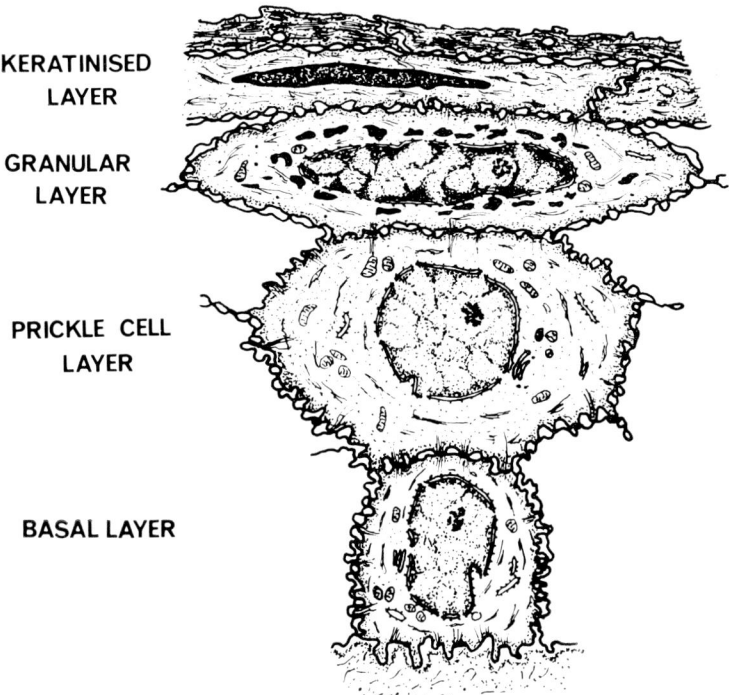

Fig. 1.3. Diagram of the appearance of cells in each layer of a keratinizing squamous epithelium. Note the change in shape of the cells of succeeding layers.

waterproofing covering. The stratified epithelial cells undergoing differentiation are frequently termed *keratinocytes* to distinguish them from the dendritic pigment cells and other cell types within the epithelium which are collectively referred to as *non-keratinocytes*. These latter are described in section 1:4.

The epidermis may be divided into several layers according to the morphology of the keratinocytes (Fig. 1.3). The least differentiated cells are those cubical or columnar cells situated in contact with the basement membrane and constituting the *basal cell layer*. These cells are primarily responsible for division and replacement of cells lost at the surface, and while it is possible to classify them functionally as the germinative cell layer, this is not altogether desirable as cell divisions in some epithelia do occur suprabasally (see section 1:3:1). Above the basal cell layer are

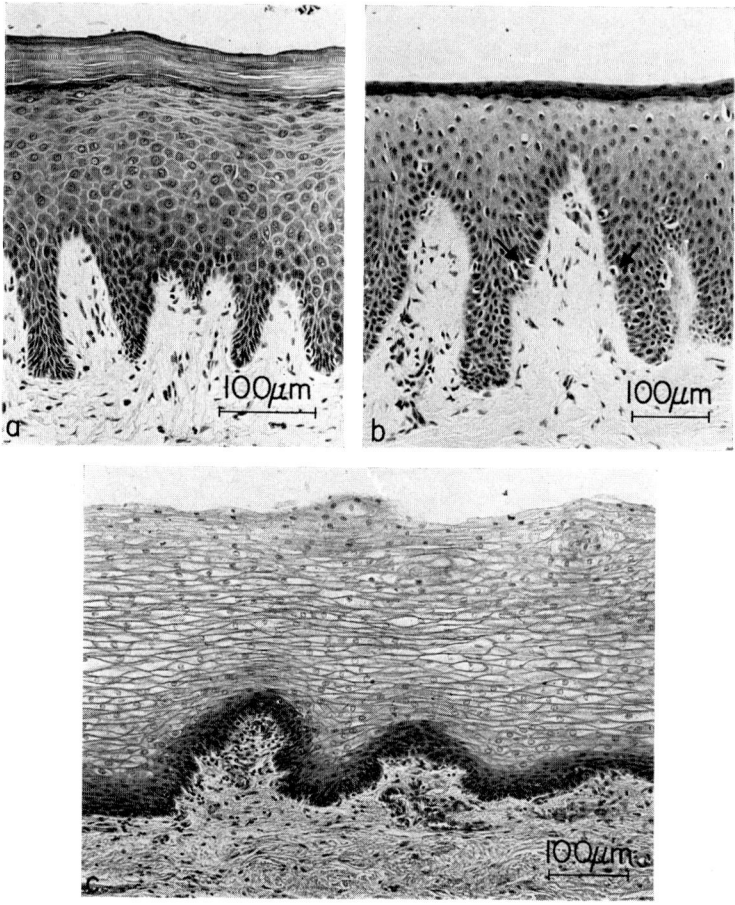

Fig. 1.4. (a) Ortho-keratinized epithelium from human hard palate. A prominent granular layer is present.

(b) Para-keratinized epithelium from human gingiva; a granular layer is not readily apparent. Several 'clear cell' (arrows) are present.

(c) Non-keratinized epithelium from human buccal mucosa. Bar represents 100 μm.

All sections stained with haematoxylin and eosin.

several layers of larger isodiametric cells which, because of the spiny appearance of their intercellular attachments in histological preparations, are called *prickle cells*. These cells differentiate to form larger but flattened cells which contain numbers of basophilic keratohyalin granules in their cytoplasm and so constitute the *granular layer*. All the cell layers so far described contain nucleated cells in which the cytoplasm becomes increasingly eosinophilic towards the surface; the term Malpighian layer has sometimes been used to describe these strata, but as there is no general agreement as to exactly which layers are included, it is best avoided. The most superficial cell layer is the *ortho-keratinized, cornified* or *horny layer*. The cells are markedly flattened and appear as hexagonal discs or squames, which lack nuclei, keratohyalin granules or other organelles and are entirely filled with eosinophilic material representing epidermal keratin. In certain areas of thick skin an intermediate light layer or *stratum lucidum* may be recognized between the granular and keratinized layers.

The surface of the oral mucosa differs from the skin not only in being smooth and moist but by having a surface epithelium that varies in its pattern of keratinization. In those regions most subject to mechanical stimulation, a keratin layer similar to that of the epidermis is found; in other regions the flexibility of a non-keratinized surface layer offers adequate protection. Such variation means that it is only possible to divide the oral epithelium into the same layers as the epidermis where there are recognizable keratohyalin granules and keratin in the surface layers. Despite some regional morphological differences, a basal and prickle cell layer can be recognized in all areas of human oral epithelium. In those areas showing a keratinized surface there is a recognizable granular layer although this and the keratinized layer are rather thinner than in the epidermis and a stratum lucidum cannot usually be identified (Fig. 1.4a).

In *para-keratinized* epithelium (Fig. 1.4b) the surface cells, while staining like keratin with eosin and other dyes, retain pyknotic nuclei and keratohyalin granules are sparse in the granular layer.

Non-keratinized oral epithelium rarely shows keratohyalin granules in histological preparations, and the superficial cells retain apparently normal nuclei, are less flattened, and show less eosinophilia than in keratinized epithelium (Fig. 1.4c). It is therefore not possible to identify a true granular or keratinized layer, but the outer third of the epithelium may be divided rather arbitrarily into '*intermediate*' and '*superficial*' layers. As will be mentioned in section 1:3:2 there may be a justification at the ultrastructural level for distinguishing these layers in non-keratinized oral epithelium.

1:2:4 Components of the dermis and lamina propria

Despite the importance of the epithelium as a barrier layer, many of the mechanical properties of the skin and mucosa depend on the underlying connective tissue, which serves to anchor the epithelium to deeper structures, usually the hypodermis or submucosa, but sometimes directly to muscle or bone.

The bulk of the dermis and lamina propria consists of a three-dimensional network of collagen, the organization of which determines the mechanical stability and resistance to deformation and extensibility of the tissue. Present in smaller amounts are elastic fibres, which serve to restore deformed collagen to its relaxed state, and reticulin fibres which enmesh bundles of collagen fibres and are predominant in the basement membrane region (see section 1:5). This fibre system is permeated by a highly hydrated matrix or ground substance composed of carbohydrate–protein complexes and contains the cells responsible for secreting both fibres and matrix, the fibroblasts, together with cells concerned with normal tissue maintenance and defence, such as plasma cells, histiocytes and mast cells. Both the dermis and lamina propria are penetrated by elements of the nervous system, sensory branches of which enter the epithelium, and the vascular system and lymphatic systems which run close to, but never enter, the epithelium. These elements are considered in more detail in section 1:6.

The subdivisions of the lamina propria and dermis have already been mentioned (section 1:2:1; Fig. 1.1) and it is in terms of the relative concentration and arrangement of fibres rather than in absolute differences that these regions are distinguished. The *papillary layer* contains predominantly fine collagen fibres, between 0·3 and 3 μm in diameter, arranged as a loose open network. In the region of the basement membrane these fibres are associated with reticulin while at the junction with the subjacent reticular layer they merge into thicker bundles. Where appendages are present the papillary layer is reflected deeply so as to surround them. In the *reticular layer* the collagen fibres are coarser, ranging from 10 to 40 μm in diameter, and are closely packed. They are often arranged in laminae in the plane of the surface, the horizontal plane, while in the vertical plane they may be aligned in the direction of minimum extensibility (Brown 1972). On the basis of fibre density, Brown (1972) has suggested that two separate regions may be recognized within the reticular layer in human dermis—a mid-zone occupying the superficial two-thirds in which fibres are compactly arranged and a deep zone with a loose arrangement of fibres and aggregations of fat cells.

During the embryological development of skin and mucous membrane there are important interactions between epithelium and connective tissue and there is evidence to suggest that it is primarily the connective tissue that determines the nature of the overlying epithelium (see section 1:5:4). These interactions give rise to important regional differences in structure.

1:2:5 Regions showing specialized functions

Skin

As well as differences between regions of the skin, such as thickness of the horny layer or frequency of hairs, there are many more subtle differences, obvious only on histological or histochemical examination. The epidermis, which everywhere shows a keratinized surface layer, differs greatly in thickness, both in terms of its total thickness and in the thickness of the horny layer. Within the epidermis there is wide variation in the number and activity of the melanocytes which produces corresponding variations in skin pigmentation. The dermis likewise shows differences in both its thickness and structure and at its junction with the epidermis presents profiles ranging from deeply interdigitated ridges and papillae to an almost smooth contour. Within the dermis the blood and nerve supply also vary and there are differences in the distribution of hair follicles and sebaceous glands. Associated with these morphological differences are functional differences such as variation in mechanical properties, percutaneous absorption, sensitivity and thermal regulation. As in the oral mucosa, one of the most obvious functional differences is in those regions of skin adapted to pressure bearing, such as the palms and soles, and regions capable of being stretched. It is not within the scope of this chapter to consider regional differences of the skin in detail, but one major variation is that between non-hairy (glabrous) and hairy skin. This coincides with the alternative classification into thick and thin skin, although this latter approach is somewhat misleading as the thickness refers to the epidermis alone, which in turn largely reflects the great differences between the keratinized layer of thick and thin skin. In Table 1.1 is set out a list of the main structural differences between glabrous and hairy human skin.

Muco-cutaneous junctions

The skin is continuous with mucous membrane in several regions—in the nose, lips, eyelids, urogenital openings and anus. The only muco-cutaneous junction to be considered here is that of the lips, where the skin meets the oral mucous membrane. At this junction the skin, containing hairs, sebaceous and sweat glands, passes into a transitional zone in which hairs and sweat glands are lacking, although occasional sebaceous glands are present, especially at the angle of the mouth (Miles 1963). The epithelium of this region is keratinized but thin and there are long connective tissue papillae, containing capillary loops close to the epithelium. This vascular pattern is responsible for the strong red coloration of the area, which is often called the red zone or vermilion border of the lip. Continuous with

Table 1.1. Differences between glabrous and hairy skin

	Location	Epidermis	Dermis
Non-hairy (glabrous) skin	Palms and soles	Thick with marked horny layer and usually a stratum lucidum. Characteristic grooved surface	Thin with no hair follicles or sebaceous glands. Large numbers of sweat glands. Where rete ridges are well developed there is a rich blood supply. Encapsulated sensory endings present
Hairy skin	Remainder of body	Thin with narrow horny layer; rarely a stratum lucidum	Thick, but varies considerably in different regions. Hair follicles and sebaceous glands present. Apocrine glands found in some areas. Where rete ridges are poorly developed the vascular supply is scant. No encapsulated sensory nerve endings

this zone on the oral side is non-keratinized oral mucosa. In a histological study of this region, Binnie & Lehner (1970) have described an intermediate zone between the vermilion border and the oral mucosa of adults, which is covered by a para-keratinized epithelium. In infants this region is thickened as an adaptation to suckling.

The oral mucosa

The oral mucosa, like the skin, shows regional differences and varies not only in the nature of the submucosa or other underlying structure, and in the composition of the lamina propria and the form of the epithelial-connective junction, but also in the type of covering epithelium, which can show a wide variation in thickness and in its pattern of keratinization. It is commonplace to regard these regional differences as representing functional adaptations and to classify oral mucosa accordingly into three functional types, namely *masticatory mucosa*, *lining mucosa* and *specialized mucosa*. Lining mucosa is strictly speaking only a 'functional adaptation' by virtue of its non-specialization, i.e. both masticatory and specialized oral mucosae represent variations of this basic lining tissue. The regions

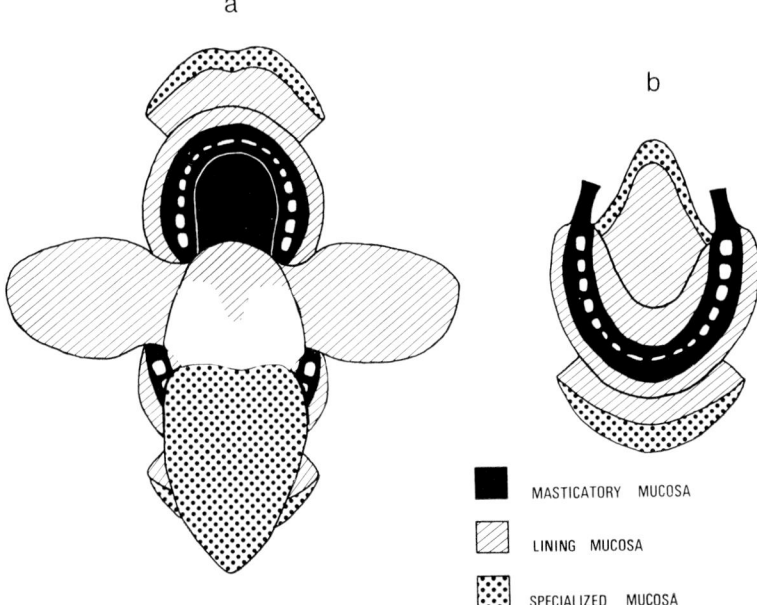

Fig. 1.5. Diagrammatic representation of the oral cavity to show the regions occupied by masticatory, lining and specialized mucosae.
(a) includes the upper lip, gingiva, hard and soft palate, cheek and dorsum of tongue;
(b) includes the underside of tongue, floor of mouth, gingiva and lower lip.

of the oral cavity occupied by each type of mucosa are illustrated diagrammatically in Fig. 1.5.

Masticatory mucosa is present in those areas of the oral cavity that are subject to the mechanical forces of mastication and in general is characterized by a keratinized epithelium overlying a thick and dense lamina propria that is bound tightly to underlying bone. The submucosa varies in different regions, being absent in gingiva but present in most areas of the palate, where it contributes to a tightly bound but resilient tissue comparable to palmar and plantar skin. *Lining mucosae* typically have a thick,

Table 1.2. Structure of mucosae lining the oral cavity

Region	Covering epithelium	Mucosa Lamina propria	Submucosa
1. Lining mucosa			
Soft palate	Thin, non-keratinized stratified squamous; taste buds present	Thick, numerous short papillae; elastic fibres forming an elastic lamina; highly vascular with well-developed capillary network	Diffuse tissue containing numerous minor salivary glands (mucous)
Ventral surface of tongue	Thin, non-keratinized stratified squamous	Thin with numerous short papillae and some elastic fibres. A few minor salivary glands (mucous, serous and mixed); capillary network in papillary layer, reticular layer relatively avascular	No distinct layer. The mucosa is bound to the connective tissue surrounding the tongue musculature
Floor of mouth	Thin, non-keratinized stratified squamous	Short broad papillae; some elastic fibres; extensive vascular supply with short, anastomosing capillary loops	Loose fibrous connective tissue containing fat, the sublingual and minor salivary glands (predominantly mucous)
Labial and buccal mucosa	Thick, non-keratinized stratified squamous (often parakeratinized in occlusal plane)	Short, irregular papillae; dense fibrous connective tissue containing collagen and some elastic fibres; rich vascular supply giving off anastomosing capillary loops into papillae	Dense collagenous connective tissue with fat, minor salivary glands, sometimes sebaceous glands, firmly attached to underlying muscle
Alveolar mucosa	Thin, non-keratinized stratified squamous	Papillae are short or absent; connective tissue containing many elastic fibres; capillary loops close to the surface supplied by vessels running superficial to the periosteum	Loose connective tissue, containing thick elastic fibres and minor salivary glands (mixed), attached to periosteum of alveolar process

2. Masticatory mucosa

Gingiva	Thick, ortho-keratinized and para-keratinized stratified squamous, often showing a stippled surface	Long narrow papillae; dense collagenous connective tissue; not highly vascular but long capillary loops with numerous anastomoses particularly on crevicular aspect	Firmly attached by collagen fibres to cementum and periosteum of alveolar process; no glands, fat or muscle
Hard palate	Thick, ortho-keratinized stratified squamous thrown into transverse palatine ridges (rugae)	Long papillae; thick dense collagenous tissue, especially under rugae; moderate vascular supply with short capillary loops	Dense collagenous connective tissue attaching to periosteum; anteriorly fat, posteriorly minor salivary glands are packed into the connective tissue

3. Specialized mucosa

Lips, vermilion border	Thin, ortho-keratinized stratified squamous	Long narrow papillae; capillary loops in papillary layer close to surface	Some sebaceous glands, minor salivary glands and fat; firmly attached to underlying muscle
Intermediate zone	Thin, para-keratinized stratified squamous	Long irregular papillae; elastic and collagen fibres in connective tissues	
Dorsal surface of tongue	Thick, keratinized stratified squamous forming three types of lingual papillae bearing taste buds	Long papillae; mucous and serous glands (von Ebners glands); lymphoid tissue (lingual tonsils); posteriorly rich innervation, especially near taste buds; capillary plexus in subpapillary layer, large vessels lying deeper	No distinct layer, the mucosa is bound to the connective tissue surrounding the masculature of the tongue

non-keratinized epithelium over a thin lamina propria. However, it is worth while remembering that in other species such as the rat and mouse, mucosa lining regions of the oral cavity corresponding to the human cheek are actually ortho-keratinized (Osmanski and Meyer 1967; see section 1:3:2); such variation would seem to justify a classification of oral mucosa in function rather than morphological terms. The lamina propria in lining mucosa is elastic (see Fig. 1.22) and variously bound to underlying structures by a sub-mucosa so that there are differences in texture and elasticity ranging from the highly elastic and tightly bound mucosa of the lips, cheeks and ventral surface of the tongue, to the soft palate, the vestibular and alveolar mucosa and to the floor of the mouth which is more loosely bound and flexibly attached.

Specialized mucosae are represented by the dorsum of the tongue where there are four types of lingual papillae; anteriorly, the filiform and fungiform, posteriorly foliate and vallate papillae. The epithelium is keratinized and tightly bound to underlying muscle by a thin but densely fibrous lamina propria. It is also convenient to include the vermilion border and transitional zone of the lips under the heading specialized mucosa, as they are neither truly masticatory nor lining mucosae.

The general structural organization of these tissues is set out in Table 1:2.

1:3 The Epithelium: Keratin-producing Cells

The epithelial lining of oral mucosa, like that of the rest of the gastrointestinal tract and the epidermis, is composed of a constantly renewing cell population so that under normal circumstances the number of new cells produced is just sufficient to match those lost from the surface due to normal wear and tear. Cell division takes place in or near the basal layers, the daughter cells either remaining as progenitor cells or entering upon the process of differentiation which gives rise to the characteristic surface cells of the particular region.

1:3:1 Cell division and tissue turnover

The rate of cell division in oral epithelium has been studied by the traditional methods of counting mitotic figures in histological sections, by mitotic arrest techniques, and by premitotic labelling with the DNA precursor thymidine usually tagged with tritium (^{3}H-T). The latter methods, which usually involve systemic administration of a drug or radioactive substance are normally precluded from use in humans and, as a result, much of the available data are derived from laboratory animals.

1:3:1a THE SITE OF CELL DIVISION IN ORAL EPITHELIA

There is considerable difference of opinion as to what really constitutes the germinative layers or progenitor cell compartment of various lining epithelia. Many authors have assumed that, in skin, mitosis can only take place within the basal layer and Cutright & Bauer (1967) were unable to observe labelled cells in other than the basal layer shortly after administration of ^{3}H-T. Other studies have claimed however that as many as two-thirds of the total mitotic figures observed in skin are suprabasal, mostly in the deep third of the stratum spinosum (Cowdrey & Thompson 1944; Thuringer & Katzberg 1959; Penneys et al 1970). Similar conflicts have been reported for oral mucosa. Cameron (1966) found thymidine labelled nuclei initially restricted to the basal layer of epithelium on the ventral surface of rat tongue, the same being true for numerous regions of the rat mouth according to Cutright & Bauer (1967). In direct contrast up to 40% of DNA synthesizing or dividing cells have been reported to be suprabasal in the oral mucosa of the rat (Sharav & Massler 1967), rabbit (Henry et al 1952), and of man (Kaidbey & Kurban 1971). For the masticatory mucosa of human gingiva, there are numerous reports of as many as two-thirds of the mitoses appearing in the spinous layer (Hayes et al 1964; Meyer, Marwah & Weinmann 1956; Marwah, Weinmann & Meyer 1960; Soni et al 1967; Kittler, Lauckner & Mieler 1969).

The problem has recently been re-examined by Löe, Karring & Hara (1972), who applied serial section and reconstruction techniques to a variety of rat oral epithelia and to human gingiva and showed that almost all dividing cells do in fact lie on the basement membrane and that all are within three cell layers of it. The greatest number of suprabasal mitoses was found in rat tongue but their data do not permit calculation of the actual proportions.

Difficulty in interpreting the level of mitosis is obviously greatest in tissues with a complex basement membrane morphology, as an apparently suprabasal nucleus may in fact be bordering on a connective tissue papilla in another plane of section. It remains possible however that there are genuine site and species differences in the distribution of the *progenitor compartment*. For example in the junctional epithelium against the tooth surface labelled cells may be seen, shortly after administration of ³H-T, at any level between the basement membrane and hard tissue interface.

It was thought for many years that the distribution of mitoses along the basement membrane was random, but it is now clear that they occur in characteristic clusters (Cameron, Gosslee & Pilgrim 1965; Rowe & Dixon 1972; Mackenzie 1973a) and that in tissue with a complex connective tissue interface, such as the oral aspect of the gingiva, mitoses are more numerous at the tips of the rete ridges (Löe, Karring & Hara 1972).

1:3:1b PHASES OF THE CELL CYCLE IN ORAL EPITHELIA

It is customary to divide the life span of mitotic cells into a number of phases (Fig. 1.6). A period of actual mitotic division, M, is followed by a post-mitotic resting period or gap, G1. In preparing for further division a cell must spend time synthesizing the extra DNA required, and this is

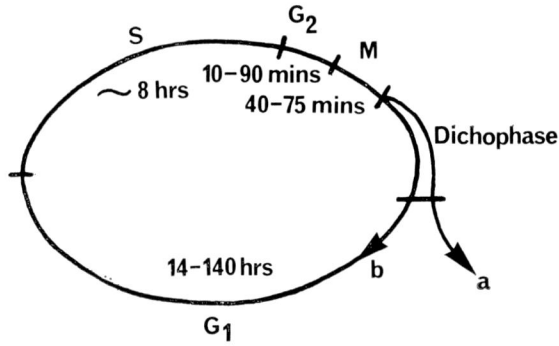

Fig. 1.6. Phases of the cell cycle:
(a) Daughter cell proceeding to differentiation;
(b) Daughter cell remaining as part of progenitor population.

termed the S phase. This is separated from the period of mitosis proper by a premitotic gap, G2.

The length of these phases can be determined by mitotic arrest, double DNA labelling or labelled mitosis techniques. A so-called *dichophase* is sometimes postulated between M and G1, this being a period of indeterminate length during which each daughter cell 'makes the decision' to remain part of the progenitor population or to begin differentiation.

Most authors regard the duration of S phase to be about 8 hours in oral mucosa, experimental estimates varying from 7 to 12 hours (Cameron 1966; Toto & Dhawan 1966; Brown & Berry 1968; Blenkinsopp 1968; Barakat, Toto & Choukas 1969). G2 is of the order of 10–90 minutes (Toto & Dhawan 1966; Barakat *et al* 1969; MacDonald 1971) and M, 40–75 minutes (Henry *et al* 1952; Toto & Dhawan 1966; Barakat *et al* 1969; MacDonald 1971). The post-mitotic gap, G1, is apparently much more variable, figures from 14 to 140 hours having been suggested (Cameron 1966; Brown & Berry 1968; Brown & Oliver 1968; Toto & Dhawan 1966; MacDonald 1971).

Comparable figures for skin appear to be somewhat longer; 10 hours or 16 hours having been proposed for S (Heenen & Galand 1971; Weinstein & Frost 1971).

1:3:1C THE CONCEPT OF TISSUE
TURNOVER TIME

The ratio of the number of cells in any given phase of the cell cycle to the time spent in that phase is clearly equal for each phase of the cycle and equal to the ratio of the total number of germinative cells in the tissue divided by total cycle time (T). During time T all germinative cells in the tissue will have returned to the same point in the cycle with a doubling of the number of cells. There has been thus a complete turnover of the 'compartments', and if the tissue has not altered in thickness an equivalent number of cells must have been shed. These ratios, as means of determining turnover time, apply with accuracy only to the progenitor compartment.

If turnover of the whole thickness of a stratified squamous epithelium is to be considered it is necessary to add the time taken for the passage of cells through the remaining layers (Halprin 1972). This factor is frequently overlooked and partly accounts for the discrepant values of turnover times found in the literature. Similar computations of total issue turnover time are frequently made by utilizing the ratio of cells in a particular phase to the total number of cells in the tissue. This however assumes a uniform behaviour of all cells and we have already seen that the progenitor compartment is limited in distribution; turnover times for whole epithelia derived in this way are thus only approximate.

1:3:1d RATE OF CELL DIVISION IN ORAL EPITHELIA

Evaluation of the evidence concerning rate of cell division in oral epithelia is confused by the variety of experimental approaches used and particularly by the variation in the methods of expressing findings.

Mitotic and radioactive label indices

The number of labelled or visibly dividing cells counted in sections variously has been expressed as a proportion of the total number of nucleated cells in the area assessed; as a proportion of the number of basal cells, assuming this to represent the progenitor compartment, or as a proportion of 'basal-looking' cells. It is not always made clear which system has been adopted. Number per unit length of the basement membrane has occasionally been employed. Recently Karring & Löe (1972) have argued that relation to unit area of desquamating surface is most meaningful, as under steady state conditions cell division must be just sufficient to replace shed cells and this latter is clearly a function of surface area. This latter approach probably provides the best method for comparing regional variations in normal activity and changes in mitotic rate associated with hyperplasia, atrophy, inflammatory or other disease states.

In an attempt to compare various studies on gingival epithelium Skougaard (1970) recalculated the original data from the literature and expressed all the results in terms of tissue renewal or turnover time. This is defined as the time taken for the total number of cells in the tissue to be shed and replaced by the same number through cell division. It is assumed that with steady state conditions one of the two daughter cells following division remains part of the progenitor compartment and the other begins the process of maturation and migration towards the surface. As explained earlier, the ratio of total cells in a tissue compartment to the turnover time (T) will be equal to the ratio of the number of cells in any particular phase of the mitotic cycle divided by the time spent in that phase. Experiments using mitotic counts, metaphase block, or DNA labelling methods can thus be compared on this basis. This approach has been adopted in Table 1.3 in which the available data for turnover in various regions of oral mucosa are compared with each other and with some of the data for epidermis. The figures can be approximations only, largely because, as mentioned above, transit time is often ignored when counts are restricted to basal or parabasal layers. Computations based on mitotic indices are also likely to vary widely because of the low numbers of mitotic figures present in normal tissues and because the duration of mitosis is not known with sufficient accuracy. Computations based on uptake of radioactive thymidine will be affected by the increase in mitotic activity stimulated by the injection of thymidine (Greulich, Cameron & Thrasher 1961; Blenkinsopp 1967; Beagrie 1970) and by possible variations in the length of S phase.

1:3:1e REGIONAL VARIATIONS

In general, oral epithelium turns over faster than epidermis, but slower than gut epithelium. The more recent estimations put epidermal turnover time in the range 12–75 days with an average of approximately 25 days. Comparable figures for oral epithelium vary from 2 to 40 days, most being of the order of 4–14 days. The exceptionally long turnover times of approximately 100 days calculated for human gingiva on the basis of mitotic counts should be interpreted with caution.

Keratinized and non-keratinized oral mucosa

No clear-cut variations from site to site can be derived from the pooled data listed in Table 1.3, because of variation in experimental method. Although regional differences are revealed when the same method is applied to different sites, the available data are almost entirely derived from rodents in which the keratin distribution differs markedly from man. It is however clear that the non-keratinized lining mucosa of the cheek and oral vestibule in primates turns over much faster than the keratinized masticatory mucosa of the attached gingiva. Thymidine labelling studies reveal a turnover time of 4–8 days for the former (McHugh & Zander 1965; Gillespie 1969; Toller 1971; Kaidbey & Kurban, 1971) and 7–15 days for the latter (Beagrie 1963; Engler, Ramfjord & Hiniker 1965a; McHugh & Zander 1965; Skougaard 1965; Demetriou & Ramfjord 1972). This difference would be further increased if the time taken for passage of cells through the stratum corneum was to be considered.

Gingiva

A great deal of work has been done on cell proliferation in the different component parts of gingiva. Again much of this has been on rodents in which the structure of the crevice and epithelial attachment is different from that found in man. This discussion will therefore be restricted to observation of mitoses in human gingiva and to kinetic studies in non-human primates.

Thymidine labelling has been used in a number of studies to investigate regional variations in monkey gingiva, but not all authors have compared the same anatomical divisions and slightly different concepts of epithelial attachment and sulcular epithelium have been employed. When cell proliferation is expressed in terms of number of ^{3}H-T labelled nuclei per total number of cells in the region studied, all of these workers (Table 1.3) agree that oral sulcular epithelium has the highest turnover, followed by the oral aspect of attached gingiva, with junctional epithelium having an extremely low turnover. Junctional epithelium also has a low labelling index when expressed in terms of unit length of basement membrane. If however the desquamating surface is taken to be a small area on the floor of the gingival sulcus, labelling index per unit of surface would produce figures well above those for any other part of the oral mucosa (Listgarten 1972; Johnson & Hopps 1974).

Whilst proportional differences between regions of the gingiva are similar in most of the published studies, the actual tissue renewal times calculated from the various labelling indices vary widely (Table 1.3). Thus the renewal time for oral sulcular epithelium apparently varies between 4·1 and 10·1 days, for attached gingiva between 7·9 and 15·4 days and for junctional epithelium between 40·5 and 145 days. Variations in species, in experimental design, degree of inflammation and any of the factors influencing mitotic rate considered below may contribute to this wide spread of results.

1:3:1f CONTROL OF MITOTIC ACTIVITY

It is now generally accepted that mitosis is largely under the control of locally produced tissue hormones termed *chalones* (Bullough & Laurence 1966a). These are thought to be produced by post-mitotic epithelial cells and to have the dual property of stimulating cell maturation and inhibiting mitosis. Cell division is thus highest in regions of low chalone concentration, e.g. when a wound is created chalone diffuses from cells at the wound margin, thus permitting the increased mitoses necessary for healing. Some systemic component is apparently essential for adequate chalone action. Bullough has proposed that this is adrenalin (Bullough & Laurence 1966b) and its absence from mucosa in organ culture may explain the rapid increase in mitosis which takes place there in the first few days after explantation. Glucocorticoid hormones enhance the chalone–adrenalin effect (Bullough & Laurence 1968). The concept is supported by studies of the effect of adrenalectomy on oral epithelial turnover (Hansen 1967a, b).

Numerous other factors influence mitotic action (Bullough 1962). Some of these are discussed below, the effect in each case being explicable in terms of alteration in chalone–adrenalin–corticosteroid action.

1:3:1g FACTORS INFLUENCING RATE OF EPITHELIAL PROLIFERATION

Diurnal rhythm

The effect of diurnal rhythms on mitotic, as on most physiological activity is marked. It is essential to account for this in any experimental design either by quoting mean daily figures of mitotic or labelling indices, or by always sampling at the same time of day. In oral tissues the proportion of cells which take up ^{3}H-T varies by a factor of 4 or 5 during a 24-hour period (England & Burke 1968, 1969, 1971).

Stress

Any condition of stress, with raised adrenalin and corticosteroid output, will depress cell turnover. It has been suggested (Skougaard 1970) that the very low mitotic counts, compared to monkey experiments using ^{3}H-T, found by Hayes *et al* (1964) in children's gingiva which was excised at the time of tooth extraction, may be explained in this way. However, the effects of handling, anaesthesia and intravenous thymidine injection on monkeys is likely to have a similar effect. This re-emphasizes the difficulty of arriving at comparative figures for epithelial turnover using different experimental techniques.

Age

Numerous studies have shown that the mitotic index, expressed as proportion of nucleated cells, increases with age in skin and mucosa in spite of the tendency of all tissues to atrophy. Hayes *et al* (1964) found a mean mitotic index of approximately 0·043% for the gingiva of 5–12-year-olds and 0·067% for 14–24-year-olds and this may be compared with 0·098% for 25–35 age group and 0·156% for 55–78 age groups reported by Meyer *et al* (1956). The figures of Soni *et al* (1967) and Kittler, Lauckner & Mieler (1969) are comparable. Similar trends have been shown for skin (Thuringer & Katzberg 1959).

Several authors have commented on the possible significance of this apparent increased epithelial turnover with age, in relation to the increasing prevalence of neoplastic disease with age, suggesting that there may be a progressive decrease in the efficiency of the controls acting on cellular proliferation. However, as Miles (1961) and Löe & Karring (1969) have pointed out, raised mitotic counts may simply reflect increased desquamation or thinning of the epithelium. Studies using DNA-labelling methods have generally tended to show a reduced mitotic activity with advancing age in oral mucosa (Dhawan & Toto 1965; Toto & Dhawan 1966; Sharav & Massler 1967; Barakat, Toto & Choukas 1969) and in other tissues, for example in duodenal epithelium (Lesher, Fry & Kohn 1961a, b; Fry, Lesher & Kohn 1961). Recently Karring & Löe (1973) have sought to explain this discrepancy by comparing mitotic index, expressed in terms of mitoses per unit of surface area (see above), and mitotic duration in old and young rats using colchicine blocking techniques. They found mitotic duration in tongue epithelium increased from 41 to 48 minutes. The mitotic INDEX was relatively constant and thus they conclude mitotic ACTIVITY decreases with increasing age. Such a change would be more in keeping with the general slowing down of metabolic events as a function of age (see section 1:7).

Sex

The series of papers by Soni and collaborators have correlated mitotic counts of human gingiva with both age and sex. Their data show a tendency for the mitotic index to be higher in males, but no statistical evaluation is presented and they appear to regard the differences as not significant (Hayes *et al* 1964; Soni *et al* 1967). A similar study by Kittler, Lauckner & Mieler (1969) and Kittler and Mieler (1969) shows consistently higher activity in males than females when paired for both age and histologic degree of inflammation, the differences frequently being statistically significant, and of the order of 10%.

Endocrine status

Beagrie (1966) has shown that oestrogen stimulates mitosis in the oral tissues of mice and Bullough (1962) has shown that androgens have a similar effect on epidermis. The rate varies during the oestrus cycle in rodents (Bullough 1950; Ebling 1954) but attempts to show changes in human oral epithelia throughout the menstrual cycle have not brought consistent results (Main & Ritchie 1967; Van Mens 1972). Evaluation of the effect of hormonal fluctuations during puberty and pregnancy are complicated by the increased inflammation, particularly gingivitis, which is so common at these times and which would itself stimulate mitotic rate.

The depressant effect of adrenaline and corticosteroids has already been mentioned. Apart from these there is little direct evidence of hormonal effects on epithelial turnover. For a general discussion of tissue changes the reader is referred to Waterhouse (1969).

Inflammation

Epithelial thickening is a common accompaniment of chronic inflammation in the oral mucosa. This is well seen in lesions of non-specific origin such as the common fibro-epithelial polyp and denture-induced granuloma where epithelial hyperplasia is expressed as both acanthosis and rete peg proliferation. The latter presumably follows damage to basement membrane and the fibres and ground substance of the lamina propria by the inflammatory process and is brought about by increased cell division. Acanthosis on the other hand could equally well result from a reduced rate of keratinocyte maturation and desquamation. It is therefore worth noting the results of Mackenzie & Miles (1973), who studied the effects of frictional stimulation on skin and oral mucosa in rodents. They found increased mitotic activity accompanied by an accelerated passage of progeny to the surface with an increased epithelial thickness due to an increase both in number and size of cells. As a result of increased rate of passage, the keratin was less well formed. It seems likely that a similar mechanism would operate in many oral lesions such as those mentioned above where chronic mechanical irritation is a cause of inflammation.

Other authors using ^{3}H-T techniques in monkey gingiva have found no consistent relationship between epithelial cell labelling and inflammation. It seems logical however that inflammation would stimulate mitosis up to a threshold beyond which direct damage would result in depressed cell activity and ultimately cell death.

1:3:2 Cell differentiation and keratin synthesis

The epidermis and oral epithelium consist of epithelial cells arranged as a stratified squamous epithelium, and it is these cells that constitute both a mechanical and permeability barrier. As the surface cells are lost by desquamation, there is a constant replacement by divisions in the basal or suprabasal layer so that the epithelium maintains a constant thickness (see section 1:3:1). By a process of differentiation a relatively impermeable surface layer is produced which may be tough such as in the epidermis and oral masticatory mucosa, or flexible as in an oral lining mucosa.

1:3:2a KERATIN AND THE PROCESS
OF KERATINIZATION

In a series of studies in which they investigated changes in cell shape, volume, dry weight and enzyme activity during the differentiation of a variety of oral epithelia, Meyer and co-workers (summarized in Alvares & Meyer 1971) showed that there were differences between different types of ortho-keratinized epithelium, such as that from rat cheek and rat palate, almost as great as those between keratinized and non-keratinized epithelium. This reinforced a suggestion made earlier by Weinmann (1940) that keratinization might be considered as a spectrum, varying in small steps between the extremes of full ortho-keratinization and non-keratinization, rather than being an all-or-none process. Thus during differentiation a number of different processes such as synthesis, breakdown, and dehydration are proceeding, the rate and extent of which determine whether the epithelium is classified on a morphological basis as keratinized, non-keratinized or intermediate in form.

As morphological appearance is the principal means of characterizing the state of keratinization of an epithelium, it is not surprising that most theories of keratin formation are based on the sequence of events seen in histological and electron microscope preparations. The superficial acidophilic layer of keratinized epithelium consists largely of insoluble fibrous protein with a high proportion of the sulphur-containing amino acid cystine. This protein is termed keratin, although it is important to remember that keratins differ widely in composition between tissues and between species and the term refers to a family of proteins (Iqbal & Gerson 1971; Baden & Goldsmith 1972). Electron micrographs show that keratin consists of aggregates of fine fibrils, essentially similar to the tonofilaments in the deeper cells of the epithelium but appearing as light structures against the darker background of the matrix in fully keratinized cells, an appearance that has been called the 'keratin pattern' (Brody 1964). The filaments are probably bound together by the same attractive forces which operate between all polypeptide chains, although the presence of appreciable numbers of disulphide linkages is an important characteristic. The keratohyalin granules present in the granular layer have been proposed as the precursor of the matrix (Brody 1959) and it is of interest that in the rabbit palate, where there are no keratohyalin granules, a keratinized layer is found which apparently lacks a matrix between the fibrils (Chen & Meyer 1971). This system of filaments within a matrix is contained within the original cell membrane which has become thickened and extremely resistant to most chemical agents (Matoltsy & Parakkal 1967). The entire structure represents a squame of which the keratinized layer is made up.

The description above refers to the keratin found in the epidermis or ortho-keratinized regions of human oral epithelium (Fig. 1.4a) but it is apparent that there are many variations on the basic theme in the spectrum of keratinization found in mammalian oral mucosa. Para-keratinization is commonly found in the human oral epithelium where 75% of the gingiva may show this pattern (Sicher & Bhasker 1972), but is never seen in normal human epidermis although aquatic mammals, such as the dolphin and whale, are reported to have a para-keratinized epidermis (Spearman 1972). In para-keratinization it seems likely that the formation of keratin proceeds in the normal way but is not accompanied by the removal of all cell organelles, in particular the nuclei, which persist in the surface cells (Fig. 1.4b). In the 'incomplete' variants of ortho- or para-keratinization (Weinmann & Meyer 1959) the surface keratin is probably susceptible to the solvent action of saliva; this may be the result of an incompletely modified cell membrane allowing the entry of fluid (Osmanski & Meyer 1971). Other variants of mammalian oral epithelium show not only partial loss of organelles, but different degrees of packing of the tonofilaments and in some cases no matrix formation. The extreme variant is non-keratinization such as in human buccal epithelium (Fig. 1.4c), where there is neither packing of tonofilaments nor matrix formation and most of the cell organelles, including the nuclei, remain in the surface cells.

In the following section the way in which these extreme differences arise in successive cell layers will be described by comparing the differentiation of keratinized and non-keratinized oral epithelium.

1:3:2b THE BASAL CELLS

The basal cells of epidermis and oral epithelium represent the least differentiated cells of the tissue. While they cannot be considered structurally or functionally undifferentiated in the same way as the free stem cells of blood or undifferentiated mesenchyme cells are, they do contain all the organelles present in most other tissue types. In electron micrographs of basal cells (Fig. 1.7) we can recognize a prominent nucleus with one or more nucleoli, numbers of small mitochondria, a Golgi complex, lysosomes,

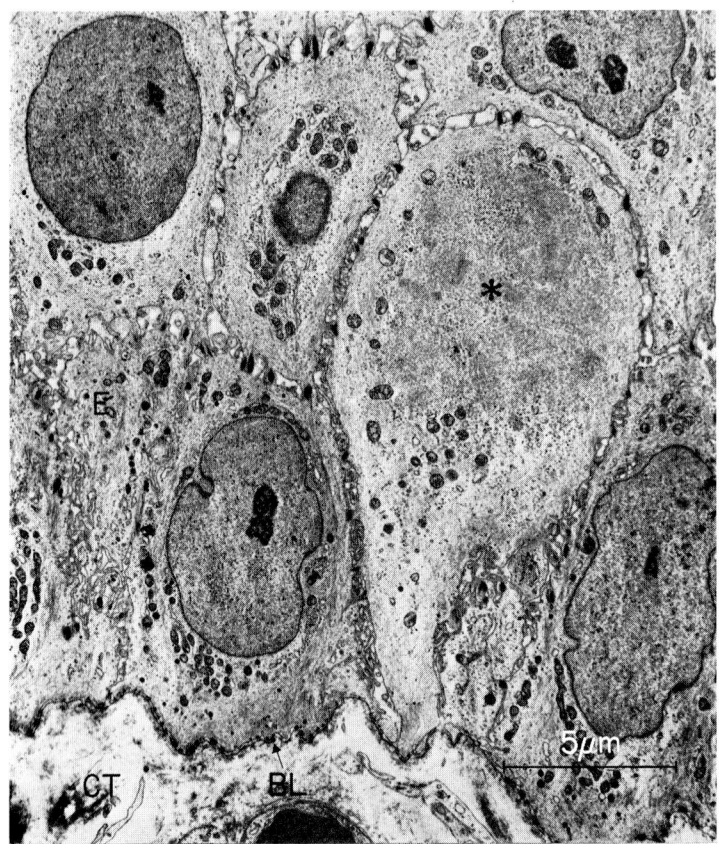

Fig. 1.7. Electron micrograph of basal cells from human buccal epithelium. The basement lamina (BL) separating the epithelium (E) from the connective tissue (CT) is clearly seen. One of the basal cells (asterisk) is beginning to divide and has lost its nuclear membrane. Mitochondria are visible in all cells. All electron micrographs are of tissue fixed in osmium tetroxide and stained with lead citrate and uranyl acetate unless otherwise stated. Bar represents 5 μm.

small amounts of granular endoplasmic reticulum and abundant free ribosomes. However, there are structures already present that distinguish these cells from the cells of most other tissues. These are the fine protein strands, some 6 nm in diameter, which may appear singly as *tonofilaments* or be arranged together in bundles to form the *tonofibrils* visible with the higher powers of the light microscope; the tonofilaments represent a synthetic product that is retained within the cell as structural protein.

The effectiveness of the epithelium as a barrier is also dependent on the cohesion between cells and the adhesion of the whole epithelium to underlying tissues. Cohesion is maintained by the presence of cement substance in the intercellular spaces, presumably secreted by the epithelial cells themselves. In addition there are characteristic structural modifications of the plasma membranes of the epithelial cells to form several types of intercellular junction. The most common of these is the *desmosome*

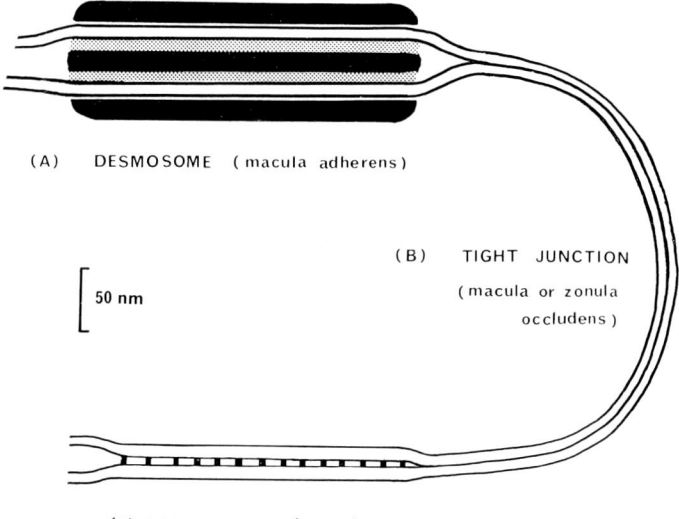

Fig. 1.8. Diagram of the three main types of intercellular junction found in oral epithelium and epidermis.

(Fig. 1.8), which occupies oval or circular areas of adjacent plasma membranes, on the cytoplasmic aspect of which the unit membrane is thickened to form an attachment plaque into which tonofilaments are inserted. Between these plaques are alternating light and dark laminae, which may represent orientated intercellular cement. At the level of the light microscope these structures and cytoplasmic extensions resulting from irregular shrinkage of the cell body, appear as the intercellular bridges although it is clear that no true cytoplasmic continuity exists between epithelial cells. Desmosomes may, however, represent a mechanical link so that forces applied to an epithelial surface will be transmitted via the cytoplasmic tonofilaments inserted in the attachment plaques and distributed over a

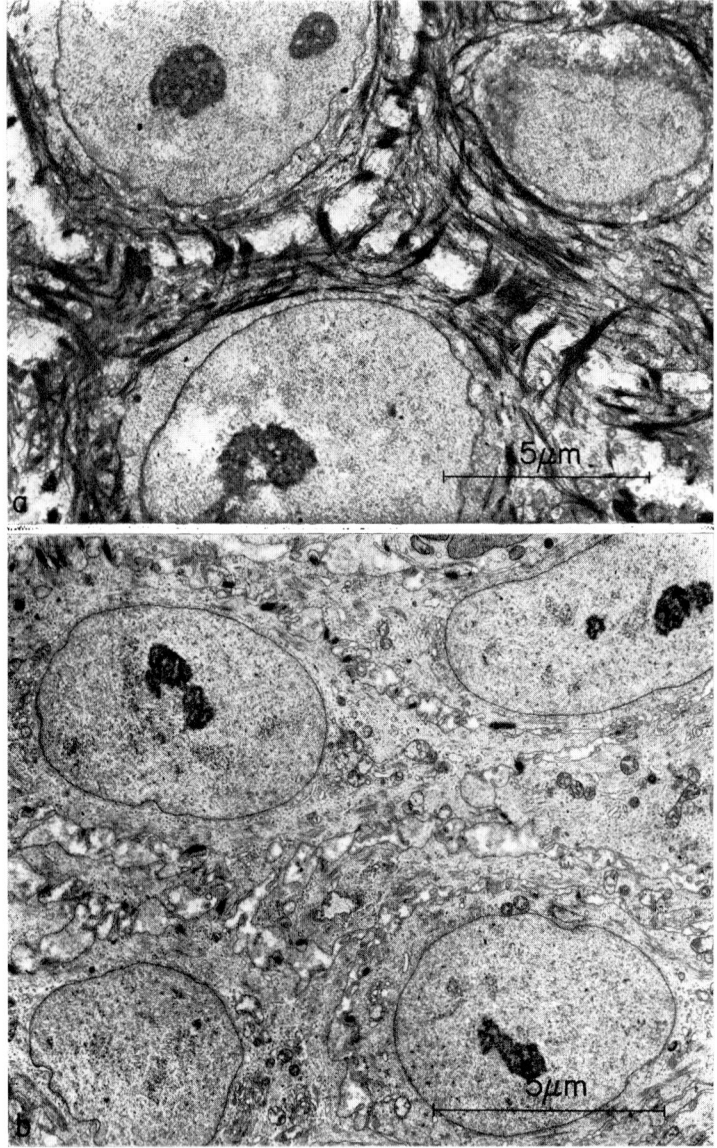

Fig. 1.9. (a) Electron micrograph of prickle cells from human gingival epithelium. Tonofilaments are gathered into bundles which are very conspicuous. Bar represents 5 μm.

(b) Electron micrograph of prickle cell from human buccal epithelium. Tonofilaments are sparse although other organelles are abundant. Bar represents 5 μm.

wide area (Scapino 1971). *The tight junction* (Fig. 1.8) is another intercellular attachment recognized morphologically by the close apposition of adjacent plasma membranes so that apparently no intercellular space remains. While these junctions may have a mechanical function, it is likely that they provide a low-resistance pathway across which ions can pass from cell to cell (Farquhar & Palade 1965). Depending on whether the tight junctions have the form of spot junctions or exist as continuous belts around the cells, they could serve to divide up the intercellular space and so act as intercellular barriers. This role has been suggested by Thilander & Bloom (1968) for tight junctions in oral epithelium, but is not substantiated by other work (see section 1:3:3). The existence of true tight junctions has been questioned in human gingival epithelium by Barnett & Szabo (1973), who claim that they are in fact *gap junctions* (Fig. 1.8) in which apposing plasma membranes are separated by an intercellular gap of approximately 2 nm.

Adhesion between the basal cell layer and the underlying connective tissue is mediated by *hemi-desmosomes* arranged along the basal plasma membrane (see Fig. 1.16). These also possess intercellular attachment plaques into which tonofilaments are inserted; direct continuity between these tonofilaments and fine filaments traversing the basal lamina has been suggested (Susi 1971; see section 1:5).

Although the basal layer contains the least differentiated cells of the epithelium, there are some differences between the basal cells of keratinizing and non-keratinizing epithelium. Meyer & Gerson (1964) reported a cross-sectional area for basal cells from keratinizing human palatal epithelium 25% greater than those of non-keratinizing buccal epithelium. The concentration of some organelles such as ribosomes, tonofilaments and desmosomes is also slightly higher in basal cells from the palate, which is keratinized, than in non-keratinizing buccal epithelial cells (Silverman 1971).

1:3:2C PRICKLE CELL LAYER

As the cells migrate into the prickle cell layer, the slight differences apparent between different epithelia in the basal layer are accentuated (Fig. 1.9). Tonofilaments and ribosomes become more concentrated in keratinizing epithelia (Fig. 1.9a), whereas in non-keratinizing regions the increase in the number of these organelles has not kept up with the increase in cell volume and so they appear sparser (Fig. 1.9b). There is also a difference in the organization of the tonofilaments which tend to be

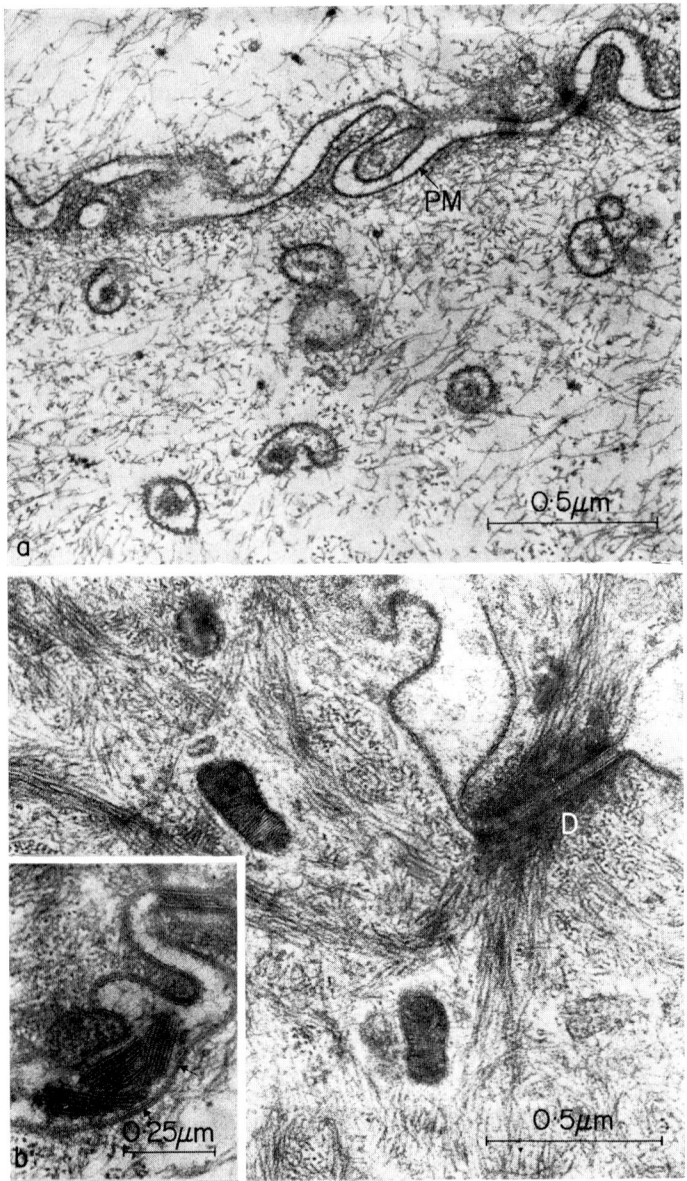

Fig. 1.10. (a) Electron micrograph of a portion of a cell from non-keratinized human oral epithelium. A number of 'membrane coating granules' are present, each with a bounding membrane and central dense core. PM = plasma membrane. Bar represents 0·5 μm.

(b) Electron micrograph of a portion of a cell from keratinizing human oral epithelium. Two lamellated membrane coating granules are apparent (arrows). D = desmosome. Bar represents 0·5 μm.

Inset. Lamellae, presumably derived from membrane coating granules, lying in the intercellular space. Note the thickening on the intracellular aspect of the plasma membrane (arrows). Bar represents 0·25 μm.

randomly distributed throughout the prickle cells of non-keratinized epithelium, but gathered together in bundles so as to form tonofibrils in keratinized tissue. Desmosomes are numerous in keratinized epithelium, but fewer in non-keratinized epithelia where the intercellular spaces are more irregular and contain abundant cement substance (Meyer & Gerson 1964).

In the superficial cells of the prickle layer, a new organelle makes its appearance; the *membrane coating granule*, Odland body, or keratinosome (Matoltsy & Parakkal 1967). These appear in groups in the superficial portion of the cell and may possibly develop in the Golgi system (Weinstock & Wilgram 1970) although the evidence is equivocal and other origins have been proposed (Odland 1960; Squier 1968). By the time the cell enters the next layer, these granules are arranged along the superficial plasma membrane. Two sorts of granules can be recognized, the morphology depending generally on whether the epithelium is keratinized or not. Thus granules from non-keratinized epithelium (Fig. 1.10a), be they from the cheek or uterine cervix, are predominantly circular membranous vesicles approximately 0·1–0·3 μm in diameter with a central dense core (Grubb, Hackemann & Hill 1968; Silverman, 1971); in epidermis and keratinized oral epithelium (Fig. 1.10b) they appear circular or elongate, up to 0·4 μm in length, and invariably contain a series of parallel lamellae that give them a striated appearance (Odland 1960; Frithiof & Wersäll 1965). Both types have been shown to contain acid phosphatase and so have been classified as lysosomes (Wolff & Holubar 1967; Silverman 1971).

1:3:2d GRANULAR OR INTERMEDIATE LAYER

In the epidermis and in all human ortho-keratinized oral epithelium a distinct granular layer is seen (Fig. 1:11a). The cells in this layer have increased in volume and dry weight and appear flattened and, although all the organelles already mentioned are still present in the deeper cells of this layer, the cytoplasm is predominantly occupied by tonofilaments. In the superficial cells of this layer, the membrane coating granules which are gathered along the plasma membrane seem to fuse with it, and their lamellae appear in the intercellular space (Frithiof & Wersäll 1965). At the same level, but unassociated with the discharge of granules an intracytoplasmic thickening develops on the plasma membrane (Fig. 1.10 inset), which is continuous with, and obscures, the attachment plaque of the desmosomes (Farbman 1966). This layer probably represents the first stage in the formation of the highly resistant membrane enclosing the keratinized squame.

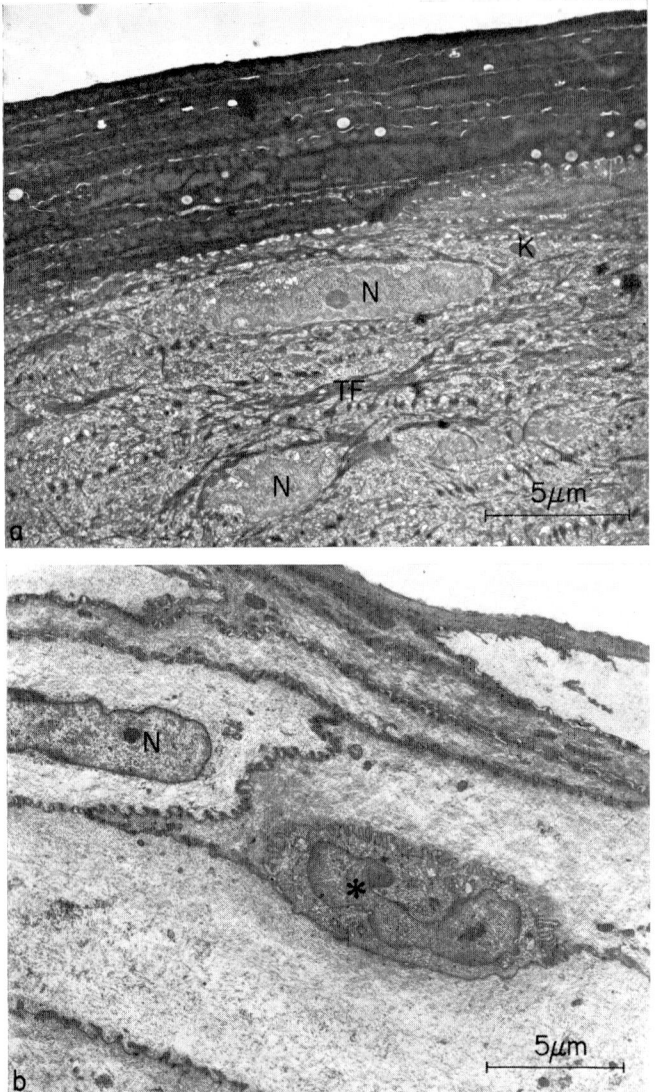

Fig. 1.11. (a) Electron micrograph of granular and keratinized layers of human gingival epithelium. There is a dramatic change at the junction of these layers: nuclei (N), tonofibrils (TF) and a keratohyalin granule (K) are visible in the granular cells. No organelles are apparent in the keratinized layer. Bar represents 5 μm.

(b) Electron micrograph of the intermediate and superficial layers of non-keratinized human buccal epithelium. Tonofilaments are sparse and not gathered into bundles, a nucleus (N) and other organelles are present in the superficial layers (compare with (a)); there is also a non-epithelial cell visible (asterisk), probably a Langerhans cell. Bar represents 5 μm.

Structure and Function

The characteristic intracellular feature of this layer is the presence of the *keratohyalin granules*, which show considerable morphological differences between various keratinizing epithelia. On the basis of their histological staining affinities and ultrastructural appearance, keratohyaline granules have been divided into two types (Weinmann, Meyer & Medak 1960; Jessen 1970). Granules which are irregular in size and shape, show an intimate association with tonofilaments and are usually surrounded by ribosomes are commonly seen in the epidermis and the keratinized regions of human oral epithelium and have been designated '*epidermal type*'

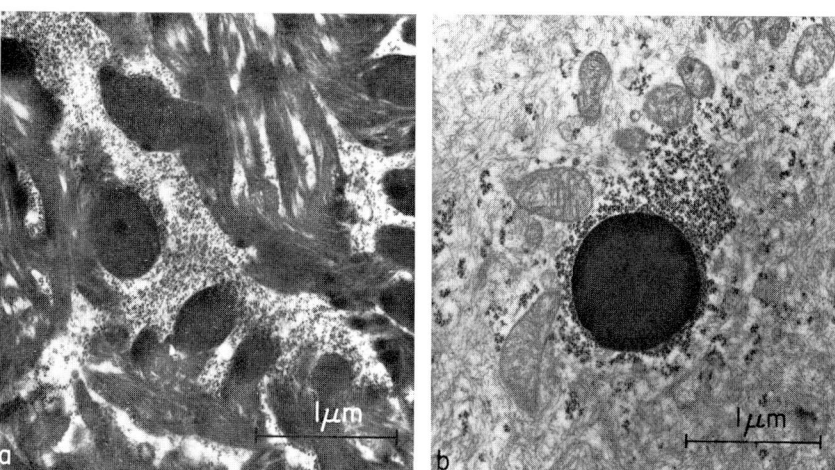

Fig. 1.12. (a) Electron micrograph of the keratohyalin granules found in epidermis and certain keratinized oral epithelia. These show close association with tonofilament bundles and numerous ribosomes are also present. Bar represents 1 μm.

(b) 'Cheek type' keratohyalin granules are not associated with tonofilaments, although ribosomes surround the granule. Bar represents 1 μm.

keratohyalin (Fig. 1.12a). In para-keratinized human oral epithelium, the granules are of the same type but fewer are present and they appear as smaller more regular structures (Silverman 1971). The second type of keratohyalin granules, the so-called '*cheek type*', are seen typically in the keratinized buccal epithelium of rodents. These granules are more regular in shape than epidermal keratohyalin but may be very variable in size, ranging from 0·5 μm to 8 μm or more in diameter; they are usually surrounded by ribosomes, but do not appear to be associated with tonofilaments (Fig. 1.12b). There is no clear evidence as to the origin of keratohyalin granules; biochemical analyses suggest that they contain protein (Matoltsy & Matoltsy 1972), and they have been shown to incorporate labelled amino acids (Fukuyama & Epstein 1967). It thus seems likely that they are synthesized by the ribosomes so frequently seen associated with them.

Dramatic changes take place in the superficial layers of the granular layer; virtually all organelles including the nuclei and keratohyalin granules disappear and the adjacent cells of the keratinized layer are filled entirely with closely packed fibrils. A *transition layer* is apparent in some regions of the epidermis (Brody 1964), but is less common in keratinized human oral epithelium (Silverman 1971); this layer shows dense concentrations of tonofilaments interspersed with amorphous masses of keratohyaline and constitutes the *stratum lucidum* of histological preparations.

In the non-keratinized regions of the human oral cavity, a typical granular layer is not distinguished. However, at the same relative level, that is in the deeper portion of the outer third of the epithelium, ultrastructural changes are seen that distinguish the cells from basal and prickle cells. These include the presence of membrane coating granules which, while differing structurally from those of keratinized epithelium, behave in a similar manner, fusing with the plasma membrane and contributing an amorphous material to the intercellular space, and a slight intracellular thickening of the plasma membrane (Frithiof 1970). At the same level, keratohyalin granules are occasionally seen both with the electron microscope (Silverman 1971) and the light microscope (Meyer, Daftary & Pindborg 1967); these granules are of the cheek type. Tonofilaments are present, but are sparse and not gathered into bundles, and there are reduced numbers of other organelles such as ribosomes and mitochondria. However, in contrast to the events occurring at this level in keratinized epithelia, these organelles, together with keratohyalin and the cell nuclei, persist in the surface layer.

1:3:2e KERATINIZED OR SUPERFICIAL LAYER

In the epidermis and keratinized regions of oral epithelium, the superficial layers consist of flattened cells filled with fibrils showing the typical keratin pattern, all other cytoplasmic organelles having disappeared (Fig. 1.11). The cell margin forms villous processes which interdigitate with adjacent cells; the plasma membrane, while showing the intracellular thickening laid down in the granular layer, also develops an additional external thickening (Frithiof 1970) which may be derived from the membrane coating granules (Martinez & Peters 1971; Hayward &

Hackemann 1973). Desmosomes are sometimes visible, but have lost their connection with the tonofilaments and rarely show the typical arrangement of intercellular laminae present in the deeper layers. In para-keratinized oral regions, the nuclei persist as condensed electron opaque zones and the rest of the cell is occupied by fibrillar material (Silverman 1971).

The superficial region of non-keratinized epithelium differs little from the preceding layer (Fig. 1.11b). There is no marked flattening of the cells and although cytoplasmic organelles are few, nuclei and, on occasions, keratohyalin granules are present in the surface layer (Rubinstein, Medak & Meyer 1970). The cell membrane shows numerous infoldings and desmosomes are reduced in number and associated with sparse tonofilaments; the intercellular space is filled with finely fibrillar material.

Studies of the surface of epidermis and oral epithelia by exfoliative cytology show the desquamating cells to be flattened hexagonal plates which, in certain areas of the epidermis, but not apparently in oral epithelium, are stacked vertically as columns (Mackenzie 1969). These columns can be traced as far as the superficial prickle cell layer, and it has been shown that they are the result of cell division consistently occurring at fixed sites in the basal layer (Mackenzie 1970, 1973a). In terms of area the superficial cells from oral epithelium are significantly larger (60–70 μm diameter) than the largest epidermal squames (34–44 μm diameter), and this relationship does not vary with the age of the individual (Plewig 1971).

Many workers have tried to correlate the cytological appearance of desquamating oral epithelial cells with systemic influences, particularly the menstrual cycle. The results are conflicting and have been summarized recently by Van Mens (1972), who claimed that while a clear sexual difference exists, and a certain 'unrest' may be observed in human palatal squames during menstruation, no real correlations between cell size or stainability and the phases of the menstrual cycle can be demonstrated.

1:3:2f GLYCOGEN

Glycogen may be recognized in most routine electron microscope preparations and can be detected by specific staining reactions in the light microscope. It is invariably seen in non-keratinized oral epithelium, in cells between the parabasal and superficial layers (Silverman 1971). In keratinized oral epithelium, glycogen is less commonly found, small amounts sometimes being seen in the upper prickle cells and granular layer of normal keratinized human gingival epithelium (Weiss, Weinmann

& Meyer 1959; Schroeder & Theilade 1966), but it is not normally found in the epidermis.

Glycogen in oral tissues may serve as a precursor for the synthesis of intercellular ground substance, which is abundant in non-keratinized epithelium (Iqbal & Gerson 1971). Silverman, Barbosa & Kearns (1971) have found an inverse relationship between the amount of glycogen and the degree of keratinization in hyperkeratotic lesions, which they interpret as being indicative of its role as a source of energy for keratin formation. The glycogen context of oral epithelium and of epidermis tends to increase in aged individuals (see section 1:7).

1:3:3 Barrier function: the structural basis of permeability

1:3:3a THE PERMEABILITY OF SKIN

The role of the skin in providing a barrier both to the entry of foreign materials and to the loss of interstitial fluid is well accepted. From a structural point of view the epidermis is an impressive barrier composed of a resistant keratinized surface, overlying several layers of closely apposed cells and, at its junction with the dermis, a basement membrane that serves to filter out all but small particles (see section 1:5). Within the connective tissue of the dermis, molecules of all sizes can circulate, although as Day (1952) has pointed out, a degree of impermeability is conferred on this tissue by the interfibrillar material (see section 1:6:2).

It is clear that under normal conditions all the components mentioned above contribute to the barrier function of the skin. Relatively large objects such as micro-organisms do not penetrate further than the superficial squames of normal intact epidermis; similarly, once embryological development is complete, cells are not normally seen traversing the basement membrane. However, at a molecular level there are a number of potential routes for the passage of substances which will depend on the size and nature of the material. Thus a substance may traverse the epidermis by passing through the intercellular spaces around the cells, by passing into and across the cells, or by passing through the follicles of hairs or the ducts of eccrine glands. The latter structures represent epidermal shunts and may be important routes for substances to which the epidermis proper is impermeable (Scheuplein & Blank 1971). The intercellular spaces represent a series of channels that link the surface of the epidermis with the connective tissue; they are filled with intercellular substance, essentially a hydrophilic mucosubstance. The epidermal cells, enclosed by lipoprotein membranes, together constitute what is essentially a multiphase membrane system across which material must pass. Although material has been shown to enter the epidermis by being taken up into basal cells by pinocytosis (Nordquist, Olson & Everett 1966; Wolff & Hönigsmann 1971) whence it might be passed on by reverse pinocytosis, this process does not seem likely to account for transport across an entire stratified and keratinized tissue. Most substances pass across epithelium either between the cells or through the cells by simple diffusion and the route taken by a particular substance will depend largely on its molecular weight and characteristics such as its oil/water solubility.

Much work has been concerned with the site of barriers to water and water-soluble substances and there is little information on the pathways taken by lipid-soluble materials. Measurements of transepidermal water loss show that this rises dramatically when the stratum corneum is removed, but that the stripping of the deeper epidermal layers has little further effect (Spruit 1970). If these measurements are continued during regeneration of the epidermis, it is found that the rate of loss decreases as soon as keratinized cells appear and that only two layers of keratinized squames constitute a reasonable barrier (Eriksson & Lamke 1971). Such results are confirmed by the use of tracer substances injected subepidermally. Horseradish peroxidase is a water-soluble protein that can be detected with the electron microscope; after being injected intradermally this substance passes freely across the basement membrane and enters the intercellular space of the epidermis (Schreiner & Wolff 1969). Here it penetrates as far as the upper granular layer, stopping at the level where the membrane coating granules are extruded into the intercellular space. Schreiner & Wolff (1969) have suggested that it is these granules that are responsible for the formation of the barrier. The barrier material probably persists throughout the intercellular spaces of the keratinized layer, so that the whole superficial layer constitutes an impermeable covering. Whether the same system also provides a barrier to compounds with a high lipid/water-solubility or whether such compounds pass predominantly through cells is unknown.

1:3:3b THE PERMEABILITY OF ORAL EPITHELIUM

Although the need to prevent transepithelial water loss would seem less important in the oral mucosa than in the epidermis, it is still necessary to restrict the entry of micro-organisms and their toxic products that are a constant feature of the oral cavity. However, in view of the ease with which many drugs can be administered orally it has become common to regard the oral mucosa as a highly permeable membrane and to suggest that this permeability is a reflection of oral keratinization being less complete than in the epidermis, or absent, so that a uniform barrier layer is missing (Malkinson 1964; Winkelmann 1969). This is an oversimplification and it is worth noting again that despite the presence of areas of non-keratinized epithelium in the human oral cavity, there are also areas of ortho-keratinization resembling in most respects that seen in the epidermis (see section 1:3:2). Unfortunately, there is little information available as to the relative permeability of these different regions, largely because methods of testing permeability in human subjects, such as the 'buccal absorption' test do not permit accurate regional discrimination (Siegel, Hall & Stambaugh 1971).

Investigations of oral mucosa using the ultrastructural tracer horse-radish peroxidase (McDougall 1970; Squier 1973) have shown that keratinized oral epithelium behaves in a very similar way to the epidermis and that a barrier to penetration exists at the same level as the membrane coating granules appear in the intercellular space. Surprisingly, non-keratinized mucosa shows a similar barrier, again corresponding with the extrusion of the membrane coating granules; in non-keratinized tissue these granules are not lamellated (see section 1:3:2) but appear to secrete an amorphous component into the intercellular space which apparently constitutes an effective barrier material (Squier 1973). Such findings have limited applicability as they only reflect the behaviour of one particular water-soluble substance, whereas in drug absorption tests the importance of a high oil/water solubility has been claimed to facilitate penetration of a given compound (Siegel, Hall & Stambaugh 1971).

1:3:3C THE GINGIVAL SULCUS

The epithelium applied to the tooth surface differs considerably from that in other parts of the mouth. Controversy has existed for decades as to whether there is structural organic union between the epithelium and the dental hard tissue or whether it is merely held in close apposition to the tooth by pressures within the connective tissue.

Recent extensive ultrastructural studies, in particular those of Schroeder, of Listgarten and of Frank, have now substantially resolved the issue (Schroeder & Listgarten 1971; Listgarten 1972; Frank & Cimasoni 1970). In health the human gingival sulcus is of the order of only 0·1 mm

Structure and Function 43

in depth. Its floor and the epithelium applied to the tooth surface, frequently referred to in the past as the 'epithelial attachment', has been designated *junctional epithelium* by Schroeder & Listgarten (Fig. 1.13).

The walls of the sulcus are lined by epithelium derived from, and continuous with that of the rest of the oral mucosa. This has been designated *oral sulcular epithelium* and has the same basic structure as non-keratinized oral epithelium, the ortho- or para-keratinized surface of the free gingiva stopping in the region of the gingival crest.

Junctional epithelium is derived from the reduced enamel epithelium of the tooth germ and consists of 2–15 cell layers with a smooth connective

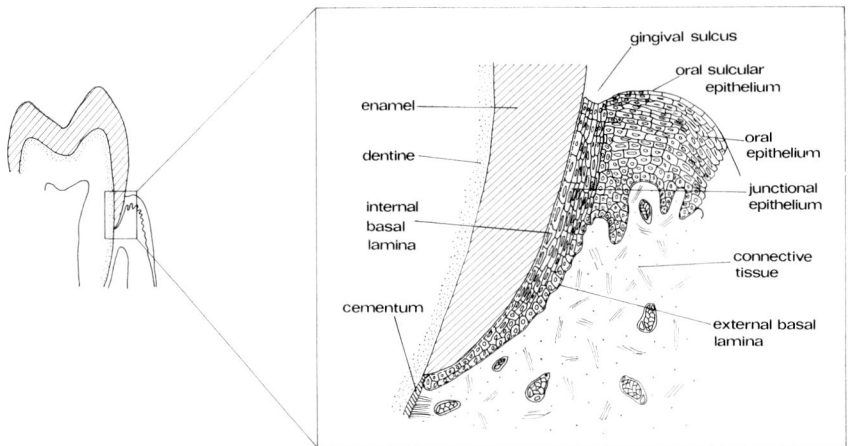

Fig. 1.13. Diagram to show the organization of epithelium at the gingivo-enamel junction. (Based on Schroeder and Listgarten 1971.)

tissue interface and a normal basal lamina, designated the *external basal lamina*, with associated hemi-desmosomes (Fig. 1.16). Between the plasma membrane of the junctional epithelial cells and the enamel surface a similar *internal basal lamina* is present, again with hemi-desmosomal attachments.

In view of the importance of this area in the development of periodontal disease it has been extensively studied and a great variety of substances have been shown to be capable of traversing the epithelium of the gingival sulcus. Tissue fluid and cells as well as dyes, carbon particles and horseradish peroxidase have been shown to pass from the connective tissue into the sulcus (Brill & Björn 1959; Egelberg 1963b; McDougal 1970), while albumin, histamine, horse-radish peroxidase, bacterial endo-toxin and carbon particles have been traced in the opposite direction (Tolo 1971; Egelberg 1963a; McDougall 1971; Schwartz et al 1972; Fine, Pechersky & McKibben 1969; Gibson & Shannon 1965). Attempts have been made to try to determine the ultrastructural pathways by which materials traverse the epithelium (McDougall 1970, 1971) and results from these studies suggest that the junctional epithelium may be more permeable than most other epithelial tissues.

Junctional epithelium is not simply an area of non-keratinized epithelium; it has particularly wide intercellular spaces and membrane coating granules seem to be absent from the cells. These features more than any other could account for the ready permeability of the tissue, although it is difficult to assess what effect inflammatory cells may also be having, as neutrophil leucocytes and mononuclear cells are such a common constituent of the region (Schroeder 1970, 1973).

1:4 The Epithelium: Non-keratinocytes

1:4:1 Types of non-keratinocytes

Histological sections through epidermis and oral epithelium frequently reveal cells at various levels that differ quite markedly from the majority of epithelial cells in possessing a clear halo around the nucleus. Such *clear cells* (Fig 1:4b) have been variously classified as pigment cells, Langerhans cells, Merkel cells or lymphocytes depending on their distribution in the epithelium and the prejudices of the observer. Ultrastructurally it is apparent that these cells all differ morphologically from a typical epithelial cell and that all of them except the Merkel cell lack desmosome attachments to adjacent cells. As Breathnach (1965) has pointed out, it is probably this absence of desmosomes which allows the cytoplasm of these cells to shrink around the nucleus during histological processing and so produce the typical 'clear' perinuclear halo that gives them their name.

Under the electron microscope it is now possible to distinguish between the various clear cells and to assign a definite function to most of them; none of these cells shows any tendency to keratinize which justifies their classification as non-keratinocytes. Table 1.4 lists the different types of non-keratinocytes found in epithelium with their histochemical and ultrastructural characteristics; a more detailed description of each cell is given below.

1:4:1a THE MELANOCYTE

Although various names such as melanoblast, melanophore, melanodendrocyte and melanocyte have been applied to the epithelial pigment

Table 1.4. Characteristics of non-keratinocytes

Cell type	Level in epithelium	Specific staining reactions	Ultrastructural features
Melanocyte	Basal	DOPA positive; tyrosinase positive; argentaffin reactive	Dendritic, no desmosomes or tonofilaments; pre-melanosomes and melanosomes present
'Amelanotic' melanocyte	Basal	DOPA negative; weakly tyrosinase positive	Dendritic, no desmosomes or tonofilaments; pre-melanosomes present
Langerhans cell	Predominantly suprabasal	Gold chloride positive; osmium iodide positive; ATPase positive; stains with quinineimine dyes	Dendritic, no desmosomes or tonofilaments; characteristic 'Langerhans granule'
Non-specific dendritic cell	Predominantly suprabasal	Unknown	Dendritic, no desmosomes or tonofilaments
Merkel cell	Basal	Probably paS positive	Non-dendritic; sparse desmosomes and tonofilaments; characteristic electron dense vesicles and associated nerve
Lymphocyte	Variable	None	Non-dendritic; large circular nucleus; scant cytoplasm with few organelles; no desmosomes or tonofilaments

cell, the term *melanocyte* has now been universally adopted (Della Porter & Mühlbock 1966) to describe the melanin-producing dendritic cell situated in the basal region of both epidermis and oral epithelium. Melanocytes lack the tonofilaments and desmosomes of epithelial cells and synthesize melanin pigment on small organelles called *melanosomes*; in pigmented individuals these cells are recognizable by their abundant content of melanin (Fig. 1.14a). The cells are less active in the production of melanin in light-skinned persons and they may thus be more easily mistaken for other types of clear cells. A more detailed account of the role of the melanocyte in pigmentation is given in section 1:4:2.

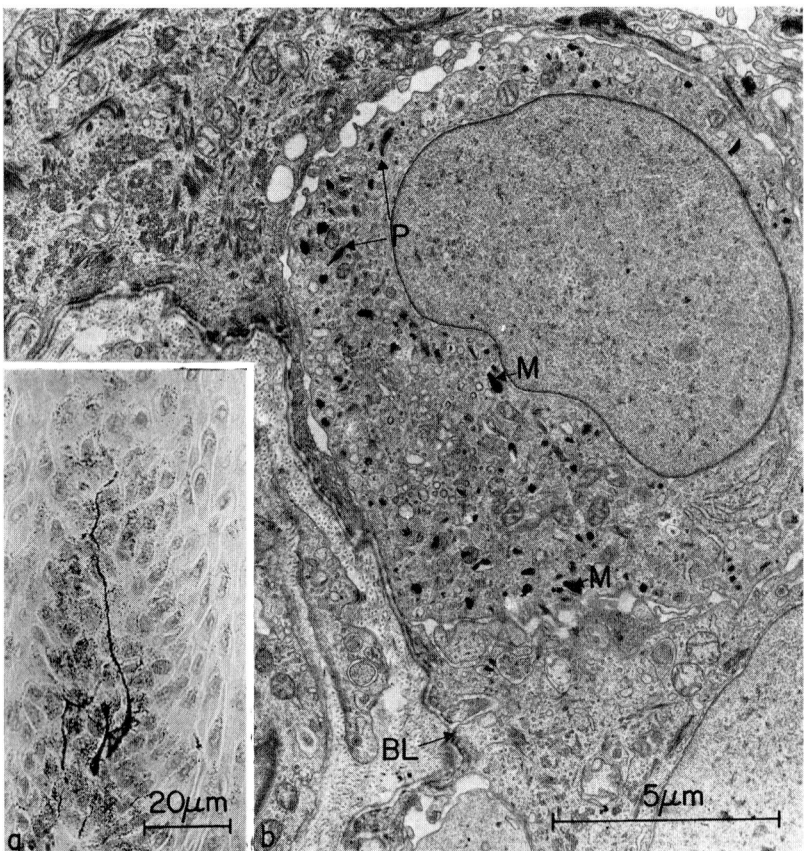

Fig. 1.14. (a) Light micrograph of a melanocyte in human gingival epithelium stained by the Masson–Fontana silver method. The cell body is situated basally although a dendritic process extends well into the prickle cell layer. Bar represents 20 μm.
(b) Electron micrograph of a melanocyte in human buccal epithelium. The cell is situated adjacent to the basal lamina (BL) and pre-melanosomes (M) and melanosomes are present in the cytoplasm. Bar represents 5 μm.

1:4:1b THE LANGERHANS CELL

This cell was first described by Paul Langerhans in 1868 during a study of sections of human epidermis impregnated with gold chloride where they were seen in the upper layers of the epidermis, a distribution which has led to their being designated 'high level' clear cells. Ultra-structural studies by Birbeck, Breathnach & Everall (1961) and Breathnach (1964)

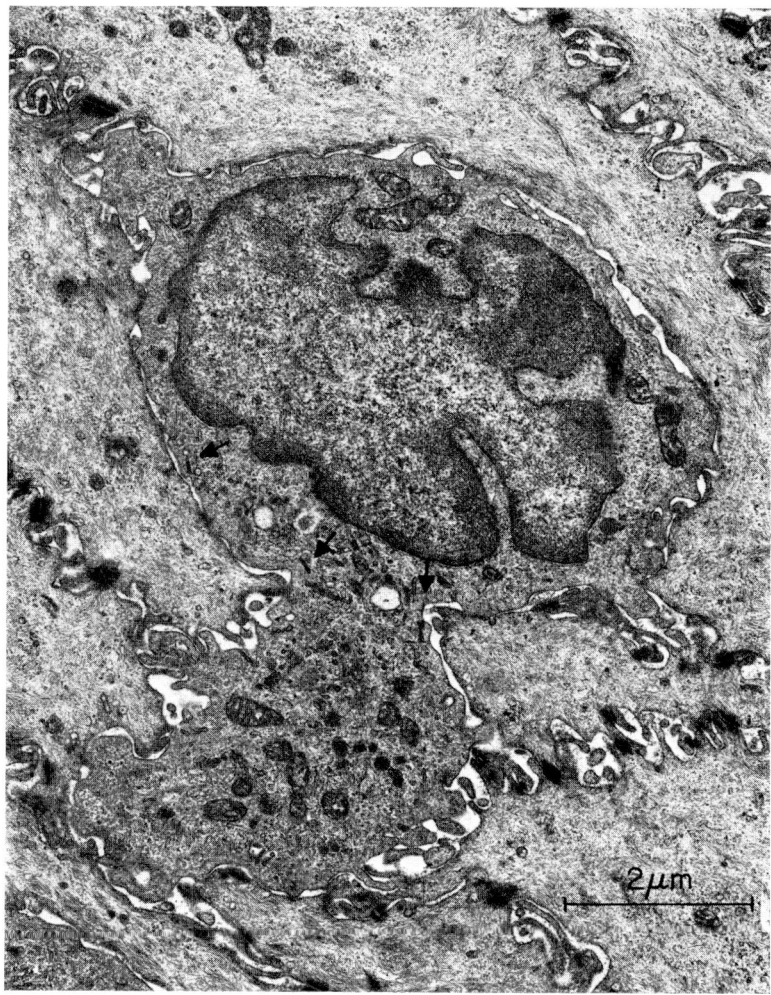

Fig. 1.15. Electron micrograph of a Langerhans cell in human buccal epithelium. The cell is dendritic with a deeply indented nucleus and several characteristic granules (arrows) may be seen. Bar represents 2 μm.

showed that these cells, like the melanocyte, are dendritic, lack tonofibrils and desmosomes but contain a characteristic granule, only visible at the electron microscope level and variously called a *Langerhans* or *Birbeck granule*. This granule usually appears as a rod-shaped body approximately 0.2 μm long which is sometimes expanded into a vesicle at one end (Sagebiel & Reed 1968). Langerhans cells with the same features have been found in human oral epithelium (Fig. 1.15) (Schroeder & Theilade 1966; Waterhouse & Squier 1967) and it is now apparent that these cells are not invariably situated at high levels in the epithelium but may be seen in deeper layers.

Despite numerous investigations of the histology, histochemistry and ultrastructure of Langerhans cells, there is no agreement as to their origin or function. This is in part due to the difficulty of reliably demonstrating the cell, for staining methods such as gold chloride or osmium iodide are capricious and at the ultrastructural level the chance of a characteristic granule appearing in every ultra-thin section is unlikely. As a consequence, some workers have chosen to establish yet another series of 'indeterminate' or 'non-specific' dendritic cells; these are considered briefly in the next section. The most reliable histochemical method of detection so far seems to be the use of the ATPase reaction (Wolff & Winkelmann 1967). The main theories put forward to explain the role of the Langerhans cell will now be briefly mentioned.

One of the earliest suggestions as to the origin of the Langerhans cell was that of Billingham & Medawar (1953), who proposed that they represented effete melanocytes. While this accounted for the similar appearance of the two cells and, in many cases, for their relative positions in the epithelium, it has not been supported by subsequent work. Ultrastructurally the cells do not appear to be effete and in fact are capable of division (Mackenzie 1973b; Konrad & Hönigsmann 1973). Moreover they appear in the developing epidermis before, or at the same time as, the melanocytes (Breathnach 1971) and have been shown to be present in the epidermis of animals from which the melanocyte-producing neurectoderm has been experimentally removed at the embryonic stage (Breathnach et al 1968).

The presence of cells with all the characteristics of Langerhans cells, including the granule, in lesions of Histiocytosis X (Basset & Turiaf 1965), as well as in lymph nodes (Kondo 1969) and in normal dermis (Zelickson 1965; Böck 1973), led to the suggestion that these cells might represent a population of epithelial macrophages having a mesodermal origin. While such a theory has its attractions, particularly in view of the presence within the Langerhans cell of lysosomes containing hydrolytic enzymes (Campo-Aasen & Pearse 1966) there is abundant experimental evidence that the cell is not actively phagocytic. Wolff & Schreiner (1970) observed that a foreign protein (horseradish peroxidase) introduced into the epidermis was taken up more rapidly by the epithelial cells than by the Langerhans cells; similarly after the surface layers of the epidermis have been damaged by tape stripping, it is customary to see cell remnants in phagocytic vacuoles within epithelial cells (Mottaz, Thorne & Zelickson 1971) rather than in the supposedly phagocytic Langerhans cell (Mottaz & Zelickson 1970).

The idea that Langerhans cells represent part of an epithelial neural network was first proposed by Langerhans himself (1868), who was impressed by the dendritic network formed by these cells after metal impregnation. However, no association of Langerhans cells with nerves either in the connective tissue or epidermis has been observed (Breathnach 1965) and other specialized cells with a neural function, the Merkel cells, exist in oral epithelium and epidermis.

More recently the role of the Langerhans cell as a regulatory or mediator cell has been proposed. Sagebiel, Clarke & Hutchens (1971) noticed differences in the numbers of Langerhans cells in keratinized and non-keratinized oral epithelium and proposed that they might produce a chalone-like substance which could influence cell division and differentiation (see section 1:3:1). In an examination of epidermis showing a regular columnar structure (see section 1:3:2), Mackenzie & Strief (1973) have found that Langerhans cells, identified by their ATPase activity, were also regularly spaced and tended to be positioned beneath the centre of the overlying columns. This, they suggest, indicates a link between Langerhans cell function and spatial organization of the keratinocytes. Silberberg (1973), in an ultrastructural study of the epidermis in contact allergic reactions, has reported the apposition of mononuclear cells to Langerhans cells and suggests that the cell may be involved in the uptake and processing of allergenic materials.

1:4:1C NON-SPECIFIC DENDRITIC CELLS

Sections of oral epithelium and epidermis examined in the electron microscope frequently reveal dendritic cells lacking either the characteristic granule of the Langerhans cell or the melanosome of the melanocyte. Such cells have been described both in epidermis (Zelickson & Mottaz 1968) and in oral epithelium (Hutchens, Sagebiel & Clarke 1971) and have been further classified as 'high level' or 'low level' cells depending on their position in the epithelium. While such cells may represent a distinct cell type, it is more likely that they are merely portions of Langerhans cells or melanocytes from which the characteristic organelle is absent. Only serial sectioning or the application of a more or less specific cytochemical stain can resolve this problem.

1:4:1d THE MERKEL CELL AND
INTRA-EPITHELIAL NERVES

Merkel cells appear histologically as 'clear cells' situated at low level in oral epithelium and epidermis, although they do not have the dendritic form characteristic of the melanocyte or Langerhans cell. Despite the fact that Merkel cells were probably first described in gingiva by Merkel in 1875 (see Hashimoto 1972) they have only recently been reported in other regions of oral epithelium (Kutuzov & Sicher 1952; Chen 1970; Nikai, Rose & Cattoni 1971; Hashimoto 1972). They are found in the epidermis of both hairy and glabrous skin where they may be associated in groups to form the Merkel disc or Haarscheiben, a touch receptor located in the basal layer overlying dermal papillae and associated with intra-epithelial nerve endings (Iggo & Muir 1969; Winkelmann & Breathnach 1973).

Ultrastructurally (Hashimoto 1972; Winkelmann & Breathnach 1973), the Merkel cell is seen to have desmosome attachments to adjacent cells although these are not as numerous or as obvious as those between epithelial cells; hemi-desmosomes are lacking but a nerve fibre is usually associated with the basal aspect of the cell. Within the cytoplasm there may be tonofilaments but the most characteristic findings are small membrane-bounded electron dense granules 80–200 μm in diameter which are usually situated on the opposite side of the cell to the Golgi complex and adjacent to the external nerve fibre. These granules are similar to the nor-adrenalin-containing vesicles of the adrenal medulla and other chromaffin cells and could act to liberate a transmitter across the cleft between the Merkel cell and adjacent nerve (Hashimoto 1972). Such an arrangement would be in accord with the proposed function of the cell as an epithelial sensory receptor. Merkel cells have been identified in biopsies of a patient with aphthous stomatitis by Wilgram (1972), who speculated that the release of catecholamine from the specific granules *might* contribute to the necrosis which accompanies the development of aphthous ulcers.

While the presence of desmosomes and tonofilaments might indicate an ectodermal origin, the Merkel cell does not appear in the human epidermis until 16 weeks (Breathnach 1971). Merkel cells have been observed in the connective tissue and also traversing the basement membrane of human embryonic skin (Winkelmann & Breathnach 1973), suggesting that they are probably an immigrant cell of mesodermal origin.

There have been many histological descriptions of intra-epidermal nerve fibres; the majority have been free endings and Weddell *et al* (1965) claim that Schwann cells and perineural cells are never found in the epidermis of normal skin. Intra-epidermal nerve fibres have never been convincingly demonstrated with the electron microscope in interfollicular regions of hairy human skin (Breathnach 1971) but they are present in glabrous skin, usually associated with Merkel cells.

In the oral mucosa, intra-epithelial nerve endings have been frequently demonstrated (Fig. 1.19), particularly in the human gingiva. As in the epidermis, they are never associated with specialized perineural cells except Merkel cells; when these cells are lacking the nerves run between epithelial cells which often ensheath or completely enclose the nerve to form a mesaxon. The nerves terminate as simple endings, usually packed with mitochondria (Farbman & Allgood 1971).

1:4:1e OTHER CLEAR CELLS

Under normal conditions the epidermis and most areas of the oral epithelium are free from inflammatory cells. However, the junctional and oral sulcular epithelium of the gingiva is often infiltrated with neutrophilic granulocytes and mononuclear cells (Schroeder 1973). Lymphocytes are frequently seen elsewhere in the gingival epithelium (Cattoni 1951) and in other regions of oral epithelium in patients with clinically normal oral mucosa (Schroeder 1973). While it is possible to obtain gingival epithelium that is effectively free from inflammatory infiltrate by a rigorous oral hygiene regime (Schroeder & Theilade 1966) it must be accepted that some inflammatory cells may be present even when there are no clinical signs of inflammation and represent a normal feature of the epithelium.

Cells with metachromatic granules and the ultrastructural characteristics of mast cells of the connective tissue have been demonstrated in gingival epithelium (Angelopoulos 1970; Barnett 1973). Such reports are, however, rare and the nature and function of these cells is unknown.

1:4:2 The melanocyte and epithelial pigmentation

The colour of skin and oral mucosa is the result of a number of related factors such as thickness of the epithelium, degree of keratinization, the presence of melanin pigment, the vascularity of the underlying connective tissue and the relative amounts of reduced or oxidized haemoglobin, and the presence of subcutaneous fat. These features may all be considered as endogenous in contrast to exogenous pigmentation in which foreign material, such as heavy metals or carbon, are introduced either systemically or locally into the body and produce coloration of the skin or oral tissues (McCarthy & Skhlar 1964). In this chapter we are concerned only with the way in which endogenous factors give rise to normal pigmentation.

The two most important features in determining skin colour seem to be the degree of vascularity and the amount of melanin pigment. Wasserman (1971) claims that in all races a red hue is present due to haemoglobin and the observed differences result from melanin in the epidermis acting as a filter interposed between the observer and this red vascular coloration. In the oral cavity the epithelium, which is non-keratinized in many areas and possesses only a thin keratin layer in other areas, overlays an extensively vascularized connective tissue. The resulting appearance is that of a brighter red coloration than is seen anywhere in the skin except at the muco-cutaneous junctions.

The effect of the melanin content of the epidermis in determining overall skin colour is thus important and melanin pigmentation has often been used as a criterion for anthropological distinction between ethnic groups. However, a major difficulty in studying pigmentation is to unambiguously classify the individual under investigation, and much confusion has been created by the use of arbitrary divisions such as 'light-skinned' or 'dark-skinned'.

There is far less information available about the melanin pigmentation of the oral mucosa than about the skin, although Dummett & Barens (1971) state that there is a direct relationship between the degree of pigmentation seen in the skin and that found in the oral mucosa. Within the oral cavity the areas most commonly pigmented are the mucosal surface of the lips, the gingiva, the buccal mucosa and the soft palate. However, the degree of pigmentation varies in all these areas with race, the greatest differences probably being seen in the buccal mucosa, which is pigmented in only 5% of 'Europeans' but in 38% of 'coloureds' (Fry & Almeyda 1968).

1:4:2a THE ROLE OF THE MELANOCYTE

Despite our ignorance of the prevalence of oral pigmentation, the mechanism by which melanin is produced and distributed through the epidermis and oral epithelium is well understood. The cell responsible for producing melanin, the melanocyte, is embryologically derived from neural crest ectoderm and in the human foetus enters the epidermis and presumably the oral epithelium from the eleventh week onwards (Breathnach 1971). Once in the epithelium these cells constitute a self-producing population normally situated within the basal layer of the fully developed human epidermis (Breathnach 1971) although they have been observed suprabasally in human oral epithelium (Squier & Waterhouse 1967; Schroeder 1969). Cells containing melanin may be seen in the connective tissue of normal pigmented human skin and mucosa; electron microscopical examination of such cells does not reveal any of the characteristics of the epithelial melanocyte and it is likely that they represent macrophages containing melanin that must have originated in the epithelium (Fig. 1.19) (Breathnach 1971). The term *melanophage* is sometimes applied to these cells.

One of the most significant findings to come out of studies of the number of melanocytes in human epidermis is that individuals, regardless of race, who show widely differing degrees of pigmentation have approximately the same number of melanocytes in any given region of the skin (Szabo 1954). Thus the ratio of melanocytes to basal epidermal cells in caucasoids and negroids varies from approximately 1:4 on the cheek to 1:11 over the thighs and arms (Fitzpatrick & Szabo 1959). Little data are available for the oral mucosa, although Fitzpatrick & Szabo quote an overall figure of 1 : 7. In the oral mucosa of Rhesus monkey, Hutchens, Sagebiel & Clarke (1971) report a ratio of melanocytes to epithelial cells ranging from 1 : 18 in pigmented buccal epithelium to 1 : 4 in the external lip; a ratio of 1 : 15 has been found in human gingival epithelium (Barker 1967).

Differences in pigmentation of a given region are thus a function of the activity, rather than the number, of melanocytes and even in conditions of hypo-pigmentation such as albinism (Becker, Fitzpatrick & Montgomery 1952) or piebaldism (Breathnach, Fitzpatrick & Wyllie 1965) this remains true and 'amelanotic' melanocytes are still present. The effect of ultraviolet radiation on pigment cells appears to be twofold; while there is an increase in the production of melanin within existing melanocytes after a single dose of radiation (Pathak, Sinesi & Szabo 1965), after multiple exposures there is an increase in the number of melanocytes giving a positive reaction when incubated with DOPA (see below) as well as in melanin production (Szabo 1967). It is now appropriate to consider how the melanocyte produces melanin and determines the pigmentation of the surrounding epithelium.

Examination of human melanocytes with the electron microscope has shown these cells to be similar in epidermis and oral epithelium (Fig. 1.14) (Birbeck 1962; Squier & Waterhouse 1967; Schroeder 1969). The cells differ from adjacent epithelial cells in being dendritic, lacking desmosomes and tonofibrils and in having a well-developed Golgi region and large areas of rough endoplasmic reticulum. These latter features are consistent with the secretory role of the cell; in the production of melanin, tyrosinase is synthesized on the ribosomes and passed via the endoplasmic reticulum to the Golgi system, where it accumulates in vesicles. These vesicles develop a matrix, apparently consisting of either helical protein fibrils (Schroeder 1969) or a rolled membranous sheet (Birbeck, Breathnach & Everall 1961) which gives the structure a striated appearance in certain planes of section; this organelle is known as a *pre-melanosome* (Fig. 1.14). The result of the oxidation of tyrosine via a number of intermediate components, including di-hydroxy phenyl alanine (DOPA), is the formation of the dense pigment melanin, which obscures the striations seen on the pre-melanosome to form the homogeneous, opaque melanosome. Melanosomes are ellipsoid bodies, approximately 0.4 μm in size, which makes them difficult to identify with the light microscope unless they are present in groups. There may be differences in melanosome size and structure in different tissues, but those described in human oral epithelium are similar to the melanosomes of the epidermis (Schroeder 1969).

As mentioned already, the degree of melanin pigmentation seen in an individual is largely determined by the activity of the melanocyte, so that in lightly pigmented tissue there are greater numbers of pre-melanosomes than melanosomes. In albinos, pre-melanosomes are formed in the melanocytes, but these do not become melanized, probably because of a low level of synthesis of melanin from its precursors rather than a total failure of the pathway (Breathnach 1971).

Melanosomes and, in lightly pigmented individuals and albinos, pre-melanosomes (Parakkal, 1967) are transferred to adjacent keratinocytes by what has been termed 'innoculation' (Masson 1948), and many studies have shown that this is a process in which the keratinocyte plays an active phagocytic role (Cruickshank & Harcourt 1964; Mottaz & Zelickson 1967). Portions of melanocyte processes containing melanosomes are pinched off and engulfed by the keratinocyte so that melanosomes are present enclosed by a plasma membrane either singly or in groups (*melanosome complexes*). This structural and functional relationship between a melanocyte and its surrounding epithelial cells has given rise to the concept of the 'epithelial (or epidermal) melanin unit' (Fitzpatrick & Breathnach 1963).

Recently it has been shown that the distribution and fate of the melanosomes within the keratinocyte is also an important factor in determining visible pigmentation, and just as the expansion or contraction of the pigment cells of amphibians produces changes in colour, so the degree of dispersion of the melanosomes in the keratinocytes differs in differently pigmented races. Thus in caucasoids the melanosomes are gathered together as melanosome complexes in membrane enclosed groups, while in negroids there is a tendency for melanosomes to be dispersed throughout the epithelial cell (Hori *et al* 1968). These workers also showed hydrolytic enzymes to be present within the membrane enclosing the melanosomes, so that they represent a form of lysosome which can presumably degrade the melanosomes (Wolff & Hönigsmann 1972). The rate of breakdown of melanosomes in keratinocytes also determines the level of clinical pigmentation, for in negroid epidermis melanosomes frequently persist even in the stratum corneum (Olson, Nordquist & Everett 1970).

We can thus summarize by saying that melanin pigmentation is dependent not upon the number of melanocytes present in a given area, but on their activity in producing melanosomes and on the subsequent degree of aggregation and extent of breakdown of these organelles within the recipient keratinocytes.

1:5 The Boundary between Epithelium and Connective Tissue

The junction between the epithelium and connective tissue in skin and oral mucosa is an irregular interface at which projections of connective tissue papillae interdigitate with the epithelial ridges. Although the morphology of this region can be studied from serial sections (Karring & Löe 1970) it is often more convenient to study whole mounts of the tissue in which the epithelium has been separated from the connective tissues by means of enzymatic digestion or chemical agents (Riley 1965; Scapino 1967); this provides a true three-dimensional specimen. More recently, scanning electron microscopy has provided a means of obtaining even more information from such preparations (Scaletta & Simmelink 1973).

The frequency, depth and shape of the interdigitations vary from region to region in both skin and oral mucosa (see Table 1.1) but in all areas are sufficient to provide a greater area of interface between the epithelium and connective tissue than is present between the surface of the epithelium and the exterior. This configuration therefore plays an important role in distributing mechanical stresses acting on the epithelium over a wide area of the supporting tissues. Furthermore, the surface layers of the epithelium are relatively impermeable so that most gaseous and metabolic exchange takes place across this junction. Thus a given configuration serves both metabolic and mechanical functions and it is difficult to separate individual structure–function relationships. Nevertheless, there are quite clear differences between the junction in masticatory and lining oral mucosa which, as we have seen, probably have different mechanical properties; in the former tissue, the ridges are numerous, tall and narrow, while in lining mucosa they are less numerous, broader and shorter. As a consequence, the area of interface between the epithe-

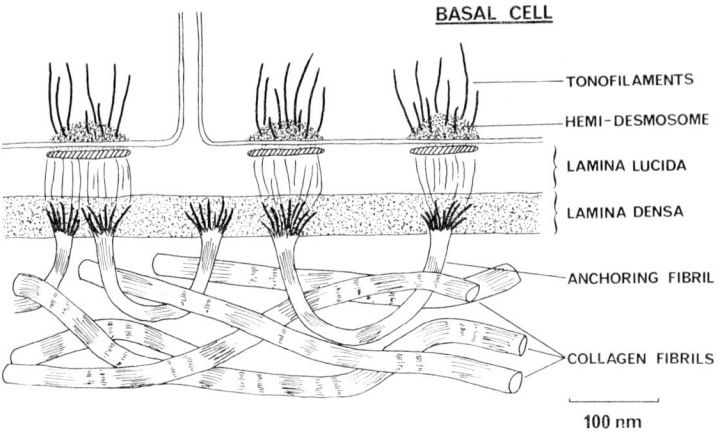

Fig. 1.16. Diagram of the ultrastructure of the junction between epithelium and connective tissue.

lium and connective tissue per unit of epithelial surface is much greater in masticatory mucosa than in lining mucosa, and so provides a stronger junctional attachment (Scapino 1971).

1:5:1 The structure of the basement membrane

The term *basement membrane* has been used at a histological level to describe the junction between epithelium and connective tissue that appears as a distinctly stained zone after treatment with periodic acid-Schiff (paS) or silver stains. The basement membrane appears as a continuous but relatively structureless layer some 1–2 μm thick (Gersh & Catchpole 1960) although Melcher (1965) has claimed that subepithelial reticulin fibres are associated with it.

Ultrastructural examination of the basement membrane in a number of tissues, such as skin (Odland 1958), oral mucosa (Kurahashi & Takuma

1962), uterine cervix (Younes *et al* 1965) and vagina (Burges & Vargas-Linores 1970) has revealed an essentially similar structure in each site; this is illustrated in Fig. 1.16. Running parallel with the basal plasma membranes of the basal epithelial cells, and separated from them by a relatively clear zone some 20–80 μm wide, is a moderately dense layer, 20–70 μm thick, appearing as a granular or finely fibrous structure. Because of their

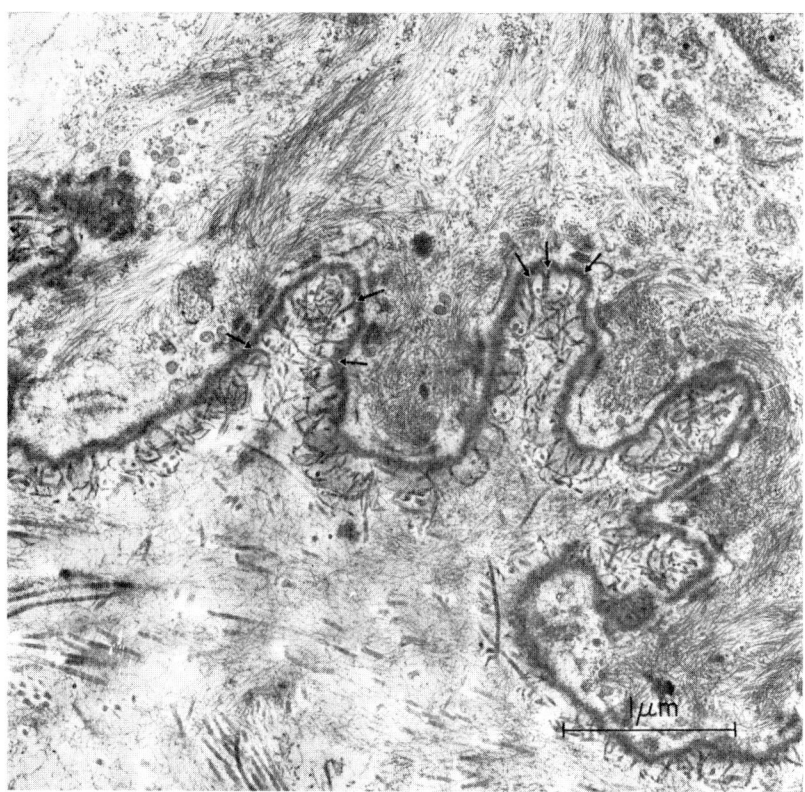

Fig. 1.17. Electron micrograph of the epithelial–connective tissue junction in human buccal epithelium. Numbers of anchoring fibrils (arrows) can be seen, inserted into the lamina densa. Bar represents 1 μm.

differing electron opacities, these two layers have been called the *lamina lucida* or light layer and the *lamina densa* or dense layer, respectively. Associated with the lamina densa are striated fibrils called *anchoring fibrils* (Palade & Farquhar 1965) which form loops through which run the collagen fibrils of the connective tissue (Fig. 1.17). Where each end of the loop enters the lamina densa it fans out to form a spray of finer filaments; it has been suggested that these filaments traverse the lamina lucida and terminate at the intercellular plaque of the hemi-desmosomes (Thilander & Bloom 1968), or continue and actually penetrate the basal plasma membrane so as to become contiguous with the tonofilaments of the epithelial cell (Susi, Belt & Kelly 1967). Even though the evidence for these latter arrangements is equivocal, it is clear that the network of anchoring fibrils provides a system which interlocks the larger collagen fibres of the connective tissue with the lamina densa and possibly even with the epithelium.

From the foregoing account of the ultrastructural appearance of the basement membrane, it is apparent that the structure is not a true membrane at all but a complex of fibrils and matrix. It is therefore more usual to use the terms *basal lamina* or *basal lamina complex* when referring to the elements observed in the electron microscope. The basement membrane seen in the light microscope is obviously a very much larger structure than the electron microscopist's basal lamina (which would not be resolved) and probably includes the associated anchoring fibrils and even some subepithelial reticulin and collagen. In an attempt to determine which structures in fact represented in light microscopic basement membrane, Swift & Saxton (1967) used a modified paS stain (pa-silver) visible in the electron microscope and found the reaction to be located in the subepithelial collagen and anchoring fibrils. However, other workers have described a staining reaction not only in the subepithelial fibres but also in the lamina densa and the cell coat of the basal epithelial cells and have suggested that all these structures contribute to the light microscopic basement membrane (Rambourg & Leblond 1967; Susi 1971).

1:5:2 The origin of the basement membrane

The basement membrane was originally thought to be a product of the connective tissue formed by the condensation of polymerized ground substances and reticulin fibres (Gersh & Catchpole 1949, 1960). However, if the basal lamina did arise from polymerized ground substance it might be expected to be composed of proteoglycans (see section 1:6:2e), whereas analyses have shown that it is composed of protein with small amounts of carbohydrates and glucosamine (Mukerjee, Sri-Ram & Pierce, 1965, Spiro 1967). Moreover a basal lamina is formed at epithelial surfaces which are not adjacent to connective tissue, such as at the enamel surface (Schroeder & Listgarten 1971) and against support films in tissue culture (Flaxman, Lutzner & Van Scott 1968). Experimental evidence from autoradiographic studies (Hay & Revel 1963) and immunochemical reactions (Pierce 1971) gives direct support to the idea that the basal lamina is a product of the epithelial cells, and experiments in which epidermis and dermis are recombined in tissue culture suggest that the lamina densa does have an epithelial origin, although the anchoring fibrils are probably products of the connective tissue (Briggaman, Dalldorf & Wheeler 1971).

1:5:3 Functions of the basement membrane

The two functions that have been consistently ascribed to the basement membrane are those of a barrier, capable of ultrafiltration, and a mechanical attachment between epithelium and connective tissue.

1:5:3a BARRIER FUNCTION

Although a structure with the characteristic appearance of the lamina densa can be seen in the skin of human embryos as early as 6 weeks, the complete basal complex is not developed until 16 weeks (Breathnach 1971), by which time the migration of cells such as the melanocyte and Langerhans cell from the mesoderm is complete and the epithelium constitutes a self-perpetuating cell population. The subsequent movement of cells such as lymphocytes or polymorphs across the junction is not unusual in oral mucosa and is associated with a local breakdown in the organization of the basal complex (Frithiof 1969); a similar disruption is seen on malignant invasion by epithelial cells (Woods & Smith 1969; Frithiof 1969).

While the majority of metabolites entering or leaving the epithelium must cross the basement membrane, it is evident that at a molecular level the basal lamina can exert a filtering effect so that only particles of a certain size can pass through. Thus while horseradish peroxidase (diameter approximately 5–6 nm) passes freely across into the intercellular spaces of the epidermis (Schreiner & Wolff 1969) or oral epithelium (McDougall 1970; Squier 1973) the passage of the larger molecules of thorotrast (diameter approximately 5–12·5 nm) is to a great extent restricted (Wolff & Hönigsmann 1971). It has also been suggested that a similar mechanism operates in the opposite direction, for when labelled albumin is applied to the surface of the oral epithelium of sensitized animals, immune complexes are formed in the epithelium and trapped above the basement membrane (Tolo 1974). In this way the basement membrane supplements the barrier function of the superficial layers of the epithelium.

1:5:3b MECHANICAL FUNCTION

All basement membranes appear to function for the attachment of epithelium to connective tissue. Two factors appear to be largely responsible for this union, one is the adhesion between the epithelial cells and the lamina densa and the other is the attachment of the basal lamina to the adjacent connective tissue. The material constituting the basal lamina has many similarities to the intercellular cement substance found between epithelial cells so that the same sort of adhesion may exist between the basal cells and the basal lamina as between epithelial cells. This does not rule out the possibility that filaments running between the basal lamina and the hemi-desmosomes provide some direct physical attachment (see section 1:5:2). There is good evidence that the basal lamina is attached to the underlying collagen of the connective tissue by the system of anchoring fibrils. Experiments in which oral epithelium or epidermis are separated from the connective tissue by suction show that the separation of epithelial cells from the basal lamina is initially restricted principally at the sites of hemi-desmosomes (Frithiof 1971). Eventually a suction blister is created by separation of the epithelium at the level of the lamina lucida, the lamina densa usually remaining attached to the connective tissue by means of the anchoring fibrils, whose loops seem to allow some sliding of the collagen fibrils and so provide for some distensibility without rupture (Grover, personal communication).

The structure of the basal lamina complex, particularly the thickness of the lamina densa, varies slightly with region and age (Frithiof 1969). These differences probably reflect functional demands, and it is likely that just as the gross configuration of the epithelial–connective tissue junction varies from region to region, so there will be differences, such as in the numbers and concentration of anchoring fibrils (Scapino 1971), that reflect these functional differences at an ultrastructural level.

1:5:4 Epithelial–mesenchymal interaction

Since all cells of a given embryo must carry the same genetic information, any signs of differentiation among the cells must be preceded by some kind of inductive mechanism which *determines* the pathway of differentiation of each cell by blocking all but the relevant parts of its genetic information. This blocking of nuclear DNA in terms of capacity to support alternate forms of development may well be a gradual one which begins very early in embryonic life until a point is reached where relatively few or merely one pathway of differentiation is left open. At this stage the cell may be said to be 'determined' towards a specific course of differentiation. Viewed in this way determination simply represents the final step in a sequence of restrictive stages (Wessells 1970).

Most of the information available on embryonic inductive phenomena has been gained from organ culture experiments and epithelial grafts and is of necessity restricted to animal tissues. This section will be limited to some of the basic observations in this field and the reader is referred to more detailed reports on the subject (Fleischmeyer & Billingham 1968; Hodges 1969; Krikos 1971; Kollar 1972) for a thorough review of the literature.

Early experiments were carried out with embryonic chick skin which differentiates normally when grown in organ culture (Fell 1964). If the dermal component is separated from the epidermis by means of trypsin, the epithelium not only fails to differentiate but eventually dies (Wessells 1962). Recombination of the separated components produces normal differentiation as in the case of whole cultured skin. McLoughlin (1961a, b), using similar techniques, recombined limb-bud epidermis of 5-day-old chick embryo with mesenchyme from limb-buds, heart and stomach and found that in all cases the mesenchyme determined the pathway of differentiation of the epithelium.

The question arises as to whether or not the conservation of specificity of the various epidermal derivatives in the adult are dependent upon the continuous action of specific inductive stimuli of the dermis. To this end, Billingham & Silvers (1968) carried out recombinations of the dermal and epidermal components of the sole of the foot, ear and trunk skin of adult guinea-pigs and transplanted these to suitable sites of isogenic host animals. After several months, they observed that in each case it was the dermis which determined the type of epidermis which was formed at the site of grafting. As in embryonic skin, therefore, the direction of the course of differentiation of adult epidermis is controlled by the underlying connective tissue. While Billingham & Silvers concluded from such findings that in skin the basal epithelial cells are 'equipotential' or undetermined, depending on the constant influence of their underlying dermis for the expression of their specific epidermal trait, Gillette (1971) prefers the idea that embryonic determination is to a certain extent flexible in that it can be changed or *modulated* under certain conditions.

Different results were, however, obtained by Billingham & Silvers (1968) with some keratinizing mucosal epithelia. When isolated epithelia of the tongue, oesophagus and hamster cheek pouch were recombined with the dermis from the sole of the foot, the mucosal epithelia retained their specificity and did not change to the type of epithelium normally associated with the type of dermis with which they were recombined.

In order to ensure, however, that there exists such a fundamental difference in the degree of flexibility of determination of the skin and mucous membranes, it is necessary to carry out reciprocal experiments by recombining mucosal connective tissue with various types of epidermis as well as different mucosal epithelia. It is possible that the connective tissue components of mucosal origin could influence the differentiation of closely related mucosal epithelia but not those of epidermal origin. Such grafts are technically difficult and meaningful results are not yet available (Billingham & Silvers 1968). It is of interest in this context that Billingham & Silvers (1967) have found that tongue epithelium, although unchanged when combined with sole of foot dermis, is able to modulate when recombined with trunk dermis, suggesting that its embryonic determination is not as fixed as might appear from other experiments.

Because signs of differentiation are more apparent in the epithelium than in the connective tissue, the latter is usually considered as exercising the determinative influence. We cannot, however, discard the possibility that the epithelium also determines the connective tissue either simultaneously or primarily. Bernfield (1970) has demonstrated the influence of epithelium on collagen synthesis early in development. Mutual determination has been shown by Koch (1967), who separated epithelium from connective tissue in embryonic tooth germs of mice and found that neither component differentiated further when cultured separately. On recombination, however, the epithelium differentiated into ameloblasts while the mesenchymal component showed the development of odontoblasts, suggesting that in this case the connective tissue depends upon the epithelium for its differentiation as much as the epithelium depends on the connective tissue. The distinctive nature of the connective tissue differentiation in this experiment has made it possible for the epithelial influence to be demonstrated. Whether it is the epithelium or the connective tissue which exerts the *initial* determining influence is of course impossible to say, even if the onset of differentiation of one component has preceded that of the other. A determined tissue or cell does not necessarily show immediate differentiation as demonstrated by Holtzer (1961), who showed that cultured, undetermined mesenchyme from the spinal chord area of salamander could be determined by 10 hours' contact with the spinal cord but showed no signs of differentiation into cartilage until four days later.

What is the possible nature of these inductive influences? It should perhaps be mentioned at this point that determination represents the first in a series of responses to induction. Mitotic activity and morphogenesis, although invariably part of the overall response, appear to be the result of separate inductive stimuli (Wessells 1970). No attempt will be made here, however, to differentiate between these three kinds of response, as the results to be discussed are all dependent on morphological differentiation as a sign of induction.

It is generally accepted that direct contact between epithelium and connective tissue is not necessary for interaction to occur. The inductive factor has been shown to pass through micro-millipore membrane filters in the case of salivary gland (Grobstein 1953), skin (Wessells 1962) and teeth (Koch 1967). Furthermore Fell (1964), Wessells (1964) and Dodson (1967) have shown that the presence of living mesenchymal cells is not required for the differentiation of embryonic chick epidermis provided the epithelium has a suitable substrate and that chick embryo juice is present in the culture medium. The inductive factor appears to be trypsin- and heat-labile (Fell 1964). Macromolecules such as "mucopolysaccharide" (McLaughlin 1961b) and RNA (Slavkin et al 1970) have been implicated as possible transmitters of inductive information.

Collagen may also play an important role in epithelial differentiation by providing a suitable substratum (Dodson 1963; Wessells 1964). Grobstein & Cohen (1965) have shown that collagenase will prevent the characteristic branching of epithelium in salivary gland histogenesis. The work of Wessells & Cohen (1966), however, indicates that collagen, although present in the chick embryo fractions which are required for differentiation in the absence of connective tissue, does not actively participate in inductive interactions, but merely exerts an organizing influence during epithelial–mesenchymal interaction. Sophisticated autoradiographic studies (Kallman & Grobstein 1965, 1966) have shown that polymerization of tropocollagen, synthesized in the mesenchyme, takes place at the epithelial surface probably under the influence of glycosamine-containing material produced by the epithelium. Such findings have prompted postulations that both the epithelium and mesenchyme produce materials which interact at the tissue interface to produce new macromolecular complexes which affect the subsequent developmental behaviour of the cells. Mercer (1964) believes that the lamina densa of the basement membrane represents such a reaction precipitate with unique characteristics for each epithelial–connective tissue complex. His opinion is not supported by immunohistochemical studies however (Midgely & Pierce 1963; Pierce

1966), which have indicated that the antigenic component of different laminae densa of mice are chemically similar to each other. The findings of Hay & Revel (1963) and Pierce *et al* (1962, 1963) further prove the lamina densa to be of epithelial origin (see section 1:5:2).

There is little doubt that the basement membrane can act as a protein filtration barrier (see section 1:5:3a) and thereby affect both epithelial and mesenchymal cells. In this context it may affect the sequence of events leading to differentiation although its possible role as a primary factor in the inductive process has been eliminated (Kallman *et al* 1967).

1:6 The Connective Tissue

The way in which the dermis of the skin and the lamina propria of the oral mucosa are organized in recognizable histological layers has already been described in section 1.2. In this section the various components of these layers, the cells, fibres and ground substance, blood vessels and nerves are considered in more detail. From a structural point of view it must be remembered that the various elements of the connective tissue of skin and mucosa do not differ greatly from those of connective tissues elsewhere in the body; functionally there are sometimes greater differences, as for example in the circulatory system. However, our knowledge of both structure and function of this region is scant.

1:6:1 Cells of the connective tissue

From a functional point of view the connective tissue components of skin and oral mucosa must contain cells responsible for:
1 the synthesis, secretion and maintenance of fibres and ground substance—the fibroblasts or fibrocytes;
2 the synthesis and storage of fat—adipose or fat cells;
3 the defence of the tissue (and of the organism)—the macrophage or histiocyte; the mast cell; variable numbers of 'inflammatory cells' derived from circulating leucocytes;
4 undifferentiated mesenchymal cells which, because of their dormancy, cannot be assigned to one of the above functional groups;
5 the constituent cells of vascular and lymphatic channels—endothelial cells and pericytes, and fibroblasts in vessels with a collagenous or elastic component;

6 the constituent cells of the neural element—the axons of neurones with distant cell bodies, the Schwann cells forming myelin and the fibroblasts of the collagenous sheaths of nerves;

7 the constituent epithelial cells of salivary and sebaceous glands and their ducts.

These cells are fundamentally the same as their counterparts in connective tissue elsewhere in the body, differing only in numbers and in degree of function. Within the oral mucosa there are marked differences between both the absolute and relative numbers of each cell type from area to area, reflecting the different function of the various regions (see section 1:2).

Nerves, blood vessels and glands are dealt with in later sections; here the distribution and morphology of the remaining cell types will be described but it should be realized that because structure and function are so closely related, the appearance of any cell will depend not only on the major functional group to which it belongs but also on its precise level of activity at the moment of tissue fixation. Furthermore the subsequent stages of specimen preparation naturally have a profound influence on the appearance of any cell.

1:6:1a FIBROBLASTS AND FIBROCYTES

In standard histological preparations for light microscopy the fibroblast appears as an elongated, fusiform or stellate cell with an elliptical nucleus usually aligned parallel to the neighbouring collagen fibre bundles; the nuclear outlines will thus be oval, elongate or circular, depending on the plane of section. The nucleus is lightly staining with a fine chromatin pattern and contains several prominent nucleoli.

Quiescent cells, usually termed fibrocytes, have relatively little cytoplasm which may be difficult to detect in routine preparations. Cytoplasmic stains, however, reveal numerous long branching cell processes (Fig. 1.18). In active cells, the nucleus is more densely staining, the cytoplasm is increased both in volume and in stain intensity—an increased basophilia arising principally from the increase in cytoplasmic RNA associated with protein synthesis.

The ultrastructure of a fibroblast (Fig 1.18) is directly related to its level of metabolic activity (Breathnach 1971). Cells active in the synthesis of collagen and other extracellular products have an abundant rough endoplasmic reticulum aligned parallel to the cell membrane within cytoplasmic extensions. Randomly dispersed cytofilaments, or small loose bundles of

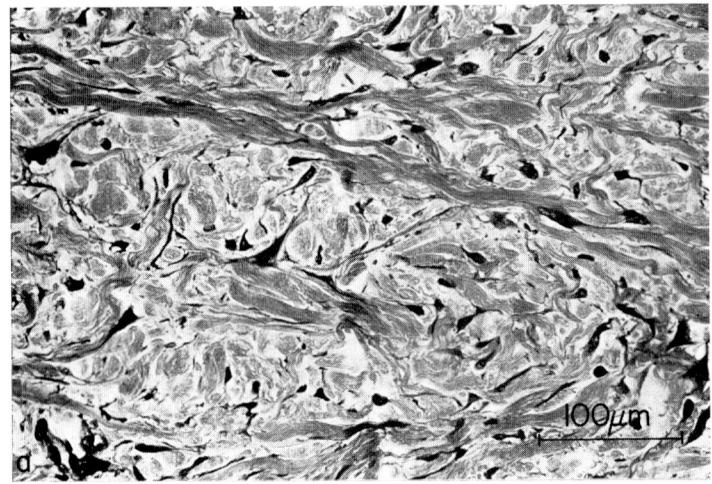

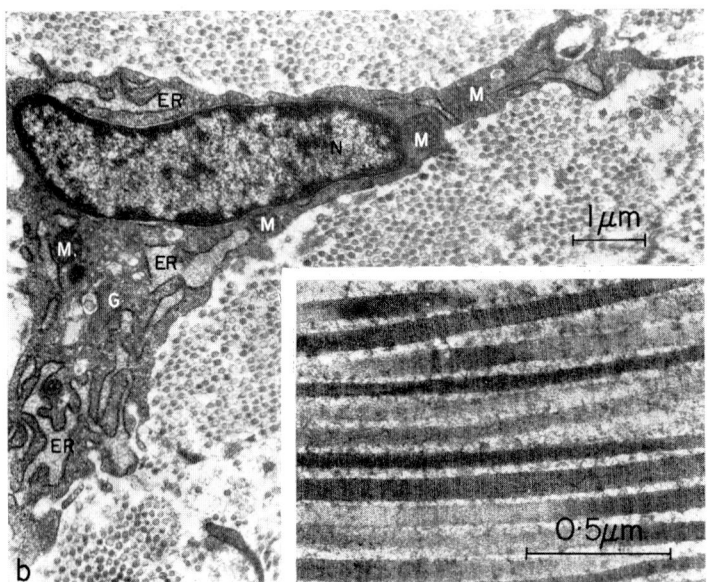

Fig. 1.18. (a) Lamina propria of human oral mucosa stained with Held's molybdic acid–haematoxylin to demonstrate cell cytoplasm. Most of the cells are fibroblasts and are elongate or stellate with long cytoplasmic processes. Processes of cells whose bodies are not in the plane of section are aligned along and between collagen fibre bundles. Bar represents 100 μm.

(b) Electron micrograph of a fibroblast in human gingiva. The cell body is stellate and contains the nucleus (N), numerous mitochondria (M), a Golgi apparatus (G), and a rough-surfaced endoplastic reticulum (ER), with dilated cisternae containing finely granular material. Portions of several narrow cytoplasmic processes can be seen in close association with transversely sectioned collagen fibrils. Preparation fixed in glutaraldehyde–formaldehyde, post-osmicated and stained with uranyl acetate and lead citrate. Bar represents 1 μm.

Inset. Longitudinally sectioned collagen fibrils prepared as above, revealing the characteristic crossbanding. Bar represents 0·5 μm.

such filaments, are common, particularly in cells in healing wounds for example; these are sometimes composed of microtubules suggesting that such cells may have contractile properties and the term myofibroblast has been coined by Montandon *et al* (1973). Others believe that such filaments are solely concerned with an internal supportive or 'skeletal' role.

The Golgi apparatus is well developed and contains numerous small membrane-bound vesicles which are also located near the cell boundaries. Current opinion is that newly synthesized tropocollagen aggregates within the cisternae of the endoplasmic reticulum, and probably within Golgi vesicles, from which it is secreted after fusion with the plasma membrane. Further aggregation to typically banded fibrils takes place extracellularly in association with the protein–polysaccharide complexes of the ground substance also secreted by the fibroblast (see section 1:6:2). Mature collagen fibrils are frequently seen in close apposition to the plasma membrane, but differential shrinkage of tissue components during electron microscopy processing may exaggerate the space between collagen and its formative cells.

Fibroblasts contain moderate numbers of mitochondria; lysosomes and autophagic vacuoles are occasionally seen, as these are a normal component of all cells. In tissues loaded with foreign material, such as after the intravenous, intradermal or intramucosal injection of carbon or vital colloidal dyes like Trypan blue, cells with the morphological characteristics of fibroblasts may phagocytose significant amounts, leading to confusion as to whether such cells should be regarded as fibroblasts or as macrophages. It is our view, however, that the fundamental criterion for cell identification ought to be a functional one. Thus a connective tissue cell with marked phagocytic properties ought to be regarded as a macrophage: morphological criteria alone, particularly at the light microscope level, are frequently inadequate for unequivocal cell identification.

1:6:1b MACROPHAGES AND HISTIOCYTES

Cells of the macrophage series are chiefly characterized by their potential for extensive phagocytosis. Their function is to ingest and break down micro-organisms, foreign material and fragments of damaged tissue following injury. In addition, important immune functions have recently been discovered which involve the recognition, ingestion and 'processing' of antigen for subsequent presentation to cells of the lymphoid series in which antibody synthesis takes place (see below and Chapter 3).

Origin and terminology

It follows from the summary of macrophage function given above that these cells will be particularly numerous and active in inflammatory foci. In this situation it has been clearly established that macrophages in inflamed mucosa or skin are derived from bone-marrow stem cells which travel in the circulation as blood monocytes and migrate into the tissue as required (Spector 1969). Further division may take place in the tissue. Both monocytes and macrophages in various stages of differentiation will thus be found in the dermis, lamina propria or deeper connective tissue if inflammation is present, the proportion of macrophages depending on the nature of the injurious stimulus.

Normal, non-inflamed tissues, however, contain 'fixed' or stationary cells which, given a suitable stimulus, show marked phagocytic ability and become indistinguishable from the macrophages present in inflammation. These have long been known as fixed tissue macrophages of 'histiocytes' and are related to other 'fixed' phagocytes in the reticulo-endothelial system.

Morphology

There is a wide variety of morphological types amongst cells of the macrophage series. Once the cytoplasm contains large amounts of ingested material, particularly if this is pigmented (like haemosiderin, carbon or vital dyes), or distinctive in shape (like bacteria or fungi), identification is easy. Such cells are usually large (up to 50 μm or more) and spherical with the dense, sometimes kidney-shaped nucleus compressed to one side. Intracytoplasmic acid hydrolytic enzymes are detectable histochemically.

Quiescent histiocytes are more difficult to identify and closely resemble fibroblasts in most light microscope preparations. They are frequently very complex stellate cells with long branching cytoplasmic extensions. Stimulation leads to withdrawal of these processes and a rounding up of the cell, but as stimulated macrophages are actively motile they may be fixed in a wide variety of shapes. The nucleus is usually regarded as being smaller and denser than that of the fibroblast with inconspicuous nucleoli. It is often indented, similar to the classical blood monocyte, but this is not a universal feature and, in any event, its visualization depends on the plane of section.

Macrophage identification is more straightforward in the electron microscope (Fig. 1.19) because the large numbers of phagosomes, which

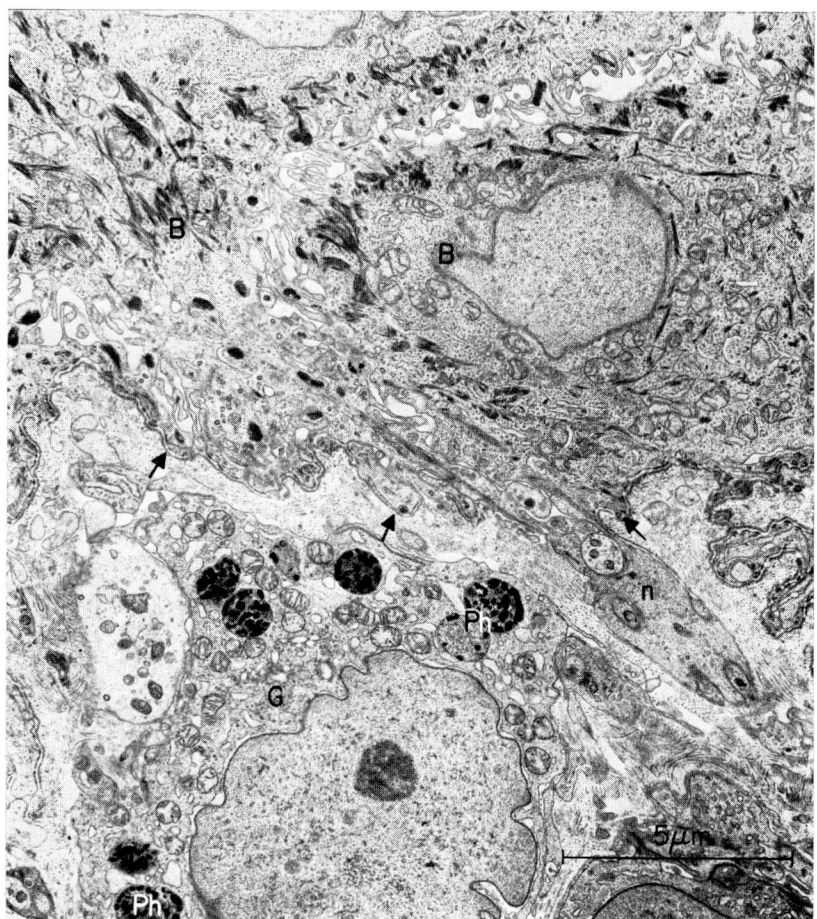

Fig. 1.19. A macrophage beneath oral epithelium containing electron-dense melanosomes within phagosomes (Ph). Numerous mitochondria and Golgi vesicles (G) are visible and the plasma membrane shows a number of infoldings. This cell can be termed a melanophage. A non-myelinated nerve (n) penetrates the basal lamina (arrows) and passes into the epithelium between the basal cells (B). Bar represents 5 μm.

they characteristically contain, can be seen easily. The cell membrane is often convoluted and material may be seen entering into the cell via phagocytic vacuoles or smaller pinocytic vesicles.

1:6:1c MELANOPHAGES AND SIDEROPHAGES

Macrophages in dermis and lamina propria may ingest melanin granules shed from within the epithelium and are common in skin and beneath pigmented oral epithelium. They contain mature melanin granules undergoing degradation (Fig. 1.19) and are not capable of melanin synthesis.

Haemosiderin, derived from red cells spilled into the tissue following vascular injury, is taken up by cells of the macrophage line and ultimately degraded *in situ* or carried away to other parts of the reticulo-endothelial system. This can be identified readily by its characteristic staining in the light microscope, and ultrastructure in the electron microscope. Siderophages may persist for many weeks at the site of injured or inflamed mucosa when other signs of inflammation have faded.

Typical mast cell granules are also sometimes seen within cells which otherwise appear to be macrophages, presumably because the granules were shed by mast cells proper and have subsequently been phagocytosed.

1:6:1d MAST CELLS

Mast cells were originally described by Ehrlich in 1877 and are still identified on the basis of the highly distinctive metachromatic granules with which their cytoplasm is filled (Selye 1965). The metachromasia of these granules is due to the presence of negatively charged, acidic, sulphated polysaccharide–protein complexes which are now known to be largely heparin. In addition, mast cells contain histamine and, in some animals but not apparently in man, 5-hydroxy tryptamine.

In functional terms, therefore, mast cells may be defined as those cells responsible for the synthesis, storage and secretion of these important pharmacological agents. They may play a role in maintaining tissue and vascular homeostasis by the controlled liberation of these anticoagulant and vasoactive substances. However, degranulation is rarely observed in normal tissues and their primary role appears to be in defence and repair. Mast cells are the primary effectors in certain types of immediate hypersensitivity reactions in which the active agents are released following interaction of cell-bound 'reaginic' antibody with its specific allergen (Keller 1966). As mentioned earlier, shed granules may be taken up by macrophages.

The characteristic human mast cell is a large, spherical or elliptical cell, up to 40 μm in length, with a relatively small centrally placed nucleus, often with a distinct clumped chromatin pattern. If related to dense collagen bundles and particularly if there has been much shrinkage during

Structure and Function

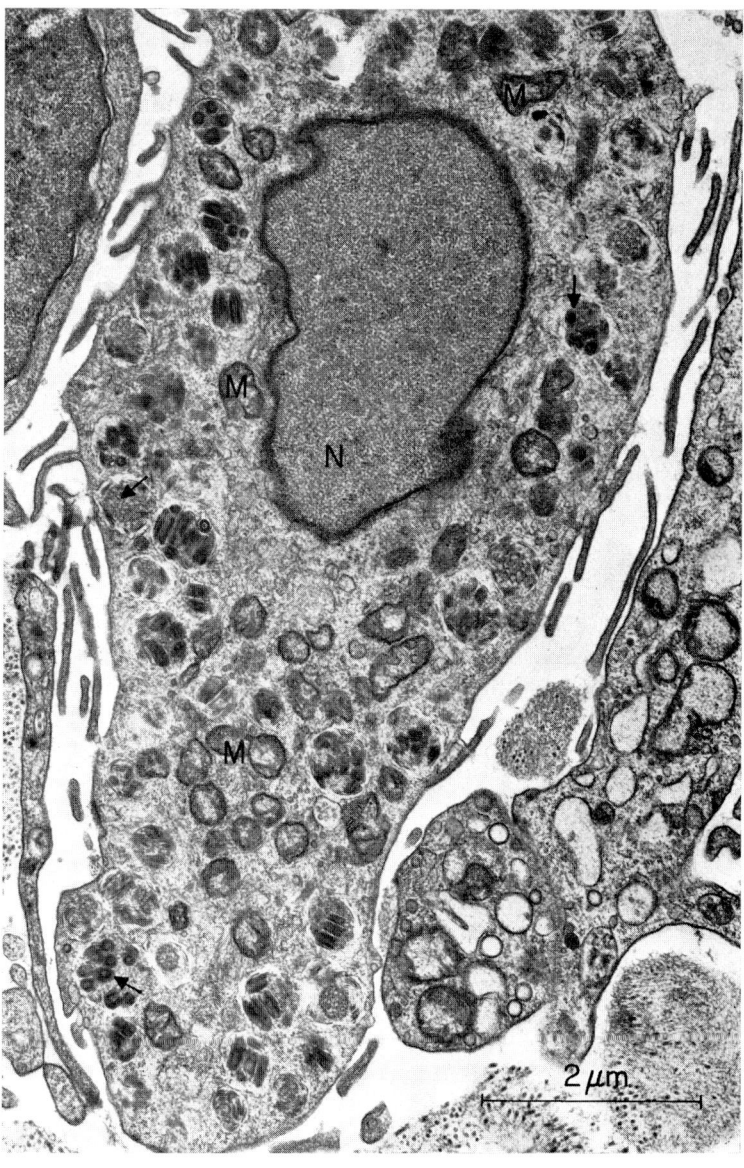

Fig. 1.20. Mast cell. Numerous long microvilli project from the cell surface and the cytoplasm contains many specific granules. These granules are composed of parallel membranes 5–10 nm thick which are frequently concentrically arranged. Such lamellated particles occur in groups of up to 10, in association with a less electron-dense granular matrix (arrows). N = nucleus, M = mitochondria. Bar represents 2 μm.

processing of the tissue, the cells may appear rather spindle-shaped. In routine preparations, the cytoplasm stains fairly intensely with both acidic and basic dyes, and dyes such as toluidine blue, thionine or methylene blue are converted to a purple metachromatic hue within the granules.

In the electron microscope, mast cells are highly distinctive (Fig. 1.20), the two main distinguishing features being the presence of numerous fine microvilli projecting from the plasma membrane and large numbers of cytoplasmic granules. These latter are membrane bound with a light or electron dense homogeneous content, or with a dense crystalline or multi-lamellar content. Granules with mixed contents also appear. Endoplasmic reticulum is sparse but there are moderate numbers of mitochondria and usually a well-developed Golgi apparatus (Breathnach 1971).

In skin and oral mucosa, mast cells tend to be distributed in perivascular and perineural locations. Pohto and Antila (1969) have shown that mast cells are common in the tongue and lining mucosa of the human mouth, and in the gingiva. Much interest has been shown in recent years in the density and distribution of mast cells in gingiva because of the possible role played by their pharmacologically active contents in sustaining the inflammatory process during chronic gingivitis (Carranza & Cabrini 1955; Zachrisson, 1968, 1969; Shapiro *et al* 1969; Sorenson *et al* 1970; Angelopoulos 1972; Robinson & de Marco 1972). Most authors are of the opinion that the mast cell population of gingiva decreases with increasing degree of inflammation; certainly mast cells are rarely observed within an inflammatory focus and, in inflamed gingiva, are preferentially located beneath the rete pegs of the free and attached gingiva. It is possible that total mast cell numbers increase with moderate degrees of inflammation but that close to the centre of the focus, particularly if this contains substantial numbers of lymphocytes, they are caused to degranulate (Angelopoulos 1973).

Whilst the granules of tissue mast cells are very similar to those of the circulating blood basophil, there is no conclusive evidence that mast cells are derived from these granulocytes. Within the oral mucosa they appear to form a relatively stable, long-lived population.

1:6:1e CELLS OF THE LYMPHOCYTIC SERIES:
LYMPHOCYTES, 'BLAST' CELLS
AND PLASMA CELLS

Lymphocytes of various types and their progeny are the fundamentally immunocompetent cells of the body and there has been an explosion in

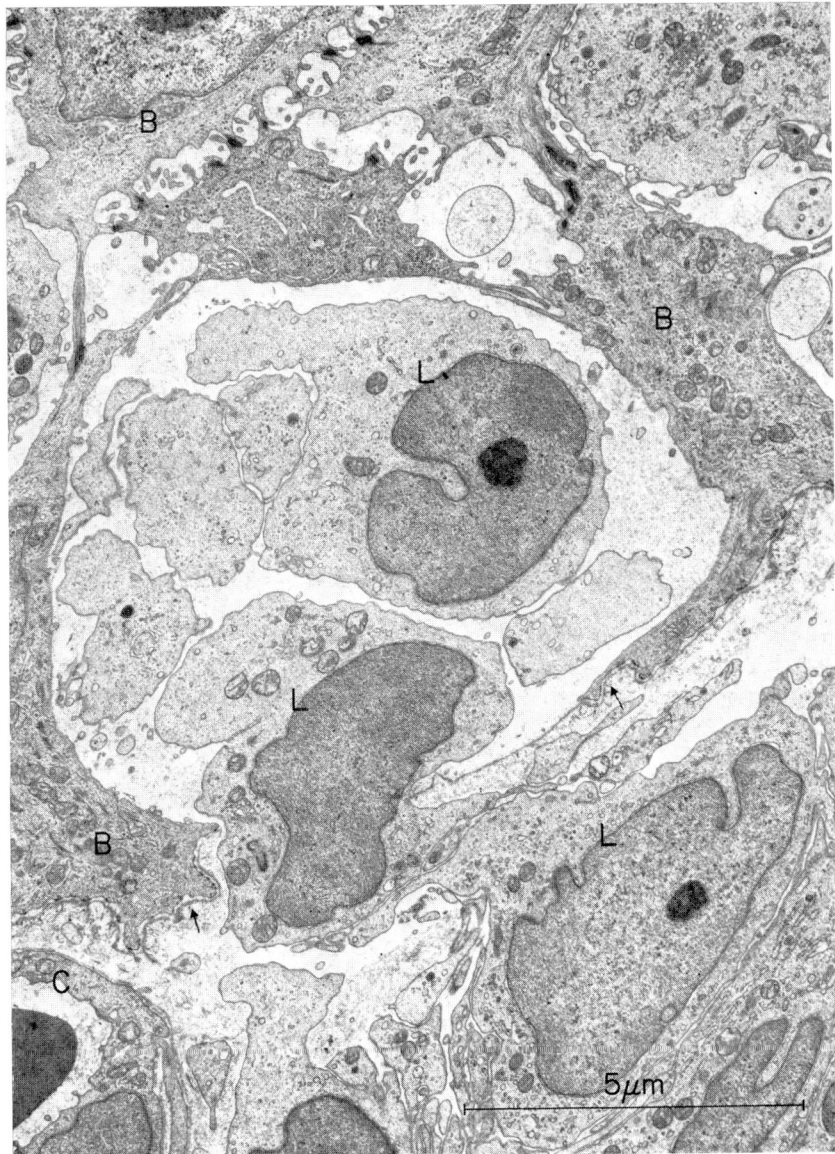

Fig. 1.21. Mononuclear inflammatory cells—small and medium lymphocytes (L)—infiltrating clinically normal human buccal epithelium through a break in the basal lamina (arrows). B = basal epithelial cells; C = capillary. Bar represents 5 μm.

knowledge of their cytology, life span and functions in the past decade. A comprehensive survey of these matters is beyond the scope of this chapter, partly because we are primarily concerned with normal mucosa. Lymphocytes and plasma cells are normally only present in significant numbers as part of a defence reaction or disease process, but as this is so common in oral mucosa, particularly in the gingiva, some account of their structure is necessary. Furthermore, lymphocyte aggregations are a normal component of some regions of the oral mucosa, the major site being the lingual tonsil. Their role in mediating the immune response of oral mucosa is described in Chapter 3.

The small lymphocyte

The small lymphocyte present in circulating blood and lymph, in lymph nodes and spleen, the thymus and the lymphoid tissue associated with the gastrointestinal tract is, at the light microscope level, a simple round cell approximately 6–10 μm in diameter with a dense nucleus and minimal cytoplasm. Cells of this appearance are present in inflammatory foci in oral mucosa and skin and in small numbers in both the connective tissue and epithelial components in apparently healthy tissue. In the electron microscope (Fig. 1.21), the cytoplasm contains a few mitochondria and scattered ribosomes but little rough endoplasmic reticulum.

Small lymphocytes, indistinguishable by routine microscopy, fall into populations with two distinct life spans—one of possibly hundreds of days, the other of the order of only a few days. All are derived initially from bone-marrow stem cells and circulate widely throughout the body. Cells of both life spans also fall into one of two major functional groups:
1 the *T lymphocyte* which is derived from, or processed by and remains dependent on, the thymus gland for its function (T = thymus)
2 the *B lymphocyte* which is dependent on certain peripheral lymphoid tissue for its function. This is the bursa of Fabricius in birds (B = bursa) and probably gastrointestinal tract associated lymphoid tissue in man, i.e. the Peyers patches and possibly also the tonsils of the oropharyngeal region.

T lymphocytes are responsible for cell mediated immunity—processes such as graft rejection and delayed hypersensitivity. Many diseases of the oral mucosa and skin have a large cell mediated immune component.

B lymphocytes are responsible for the second arm of the immune response, humoral immunity. When stimulated by specific antigen, a clone of B lymphocytes will proliferate and differentiate into plasma cells which synthesize and secrete soluble immunoglobulin (see Chapter 3). Recently it has been claimed that B and T cells may be distinguished on morphological grounds by differences in the configuration of their cell membranes which can be visualized by scanning electron microscopy (Polliack et al 1973; Lin, Cooper & Wortis 1973).

Medium and large lymphocytes

These terms are frequently used to describe lymphocytes with similar overall morphology to the small lymphocyte but with diameters of up to 16 μm and increased amounts of cytoplasm. They may be precursor cells of small lymphocytes in a lymphoid follicle somewhere in the body or 'transformed' B or T cells stimulated by contact with a specific antigen or non-specific mitogen. The terms have no clear connotation and are best avoided.

Blast cells

A number of substances, e.g. phyto-haemagglutannin, Poke-weed mitogen, stimulate the multiplication of lymphocytes in a relatively non-specific fashion. In addition, contact with its specific antigen will cause the appropriate B or T lymphocyte in the body to proliferate to form a clone of cells which will then manufacture specific antibody. Such cells are said to be 'transformed' and become 'blast' cells. The designation *immunoblast* is usually taken as a blanket term covering the transformation of both B and T cells. (WHO Tech Report 448, 1970). Immunoblasts are occasionally found in sections of relatively normal oral mucosa and skin and are common in inflammatory foci (Schroeder, Münzel-Pedrazzoli & Page 1973).

Apart from cell division or the preparation for it—detectable by visualizing mitotic figures or by the incorporation of isotope-labelled DNA precursors—the nucleus becomes larger with a looser chromatin pattern and more distinct nucleoli and the cytoplasm of such cells enlarges in preparation for the synthesis of antibody and other effector molecules. This primarily requires an increase in the amount of endoplasmic reticulum, which readily can be detected in the electron microscope and in the light microscope by the increased volume and basophilia of the cytoplasm. Methyl green–pyronin staining has recently become popular as an aid in the differentiation of cells of the immune system; the reaction depends on competition between the two dyes which have different affinities for DNA and RNA. DNA, and hence the nucleus, is stained by methyl green and RNA red by pyronin; cells with a high cytoplasmic ribosome content are thus pyroninophilic, be they lymphoid blast cells, plasma cells, or other types of actively synthetic cell.

Plasma cells

The mature plasma cell is readily identifiable as a round or oval cell up to 20 μm in diameter with an eccentrically placed nucleus containing descrete chromatin granules arranged in the so-called 'clock-face' or 'spoked wheel' fashion. The plentiful cytoplasm is basophilic and intensely pyroninophilic due to the extensive RNA content.

Electron microscopy reveals an extensive rough endoplasmic reticulum and there is also a well-developed Golgi zone. Antibody production can be demonstrated by fluorescent tracer techniques with the light microscope and comparable methods with labelled antisera in the electron microscope. It is possible to determine the class of immunoglobulin being synthesized by a particular plasma cell or clone of cells and to show specific antibody (see Chapter 3).

Various stages in the maturation of these cells can be recognized and in long-standing foci of chronic inflammation spherical aggregations of immunoglobulins—Russell bodies—may be seen both within and between plasma cells. Because inflammation is so common in the oral cavity, plasma cells are frequently seen—again in particularly large numbers in chronic gingivitis and in lingual tonsils.

1:6:1f GRANULOCYTES

Granular polymorphonuclear leucocytes are of course common components of certain types of inflammatory reaction in skin and oral mucosa, as elsewhere. Neutrophils are most commonly encountered and may occasionally be found in apparently healthy tissue. There are almost always significant numbers in gingival exudate (Attström 1971) even in the absence of clinical gingivitis and, in gingiva, they are mostly observed within blood vessels, in the process of traversing vessel walls, or within the sulcular and junctional epithelium; within the epithelium they are apparently accompanied by approximately equal numbers of mononuclear cells, mostly small lymphocytes, immunoblasts or macrophages (Schroeder 1973). The connective tissue is relatively free of such cells although free lysosomal bodies probably derived from disintegrated polymorphs have been described (Freedman, Listgarten & Taichman 1968; Gavin 1970; Garant & Mulvihill 1971).

In the electron microscope the shape of neutrophils is variable as, being motile, they can be fixed in any position. The lobed nucleus is apparent and may appear in section as separate nuclei. The cytoplasm is chiefly characterized by neutrophilic granules representing various types of lysosome and peroxisomes; phagocytosed material may be seen.

1:6:2 Fibre types and ground substance

The extracellular component of the loose connective tissue of the dermis and lamina propria consists of two main fibre types, collagen fibres and elastic fibres, which are embedded in a ground substance or matrix. The general arrangement of the fibres and the matrix has been adequately dealt with in section 1:2:4 and it is their microscopical appearance and their chemical properties which will be discussed here.

1:6:2a COLLAGEN

Collagen fibres consist of a specialized protein, collagen, which contains the unusual amino acid residues hydroxyproline and hydroxylysine. The fibres have almost identical physical properties in all mammals and show only minor variations in composition among mammalian species.

The basic component of collagen is the *tropocollagen* molecule which is composed of three intertwined helical polypeptide chains (Ramachandran & Kartha 1954, 1955). The tropocollagen molecule is rod-shaped, measuring 290 nm in length and 1·36 nm in width with a molecular weight of 300,000. These are synthesized by fibroblasts and immediately subsequent to their secretion parallel alignment takes place (Fitton-Jackson 1956, 1959). This alignment, followed by intra- and inter-molecular cross-linking, results in the formation of fibrils which in the electron microscope exhibit a characteristic band pattern that repeats every 64 nm (Fig. 1.18 inset). This distinguishing feature of collagen fibrils only becomes apparent when the thickness of the fibril approaches a diameter of 10 nm. These fibrils are gathered into bundles approximately 0·2 μm thick which are then apparent as collagen fibres in the light microscope. These, in turn, form bundles of collagen fibres which frequently branch although the fibres and their component fibrils do not.

The most abundant amino acid in the tropocollagen molecule is glycine, which constitutes about one-third of the total amino acid composition of collagen and is thought to be uniformly spaced throughout the polypeptide chain. The amino acids which are almost totally confined to collagen proteins are hydroxyproline and hydroxylysine. It is generally thought that these are incorporated into the polypeptide chain as proline and lysine and are subsequently hydroxylated (Kivirikko & Prockop 1967). Vitamin C (ascorbic acid), as well as ferrous ions, α-ketoglutarate and molecular oxygen are essential for this oxidation (Hutton *et al* 1967). If oxygen is excluded from embryonic cartilage in tissue culture, biosynthesis of collagen is arrested at the protocollagen stage, i.e. tropocollagen is not formed and no extracellular fibrils are produced. Instead protocollagen accumulates within the fibroblasts until oxygen is restored to the culture, thus enabling the oxidation of proline to hydroxyproline to proceed.

A large proportion of the amino acids besides hydroxyproline and hydroxylysine have hydroxyl groups in their side chains which contributes to the hydrophilic property of the collagen protein. When in contact with water, it therefore tends to remain straight. Since there is an excess of amino acids which possess basic groups on their side chains, collagen is a basic protein.

Fibrilogenesis

When collagenous tissues in an actively developing state are extracted with various cold electrolyte solutions, a proportion of the total collagen of the tissue dissolves as soluble collagen. However, with age progressive inter- and intra-molecular cross-linking occurs, thus reducing the solubility of collagen, so that more vigorous methods have to be employed for its extraction.

Although initially the triple helix is held together by hydrogen bonds, and the fibrillar aggregate of macromolecules by electrostatic bonds, the process of maturation involves the gradual formation of covalent bonds both within and between tropocollagen molecules. The diameter of the fibrils thus formed varies considerably.

The mechanical properties associated with the dermis and lamina propria could not be achieved merely by further collagen–collagen interaction. It is now clearly established that small amounts of the hexose sugars glucose and galactose form an integral part of the collagen macromolecule and account for 0·3–0·5% by weight of insoluble collagen. Cohesive forces between fibrils (Jackson 1969) probably also involve glycoprotein and proteoglycans such as dermatan sulphate.

Periodicity

A number of theories have been proposed concerning the arrangement of tropocollagen molecules so as to account for the periodicity of 64 nm usually observed in electron micrographs. A modified version of the so-called quarter-stagger hypothesis put forward by Hodge & Petruska (1962) can account for such an appearance. According to these authors each tropocollagen molecule overlaps the next by one-quarter of its length, leaving a gap of approximately 38 nm (three-fifths of the total period) between the ends of the linearly arranged macromolecules. Grant *et al* (1965) believe, however, that a more random aggregation is statistically more probable and propose that any one of five possible degrees of overlap may occur between adjacent macromolecules. More recently Veis *et al* (1967) suggested a quarter-stagger arrangement within each tropocollagen molecule in order to maintain bonding contacts in three dimensions.

While the above hypotheses to a large extent account for the 64 nm periodicity, repeating units within the tropocollagen molecule itself are partly responsible for the finer cross-banding seen between the main 64 nm bands.

Staining reactions of collagen

Although collagen fibrils are readily identifiable at the ultrastructural level, there is, as yet, no histochemical procedure by which they can be specifically demonstrated at the light microscopic level. While the presence of hydroxyproline is the basis of standard biochemical assays for collagen, they cannot be adapted to histochemistry without losing the structural entity of collagen. There are, however, a number of stains by means of which collagen can be visualized more readily; these include van Gieson's picrofuchsin (see Fig. 1.2) and the methods of Masson and Mallory which employ aniline blue and light green.

1:6:2b RETICULIN FIBRES

The term reticulin denotes a system of fibres which is characteristically argyrophilic in that it has the capacity to adsorb metallic silver when treated with alkaline solutions of reducible silver salts. Such fibres are most apparent in developing connective tissue where they represent the earliest visible fibrous material, usually in the form of a fine, branched network. At a later stage of development, thicker, wavy and unbranched argyrophilic fibres predominate which ultimately develop into non-argyrophilic mature collagen fibres. Although not easily recognized, the original network can be demonstrated in mature connective tissue of skin and of gingiva where it surrounds the mature collagen fibres, wavy unbranched argyrophilic fibres being absent at this stage.

In order to distinguish between these two types of argyrophilic elements described by light microscopists, Melcher & Eastoe (1969) have suggested that the term 'reticulin' should be restricted to the branched network of fine fibres while the wavy argyrophilic fibres, which are soluble in neutral and acid solvents, should be referred to as 'argyrophilic developing collagen fibres'.

Both these transient argyrophilic fibres and the reticulin fibres are indistinguishable in the electron microscope from collagen, although they do not always show the banded structure. Melcher & Eastoe (1969) point out, however, that in the electron microscope reticulin fibres are associated with significant amounts of matrix. In the light microscope the outer part of the matrix may be the only component which is stained, so that the term 'fibres' is strictly incorrect in describing this system.

Since the argyrophilic network is present in both developing and mature connective tissue, it is unlikely that it is a precursor of argyrophilic developing collagen fibres. Robb-Smith (1958) has suggested that these two components are synthesized independently by fibroblasts and that only the thicker, unbranched fibres develop further into collagen fibres. Melcher (1966) has attributed to reticulin the function of providing a suitable environment for the assembly of collagen building blocks so that collagen is formed within, but not by direct conversion of, the reticulin 'fibres'.

Biochemical analysis indicates that the argyrophilic property of both the permanent reticulin network and the transient developing collagen fibres is due to considerable amounts of carbohydrate (4·2%) which are intimately associated with them. These carbohydrate components are also responsible for their stainability with periodic acid–Schiff (see section 1:6:2e) and their metachromasia with certain dyes. Unlike collagen, reticulin contains 11% lipid which to some extent also accounts for different staining properties. The main constituent of reticulin (85%) is a protein having a composition identical with that of collagen. The fact that highly specific collagenases will attack both collagen and reticulin is further evidence of their similarity in composition.

1:6:2C ELASTIC FIBRES

Elastic fibres consist largely of the protein elastin which, of all fibre proteins, is the most resistant to change. The elastin content of both skin and oral mucosa is very low compared with collagen, yet it confers an important elastic property on these tissues. Elastic fibres are less well represented in masticatory mucosa which is correspondingly less flexible than the highly deformable lining mucosa which has relatively more fibres (Fig. 1.22). Unlike collagen fibres, elastic fibres branch and anastomose and run singly rather than in bundles. Mature elastic fibres in skin measure 1·3–3·5 μm in diameter and can be 0·5 mm or more in length. They can be streched to 150% of their original length before the breaking point

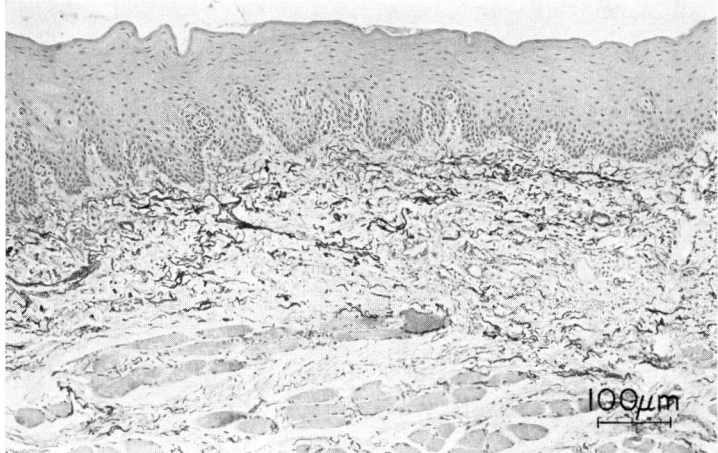

Fig. 1.22. Numerous elastic fibres in the lamina propria of human alveolar mucosa. Hart's elastin stain. Bar represents 100 μm.

is reached and will return to their original state after being stretched. In young elastic fibres groups of hollow filaments, 10–14 nm thick, termed elastic fibre microfibrils, can be seen. Like tropocollagen these are produced by fibroblasts but may also be secreted by smooth muscle cells. As the fibre matures, central finely granular areas develop, consisting of the protein, elastin. The fibre increases in size by addition of newly synthesized elastin to the homogeneous or finely granular region. Mature elastic fibres thus consist of two morphological components, a central granular area surrounded by a thin layer of hollow fibrils which display no periodicity although they occasionally have a beaded appearance. Greenlee et al (1966) found the central region to show an affinity for phosphotungstic acid stains while the fibrils are clearly demonstrated by lead salts and uranyl acetate. Amino acid analyses of elastin show a high proportion of glycine and of amino acids, with hydrocarbon side chains. Owing to the large number of hydrocarbon side chains and the small proportion of hydrophilic groups (ionizable and hydroxyl), elastin is a lipophilic protein in contrast to collagen which is hydrophilic. Hydroxyproline is also present in far lower quantities (2%) than in collagen. It is possible, however, that this may represent contamination by collagen which is always closely associated with elastic fibres.

1:6:2d OXYTALAN FIBRES

The term oxytalan describes the resistance of these fibres to acid; they stain with elastic stains only after oxidation with peracetic acid or performic acid, when they can be digested with elastase. In the oral mucosa they have been described only in the periodontal tissues where they are considerably more numerous than elastic fibres, while in skin they occur only around the appendages. Electron microscopically they consist of bundles of fibrils, 15–16 nm thick, which closely resemble immature elastic fibres. Although it has been suggested that they represent degenerate collagen (Selvig 1966), their chemical composition has not been investigated.

1:6:2e THE GROUND SUBSTANCE

The ground substance or matrix of loose connective tissue is a colloidal complex which embeds all other connective tissue components. Since no structural features are apparent at the light or electron microscope levels, it is frequently described as amorphous, but evidence is accumulating which indicates that it has a high degree of macromolecular organization.

The structural components of ground substance consist basically of carbohydrate–protein complexes which are permeated by tissue fluids. The latter contain plasma proteins, vitamins, hormones, enzymes, various electrolytes, and metabolic substances. The matrix is in a continual state of flux, its exact composition being dependent to a large extent on the general metabolic state of the surrounding cells and of the organism as a whole.

Carbohydrate–protein complexes

Initially the 'amorphous' ground substance of connective tissue was thought to belong to a chemically ill-defined group of substances called mucoids. It subsequently became apparent that this intercellular and interfibrillar substance consisted chiefly of carbohydrate and was from then on referred to as mucopolysaccharide. More recent research led to the awareness that in these substances carbohydrates were in most cases covalently linked with proteins to a greater or lesser degree. Subsequent terminology has been confused but it is now common to divide carbohydrate–protein complexes into two main groups, proteoglycans and glycoproteins.

(i) *Proteoglycans*. These are characterized by their constituent glycosaminoglycan, an acid mucopolysaccharide which has a high molecular weight and a large number of negatively charged carboxyl groups. Uronic acids are also a characteristic component of this group of macromolecules.

There are two prominent glycosaminoglycans in the loose connective tissue of skin and the oral mucosa, namely hyaluronic acid and chondroitin sulphate B, more recently known as dermatan sulphate. Hyaluronic acid consists of the hexosamine *N*-acetyl glucosamine and glucuronic acid. It is loosely complexed with 25–30% of protein and the resulting proteoglycan provides the physical structure for the ground substance and is responsible for the water-holding capacity of connective tissue. The molecule is very long, thin and flexible and occupies a relatively large amount of space or 'domain' due to its tangled configuration. These large domains confer on this polysaccharide the ability to control the passage of molecules through the tissue.

Dermatan sulphate (chondroitin sulphate B) is made up of sulphated *N*-acetyl galactosamine and iduronic acid. In the proteoglycan complex, these long polysaccharide chains are covalently attached to a protein core from which they radiate in a straight configuration due to mutual repulsion of the charged groups on the carbohydrate chains. This gives the molecule a rigid, rod-like structure.

(ii) *Glycoproteins*. These represent a chemically rather ill-defined group. The carbohydrate components, unlike those of proteoglycans, are of low molecular weight and lack a serially repeating unit. The total carbohydrate content is generally lower than in proteoglycans. They contain the hexosamines *N*-acetyl glucosamine and *N*-acetyl galactosamine, a feature they share with proteoglycans, but uronic acids are absent. The hexose sugars mannose, fucose and galactose are commonly present. Sialic acid (neuraminic acid) is perhaps the most characteristic component of glycoproteins, and is usually situated at the terminal portion of the carbohydrate chains, distal to the protein core. When present in sufficiently high numbers, they impart an acidic property to the glycoprotein molecule.

Staining reactions of the ground substance

In the periodic acid-Schiff (paS) reaction adjacent glycol groups are oxidized with periodic acid to di-aldehydes which give a deep magenta colour on treatment with Schiff reagent. A large proportion of glycoproteins are, therefore, paS positive whereas the majority of proteoglycans are unreactive. Since many glycoproteins and proteoglycans contain dissociable acid groups they will react with alcian blue; this is therefore a stain for acidic carbohydrate–protein complexes, but lacks any real specificity as far as these components are concerned.

1:6:3 Blood vessels and lymphatics

Although both epidermis and oral epithelium can reach a thickness of more than one mm they are avascular tissues and rely for their blood supply on the capillaries present in the connective tissue. The blood supply to these tissues is greatly in excess of what is required for metabolic needs because it also has a major role in thermal regulation.

1:6:3a THE CIRCULATORY SYSTEM IN THE SKIN

Cutaneous blood vessels are commonly associated with cutaneous nerves to form a neurovascular bundle; their distribution therefore reflects to some extent that of the nerves. The arteries form two major networks, the rete cutaneum lying between the dermis and hypodermis and the superficial subpapillary system (the rete subpapillary) lying between the reticular and papillary layers of the dermis itself. This latter network gives off capillary loops that run in the dermal papillae and pass close to the basement membrane of the epidermis. The flow through these loops is controlled by precapillary sphincters and is determined by local demands such as nutritional requirements. Blood from the capillary loops drains into a network of venules beneath the papillae, and it is these vessels that are largely responsible for the dermal component of skin colour. Deeper networks carry the blood back to the veins in the hypodermis that accompany the arteries. Branches of the rete cutaneum run to the sweat glands and deep portions of the hair follicles.

An important feature of the cutaneous circulation is the presence of arterio-venous anastomoses or shunts which are important for thermal regulation; by dilation they substantially increase the total volume of blood flowing through skin.

Accompanying the blood vascular system is an extensive lymphatic system, which arises in the papillary layer as blind-ending lymphatic capillaries, the walls of which have large pores, through which foreign particulate matter enters the system (Nicholl & Cortese 1972). This represents a major protective mechanism. The superficial network of lymphatics communicates with a deeper network and finally drains into large subcutaneous lymphatic vessels.

The pattern of the cutaneous circulation varies in different regions of the skin, particularly with the thickness of the epithelium and configuration of the epithelial–connective tissue boundary. Thus where the rete ridges are poorly developed, there is a sparse vascular bed with few capillary loops, while areas with well-developed rete ridges show elaborate loops in the papillary layer. It has been suggested that there is an association between the mitotic rate and the richness of the vascular bed (Ellis 1963).

1:6:3b THE CIRCULATORY SYSTEM IN
THE ORAL MUCOSA

The blood supply to the oral mucosa has not been studied to the same extent as that of skin. Some work has been done on selected areas of experimental animals such as dog and rabbit tongue, and hamster cheek pouch, as well as on human gingiva. A comprehensive account of the vascular pattern of primate oral mucosa has been given by Cutright & Hunsuck (1970), who examined injected preparations of macaque monkey. These authors describe a vascular pattern at the vermilion border of the lip which, like that of the oral mucosa, is richer than in the skin due to a concentrated network of interconnected vessels. This is one reason for the greater coloration of the oral mucosa. Arteries run in the submucosa or, where there is a periosteum, in the deeper part of the lamina propria. They give off progressively smaller branches to form a capillary network immediately beneath the reticular layer which thus corresponds to the rete cutaneum of the skin. From this network branches rise to form a subpapillary network which in turn gives off capillary loops to the papillae. As in skin there are anastomoses between small arteries and veins, arterioles and venules and between capillaries. The subpapillary network is closer to the basal layer of the epithelium than in the skin (see, for example, Fig. 1·21) and the capillary loops from this system are also larger and more numerous. In the gingiva these loops are the longest in the body, originating at the border of the attached and free gingiva and extending to the gingival crest. The tongue has a rich capillary system running into the lingual papillae, particularly the fungiform type, and it is likely that taste sensitivity is affected by changes in blood flow (Hellekant 1972). The salivary gland ducts are served by a separate plexus, a feature not found around the ducts of the sweat glands or sebaceous glands of the skin. Blood from the capillary beds is collected by a series of veins which accompany the arteries. Lymphatic capillaries in the lamina propria drain into larger vessels in the submucosa and generally follow the course of the blood vessels.

Despite the frequent anastomoses between the arterial and venous systems it is uncertain whether these pathways have the same thermoregulatory role in the oral mucosa as do the arterio-venous anastomoses of the skin. Sicher & Du Brul (1970) state that heat exchange could occur between the anastomoses of the sublingual area and the environment, but although typical arterio-venous shunts have been described in the tongue of a number of mammals, they are rare or even absent in man (Hellekant 1972).

1:6:4 Nerves

1:6:4a NERVES IN SKIN

Myelinated and unmyelinated nerve fibres penetrate the entire dermis and, in some areas, their free ends enter the epidermis (Ryan 1973). The skin, in keeping with its sensory function, has numerous sensory nerves in the middle and upper dermis (Winkelmann 1967), while autonomic nerves (chiefly sympathetic) supply regions containing smooth muscle and glands.

The majority of sensory nerves are heavily myelinated, but tend to lose their myelin sheaths abruptly in the upper dermis, where they form two recognizable plexuses, one between the reticular and papillary layers, the other concentrated immediately beneath the basement membrane. Multiple innervation of the skin ensures that most stimuli affect more than one nerve and are transmitted by more than one axon.

All human cutaneous nerves have naked endings, i.e. no perineural or myelin sheath, and can be classified into two groups; *simple* or *free endings* occur predominantly in hairy skin while *organized* or *encapsulated endings*, such as the Meissner and Pacinian corpuscles, are found in glabrous skin. It is now generally accepted that a specific receptor is not exclusively associated with a particular sensory modality and less emphasis is placed on an elaborate classification of endings in terms of morphology.

The existence of intra-epidermal nerves has been an area of some controversy and Breathnach (1971) claims that they have never convincingly been demonstrated in the interfollicular regions of hairy human skin. They are present in non-hairy skin, where they are frequently associated with Merkel cells (see section 1:4).

1:6:4b NERVES IN ORAL MUCOSA

As in skin, sensory nerves supplying the oral mucosa lose their myelin sheath as they enter the lamina propria where they branch to form a network within the reticular layer; a fine subepithelial plexus can also be recognized. Thin unmyelinated fibres are also seen in the adventitia of larger blood vessels and free in the connective tissue, these are thought to be part of the autonomic system (Plenk & Raab 1969).

In the case of sensory fibres, both free and organized endings are distinguished as in skin. Free endings are recognized as simple terminations of the nerve fibres either in the connective tissue of the lamina propria or intra-epithelially (Farbman & Allgood 1971); some free endings may be closely coiled so as to resemble an organized ending. Frequently more than one fibre can contribute to a simple ending. As in skin, some intra-epithelial nerve endings seem to be associated with Merkel cells (see section 1:4). Organized nerve endings consist of a coiled fibre or group of fibres that may be enclosed in a connective tissue capsule to form Meissner, Ruffini, or Pacinian corpuscles, Krause end-bulbs and muco-cutaneous end organs. Sensory endings and the mucosal nerve plexuses tend to be more concentrated in the anterior part of the oral cavity, particularly at the tip of the tongue and on the incisive papilla and the rugal crests of the hard palate (Farbman & Allgood 1971). In a study of nerve endings in the gingiva, Desjardins, Winkelmann & Gonzales (1971) found a decrease in sensory endings from incisor to molar region of the maxillary arch, and a reverse trend in the mandibular arch.

There is some uncertainty over the innervation of the mucosa of edentulous patients. Large numbers of intra-epithelial processes projecting from organized endings in the connective tissue were described by Marsland & Fox (1958) in regions where dentures were painful. Desjardins, Winkelmann & Gonzales (1971) claimed that absence of teeth did not produce qualitative differences in the type of endings and that the observed decrease in the complexity of the nervous network in the edentulous mucosa was the direct effect of a prosthesis.

Taste buds are found exclusively in the mucosa of the tongue, soft palate and pharynx. The majority are present within the epithelium of the fungiform, foliate and circumvallate papillae of the tongue. Taste buds consist of a group of 30–60 spindle-shaped cells some of which (the receptor cells) form synapses with nerve endings; the nerve endings may also be directly sensitive to taste. The basic modalities of taste—salty, sweet, sour and bitter—may each be detected by different fungiform papillae; taste buds in different regions of the oral cavity may have different sensitivities to a given modality (Farbman & Allgood 1971).

1:7 Age Changes in Oral Mucosa and Skin

All tissues undergo gradual, inexorable and cumulative changes with age. These are perhaps most easily recognized in skin, for example thinning and wrinkling of body skin, greying of hair and increasing prevalence of baldness. The oral mucosa of the aged is comparatively thin, smooth and dry and symptoms such as burning or itching, roughness and abnormal taste sensations are commonplace, particularly in post-menopausal women. It is difficult to determine to what extent these, and other more specific alterations described below, are inevitable consequences of 'programmed senescence' in the tissues themselves, are secondary to environmental 'wear and tear', or are secondary to systemic factors such as changes in hormonal, nutritional and cardiovascular status. What follows, therefore, is mainly a description of the better documented age-related alterations in skin and oral mucosa, with little reference to mechanisms.

1:7:1 Changes in epithelial structure

It is generally believed that epidermis becomes thinner with advancing age, although numerous conflicting reports appear in the literature (see review by Giacometti 1965). This conflict is partly explained by the large regional variation normally present, and partly by a greater irregularity of thickness in older persons. All layers appear to vary in thickness, there is disparity in size and shape of individual cells and their nuclei and, consequently, a less ordered packing (Montagna 1965). The basophilia of basal cells is reduced, probably reflecting reduced nucleic acid content, and glycogen tends to accumulate in the upper spinous layers. The dermo-epidermal junction becomes smoother and the basement membrane thinner and of inconsistent thickness.

Whilst scaling and flaking of the skin are commonly seen in the elderly, histological studies do not reveal any uniform trend to an increase or a decrease in the thickness of the keratin layers. Changes are most marked on exposed surfaces such as the face and dorsum of the hands (Montagna 1965) and it is difficult to differentiate true age changes from those due to environmental stimuli.

There may be an increase in the number of recognizable clear cells within the epithelium but a reduction in obvious melanocytes. The average number of melanocytes per unit area of skin surface decreases by about 11% per decade throughout life, with a consequent rise in the ratio of Malpighian cells to melanocytes (Fitzpatrick, Szabo & Mitchell 1965). The pigment distribution frequently becomes irregular, leading to the formation of pigmented patches known as 'senile lentigo'.

Detailed studies of changes in the oral epithelium with age are few and, again, contradictory (Miles 1972). Richman & Abarbanel, in 1943, reported a decrease in width of the Malpighian layers and increased keratinization, sometimes resulting in the formation of white plaques, in post-menopausal women. In most cases menopause was surgically induced, and administration of oestrogen reversed the changes. Shklar (1966) subjectively compared sections of oral mucosa from 100 individuals of mixed sex below the age of 16 with 100 similar individuals above the age of 60, and found the epithelium to be thinner and the rete ridges reduced in all parts of the mouth in the older group. A tendency to increased keratinization was detectable only on the hard palate. In contrast the more recent quantitative study of Löe & Karring (1971) indicates that the cell population of human gingiva remains relatively constant throughout life.

Somewhat different results emerge from studies employing exfoliative cytology. Papic & Glickmann (1950) found, in females, a trend towards decreased keratinization of gingiva with age beyond the third decade, though this was not noticeably accelerated after menopause. Montgomery

(1951) and Miller, Stahl & Soberman (1952) failed to detect such changes, although a similar decrease was noted in males by Pedreira (1951) and by Zimmermann & Zimmermann (1965). In the latter study, ageing was associated with a statistically significant reduction in the proportion of keratinized squames from the hard palate and gingiva but not from the tongue or buccal mucosa.

These apparently conflicting results, with clinical observation and histology suggesting increased keratinization with age, and exfoliative cytology suggesting, if anything, the reverse, may partly be explained by regional differences.

In addition to hormonal influences, nutritional deficiencies, particularly of iron and of B group vitamins, are relatively common in the aged and these are known to predispose to mucosal atrophy, particularly on the tongue, where loss of filiform papillae may be marked (Frantzell et al 1945; Miles 1972) (see Chapter 5).

1:7:2 Changes in epithelial turnover

This has been discussed in section 1:3:1a. In spite of a large number of studies showing increased mitotic index with advancing age in man and experimental animals, it now appears likely that tissue turnover actually decreases. More recent work employing thymidine-labelling techniques or studies of the distribution of the phases of mitosis indicates that the duration of the mitotic cycle is increased, with a consequent slowing of tissue turnover (see Barakat et al 1969; Karring & Löe 1973).

1:7:3 Changes in connective tissue

Although no precise figures are available, there is little doubt that the cell population of the dermis is substantially decreased in old age (Andrew & Sato 1964; Papa & Kligman 1965). All cell types appear to be involved, the fibroblasts in particular becoming shrunken with condensed elongate nuclei and scanty cytoplasm. The lamina propria of oral mucosa shows similar changes. In skin the fibroblast depletion is associated with a marked reduction in stainable acid proteoglycan and other components of the ground substance (Sobel & Marmorston 1956). A more youthful appearance is said to be induced by topical application of testosterone or progesterone (Papa & Kligman 1965).

The number and thickness of elastic fibres in the dermis appears to increase with age, particularly in exposed skin (Lee 1957; Giacometti

1965; Pearce & Grimmer 1972). This change, often referred to as 'senile elastosis', is very much more marked in exposed than in non-exposed skin (a rise from 2% to 13% by weight), and the term 'solar elastosis' is preferred by some (Troy 1968). In spite of this dramatically increased elastic content, degenerative changes seem to occur in the ultrastructure of the fibres (Danielsen & Kobayasi 1972). Apart from the study of Dependorf (1903), which suggested a similar increase in elastic content in the cheek, there is no information on variations in the elastin content of oral mucosa.

Skin collagen fibres likewise appear thicker and denser with advancing age, although not all authors agree (Giacometti 1965). However, there is a progressive decrease in the ratio of soluble to insoluble collagen with age (Sams & Smith 1965; Troy 1968), a reduction in turnover as measured by radioactive amino acid incorporation, and a progressive increase in intra- and inter-molecular cross links (Jackson 1965) leading to increased tension and a rise in shrinkage temperature (Rasmussen, Wakim & Winkelmann 1965; Troy 1968). The biophysical properties of ageing skin have recently been reviewed by Elden (1970). It is likely that similar, but less marked, changes occur in the collagen of oral mucosa. Shklar (1966) describes degeneration, fragmentation, hyalinization and basophilia in the lamina propria of aged human oral mucosa. In contrast, the chemical analysis comparing the composition of young and old guinea-pig palate carried out by Burzynski & Rogers (1965a, b) showed no significant differences in the content of collagenous or non-collagenous proteins, though there was a significant rise in the collagen-bound hexose in the older group.

It is generally agreed (see review by Winkelmann 1965) that sensory nerve endings in skin decrease significantly with advancing age, but a careful study by Cauna (1965) reveals that different functional endings respond in different ways. For example the density of myelinated endings in the skin of the finger tip decreases in the elderly but individual endings may enlarge. These changes are thought to reflect a response to changing functional requirements rather than to represent a true process of senescence. Free nerve endings appear to remain relatively stable in distribution and structure. The oral mucosa shows a similar spectrum of change (Winkelmann 1965), particularly in the gingiva and tongue, though apparently not affecting taste buds. Within the mouth the interpretation of these changes must be complicated by functional alterations related to the high prevalence of tooth loss, the wearing of prostheses and consequent variations in masticatory efficiency, and by disease, particularly periodontal disease.

The vascular pattern of aged skin is not remarkably different from that of younger individuals. In the scalp, for example, a significant reduction in capillary density occurs only in association with hair loss (Giacometti 1965). Vessels may, however, become more 'fragile' in the elderly, as evidenced by the incidence of so-called 'spider naevi'. Unusually long dilated capillaries have been described in conjunctiva and nail bed in aged individuals (Nicola 1965). The only documented changes in the vasculature of oral mucosa with age are the increasing prevalence of sublingual varicosities, or 'caviar tongue', which may be seen in 60% or more of individuals beyond the age of 60 years (Bean 1955, 1956), and similar varicosities in the lips and cheeks (Miles 1972).

1:7:4 Changes in appendages and glands

Eccrine sweat glands are reduced in number with age and many of those remaining appear atrophic. These changes are less marked in the apocrine glands (Montagna 1965).

The minor salivary glands of the oral cavity of ageing individuals contain relatively fewer functional acini with a concomitant increase in fibrous tissue. Diffuse infiltrations of lymphocytes are common in persons over 45 years of age, up to 70% of glands showing such changes, although the prevalence does not increase further with advancing age (Chisholm, Waterhouse & Mason 1970). Similar changes occur in the major salivary glands and in both situations dense focal aggregations of lymphocytes are indicative of Sjögren's syndrome (see Chapter 10). Taste buds appear to become reduced in number (Kaplan 1971; Miles 1972).

Sebaceous glands of skin do not obviously atrophy with age (Montagna 1965), though their functional activity may fall off as evidenced by the reduced lipid found on the skin surface of the aged (Pochi & Strauss 1965). There may even be histological signs of hyperplasia, particularly in the balding scalp. Miles (1958, 1963, 1972) has clearly shown that sebaceous glands in the lips and buccal mucosa increase in number with advancing age.

1:8 Further Reading

1:8:1 Skin

There is a large literature dealing with the structure and function of skin.

Good general accounts of skin structure are to be found in:

MONTAGNA W. and PARAKKAL P. F. (1974) *The Structure and Function of Skin* 3rd edition. Academic Press, London.

MONTAGNA W. & LOBITZ W.C. (eds) (1964) *The Epidermis*. Academic Press, London.

Various aspects of structure and function are dealt with in the series of volumes, Advances in Biology of the Skin. These include:

Volume VI   MONTAGNA W. (ed.) (1965) *Ageing*. Pergamon Press, Oxford.
Volume VIII   MONTAGNA W. & HU F. (eds) (1967) *The Pigmentary System*. Pergamon Press, Oxford.
Volume X   MONTAGNA W., BENTLEY J.P. & DOBSON R.L. (eds) (1970) *The Dermis*. Appleton-Century Crofts, New York.
Volume XI   MONTAGNA W. & BILLINGHAM R.E. (eds) (1971) *Immunology and the Skin*. Appleton-Century Crofts, New York.

Comprehensive accounts of the ultrastructure of the skin, including development and differentiation, are provided by:

ZELICKSON A.S. (1967) *Ultrastructure of Normal and Abnormal Skin*. Henry Kimpton, London.

BREATHNACH A.S. (1971) *An Atlas of the Ultrastructure of the Human Skin*, J. & A. Churchill, London.

Keratinization is considered from a general biological viewpoint in MERCER E.H. (1961) *Keratin and Keratinisation; an essay in molecular biology*. Pergamon Press, Oxford, while the subject has recently been discussed in FRASER R.D.B., MACRAE T.P. & ROGERS G.E. (1972) *Keratins; their composition, structure and biosynthesis*. Charles C. Thomas, Springfield, Illinois.

Specialized tissue cells are described in the following texts:

WEISS L. (1972) *The Cells and Tissues of the Immune System*. Prentice-Hall, Englewood Cliffs, New Jersey.

SELYE H. (1965) *The Mast Cells*. Butterworths, Washington.

KELLER R. (1966) *Tissue Mast Cells in Immune Reactions*. Monographs in Allergy 2, Elsevier, New York.

VERNON-ROBERTS B. (1972) *The Macrophage*. Cambridge Univ. Press, London.

PEARSALL N. & WEISER R.S. (1970) *The Macrophage*. Lea & Febiger, Philadelphia.

NELSON D.S. (1969) *Macrophages and Immunity*. North Holland, Amsterdam.

KULONEN E. & PIKKARAINEN J. (eds) (1973) *Biology of the Fibroblast*. Academic Press, London.

The following texts deal with other selected aspects of skin structure or function:

SINCLAIR D. (1967) *Cutaneous Sensation*. Oxford University Press, London.

SINCLAIR D. (1973) Normal anatomy of sensory nerves and receptors. In JARRETT A. (ed.) *The Physiology and Pathophysiology of the Skin*, 347–420. Academic Press, London.

RYAN T.J. (1973) Structure, pattern and shape of the blood vessels of the skin. In JARRETT A. (ed.) *The Physiology and Pathophysiology of the Skin*, 577–651, Academic Press, London.

The principles involved in cell proliferation studies and the methods in current use are well considered in:

CLEAVER J.E. (1967) *Thymidine Metabolism and Kinetics*. North Holland, Amsterdam.

FEINENDEGEN L.E. (1967) *Tritium Labelled Molecules in Biology and Medicine*. Academic Press, New York.

Various aspects of epithelial connective tissue interactions appear in:

FLEISCHMEYER R. & BILLINGHAM R.E. (eds) (1968) *Epithelium Mesenchymal Interactions*. Williams & Wilkins, Baltimore.

SLAVKIN H.E. & BAVETTA I.A. (ed.) (1972) *Developmental Aspects of Oral Biology*. Academic Press, New York.

1:8:2 Oral Mucosa

There are comparatively few works dealing exclusively with the structure and function of the oral mucosa. Many of the aspects discussed in this chapter are considered in:

SQUIER C.A. & MEYER J. (eds) (1971) *Current Concepts of the Histology of Oral Mucosa*. Charles C. Thomas, Springfield, Illinois.

The specialized regions of the oral epithelium of the periodontium are described in:

MELCHER A.H. & ZARB G.A. (eds) (1972) *Gingival Epithelium, Oral Sciences Reviews*. Vol. 1. Munksgaard, Copenhagen.

SCHROEDER H. E. & LISTGARTEN M.A. (1971) *Fine Structure of the Developing Epithelial Attachment of Human Teeth*. S. Karger, Basel.

The normal and pathological basement membrane is illustrated in:

FRITHIOF L. (1969) Ultrastructure of the basement membrane in normal and hyperplastic human oral epithelium compared with that in preinvasive and invasive carcinoma. *Acta path. microbiol. Scand.*, Supp. 200, Munksgaard, Copenhagen.

A comprehensive account of the connective tissue is given in:
MELCHER A.H. & EASTOE J.E. Connective tissues of the periodontium. In MELCHER A.H. & BOWEN W.H. (eds) 167–344. (1969) *Biology of the Periodontium*, Academic Press, London.
FULLMER H.M. Connective tissue components of the periodontium. In MILES A.E.W. (ed.) (1967) *Structural and Chemical Organisation of Teeth*, Vol. 2, 349–414. Academic Press, New York.

Some aspects of oral physiology (particularly oral circulation) are covered in:
EMMELIN N. & ZOLTERMAN Y. (eds) (1972) *Proceedings of the International Symposium, Oral Physiology, Stockholm, 1971*. Pergamon Press, Oxford.

Acknowledgements

We are grateful to Professor A.E.W. Miles, Dr Julia Meyer, Dr Rosamund Hopps and Dr P.M. Gaylarde for advice during the preparation of this chapter and to Mr J.E. Linder and Miss J. Stennett-Wilson for the production of histological and photographic material.

1:9 References

ALVARES O.F. & MEYER J. (1971) Variable features and regional differences in oral epithelium. In SQUIER C.A. & MEYER J. *Current Concepts of the Histology of Oral Mucosa*, 97–113. Charles C. Thomas, Springfield, Illinois.

ALVARES O., SKOUGAARD M.R., PINDBORG J.J. & ROED-PETERSON B. (1972) In vitro incorporation of tritiated thymidine in oral homogeneous leukoplakias. *Scand. J. dent. Res.*, **80**, 510–514.

ANDREW W. & SATO T. (1964) The gross and microscopic morphologic changes in ageing skin. *Proc. Sci. Sect. Toil. Goods Assocn.*, **41**, 12 (cited by Papa & Kligman 1965).

ANGELOPOULOS A.P. (1970) Metachromatic cells of the human gingival epithelium: mast cells or melanocytes? *I.A.D.R. Abstracts (North American Division)*, No. 377.

ANGELOPOULOS A.P. (1972) A method for quantitative estimation of tissue components and number of mast cells in the gingiva. *J. periodont. Res.*, **7**, Supp. 9.

ANGELOPOULOS A.P. (1973) Studies of mast cells in the human gingiva. *J. periodont. Res.*, **8**, 314–322.

ATTSTRÖM R. (1971) Studies on neutrophil polymorphonuclear leukocytes at the dento-gingival junction in gingival health and disease. *J. periodont. Res.*, **8**, Supp. 8.

BADEN H.P. & GOLDSMITH L.A. (1972) The structural protein of epidermis. *J. invest. Derm.*, **59**, 66–76.

BARAKAT N.J., TOTO P.D. & CHOUKAS N.C. (1969) Ageing and cell renewal of oral epithelium. *J. periodont.*, **40**, 599–602.

BARKER D.S. (1967) The dendritic cell system in human gingival epithelium. *Archs. oral Biol.*, **12**, 203–208.

BARNETT M.L. (1973) Mast cells in the epithelial layer of human gingiva. *J. Ultrastruct. Res.*, **43**, 247–255.

BARNETT M.L. & SZABO S. (1973) Gap junctions in human gingival keratinized epithelium. *J. periodont. Res.*, **8**, 117–126.

BASSETT F. & TURIAF M.J. (1965) Identification par la microscopie électronique de particules de nature probablement virale dans les lésion granulomateuses d'une histiocytosis 'X' pulmonaire. *C.r. hebd. Seance Acad. Sci., Paris*, **261**, 3701–3703.

BEAGRIE G.S. (1963) An autoradiographic study of the gingival epithelium of mice and monkeys with thymidine-^{3}H. *Dent. Pract.*, **14**, 18–26.

BEAGRIE G.S. (1966) Observations on the cell biology of gingival tissues of mice. *Brit. dent. J.*, **121**, 417–420.

BEAGRIE G.S. (1970) The in vivo effects of ^{3}H thymidine on the mitosis in oral epithelium of the mouse. *Archs. oral Biol.*, **15**, 205–211.

BEAGRIE G.S. and SKOUGAARD M.S. (1962) Observations on the life cycle of gingival epithelial cells of mice revealed by autoradiography. *Acta odont. Scand.*, **20**, 15–31.

BEAN W.B. (1955) Changing incidence of certain vascular lesions of the skin with ageing. In WOLSTENHOLME G.E.W. & CAMERON M.P. *Ciba Foundation Colloquia on Ageing*, Vol. 1. J. & A. Churchill Ltd, London.

BEAN W.B. (1956) The changing incidence of certain vascular lesions of the skin with ageing. *Geriatrics*, **11**, 97–102.

BECKER S.W., FITZPATRICK T.B. & MONTGOMERY H. (1952) Human melanogenesis: cytology and histology of pigment cells (melanodendrocytes). *Arch Derm and Syph.*, **65**, 511–523.

BERNFIELD M.R. (1970) Collagen synthesis during epithelio-mesenchymal interactions. *Dev. Biol.*, **22**, 213–231.

BILLINGHAM R.E. & MEDAWAR P.B. (1953). A study of the branched cells of the mammalian epidermis with special reference to the fate of their division products. *Trans. Roy. Phil. Soc., London (B)*, **237**, 151–171.

BILLINGHAM R.E. & SILVERS W.K. (1967) Studies on the conservation of epidermal specificities of skin and certain mucosas in adult mammals. *J. exp. Med.*, **125**, 429–446.

BILLINGHAM R.E. & SILVERS W.K. (1968) Dermoepidermal interactions and epithelial specificity, Chap. 17, 252–266. In FLEISCHMAJER R. & BILLINGHAM R.E. *Epithelial-Mesenchymal Interactions*. The Williams & Wilkins Co., Baltimore.

BINNIE W.H. & LEHNER T. (1970) Histology of the muco-cutaneous junction at the corner of the human mouth. *Archs. oral Biol.*, **15**, 777–786.

BIRBECK M.S.C., BREATHNACH A.S. & EVERALL J.D. (1961) An electron microscope study of basal melanocytes and high level clear cells (Langerhans cells) in Vitiligo. *J. invest. Derm.*, **37**, 51–64.

BIRBECK M.S.C. (1962) Electron microscopy of melanocytes. *Brit. med. Bull.*, **18**, 220–222.

BLENKINSOPP W.K. (1967) Effect of tritiated thymidine on cell proliferation. *J. Cell. Sci.*, **2**, 305–308.

BLENKINSOPP W.K. (1968) Cell proliferation in stratified squamous epithelium in mice. *Exp. cell. Res.*, **50**, 265–276.
BÖCK P. (1973) Langerhans Granula in Bindegewebszellen der Maus. *Cytobiologie*, **7**, 327–336.
BREATHNACH A.S. (1964) Observations on cytoplasmic organelles in Langerhans cells of human epidermis. *J. Anat.*, **98**, 265–270.
BREATHNACH A.S. (1965) The cell of Langerhans. *Int. Rev. Cytol.*, **18**, 1–28.
BREATHNACH A.S. (1971) *An Atlas of Ultrastructure of Human Skin: Development, Differentiation and Post-natal Features.* J. & A. Churchill, London.
BREATHNACH A.S., FITZPATRICK T.B. & WYLLIE L.M.A. (1965) Electron microscopy of melanocytes in human piebaldism. *J. invest. Derm.*, **45**, 28–37.
BREATHNACH A.S., SILVERS W.K., SMITH J. & HEYNER S. (1968) Langerhans cells in mouse skin experimentally deprived of its neural crest component. *J. invest. Derm.*, **50**, 147–160.
BRIGGAMAN R.A., DALLDORF F.G. & WHEELER C.E. (1971) Formation and origin of basal lamina and anchoring fibrils in adult human skin. *J. Cell Biol.*, **51**, 384–395.
BRILL N. & BJÖRN H. (1959) Passage of tissue fluid into human gingival pockets. *Acta odont. Scand.*, **18**, 95–100.
BRODY I. (1959) An ultrastructural study on the role of the keratohyaline granules in the keratinization process. *J. Ultrastruct. Res.*, **3**, 84–104.
BRODY I. (1964) Different staining methods for the electron microscopic elucidation of the tonofibrillar differentiation in normal epidermis. In MONTAGNA W. & LOBITZ W.C. *The Epidermis*, 251–273. Academic Press, New York.
BROWN I.A. (1972) Scanning electron microscopy of human dermal fibrous tissue. *J. Anat. Lond.*, **113**, 159–168.
BROWN J.M. & BERRY R.J. (1968) The relationship between diurnal variation of the number of cells in mitosis and the number of cells synthesising DNA in the epithelium of the hamster cheek pouch. *Cell Tissue Kinet.*, **1**, 23–33.
BROWN J.M. & OLIVER R. (1968) A new method of estimating the cell cycle time in epithelial tissues of long generation time. *Cell Tissue Kinet.*, **1**, 11–21.
BULLOUGH W.S. (1950) Epidermal mitotic activity in the adult female mouse. *J. Endocrinol.*, **6**, 340–349.
BULLOUGH W.S. (1962) The control of mitotic activity in adult mammalian tissues. *Biol. Rev.*, **37**, 307–342.
BULLOUGH W.S. & Laurence E.B. (1966a) Tissue homeostasis in adult mammals. In MONTAGNA W. & DOBSON R.L. *Advances in Biology of Skin*, Vol. VII, 1–36. Pergamon Press, Oxford.
BULLOUGH W.S. & LAURENCE E.B. (1966b) The duirnal cycle in epidermal mitotic duration and its relation to chalone and adrenalin. *Exptl. Cell Res.*, **43**, 343–350.
BULLOUGH W.S. & LAURENCE E.B. (1968) The role of glucocorticoid hormones in the control of epidermal mitosis. *Cell Tissue Kinet.*, **1**, 5–10.
BURGES M.H. & VARGAS-LINORES C.E.R. (1970) Cell junctions in the human vaginal epithelium. *Am. J. Obs. Gyn.*, **108**, 565–571.
BURZYNSKI N.J. & ROGERS J.B. (1965a) Observations of chemical changes in the palate of guinea pigs with relation to ageing. *J. dent. Res.*, **44**, 1410.

BURZYNSKI N.J. & ROGERS H.B. (1965b) Effects of ageing in palatal tissue of the guinea pig. *J. Geront.*, **20**, 420–422.

CAMERON I.L. (1966) Cell proliferation, migration and specialisation in the epithelium of the mouse tongue. *J. exp. Zool.*, **163**, 271–284.

CAMERON I.L., GOSSLEE D.G. & PILGRIM C. (1965) The spatial distribution of dividing and DNA synthesising cells in mouse epithelium. *J. Cell comp. Physiol*, **66**, 431–436.

CAMPO-AASEN J. & PEARSE A.G.E. (1966) Enzimologia de la célula de Langerhans. *Medicina Cutánea*, **1**, 35–44.

CARRANZA F.A. & CABRINI R.L. (1955) Mast cells in human gingivae. *Oral Surg.* **8**, 1093.

CATTONI M. (1951) Lymphocytes in the epithelium of the healthy gingiva. *J. dent. Res.*, **30**, 627–637.

CAUNA N. (1965) The effects of ageing on the receptor organs of the human dermis. In MONTAGNA W., *Advances in Biology of Skin*, Vol. VI, 63–96. Pergamon Press, Oxford.

CHEN S.Y. (1970) Comparison of the fine structure of the mucosa of cheek and hard palate in the rabbit. M.Sc. Thesis, University of Illinois at the Medical Center, Chicago, Illinois.

CHEN S.Y. & MEYER J. (1971) Regional differences in tonofilaments and kerato-hyaline granules. In SQUIER C.A. & MEYER J. *Current Concepts of the Histology of Oral Mucosa*, 114–128. Charles C. Thomas, Springfield, Illinois.

CHISHOLM D.M., WATERHOUSE J.P. & MASON D.K. (1970) Lymphocytic sialadenitis in the major and minor glands; a correlation in post-mortem subjects. *J. clin. Path.*, **23**, 690–694.

COWDRY E.U. & THOMPSON H.C. (1944) Localisation of maximum cell division in epidermis. *Anat. Rec.*, **88**, 403–409.

CRUICKSHANK C.N.D. & HARCOURT S.A. (1964) Pigment donation in vitro. *J. invest. Derm.*, **42**, 183–184.

CUTRIGHT D.E. & BAUER H. (1967) Cell renewal in the oral mucosa and skin of the rat. 1. Turnover time. *Oral Surg.*, **23**, 249–257.

CUTRIGHT D.E. & HUNSUCK E.E. (1970) Micro-circulation of the peri-oral regions in the Macaca rhesus. *Oral Surg.* **29**, 776–785, 926–934.

DANIELSEN L. & KOBAYASI T. (1972) Degeneration of dermal elastic fibres in relation to age and light exposure. *Acta. Derm.-vener. (Stockh.)*, **52**, 1–10.

DAY T.D. (1952) The permeability of interstitial connective tissue and the nature of the interfibrillary substance. *J. Physiol.*, **117**, 1–8.

DELLA PORTER G. & MÜHLBOCK O. (1966) *Structure and Control of the Melanocyte*, 1–5. Springer-Verlag, Berlin.

DEMETRIOU N.A. & RAMFJORD S.P. (1972) Premitotic labelling and inflammation in the gingiva of rhesus monkeys. *J. Peridont.*, **43**, 606–613.

DEPENDORF T. (1903) Cited by MILES A.E.W. (1972) (*Öst.-ung. Vrtljschr. Zahnh.*, **19**, 9–59, 247, 337).

DESJARDINS R.P., WINKELMANN R.K. & GONZALES J.B. (1971) Comparison of nerve ending in normal gingiva with those in mucosa covering edentulous alveolar ridges. *J. dent. Res.*, **50**, 867–879.

DHAWAN A.S. & TOTO P.D. (1965) Renewal of cell population in palate and tongue epithelia of mice. *J. dent. Res.*, **44**, 989–995.
DIMASSIMO C.A. (1963) Proliferation and migration of cells in the gingival epithelium. Thesis, University of Rochester, N.Y.
DODSON J.W. (1963) On the nature of tissue interaction in embryonic skin. *Exptl. Cell Res.*, **31**, 233–235.
DODSON J.W. (1967) The differentiation of epidermis. I. The interrelationship of epidermis and dermis in embryonic chicken skin. *J. Embryol. Exp. Morph.*, **17**, 83–105.
DUMMETT C.O. & BARENS G. (1971) Oromucosal pigmentation: an updated literary review. *J. Periodont.*, **42**, 726–736.
EBLING F.J. (1954) Changes in sebaceous glands and epidermis during oestrus cycle of albino rat. *J. Endocrinol.*, **10**, 147–154.
EGELBERG J. (1963a) Diffusion of histamine into the gingival crevice and through the crevicular epithelia. *Acta odont. Scand.*, **21**, 271–282.
EGELBERG J. (1963b) Cellular elements in gingival pocket fluid. *Acta odont. Scand.*, **21**, 283–287.
ELDEN H.R. (1970) Biophysical properties of ageing skin. In MONTAGNA W., BENTLEY J.P. & DOBSON R.L. *Advances in Biology of Skin*, Vol. X, 231–252. Appleton-Century-Crofts, New York.
ELLIS R.A. (1963) Vascular patterns of the skin. In MONTAGNA W. & ELLIS R.A. *Advances in Biology of Skin*, Vol. II, 20–37. Pergamon Press, Oxford.
ENGLAND M.C. & BURKE G.W. (1968) Diurnal variation in DNA synthesis in selected epithelial tissues of male rats. *J. dent. Res.*, **47**, 478–481.
ENGLAND M.C. & BURKE G.W. (1969) Autoradiographic demonstration of DNA synthesis in selected epithelial tissues in male rats. *J. dent. Res.*, **48**, 1219–1223.
ENGLAND M.C. & BURKE G.W. (1971) Diurnal variation in DNA synthesis in hamster oral epithelium. *J. dent. Res.*, **50**, 976.
ENGLER W.O., RAMFJORD S.P. & HINIKER J.J. (1965a) Development of epithelial attachment and gingival sulcus in rhesus monkeys. *J. Periodont.*, **36**, 44–57.
ENGLER W.O., RAMFJORD S.P. & HINIKER J.J. (1965b) Healing following simple gingivectomy. A tritiated thymidine radioautographic study. 1. Epithelization. *J. Periodont.*, **37**, 298–308.
EPSTEIN W.L. and MAIBACH H.I. (1965) Cell renewal in human epidermis. *Archs Derm.*, **92**, 426–468.
ERIKSSON G. & LAMKE L.-O. (1971) Regeneration of human epidermal surface and water barrier function after stripping. *Acta Derm.-vener. (Stockh.)*, **51**, 169–178.
FARBMAN A.I. (1966) Plasma membrane changes during keratinization. *Anat. Rec.*, **156**, 269–282.
FARBMAN A.I. (1970) The dual pattern of keratinization in filiform papillae on rat tongue. *J. Anat. Lond.*, **104**, 233–242.
FARBMAN A.I. & ALLGOOD J.P. (1971) Innervation, sensory receptors and sensitivity of the oral mucosa. In SQUIER C.A. & MEYER J. *Current Concepts of the Histology of Oral Mucosa*, 250–273. Charles C. Thomas, Springfield, Illinois.

FARQUHAR M.G. & PALADE G.E. (1965) Cell junctions in amphibian skin. *J. Cell Biol.*, **26**, 263-291.
FELL H.B. (1964) The experimental study of keratinization in organ culture. In MONTAGNA W. & LOBITZ W.C. *The Epidermis*, 61-81. Academic Press, New York.
FINE D.H., PECHERSKY J.L. & MCKIBBEN D.H. (1969) The penetration of human gingival sulcular tissue by carbon particles. *Archs. oral Biol.*, **14**, 1117-1119.
FITTON-JACKSON, SYLVIA (1956) The morphogenesis of avian tendon. *Proc. R. Soc. London (B)*, **144**, 556-572.
FITTON-JACKSON, SYLVIA (1959) Connective tissue cells. In BRACHET J. & MIRSKY A.E. *The Cell*, Vol. VI, *Biochemistry, Physiology, Morphology*, 387-520. Academic Press, London.
FITZPATRICK T.B. & BREATHNACH A.S. (1963) Das epidermale Melanin—Einhat System. *Derm. Wschr.*, **147**, 481-489.
FITZPATRICK T.B., SZABO G. & MITCHELL R.E. (1965) Age changes in the human melanocyte system. In MONTAGNA W. *Advances in Biology of Skin*, Vol. VI, 35-50. Pergamon Press, Oxford.
FITZPATRICK T.B. & SZABO G. (1959) The melanocyte; cytology and cytochemistry. *J. invest. Derm.*, **32**, 197-209.
FLAXMAN B.A., LUTZNER M.A. & VAN SCOTT E.J. (1968) Ultrastructure of cell attachment to substratum in vitro. *J. Cell Biol.*, **36**, 406-410.
FLEISCHMEYER R. & BILLINGHAM R.E. (eds) (1968) *Epithelial Mesenchymal Interactions.* 18th Hahnemann Symposium. The Williams & Wilkins Company, Baltimore.
FRANK R.M. & CIMASONI G. (1970) The ultrastructure of the normal human gingivo-dental junction. *Z. Zellforsch. mikrosk. Anat.*, **109**, 356-379.
FRANTZELL A., TÖRNQUIST R. & WALDENSTRÖM J. (1945) Examination of the tongue: a clinical and photographic study. *Acta med. Scand.*, **122**, 207-237.
FREEDMAN H.L., LISTGARTEN M.A. & TAICHMAN N. S. (1968) Electron microscopic features of chronically inflamed human gingivae. *J. periodont. Res.*, **3**, 313-327.
FRITHIOF L. (1969) Ultrastructure of the basement membrane in normal and hyperplastic human oral epithelium compared with that in pre-invasive and invasive carcinoma *Acta path. microbiol. Scand.*, Supp. **200**.
FRITHIOF L. (1970) Ultrastructural changes in the plasma membrane in human oral epithelium. *J. Ultrastruct. Res.*, **32**, 1-17.
FRITHIOF L. (1971) Ultrastructural relations between the oral epithelial cell and its environment. Doctoral thesis; Karolinska Institute, Stockholm.
FRITHIOF L. & WERSÄLL J. (1965) A highly ordered structure in keratinizing human oral epithelium. *J. Ultrastruct. Res.*, **12**, 371-379.
FRY L. & ALMEYDA J.R. (1968) The incidence of buccal pigmentation in Caucasoids and Negroids in Britain. *Brit. J. Derm.*, **80**, 244-247.
FRY R.J.M., LESHER S. & KOHN H.I. (1961) Age effect on cell-transit time in mouse jejunal epithelium. *Am. J. Physiol.*, **201**, 213-216.
FUKUYAMA K. & EPSTEIN W.L. (1967) Ultrastructural autoradiographic studies of keratohyalin granule formation. *J. invest. Derm.*, **49**, 595-604.
GARANT P.R. & MULVIHILL J.E. (1971) The ultrastructure of leukocyte emigration through the sulcular epithelium in the beagle dog. *J. periodont. Res.*, **6**, 266-277.

GAVIN J.B. (1970) Ultrastructural features of chronic marginal gingivitis. *J. periodont Res.*, **5**, 19–29.

GERSH I. & CATCHPOLE H.R. (1949) The organisation of ground substance and basement membrane and its significance in tissue injury, disease and growth. *Am. J. Anat.*, **85**, 457–522.

GERSH I. & CATCHPOLE H.R. (1960) The nature of ground substance of connective tissue. *Perspectives Biol. Med.*, **3**, 282–319.

GIACOMETTI L. (1965) The anatomy of the human scalp. In MONTAGNA W. *Advances in Biology of Skin*, Vol. VI, 97–120. Pergamon Press, Oxford.

GIBSON W.A. & SHANNON I.L. (1965) Simulation with carbon particles of bacterial infiltration of human gingival tissue. *Periodontics*, **3**, 57–59.

GILLESPIE G. (1969) Renewal of buccal epithelium. *Oral Surg.*, **27**, 83–89.

GILLETTE R. (1971) On epithelial–mesenchymal interactions, in SQUIER C.A. & MEYER J. *Current Concepts of the Histology of Oral Mucosa*, 203–212. Charles C. Thomas, Springfield, Illinois.

GRANT R.A., HORNE R.W. & COX R.W. (1965) New model for the tropocollagen macromolecule and its mode of aggregation. *Nature, Lond.*, **207**, 822–826.

GREENLEE T.R. JR, ROSS R. & HARTMAN J.L. (1966) The fine structure of elastic fibres. *J. Cell Biol.*, **30**, 59–71.

GREULICH R.C., CAMERON I.L. & THRASHER J.D. (1961) Stimulation of mitosis in adult mice by administration of thymidine. *Proc. nat. Acad. Sci., U.S.A.*, **47**, 743–748.

GROBSTEIN C. (1953) Morphogenetic interaction between embryonic mouse tissues separated by a membrane filter. *Nature, Lond.*, **172**, 869–871.

GROBSTEIN C. & COHEN J. (1965) Collagenase: effect on the morphogenesis of embryonic salivary epithelium in vitro. *Science*, **150**, 626–628.

GROTH O. (1967) Cell proliferation in epidermis during the development of contact reactions as revealed by autoradiography after injection of thymidine-^{3}H. The epithelial cells. *Acta Derm.-vener. (Stockh.)*, **47**, 397–402.

GRUBB C., HACKEMANN M. & HILL K.R. (1968) Small granules and plasma membrane thickening in human cervical squamous epithelium. *J. Ultrastruct. Res.*, **22**, 458–468.

HALPRIN K.M. (1972) Epidermal 'turnover time'—a re-examination. *Brit. J. Derm.*, **86**, 14–19.

HANSEN E.R. (1967a) Mitotic activity in tongue and gingival epithelium of adrenalectomised rats. *Odont. T.*, **75**, 467–472.

HANSEN E.R. (1967b) Mitotic activity and mitotic duration in tongue and gingival epithelium of mice—effects of chalone. *Odont. T.*, **75**, 480–487.

HASHIMOTO K. (1972) Fine structure of Merkel cell in human oral mucosa. *J. invest. Derm.*, **58**, 381–387.

HAY E.D. & REVEL J.P. (1963) Autoradiographic studies of the origin of the basement lamella in Ambystoma. *Dev. Biol.*, **7**, 152–168.

HAYES R.L., SILBERKWEIT M., SONI N.N. & SIMPSON T.H. (1964) Pattern of mitotic activity and cell densities in normal gingival epithelium of children. *J. dent. Res.*, **43**, 217–223.

HAYWARD A.F. & HACKEMANN M. (1973) Electron microscopy of membrane-coating granules and a cell surface coat in keratinized and non-keratinized human oral epithelium. *J. Ultrastruct. Res.*, **43**, 205–219.

HEENEN M. & GALAND P. (1971) Cell population kinetics of human epidermis: *in vitro* autoradiographic study by double labelling method. *J. invest. Derm.*, **56**, 425–429.

HELL E. and HODGSON C. (1966) The uptake of ³H-thymidine by epidermal cells in normal and psoriatic subjects. *Brit. J. Derm.*, **78**, 262–268.

HELL E. and MAIBACH H. (1972) A comparison of *in vivo* and *in vitro* methods of identifying human epidermal cells in DNA synthesis. *Brit. J.Derm.*, **86**, 506–507.

HELLEKANT G. (1972) Circulation of the tongue. In EMMELIN N. & ZOTTERMAN Y. *Oral Physiology:* Proceedings of the International Symposium, Stockholm, 1971, 127–137. Pergamon Press, Oxford.

HENRY J.L., MEYER J., WEINMANN J.P. & SCHOUR I. (1952) Pattern of mitotic activity in oral epithelium in rabbit. *Arch. Path.*, **54**, 281–297.

HODGE A.J. & PETRUSKA J.A. (1962) Some recent results on the electron microscopy of tropocollagen structures. In BREESE S.S. *Electron Microscopy*, Proceedings of the 5th International Congress for Electron Microscopy, Philadelphia QQ-1. Academic Press, New York.

HODGES G.M. (1969) Stromal–epithelial interactions. In MELCHER A.H. & BOWEN W.H. *Biology of the Periodontium*, 27–52. Academic Press, London.

HOFFMAN J.G. (1949) Quantitative aspects of the growth of epidermis. *Arch. Path.*, **47**, 37–43.

HOLTZER H. (1961) Aspects of chondrogenesis and myogenesis. In RUDNIK D. *Synthesis of Molecular and Cellular Structure*, 35–87. Ronald Press Co., New York.

HORI Y., TODA K., PATHAK M., CLARK W.H. & FITZPATRICK T.B. (1968) A fine structure study of the human epidermal melanosome complex and its acid phosphatase activity. *J. Ultrastruct. Res.*, **25**, 109–120.

HUTCHENS L.H., SAGEBIEL R.W. & CLARKE M.A. (1971) Oral epithelial dendritic cells of the rhesus monkey: histologic demonstration, fine structure and quantitative distribution. *J. invest. Derm.*, **56**, 325–336.

HUTTON J.J., TAPPEL A.L. & UDENFRIEND S. (1967) Co-factor and substrate requirements of collagen proline hydroxylase. *Archs. Biochem. Biophys.*, **118**, 231–240.

IGGO A. & MUIR A.R. (1969) The structure and function of a slowly adapting touch corpuscle of hairy skin. *J. Physiol. (Lond.)*, **200**, 763–796.

IQBAL M. & GERSON S.J. (1971) Biochemical features of oral epithelium. In SQUIER C.A. & MEYER J. *Current Concepts of the Histology of Oral Mucosa*, 34–60. Charles C. Thomas, Springfield, Illinois.

IVERSON O.H. (1965) Kinetics of epidermal reaction to carcinogens and other skin irritants. *Advances in Biology of Skin*, Vol. VII. Edited by Montagna W. and DOBSON R. L. Pergamon Press, Oxford.

JACKSON D.S. (1965) Temporal changes in collagen—Ageing or essential maturation. In MONTAGNA W. *Advances in Biology of Skin*, Vol. VI, 219–228. Pergamon Press, Oxford.

JACKSON D.S. (1969) Biological function of collagen in the dermis. In MONTAGNA, BENTLEY & DOBSON. *Advances in the Biology of Skin*, Vol. X, *The Dermis*, 39. Appleton-Century-Crofts, New York.

JESSEN H. (1970) Two types of keratohyalin granules. *J. Ultrastruct. Res.*, **33**, 95–115.

JOHNSON N.W. & HOPPS R.M. (1974) Epithelial cell proliferation in gingiva of macaque monkeys studied by local injections of ^{3}H-Thymidine. *Archs. oral Biol.*, **19**, 265–268.

KAIDBEY K.H. & KURBAN, A.K. (1971) Mitotic behaviour of the buccal mucosal epithelium in psoriasis. *Brit. J. Derm.*, **85**, 162–166.

KANDUTSCH A.A. (1964) Sterol metabolism in skin and epidermis. In MONTAGNA W. & LOBITZ W.C. *The Epidermis*, 493–510. Academic Press, New York.

KALLMAN F., EVANS J. & WESSELLS N.K. (1967) Normal epidermal basal cell behaviour in the absence of basement membrane. *J. Cell Biol.*, **32**, 231–236.

KALLMAN F. & GROBSTEIN C. (1965) Source of collagen at epithelio-mesenchymal interfaces during inductive interaction. *Dev. Biol.*, **11**, 169–183.

KALLMAN F. & GROBSTEIN C. (1966) Localization of glucosamine-incorporating materials at epithelial surfaces during salivary epitheliomesenchymal interaction in vitro. *Dev. Biol.*, **14**, 52–67.

KAPLAN H. (1971) The oral cavity in geriatrics. *Geriatrics*, **26**, 96–102.

KARRING T. & LÖE H. (1970) The three-dimensional concept of the epithelium connective tissue boundary of gingiva. *Acta odont. Scand.*, **28**, 917–933.

KARRING T. & LÖE H. (1972) The reliability of various mitotic index systems in assessing mitotic activity in stratified squamous epithelium. *J. periodont. Res.*, **7**, 271–282.

KARRING T. & LÖE H. (1973) The effect of age on mitotic activity in rat oral epithelium. *J. periodont. Res.*, **8**, 164–170.

KELLER R. (1966) Tissue mast cells in immune reactions. *Monographs in Allergy*, Vol. 2. American Elsevier, New York.

KITTLER G., LAUCKNER H. & MIELER I. (1969) Mitosis coefficient of healthy and inflamed interdental papillae I. *Deutsch Zahn Mund Kieferheilk*, **53**, 10–18.

KITTLER G. & MIELER I. (1969) Mitosis coefficient of healthy and inflamed interdental papillae II. Mitosis coefficient in chronically inflamed interdental papillae. *Deutsch Zahn Mund Kieferheilk*, **53**, 19–27.

KIVIRIKKO K.I. & PROCKOP D.J. (1967) Partial characterization of protocollagen from embryonic cartilage. *Biochem. J.*, **102**, 432–442.

KNAPP M.J. (1970) Oral tonsils: location, distribution and histology. *Oral Surg.* **29**, 155–161.

KNAPP M.J. (1971) Lingual sebaceous glands and a possible thyroglossal duct. *Oral Surg.* **31**, 70–78.

KOCH W.E. (1967) In vitro differentiation of tooth rudiments of embryonic mice I. Transfilter interaction of embryonic incisor tissues. *J. exp. Zool.*, **165**, 155–170.

KOLLAR E.J. (1972) Histogenic aspects of dermal-epidermal interactions. In SLAVKIN H.C. & BAVETTA L.A. *Developmental Aspects of Oral Biology*, Chap. 7, 125–149. Academic Press, New York.

KONDO Y. (1969) Macrophages containing Langerhans cell granules in normal lymph nodes of the rabbit. *Z. Zellforsch*, **98**, 506–511.

KONRAD K. & HÖNIGSMANN H. (1973) Ultrastructural observation of a mitotic Langerhans cell in normal human epidermis. *Arch. Derm. Forsch.*, **246**, 70–76.

KRIKOS G.A. (1971) Dermal–epidermal interactions. *Oral Surg.*, **32**, 744–751.

KURAHASHI Y. & TAKUMA S. (1962) Electron microscopy of human gingival epithelium. *Bull. Tokyo dent. Coll.*, **3**, 29–43.

KUTUZOV H. & SICHER H. (1952) Anatomy and function of the palate in the white rat. *Anat. Rec.*, **114**, 67–84.

LACHAPELLE J.M. (1969) Isotopic labelling of cutaneous structures. A preliminary comparison of local *in vivo* and *in vitro* techniques applied to healthy and pathological human skin. *Brit. J. Derm.*, **81**, 299–305.

LANGERHANS P. (1868) Ueber die Nerven der menschlichen Haut. *Virchows Arch. Path. Anat. Physiol.*, **44**, 325–337.

LEE M.M.C. (1957) Physical and structural age changes in human skin. *Anat. Rec.*, **129**, 473–494.

LESHER S., FRY R.J.M. & KOHN H.I. (1961a) Age and the generation time of the mouse duodenal epithelial cell. *Exp. Cell Res.*, **24**, 334–343.

LESHER S., FRY R.J.M. & KOHN H.I. (1961b) Influence of age on transit time of cells of mouse intestinal epithelium. *Lab. Invest.*, **10**, 291–300.

LIEBOW A.A. (1963) Situations which lead to changes in vascular patterns. In HAMILTON W.F. *Handbook of Physiology*, Vol. 2, 1251–1276. American Physiological Society, Washington, D.C.

LIN P.S., COOPER A.G. & WORTIS H.H. (1973) Scanning electron microscopy of human T-cell and B-cell rosettes. *New Engl. J. Med.*, **289**, 548–551.

LISTGARTEN M.A. (1972) Normal development, structure, physiology and repair of gingival epithelium. *Oral Sci. Rev.*, **1**, 3–67.

LÖE H. & KARRING T. (1969) A quantitative analysis of the epithelium–connective tissue interface in relation to assessments of the mitotic index. *J. dent. Res.*, **48**, 634–640.

LÖE H. & KARRING T. (1971) The three-dimensional morphology of the epithelium–connective tissue interface of the gingiva as related to age and sex. *Scand. J. Dent. Res.*, **79**, 315–326.

LÖE H., KARRING T. & HARA K. (1972) The site of mitotic activity in rat and human oral epithelium. *Scand. J. dent. Res.*, **80**, 111–119.

MCCARTHY P.L. & SHKLAR G. (1964) *Diseases of the Oral Mucosa*, 228. McGraw-Hill, New York.

MCDONALD D.G. (1971) In SQUIER C.A. & MEYER J. *Current Concepts of the Histology of Oral Mucosa*, 61–79. Charles C. Thomas, Springfield, Illinois.

MCDOUGALL W.A. (1970) Pathways of penetration and effects of horseradish peroxidase in rat molar gingiva. *Archs. oral Biol.*, **15**, 621–633.

MCDOUGALL W.A. (1971) Penetration pathways of a topically applied foreign protein into rat gingiva. *J. periodont. Res.*, **6**, 89–99.

MCHUGH W.D. & ZANDER H.A. (1965) Cell division in the periodontium of developing and erupted teeth. *Dent. Pract.*, **15**, 451–457.

MCLOUGHLIN C.B. (1961a) The importance of mesenchymal factors in the differentiation of chick epidermis II. Modifications of epidermal differentiation by contact with different types of mesenchyme. *J. Embryol. Exp. Morph.*, **9**, 385–409.

MCLOUGHLIN C.B. (1961b) The importance of mesenchymal factors in the differentiation of chick epidermis I. The differentiation in culture of isolated epidermis of the embryonic chick and its response to excess vitamin A. *J. Embryol. Exp. Morph.*, **9**, 370–384.

MACKENZIE I.C. (1969) Ordered structure of the stratum corneum of mammalian skin. *Nature, Lond.*, **222**, 881–882.

MACKENZIE I.C. (1970) Relationship between mitosis and the ordered structure of the stratum corneum in mouse epidermis. *Nature, Lond.*, **226**, 653–655.
MACKENZIE I.C. (1973a) The ordered structure of mammalian skin In MAIBACH H.I. & ROVEE D.T. *Epidermal Wound Healing*. Year Book Medical Publishers Inc., Chicago.
MACKENZIE I.C. (1973b) Langerhans cell population kinetics. *I.A.D.R. Abstracts (North American Division)*, No. 359.
MACKENZIE I.C. & MILES A.E.W. (1973) The effect of chronic frictional stimulation on hamster cheek pouch epithelium. *Archs. oral Biol.*, **18**, 1341–1349.
MACKENZIE I.C. & STRIEF J. (1973) Relationship of Langerhans cells to ordered epithelial structure. *I.A.D.R. Abstracts (North American Division)*, No. 358.
MAIN, D.M. & RITCHIE G.M. (1967) Cyclic changes in oral smears from young menstruating women. *Brit. J. Derm.*, **79**, 20–30.
MALKINSON F.D. (1964) Permeability of the stratum corneum. In MONTAGNA W. & LOBITZ W.C. *The Epidermis*, 435–452. Academic Press, New York.
MARSLAND E.A. & FOX E.C. (1958) Some abnormalities in the nerve supply of the oral mucosa. *Proc. R. Soc. Med.*, **51**, 951–956.
MARTINEZ I.R. & PETERS A. (1971) Membrane-coating granules and membrane modifications in keratinizing epithelia. *Am. J. Anat.*, **130**, 93–120.
MARWAH A.S., WEINMANN J.P. & MEYER J. (1960) Effect of chronic inflammation on the epithelial turnover of the human gingiva. *Arch. Path.*, **69**, 147–153.
MASSON P. (1948) Pigment cells in man. In MINER W. *The Biology of Melanomas*, 28. Spec. Publications N.Y. Acad. Sci., IV, New York.
MATOLTSY A.G. & PARAKKAL P.F. (1967) Keratinization. In ZELICKSON A.S. *Ultrastructure of Normal and Abnormal Skin*, 76–104. Lea & Febiger, Philadelphia.
MATOLTSY A.G. & MATOLTSY M.N. (1972) The amorphous component of keratohyalin granules. *J. Ultrastruct. Res.*, **41**, 550–560.
MELCHER A.H. (1965) The nature of the 'Basement Membrane' in human gingiva. *Archs. oral Biol.*, **10**, 785–792.
MELCHER A.H. (1966) Gingival reticulin: Identification and role in histogenesis of collagen fibers. *J. dent. Res.*, **45**, 426–439.
MELCHER A.H. & EASTOE J.E. (1969). The connective tissue of the periodontium. Chapter 6 in MELCHER A.H. & BOWEN W.H. *Biology of the Periodontium*. Academic Press, London and New York.
MERCER E.H. (1964) Protein synthesis and epidermal differentiation. In MONTAGNA W. & LOBITZ W.C. *The Epidermis*. Academic Press, New York.
MEYER J., DAFTARY D.K. & PINDBORG J.J. (1967) Studies in oral leukoplakias XI. Histopathology of leukoplakias in Indians chewing 'pan' with tobacco. *Acta odont. Scand.*, **25**, 397–435.
MEYER J. & GERSON S.J. (1964) A comparison of human palatal and buccal mucosa. *Periodontics*, **2**, 284–291.
MEYER J., MARWAH A.S. & WEINMANN J.P. (1956) Mitotic rate of gingival epithelium in two age groups. *J. invest. Derm.*, **27**, 237–247.
MEYER J., MEDAK H. & WEINMANN J.P. (1960) Mitotic activity and rates of growth in regions of oral epithelium differing in width. *Growth*, **24**, 29–46.
MIDGELY A.R. & PIERCE G.B. JR. (1963) Immunohistochemical analysis of basement membranes of the mouse. *Am. J. Path.*, **43**, 929–943.

MILES A.E.W. (1958) Sebaceous glands in the lip and cheek mucosa of man. *Brit. dent. J.*, **105**, 235–248.
MILES A.E.W. (1960) A hair follicle in human cheek mucosa. *Proc. R. Soc. Med.*, **53**, 527–528.
MILES A.E.W. (1961) Ageing in the teeth and oral tissues. In BOURNE G.H. *Structural Aspects of Ageing*, 351–397. Pitman, London.
MILES A.E.W. (1963) Sebaceous glands in oral and lip mucosa. In MONTAGNA W., ELLIS R.A. & SILVER A.F. *Advances in Biology of Skin*, Vol. IV, 1–32. Pergamon Press, Oxford.
MILES A.E.W. (1972) 'Sans Teeth': Changes in the oral tissues with advancing age. *Proc. R. Soc. Med.*, **65**, 801–806.
MILLER S., STAHL J. & SOBERMAN A. (1952) A study of the cornification of the oral mucosa in normal males. *J. dent. Med.*, **7**, 35–39.
MONTAGNA W. (1963) The sebaceous glands in man. In MONTAGNA W., ELLIS R.A. & SILVER A.F. *Advances in Biology of Skin*, Vol IV, 19–31, Pergamon Press, Oxford.
MONTAGNA W. (1965) Morphology of the ageing skin: The cutaneous appendages. In MONTAGNA W. *Advances in Biology of Skin*, Vol. VI, 1–16. Pergamon Press, Oxford.
MONTANDON D., GABBIANI G., RYAN G.B. & MAJNO G. (1973) The contractile fibroblast. *Plastic and Reconstructive Surgery*, **52**, 286–290.
MONTGOMERY P.W. (1951) A study of exfoliative cytology of normal human oral mucosa. *J. dent. Res.*, **30**, 12–18.
MOTTAZ J.H., THORNE E.G. & ZELICKSON A.S. (1971) Lysosomes in keratinocytes after tape stripping. *Acta Derm.-vener. (Stockh.)*, **51**, 335–339.
MOTTAZ J.H. & ZELICKSON A.S. (1967) Melanin transfer: a possible phagocytic process. *J. invest. Derm.*, **49**, 605–610.
MOTTAZ J.H. & ZELICKSON A.S. (1970) The phagocytic nature of the keratinocyte in human epidermis after tape stripping. *J. invest. Derm.*, **54**, 272–278.
MUKERJEE H., SRI RAM J. & PIERCE C.B. (1965) Basement membranes V. Chemical composition of neoplastic basement membrane mucoprotein. *Am. J. Path.*, **46**, 49–51.
NICOLA P DE (1965) The small vessels of the skin and mucous membranes in presenile and senile age. *Bibl. Anat.*, **7**, 498–500.
NICOLL P.A. & CORTESE T.A. (1972) The physiology of skin. *Am. Rev. Physiol.*, **34**, 177–203.
NIKAI H., ROSE G.G. & CATTONI M. (1971) Merkel cell in human and rat gingiva. *Archs. oral Biol.*, **16**, 835–843.
NORDQUIST R.E., OLSON R.L. & EVERETT M.A. (1966) The transport, uptake and storage of ferritin in human epidermis. *Archs Derm.*, **94**, 482–490.
ODLAND G.F. (1958) The fine structure of the interrelationship of cells in the human epidermis. *J. Cell Biol.*, **4**, 529–538.
ODLAND G.F. (1960) A submicroscopic granular component in human epidermis. *J. invest. Derm.*, **34**, 11–15.
OLSON R.L., NORDQUIST I. & EVERETT M.A. (1970) The role of epidermal lysosomes in melanin physiology. *Brit. J. Derm.*, **83**, 189–199.
OSMANSKI C.P. & MEYER J. (1967) Differences in the fine structure of the mucosa of mouse cheek and palate. *J. invest. Derm.*, **53**, 309–317.

OSMANSKI C.P. & MEYER J. (1971) The oral epithelium; summary. In SQUIER C.A. & MEYER J. *Current Concepts of the Histology of Oral Mucosa*, 167–170. Charles C. Thomas, Springfield, Illinois.

OWINGS J.R. (1969) A clinical investigation of the relationship between stippling and surface keratinization of the attached gingiva. *J. Periodont.*, **40**, 588–592.

PALADE G.E. & FARQUHAR M.G. (1965) A special fibril of the dermis. *J. Cell Biol.*, **27**, 215–222.

PAPA C.M. & KLIGMAN A.M. (1965) The effect of topical steroids on the aged human axilla. In MONTAGNA W. *Advances in Biology of Skin*, Vol. VI, *Ageing*, 177–198. Pergamon Press, Oxford.

PAPIC M. & GLICKMAN I. (1950) Keratinization of the human gingiva in the menstrual cycle and menopause. *Oral Surg.*, **3**, 504–516.

PARAKKAL P.F. (1967) Transfer of premelanosomes into the keratinizing cells of albino hair follicle. *J. Cell Biol.*, **35**, 473–477.

PATHAK M.A., SINESI S.J. & SZABO G. (1965) The effect of a single does of ultraviolet radiation on epidermal melanocytes. *J. invest. Derm.*, **45**, 520–528.

PEARCE R.H. & GRIMMER B.J. (1972) Age and the chemical constitution of normal human dermis. *J. invest. Derm.*, **58**, 347–361.

PEDREIRA R.A. (1951) A study of the keratinization of the oral mucosa of aged males. *J. dent. Med.*, **6**, 88–91.

PENNEYS N.S., FULTON J.E., WEINSTEIN G.D. & FROST P. (1970) Location of proliferating cells in human epidermis. *Archs Derm.* **101**, 323–327.

PIERCE G.B. JR (1966) The development of basement membranes of the mouse embryo. *Dev. Biol.*, **13**, 231–249.

PIERCE G.B. (1971) The origin of basement membrane. In MONTAGNA W., BENTLEY J.P. & DOBSEN R.L. *Advances in Biology of Skin*, Vol. X, *The Dermis*, 173–194. Appleton-Century-Crofts, New York.

PIERCE G.B., MIDGELY A.R. JR, SRI RAM R. & FELMAN J.D. (1962) Parietal yolk sac carcinoma: clue to the histogenesis of Reichert's membrane of the mouse embryo. *Am. J. Path.*, **41**, 549–566.

PIERCE G.B. JR, MIDGELY A.R. JR & SRI RAM J. (1963) The histogenesis of basement membranes. *J. exp. Med.*, **117**, 339–348.

PINKUS H. (1965) Personal communication cited in Epstein and Maibach.

PLENK H. & RAAB H. (1969) The nerves of the human gingiva. *Z. Mikr. Anat. Forsch.*, **81**, 153–181.

PLEWIG G. (1971) Size, form and structural arrangement of mucous membrane cells. *Arch. Derm. Forsch.*, **242**, 30–42.

POCHI P.E. & STRAUSS J.S. (1965) The effect of ageing on the activity of sebaceous gland in man. In MONTAGNA W. *Advances in Biology of Skin*, Vol. VI, *Ageing*, 121–128. Pergamon Press, Oxford.

POHTO P. & ANTILA R. (1969) Histamine-storing cells in oral tissues. *Acta odont Scand.*, **27**, 519–537.

POLLIACK A., LAMPEN N., CLARKSON B.D. & DE HARVEN E. (1973) Identification of human B and T lymphocytes by scanning electron microscopy. *J. exp. Med.*, **138**, 607–624.

PROVENZA D. (1964) *Oral Histology*, 186. Pitman Medical Publishing Co. Ltd, London.

RACHMANDRAN G.N. & KARTHA G. (1954) Structure of collagen. *Nature, Lond.* **174,** 269–270.
RACHMANDRAN G.N. & KARTHA G. (1955) Structure of collagen. *Nature, Lond.,* **176,** 593–595.
RAMBOURG A. & LEBLOND C.P. (1967) Staining of basement membranes and associated structures by the periodic acid–Schiff and periodic acid–silver methenamine techniques. *J. Ultrastruct. Res.,* **20,** 306–309.
RASMUSSEN D.M., WAKEIN K.G. & WINKELMANN R.K. (1965) Effect of ageing on human dermis: Studies of thermal shrinkage and tension. In MONTAGNA W. *Advances in Biology of Skin,* Vol. VI, 151–162. Pergamon Press, Oxford.
RICHMAN M.J. & ABARBANEL A.R. (1943) Effect of estradiol and diethylstilbestrol upon the atrophic human buccal mucosa with a preliminary report on the use of estrogens in the management of senile gingivitis. *J. Clin. Endocrin.,* **3,** 224–226.
RILEY P.A. (1965) Studies of melanocyte function. Ph.D Thesis, University of London.
ROBB-SMITH A.H.T. (1958) In STAINSBY G. *Recent Advances in Gelatin and Glue Research,* 38–44. Pergamon Press, London.
ROBINSON L.P. & DE MARCO T.J. (1972) Alteration of *mast cell* densities in experimentally inflamed human gingiva. *J. Periodont.,* **43,** 614–622.
ROSENBERG H.M. & MASSLER M. (1967) Gingival stippling in young adult males. *J. Periodont.,* **38,** 473–480.
ROTHBERG S., CROUNSE R.G. and LEE J.L. (1961) Glycine C^{14} incorporation into the proteins of normal stratum corneum and the abnormal stratum corneum of psoriasis. *J. Invest. Derm.,* **37,** 497–505.
ROWE L. & DIXON W.J. (1972) Clustering and control of mitotic activity in human epidermis. *J. invest. Derm.,* **58,** 16–23.
RUBINSTEIN A., MEDAK H. & MEYER J. (1970) Early effects of smoking on surface cytology of the oral mucosa I. Regional differences in surface cytology of smokers and non-smokers. *Oral Surg.,* **30,** 131–141.
RYAN T.J. (1973) Structure, pattern and shape of the blood vessels of the skin. In JARRETT A. *The Physiology and Pathophysiology of the Skin,* Vol. 2, 577–651. Academic Press, London.
SAGEBIEL R.W., CLARKE M.A. & HUTCHENS L.H. (1971) Dendritic cells in oral epithelium. In SQUIER C.A. & MEYER J. *Current Concepts of the Histology of Oral Mucosa,* 143–166. Charles C. Thomas, Springfield, Illinois.
SAGEBIEL R.W. & REED T.H. (1968) Serial reconstruction of the characteristic granule of the Langerhans cell. *J. Cell Biol.,* **36,** 595–602.
SAMS W.M. & SMITH J.G. (1965) Alterations in human dermal fibrous connective tissue with age and chronic sun damage. In MONTAGNA W. *Advances in Biology of Skin,* Vol. VI, 199–210. Pergamon Press, Oxford.
SCALETTA L.J. & SIMMELINK J.W. (1973) Scanning electron microscopy of the epithelial connective tissue interface. *I.A.D.R. Abstracts (North American Division),* No. 353.
SCAPINO R.P. (1967) Biomechanics of prehensile oral mucosa. *J. Morph.,* **122,** 89–114.
SCAPINO R.P. (1971) Biomechanics of masticatory and lining mucosa. In SQUIER C.A. & MEYER J. *Current Concepts of the Histology of Oral Mucosa,* 181–202, Charles C. Thomas, Springfield, Illinois.

SCHEUPLEIN R.J. & BLANK I.H. (1971) Permeability of the skin. *Physiol. Rev.*, **51**, 702–747.
SCHREINER E. & WOLFF K. (1969) Die-Permeabilitat des epidermalen Intercellularraums für kleinmolekulares Protein. *Arch. Klin. exp. Derm.*, **235**, 78–88.
SCHROEDER H.E. (1969) Melanin containing organelles in cells of the human gingiva. *J. periodont. Res.*, **4**, 1–18.
SCHROEDER H.E. (1970) Quantitative parameters of early human gingival inflammation. *Archs. oral Biol.*, **15**, 383–400.
SCHROEDER H.E. (1973) Transmigration and infiltration of leucocytes in human junctional epithelium. *Helv. Odont. Acta*, **17**, 6–18.
SCHROEDER H.E. & LISTGARTEN M.A. (1971) *Fine Structure of the Developing Attachment of Human Teeth.* S. Karger, Basel.
SCHROEDER H.E., MÜNZEL-PEDRAZZOLI S. & PAGE R. (1973) Correlated morphometric and biochemical analysis of gingival tissue in early chronic gingivitis in man. *Archs. oral Biol.*, **18**, 899–923.
SCHROEDER H. E. & THEILADE J. (1966) Electron microscopy of normal human gingival epithelium. *J. periodont. Res.*, **1**, 95–119.
SCHWARTZ J., STINSON F.L. & PARKER R.B. (1972) The passage of tritiated bacterial endotoxin across intact gingival crevicular epithelium. *J. Periodont.*, **43**, 270–276.
SELVIG K.A. (1966) Ultrastructural changes in cementum and adjacent connective tissue in periodontal disease. *Acta odont. Scand.*, **24**, 459–500.
SELYE H. (1965) *The Mast Cells.* Butterworths, Washington.
SHAPIRO S., ULMANSKY M. & SCHEUER M. (1969) Mast cell population in gingiva affected by chronic destructive periodontal disease. *J. Periodont.*, **40**, 276–278.
SHARAV Y. & MASSLER M. (1967) Age changes in oral epithelia. *Exp. Cell Res.*, **47**, 132–138.
SHKLAR G. (1966) The effects of ageing upon oral mucosa. *J. invest. Derm.*, **47**, 115–120.
SICHER H. & BHASKER S.N. (1972) *Orban's Oral Histology and Embryology*, 7th edition, 244. Mosby, St Louis, Missouri.
SICHER H. & DU BRUL E.L. (1970) *Oral Anatomy*, 5th edition.
SIEGEL I.A., HALL S.H. & STAMBAUGH R. (1971) Permeability of the oral mucosa. In SQUIER C.A. & MEYER J. *Current Concepts of the Histology of Oral Mucosa*, 274–286. Charles C. Thomas, Springfield, Illinois.
SILBERBERG I. (1973) Apposition of mononuclear cells to Langerhans cells in contact allergic reactions. *Acta. Derm.-vener. (Stockh.)*, **53**, 1–12.
SILVERMAN S. (1971) Non-keratinization and keratinization; the extremes of the human range. In SQUIER C.A. & MEYER J. *Current Concepts of the Histology of Oral Mucosa*, 30–96. Charles C. Thomas, Springfield, Illinois.
SILVERMAN S., BARBOSA J. & KEARNS G. (1971) Ultrastructural and histochemical localization of glycogen in human normal and hyperkeratotic oral epithelium. *Archs. oral Biol.*, **16**, 423–434.
SKOUGAARD M. (1965) Turnover of gingival epithelium in Marmosets. *Acta odont. Scand.*, **23**, 623–643.
SKOUGAARD M. (1970) Cell renewal with special reference to the gingival epithelium. *Advances Oral Biol.*, **4**, 261–288.

SLAVKIN H.C., FLORES P., BRINGAS P. & BAVETTA L.A. (1970) Epithelial–mesenchymal interactions during odontogenesis. I. Isolation of several intercellular matrix low molecular weight methylated RNAs. *Dev. Biol.*, **23**, 276–296.
SOBEL H. & MARMORSTON J. (1956) The possible role of the gel–fibre ratio of connective tissue in the ageing process. *J. Geront.*, **11**, 2–7.
SONI N., SILBERKWEIT M., STRICKER E. & SALAMAT K. (1967) Mitotic activity in human gingival epithelium associated with dilantin sodium therapy. *Periodontics*, **5**, 70–72.
SORENSON F.M., BENNETT J.S., FUJITA D., POINDEXTER, F.R. & HALL W.B. (1970) Photoelectric method for quantitative evaluation of mast cell associated enzyme activity in human gingival tissues. *J. dent. Res.*, **49**, 480–486.
SPEARMAN R.I.C. (1972) The epidermal stratum corneum of the whale. *J. Anat.*, **113**, 373–381.
SPECTOR W.G. (1969) The granulamatous inflammatory exudate. *Int. Rev. Exp. Path.*, **8**, 1–55.
SPIRO R.G. (1967) Studies on the renal glomerular basement membrane. Preparation and chemical composition. *J. biol. Chem.*, **242**, 1915–1922.
SPRUIT D. (1970) The water-barrier of stripped and normal skin. *Dermatologica*, **141**, 54–59.
SQUIER C.A. & WATERHOUSE J.P. (1967) The ultrastructure of the melanocyte in human gingival epithelium. *Archs. oral Biol.*, **12**, 119–129.
SQUIER C.A. (1968) Ultrastructural observations on the keratinization process in rat buccal epithelium. *Archs. oral Biol.*, **13**, 1445–1451.
SQUIER C.A. (1973) The permeability of keratinized and non-keratinized oral epithelium to horseradish peroxidase. *J. Ultrastruct. Res.*, **43**, 160–177.
SUSI F.R., BELT W.D. & KELLY J.W. (1967) Fine structure of fibrillar complexes associated with the basement membrane in human oral mucosa. *J. Cell. Biol.*, **34**, 686–690.
SUSI F.R. (1971) The basal lamina and its fibrils. In SQUIER C.A. & MEYER J. *Current Concepts of the Histology of Oral Mucosa*, 173–180. Charles C. Thomas, Springfield, Illinois.
SUTTON R.L. (1948) Early epidermal neoplasia. *Arch. Derm. Syph.*, **37**, 738–780.
SWIFT J.A. & SAXTON C.A. (1967) The ultrastructural location of the periodate–Schiff reactive basement membrane at the dermo-epidermal junctions of human scalp and monkey gingiva. *J. Ultrastruct. Res.*, **17**, 23–33.
SZABO G. (1954) The number of melanocytes in human epidermis. *Brit. med. J.*, **1**, 1016–1017.
SZABO G. (1967) Photobiology of melanogenesis: cytological aspects with special reference to differences in racial coloration. In MONTAGNA W. & HU F. *Advances in Biology of Skin*, Vol. VIII, 379–396. Pergamon Press, Oxford.
THILAGARATNAM G.N. (1969) Cell cycle characteristic in epithelium of hamster cheek pouch palate (abstract). *I.A.D.R.* (*British Division*) *Abstract*, No. 52. *J. Dent. Res.*, **48**, 1113–1114.
THILANDER H. & BLOOM G.D. (1968) Cell contacts in oral epithelium. *J. periodont. Res.*, **3**, 96–110.
THURINGER J.M. & KATZBERG A.A. (1959) The effect of age on mitosis in the human epidermis. *J. invest. Derm.*, **33**, 35–39.

TIBER A., STAHL S.S. and WEINER J.M. (1972) Histologic and autoradiographic evaluations of long term gingival wound sites in adult rats. *J. Periodont. Res.*, **7**, 266–269.
TOLLER P. (1971) Autoradiography of explants from odontogenic cysts. *Brit. dent. J.*, **131**, 57–61.
TOLO K.J. (1971) A study of permeability of gingival pocket epithelium to albumin in guinea pigs and Norwegian pigs. *Archs. oral Biol.*, **16**, 881–888.
TOLO K.J. (1974) Penetration of human albumin through the oral mucosa of guinea pigs immunised to this protein. *Archs. oral Biol.*, **19**, 259–264.
TOTO P.D. & DHAWAN C.S. (1966) Generation cycle of oral epithelium in 400 day old mice. *J. dent. Res.*, **45**, 948–950.
TROTT J.R. and GORENSTEIN S.L. (1963) Mitotic rates in the oral and gingival epithelium of the rat. *Archs. oral Biol.*, **8**, 425–434.
TROY W.R. (1968) Changes in human skin in the light of current theories of ageing. *J. Soc. Cosmetic Chemists*, **19**, 829–840.
VAN MENS P.R. (1972) Quantitative aspects on exfoliated human palatal cells. Thesis, University of Amsterdam, Amsterdam.
VEIS A., ANESEY J. & MUSSELL S. (1967) A limiting microfibril model for the three-dimensional arrangement within collagen fibres. *Nature, Lond.*, **215**, 931–934.
WASSERMAN H.P. (1971) The colour of human skin. Spectral reflectance versus skin colour. *Dermatologica*, **143**, 166–173.
WATERHOUSE J.P. (1969) Effects of endocrine secretions on the periodontium and related tissues. In MELCHER A. & BOWEN W.H. *Biology of the Periodontium*. Academic Press, London.
WATERHOUSE J.P. & SQUIER C.A. (1967) The Langerhans cell in human gingival epithelium. *Archs. oral Biol.*, **12**, 341–348.
WEDDELL G., COWAN M.A., PALMER E. & RAMASWAMY S. (1965) Psoriatic skin. *Archs Derm.*, **91**, 252–266.
WEINMANN J.P. (1940) The keratinization of the human oral mucosa. *J. dent. Res.*, **19**, 57–71.
WEINMANN J.P. & MEYER J. (1959) Types of keratinization in the human gingiva. *J. invest. Derm.*, **32**, 87–94.
WEINMANN J.P., MEYER J. & MEDAK H. (1960) Correlated differences in granular oral keratinous layers in the oral mucosa of the mouse. *J. invest. Derm.*, **34**, 423–431.
WEINSTEIN G.D. & FROST P. (1971) Methotrexate for psoriasis. A new therapeutic schedule. *Archs Derm.*, **103**, 33–38.
WEINSTOCK M. & WILGRAM G.F. (1970) Fine structural observations of the formation and enzymatic activity of keratinosomes in mouse tongue filiform papillae. *J. Ultrastruct. Res.*, **30**, 262–274.
WEISS M.D., WEINMANN J.P. & MEYER J. (1959) Degree of keratinization and glycogen content in the uninflamed and inflamed gingiva and alveolar mucosa. *J. Periodont.*, **30**, 208–218.
WESSELLS N.K. (1962) Tissue interactions during skin histo-differentiation. *Dev. Biol.*, **4**, 87–107.
WESSELLS N.K. (1964) Substrate and nutrient effects upon epidermal basal cell orientation and proliferation. *Proc. nat. Acad. Sci., U.S.A.*, **52**, 252–259.
WESSELLS N.K. (1970) Some thoughts on embryonic inductions in relation to determination. *J. invest. Derm.*, **55**, 221–225.

WESSELLS N.K. & COHEN J.H. (1966) The influence of collagen and embryo extract on the development of pancreatic epithelium. *Expl. Cell Res.*, **43**, 680–684.
WILGRAM G.F. (1972) A possible role of the Merkel cell in aphthous stomatitis. *Oral Surg.* **34**, 231–238.
WINKELMANN R.K. (1965) Nerve changes in ageing skin. In MONTAGNA W *Advances in Biology of Skin*, Vol. VI, *Ageing*, 51–62. Pergamon Press, Oxford.
WINKELMANN R.K. (1967) Cutaneous Nerves. In ZELICKSON A.S. *Ultrastructure of Normal and Abnormal Skin*, 202–227. Henry Kimpton, London.
WINKELMANN R.K. (1969) The relationship of the structure of the epidermis to percutaneous absorption. *Brit. J. Derm.*, **81**, Suppl. 4, 11–22.
WINKELMANN R.K. & BREATHNACH A.S. (1973) The Merkel cell. *J. invest. Derm.*, **60**, 2–15.
WOLFF K. & HOLUBAR K. (1967) Odland–Körper (membrane-coating granules, keratinosome) als epidermale Lysosomen. *Arch. klin exp. Derm.*, **231**, 1–19.
WOLFF K. & HÖNIGSMANN H. (1971) Permeability of the epidermis and the phagocyte activity of keratinocytes. *J. Ultrastruct. Res.*, **36**, 176–190.
WOLFF K. & HÖNIGSMANN H. (1972) Are melanosome complexes lysosomes? *J. invest. Derm.*, **59**, 170–176.
WOLFF K. & SCHREINER E. (1970) Uptake, intracellular transport and degradation of exogenous protein by Langerhans cells. *J. invest. Derm.*, **54**, 37–47.
WOLFF K. & WINKELMANN R.K. (1967) Nonpigmentary enzymes of the melanocyte–Langerhans cell system. In MONTAGNA W. & HU F. *Advances in Biology of Skin*, Vol. VIII, *The Pigmentary System*, 35–167. Pergamon Press, Oxford.
WOODS D.A. & SMITH C.J. (1969) Ultrastructure of the dermal–epidermal junction in experimentally induced tumours and human oral lesions. *J. invest. Derm.*, **52**, 259–263.
WORLD HEALTH ORGANIZATION TECHNICAL REPORT SERIES NO. 448 (1970) *Factors Regulating the Immune Response.*
YOUNES M.S., STEELE H.D., ROBERTSON E.M. & BENCOSME S.A. (1965) Correlative light and electron microscope study of the basement membrane of the human ectocervix. *Am. J. Obs. Gyn.*, **92**, 163–171
ZACHRISSON B.U. (1968) Mast cells of human gingiva I. *Odont. Rev.*, **19**, 1:1.
ZACHRISSON B.U. (1969) Mast cells of the human gingiva IV. Experimental gingivitis. *J. periodont. Res.*, **4**, 46–55.
ZELICKSON A.S. (1965) The Langerhans cell. *J. invest. Derm.*, **44**, 201.
ZELICKSON A.S. & MOTTAZ J.H. (1968) Epidermal dendritic cells; a quantitative study. *Archs Derm.*, **98**, 652–659.
ZIMMERMANN E.R. & ZIMMERMANN A.L. (1965) Effects of race, age, smoking habits, oral and systemic disease on oral exfoliative cytology. *J. dent. Res.* 627–631.

CHAPTER 2
THE PHYSIOLOGICAL RESPONSIVENESS OF THE ORAL MUCOSA: THE ROLE OF SALIVA

T.W. MACFARLANE AND D.K. MASON

2:0 Introduction

The human mouth is lined with a mucous membrane which consists of a superficial epithelial layer and a deeper connective tissue layer. Although the oral mucous membrane has this basic structure in all parts of the mouth, it is modified in certain regions, according to function. Regional differences in the degree and type of keratinization, the distribution of taste, touch and pain receptors and sebaceous glands (Fordyce Spots) have been discussed in the previous chapter. The oral mucosa is interrupted by teeth if they are present and is closely related to the tooth surface by means of the epithelial attachment. In addition, the mucosal surface is pierced not only by the ducts of the parotid, submandibular and sublingual glands, but also by the numerous small ducts of the accessory salivary glands scattered throughout the oral mucous membrane. A thin film of saliva therefore bathes the surface of the mucosa during waking hours and contained in the salivary layer are polymorphonuclear leukocytes, epithelial squames and the commensal oral microflora. The general environment of the outer layer of the oral mucosa could, therefore, be described as possessing a somewhat rough surface, interrupted by teeth and the orifices of ducts coated with micro-organisms and moistened with saliva. Since this chapter deals with the role of saliva in the physiology of the oral mucosa, much of it will be concerned with the interface of saliva and the epithelial surface rather than with the deeper tissues. Before dealing with the physiology of the oral mucosa, however, it is necessary to consider the source, constitution and control of salivary production.

Chapter 2

2:1 Secretion and Composition

2:1:1 Secretion

Saliva is derived from the secretions of three pairs of large glands, the parotid, submandibular and sublingual, and numerous smaller glands located in the labial, buccal, retromolar, glossopalatine, palatine, tonsillar and lingual areas of the oral submucosa (Orban 1972). The salivary striated duct cells have a similar morphology to those associated with water transport in other parts of the body, e.g. kidney, and there is good evidence that the ducts do not play a passive role, but contribute to the composition of saliva (Henriques 1961, 1962; Tandler 1963; Junqueira 1964; Petersen 1972). It has been shown that water and several electrolytes—calcium, chloride, bicarbonate, sodium and potassium—can be secreted and re-absorbed by the duct epithelium. One well-established physiological action of the duct epithelium is the concentration of iodide and thiocyanate (Cohen *et al* 1955; Stephen *et al* 1973). The nature and mode of action of the factors controlling the physiological action of the duct epithelium is not fully understood. In addition to the salivary secretions themselves, mixed saliva contains a number of non-salivary components derived from gingival exudate, leukocytes, epithelial cells, micro-organisms and occasionally food debris.

2:1:1:a COMPOSITION

Saliva consists of a complex mixture of inorganic and organic substances. The main electrolytes in human saliva are sodium, potassium, calcium, chloride, bicarbonate, inorganic phosphate and thiocyanate with small amounts of fluoride, iodide and magnesium. The differences in the relative proportions of these electrolytes in the major salivary gland secretions have been reviewed by Burgen & Emmelin (1961) and Schneyer & Schneyer (1967).

The main organic constituents of saliva consist of salivary mucoids, amylase, albumen, lysozyme, gamma-globulins and urea with smaller amounts of blood group substances, vitamins, amino acids, ammonia, glucose, lactate, citrate, kallikrein, factors concerned in blood coagulation and various enzymes. In addition, mixed saliva contains variable amounts of organic and inorganic substances derived from gingival exudate, degenerating leukocytes and epithelial cells and the metabolic products of the very complex and varied oral microbial flora. These very variable additions to salivary secretions affect the detailed analysis of salivary components (Ellison 1967).

At the present time there are at least three types of cell capable of contributing to the composition of saliva, namely the serous and mucous acinar cells and the lining cells of the ducts. The parotid glands consist mainly of serous acini, the sublingual glands of mucous acini and the submandibular glands of roughly equal numbers of serous and mucous acini. The minor glands consist of mainly mucous acini. Although the composition of the mucous and serous acinar secretions differ qualitatively and quantitatively, both are concerned with the transportation of electrolytes from serum to saliva and elaborate amylase, and a variety of mucoid substances. Saliva derived from the different groups of salivary glands varies in composition and the relative contribution of each group to mixed saliva may vary considerably. For instance, parotid saliva is relatively low in calcium and high in phosphate as compared with submandibular secretions and most of the salivary amylase is derived from the parotid gland (Dawes 1965). It is interesting to note that the main anion in the labial minor mucous gland secretions of human is chloride and that no amylase and very little bicarbonate or phosphate is found in these secretions (Dawes & Wood 1973). Also the human lip mucous gland secretions have a very low buffering capacity in comparison with that of stimulated secretions from the major salivary glands.

Fordyce Spots

Fordyce Spots are sebaceous glands which are found in significant numbers in the oral mucosa of 60–75% of adults (Miles 1958). The composition of human skin sebum is well characterized but a similar analysis of the sebum of the labial and buccal sebaceous glands is not available, although it is likely that it is similar to that of the skin. Recent analysis of pure sebum from the human skin suggests that squalene, wax, esters and triglycerides are present in unsecreted sebum (Kellman 1967). However, the sterols or sterol esters which are found on the skin surfaces are derived mainly from the keratinizing epidermis, while free fatty acids are released from sebum triglycerides by lipolytic enzymes lining the sebaceous ducts and by lipolytic members of the commensal skin flora.

Miles (1958) suggested that buccal sebaceous glands contribute to both the lipid and cholesterol content of mixed saliva. Thus in those individuals who have significant numbers of Fordyce Spots, sebum must be regarded as a constituent of saliva, although it is not possible to state the extent, function or importance of sebum in such saliva.

2:1:2 Factors affecting composition

The effect of flow rate, duration and type of stimulus, diet, and hormones on the composition of saliva have been reviewed and discussed by Afonsky (1961), Burgen & Emmelin (1961), Jenkins (1966a) and Dawes (1970a). There are a number of important conclusions which can be drawn from the results of work in recent years into the factors which affect the composition of saliva.

Flow rate

Variation in flow rate has a marked effect on the concentration of various components in saliva. In general, as the flow rate of parotid saliva is increased slightly above the unstimulated rate, sodium, bicarbonate and pH increase; whereas potassium, calcium, phosphate, chloride, urea and protein decrease. At higher flow rates, sodium, calcium, chloride, bicarbonate, protein and pH increase; whereas phosphate decreases and potassium shows little further change (Shannon & Prigmore 1960; Dawes 1969). Unstimulated saliva shows significant circadian rhythms with regard to flow rate and in the concentrations of sodium and chloride, but not in the concentrations of protein, potassium, calcium, phosphate and urea (Dawes 1972). The effect of such rhythms on salivary flow rate and composition must influence the concept of normal values. In any study on salivary constituents, therefore, the time of day when sampling is carried out could have an important bearing on the results.

Diet

Dawes (1970a) reviewed the literature dealing with the effects of diet on salivary composition and stressed the difference between the immediate local reflex effect of diet on salivary flow rate, e.g. the relatively high flow rates elicited by highly flavoured diets that require considerable mastication and systemic effects which may take some time to develop. He concluded that there is little evidence that differences in diet can exert systemic effects on salivary flow rate and composition, although high-protein diets increase blood urea which, in turn, tend to maintain relatively high salivary urea levels.

Duration and type of stimulus

Dawes (1969, 1970b) has shown that when the flow rate of stimulated parotid saliva is maintained constantly for several minutes, the composition of saliva changes considerably with the duration of the stimulus. Total protein, calcium, bicarbonate concentrations and pH increase with duration of stimulation, whereas the chloride concentration decreases. In recent studies (Caldwell & Pigman 1966; Dawes 1970c) in which flow rate, duration of stimulation and time of day were standardized, it was found that the nature of the stimulus decidedly influenced the protein concentration of both parotid and submandibular secretions. Other studies have shown that the salivary glands respond differently to electric, pharmacologic and gustatory stimuli (Dische et al 1962; Dawes 1966; Mandel et al 1968).

Hormones

The only established hormonal effect on salivary composition is the lowering of salivary sodium concentration, by injection of adreno-corticotropic hormone or cortisone (Blair-West et al 1967).

Recently, Puskulian (1972), in an investigation into the salivary changes during the normal menstrual cycle, has shown a decrease in the calcium and sodium concentration and an increase in the potassium concentration of submaxillary saliva at the time of ovulation, compared with the time of menstruation. It was suggested that a hormone, probably oestrogen, may be directly or indirectly responsible for the changes in salivary composition.

Size of salivary gland

The most accurate method of expressing salivary flow rate would be ml/min/g of gland, since variation in salivary composition may be due to variation in salivary gland weight. The great difficulty is to weigh the salivary glands. However, Ericson (1971), using a radiographic and statistical method of estimating parotid gland size, has shown that the most important cause of individual differences in the amount of citric-acid-stimulated parotid secretions is individual differences in the size of the parotid glands.

Plasma levels

The salivary concentration of some constituents, for example iodide, calcium and bicarbonate, is dependent on their plasma concentration

(Mason et al 1966). Salivary levels can be interpreted therefore only if the plasma level is known. For example, as the concentration of iodide rises in blood plasma, the concentration of iodide in saliva also rises, but the saliva/plasma iodide ratio remains relatively constant.

2:2 The Physiology of Saliva in Relation to the Oral Mucosa

2:2:1 Mucosubstances

Salivary mucosubstances are responsible for lubricating, physically protecting, waterproofing and mechanically cleansing the oral mucosa. Mucosubstances are complex molecules consisting of protein and polysaccharide components linked together by covalent chemical bonds. The protein component is always a single chain forming, as it were, a central backbone for the molecule. Polysaccharide side chains are attached to the protein backbone and the number and nature of these determine to a great extent the properties of the molecules. Mucosubstances can be divided into glycoproteins and proteoglycans (mucopolysaccharides) on the basis of structural characteristics (Barrett 1971).

Salivary mucins are basically glycoprotein in nature and although the carbohydrate side chains comprise quite a large part of the molecule, they show some properties normally associated with polysaccharides. It is the properties of this group of glycoprotein which give saliva its lubricating properties. Salivary mucus coats foodstuffs with a lubricant layer which assists chewing and swallowing. Similarly the surfaces of the tongue, oral mucosa and teeth have a lubricant coating in order that the complex interactions of these tissues involved in the production of speech can occur. The precise nature and composition of this continuous mucous coat or sheath as it is sometimes termed, is unknown. The mucus in direct contact with the superficial epithelial cells of the oral mucosa is most likely derived from the secretions of the minor salivary glands, whose ducts open on to the mucosal surface. Little is known about the precise biochemical composition of minor gland secretions, although Klinkhammer (1968) has reported that it is isotonic compared with mixed saliva.

Recently, Adams (1973) in an investigation of the relationship of saliva and the surface of the oral mucosa described the development and appearance of a 'fuzzy' coat on the outermost surface of oral epithelial cells. This layer contained mainly acidic mucopolysaccharide, and appeared to consist of two components; the first and innermost being derived from microgranules within the cell, and the outer from salivary mucopolysaccharides and glycoproteins. It has also been shown that the survival rate of Hela cells which are subjected to changes in osmotic pressure is enhanced if the cells are protected by a 'coat' of mixed saliva (Adams 1973). The salivary layer is not stagnant but is constantly renewed by secretions from both minor and major salivary glands. Bloomfield (1921, 1922)

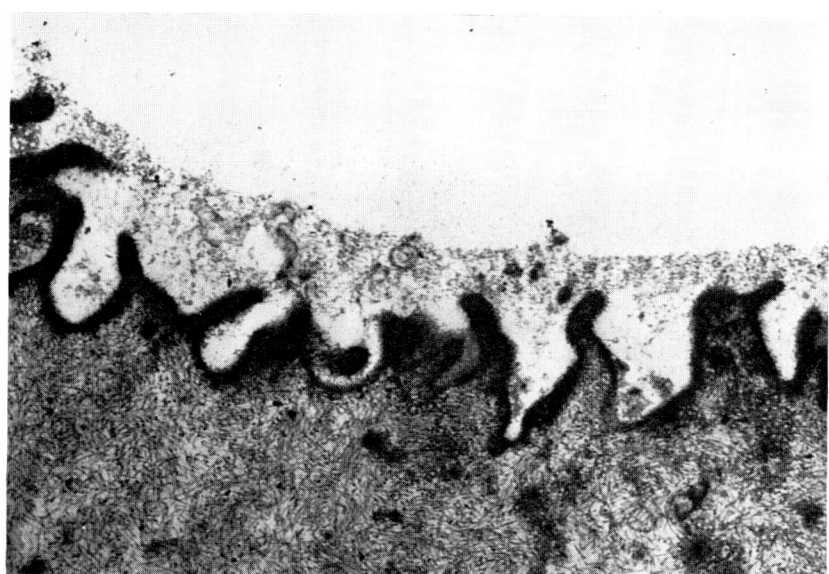

Fig. 2.1. Electron micrograph of human buccal mucosa. This surface cell is covered by 'fuzz' made up of filamentous material attached to the plasma membrane and an outer amorphous component which is probably derived from the saliva. Lead citrate and uranyl acetate. ×30,380. (By kind permission of Dr D. Adams, Senior Lecturer in Oral Biology, The Welsh National School of Medicine, Dental School, Heath, Cardiff.)

has shown that salivary mucus takes a direct and relatively constant course along specific routes towards the oropharynx and is finally swallowed. Micro-organisms and foreign particles are 'trapped' in the mucus and eventually destroyed by the gastric juice. This mechanical washing action is probably an important factor in limiting the microbial population of the mouth and preventing primary infection of the oral mucosa. In addition, it is probable that the layer of salivary mucus protects the underlying mucosa from the harmful effects of noxious chemicals, microbial toxins and minor trauma.

2:2:2 Antibacterial factors

The antibacterial activity of saliva has been investigated by Bibby et al (1938), Van Kestern et al (1942) and Kerr & Wedderburn (1958) and reviewed by Burnett & Scherp (1968) and MacFarlane & Mason (1972). It is generally agreed that human saliva consists of a number of potential antimicrobial components; lysozyme, the antilactobacillus thiocyanate-dependent factors, salivary immunoglobulins, lactoferrin, Green's factor and fluoride. A review of salivary immunoglobulins is given in Chapter 3.

Lysozyme

Salivary lysozyme, first described by Fleming (1922), is derived from a number of sources; from the parotid, submandibular and sublingual glands (Hoerman et al 1965), from the gingival exudate (Brandtzaeg & Mann 1964) and from the lysosomes of the salivary leukocytes. Jolles (1967) has shown that lysozymes from different sources have qualitatively the same biological activity but different primary structures and specific activities. Salivary lysozyme therefore is not homogeneous in nature, but a mixture of different, but closely related substances, and its specific antimicrobial activity is as a result not easily assessed. Inhibition between lysozyme and some constituents of saliva appear to occur *in vivo*, since Hoerman et al (1956) described a mucopolysaccharide present in submandibular–sublingual saliva which selectively inhibited the action of parotid lysozyme. It would appear that lysozyme has little inhibitory effect on the oral commensal flora (Gibbons et al 1966), but appears to play a role in preventing non-commensal bacteria from colonizing the oral cavity.

It is interesting to note, however, that lysozyme combined with complement and colostral IgA, was able to lyse *E. coli* (Adinolfi et al 1966). There is doubt whether this system could function in the mouth due to the anti-complementary nature of saliva, but it is possible that similar interactions may have a protective function in the gingival crevice (see also Chapter 3).

Thiocyanate-dependent factors

It has been suggested by Dogon & Amdur (1970) that two thiocyanate-dependent factors are present in human parotid saliva. The first consists of thiocyanate and an, as yet, unidentified salivary protein component (Dogon & Amdur 1965). The second system consists of a peroxidative enzyme, probably lactoperoxidase, thiocyanate and hydrogen peroxide (Klebanoff & Luebke 1965). These antimicrobial factors are effective only on actively growing micro-organisms, killing them by inhibiting some essential growth factor (Zeldow 1961). Much of the experimental work into the nature and activity of these factors has been carried out using parotid saliva, although antilactobacillus activity has been demonstrated using mixed saliva. The antibacterial activity of Klebanoff's factor *in vivo* is uncertain, since catalase, which is produced by oral micro-organisms and by the cellular activities of the host, is known to inhibit its action. The antibacterial effect of the thiocyanate-dependent factors on lactobacilli has been fully demonstrated, but the effect on the other oral commensal bacteria is unknown. There is some evidence that *E. coli* and perhaps other coliform bacilli are inhibited by thiocyanate-dependent factors (Klebanoff et al 1966).

Green's Factor

The bacteriolytic factor described by Green (1959, 1966) in the saliva of caries-free individuals was believed to be important in protecting them against dental caries. However, there has been no evidence to suggest that the factor had any role to play in the general defence of the oral mucosa. Since Geddes (1972) in a reassessment of Green's work was unable to demonstrate the factor in parotid saliva from caries-free individuals, the importance of Green's Factor is in considerable doubt.

Lactoferrin

Lactoferrin is an iron-binding protein normally present in milk. Masson et al (1966a) described lactoferrin in human saliva, other body fluids and in the lysosomes of polymorphonuclear leukocytes. It has been suggested that the iron-binding properties of this protein are of importance in protecting mucosal surfaces against infection. The precise way in which lactoferrin accomplishes its protective role is unknown. However, iron is essential for bacterial growth and if the host can deny iron to a potentially pathogenic bacterium, infection by that bacterium may be prevented. It is likely, therefore, that due to its strong iron-binding activity, lactoferrin has an important role to play in the host defence to bacterial infection. There is at the moment no experimental work dealing with the antibacterial activity of lactoferrin on the commensal oral flora although it is known that *Staph. aureus* and *P. aeruginosa* are inhibited (Masson et al 1966b).

Hydrogen ion concentration and buffering capacity

The pH of mixed saliva varies widely in any one individual; the normal range is 5·6 to 7·0 with an average value of 6·7. Many factors affect the pH and buffering capacity of saliva, the more important factors being salivary flow rate and the duration of stimulation. Although bicarbonate is the most important buffer in saliva, phosphate probably plays a small part (Lilienthal 1955). The pH and buffering capacity of saliva may protect the oral tissues in two ways. Firstly, since many bacteria require specific pH conditions for maximal growth, saliva may deny such conditions and thereby prevent potential pathogens from colonizing the mouth. It is of interest to note that the carrier rate of *C. albicans* in healthy young adults with a salivary pH 5·0 to 5·5 was 90% compared with a carrier rate of 56% in subjects with a pH of 6·5 to 7·0 (Young *et al* 1951). Secondly it is possible that a relatively steady pH of about 6·7 is necessary for maximal activity of salivary antimicrobial agents and microbial antagonisms.

2:2:3 Permeability

The oral mucosa, like the epidermis, provides a route for the transfer of solutes from the host tissues to the surface and vice versa. Whereas the permeability of the human epidermis has been studied for more than 50 years (Tregear 1966), the corresponding properties of the oral mucosa have received little or no attention. The investigations which have been carried out have concentrated mainly on the inward transport mechanism, owing to the importance of the oral mucosa in the absorption of drugs (Gibaldi & Kanig 1965; Beckett *et al* 1968; Crooks 1964). Many of these reports, however, did not measure directly the rate or amount of penetration of drugs, but rather their speed of action on patients. The outward transport system of water and solutes under physiological conditions has been studied by only a few workers (Kaaber 1971a,b,c), although a number of permeability studies have been carried out in relation to inflamed gingival epithelium (Brill 1962; Egelberg 1967; Tolo 1971). The subject of permeability of the oral mucosa has been reviewed recently by Siegel *et al* (1971).

There are many technical and theoretical difficulties involved in experiments dealing with oral mucosa permeability. The technical problems are mainly due to difficulties in collecting and quantifying the small amounts of material involved in such experiments. The theoretical difficulties are associated with the mathematics involved in calculating the amount of substance crossing a membrane per unit time.

There are at least three general processes by which substances have been shown to cross various epithelial membranes: diffusion, carrier-facilitated transport, and pinocytosis. The available data suggests that most molecules are transported across the oral mucosa by diffusion, although due to the paucity of the data this is by no means definite. In order to pass across a tissue by simple diffusion, a substance must be sufficiently lipid-soluble to dissolve in cell membranes, or be of a sufficiently small size to pass through the cell membrane pores. Other factors which may affect the rate and degree of permeability of a substance are—molecular weight, temperature, hydrogen ion concentration and molecular interactions between substance and host tissues.

Kaaber (1971b,c) has shown that in both human palatal and buccal epithelium, there is a continuous outward loss of water, but no loss of sodium or potassium. When the palate and buccal mucosa were compared, Kaaber found that more water was lost from the cheek than from the palate. There are two probable explanations for this difference in the rate of water loss. One explanation is the presence of an extracellular accumulation of fluid, sodium and potassium in the upper epithelial layers of the buccal epithelium, the other a greater continuous and steady diffusion of fluid through the buccal epithelium compared with the palatal mucosa. These results suggest that the non-cornified buccal epithelium is as effective as the cornified palatal epithelium in preventing the loss of sodium and potassium from the host tissues, but that water is lost more readily from the cheek as compared to the palate. The likely source of the fluid accumulations in the buccal epithelium is from saliva, and it is probably that there exists an equilibrium between the oral epithelium and its salivary coat. The nature and role, if any, that this equilibrium plays in the permeability or protection of the oral mucosa is not clear.

The permeability of the oral mucosa has been investigated by various *in vitro* techniques (Adams 1973). He has shown that the rate of transmission of water through the oral mucous membrane is ten to one hundred times faster than the rate through the skin. Also, transmission is higher through the sublingual mucosa compared with the buccal mucosa. It is interesting to note that both Kaaber (1971c) and Adams (1973), although using *in vivo* and *in vitro* techniques respectively, have published similar values for the transmission rate of water through human buccal oral mucosa. Adams (1973) has also shown that fluorescent dyes did not penetrate the normal keratinized oral mucosa of rabbits and rats and only penetrated non-keratinized mucosa to a limited extent. The effect of both inhibition of salivary flow and the application of mucolytic agents either alone or in combination with one another, however, caused an increase in the penetration of the dye into oral epithelium, presumably due to loss of the superficial salivary glycoprotein component of the mucus barrier.

Since we know very little regarding the mechanics underlying permeability of the oral mucosa, it is very difficult to assess the effectiveness of different areas of the oral mucosa in absorbing or blocking the absorption of any given solute. Although much work has been carried out in relation to the site and nature of the barrier zone in the skin, there is little information concerning the existence of such a zone in the oral mucosa. Bettley (1970) reported that the main barrier to water diffusion in the skin lies in the compact zone of the stratum corneum. Other workers suggested that the whole of the stratum corneum forms the barrier. It seems probable that the barrier zone for different solutes will be found at different sites of the stratum corneum, e.g. some solid or viscous substances may be stopped at the outermost layer of the stratum corneum, whereas smaller molecules may be trapped deeper in the epithelial layer. The work carried out by Kaaber (1971) suggests that the stratum corneum of the keratinized oral mucosa has some significance as a diffusion barrier.

2:2:4 Taste

The literature of taste physiology has been somewhat controversial. It has been reviewed by Jenkins (1966b) and, more recently, by Farbman & Allgood (1971). Only the role of saliva in the physiology of taste and also the influence of taste on salivary flow measurement will be considered here.

When a chemical comes into contact with the antero-dorsal area of the tongue, there are two possible routes by which neural stimulation can occur: (1) chemicals diffusing into taste pores can stimulate the cells of the taste buds and elicit a chorda tympani response, or (2) by penetrating a certain depth of dorsal tongue epithelium, chemicals can reach the free nerve endings of the trigeminal part of the lingual nerve. Due to the relative impermeability of tongue epithelium, however, the latter mechanism is probably rarely effective (Mistretta 1971).

Most workers agree that there are four basic modalities of taste—salt, sweet, sour and bitter—and some include a fifth, the water taste. Although, generally speaking, no specificity has yet been demonstrated in taste buds or in the nerves supplying them, Trefz (1972) has claimed that in the adult rhesus monkey, the taste buds associated with sweet, sour, salt and bitter tastes yield considerable enzymatic differences. He also suggested that on the basis of enzymatic activities, sweet should be grouped with salt, and sour with bitter. This is in agreement with work by Henkin *et al* (1969), who showed that in certain human diseases where taste acuity is diminished, sweet functions with salt and sour with bitter and the two subunits operate quite independently of each other during therapy.

The concentration at which solutions of sodium chloride begin to taste salty to normal human subjects varies with the sodium concentration to which their tongue has just been exposed and, if not deliberately modified, it matches the sodium concentration of mixed saliva (McBurney & Pfaffman 1963). However, the threshold does not depend exclusively on the sodium concentration of saliva; for example, it can fall during forced water intake without change in the saliva (De Wardener & Herxheimer 1957).

It is generally agreed that the sensation of taste is produced only by substances in solution. Foods with a low water content require saliva to dissolve the substances within them which have a taste so that the taste of the particular food can be perceived. In foods with a high water content, however, the requirement of saliva for taste perception is negligible. The work of Catalonotto & Sweeney (1972) is of interest in relation to the importance of saliva in taste acuity. They reported that the taste acuity of surgically desalivated rats was decreased when compared to control animals.

One of the many factors which affect the secretion and flow rate of saliva is taste. A knowledge of the extent to which taste can cause variation in salivary flow rates may be of importance in assessing the salivary gland function of a patient. Ericson (1971), in a multifactorial analysis of the salivary flow rate of the human salivary gland, concluded that individual differences in taste with one and the same stimulus can produce a small but definite stimulus to salivary flow. However, the contribution of taste to the total variance of salivary secretion is small. Speirs (1971), in an investigation of the interactions between gustatory stimuli on the reflex flow rate of human parotid saliva, used mixtures of sweet and sour substances, prepared over a range of concentration such that the taste quality masked, suppressed or enhanced another. The results showed that basically the reflex flow rate of parotid saliva in response to these mixtures was more closely related to the taste intensity than to the overall concentration of the solutions in the mixtures.

It has been shown that tactile stimulation of the oral mucosa, especially the palate, contributes to the flow of saliva elicited by a purely gustatory stimulus (Shannon *et al* 1967; Chauncey *et al* 1967). It has also been demonstrated in subjects wearing plastic mouthguards covering the palate that taste acuity, as measured by parotid salivary secretion, was diminished in response to solid foods probably due to the loss of tactile stimulation (Feller & Shannon 1970).

2:2:5 Blood coagulation

When freshly collected blood is diluted with saliva its clotting time is reduced (Nour-Eldin & Wilkinson 1957). However, saliva also decreases the maximal solidity of a blood clot and, due to the presence of salivary activators, fibrinolysis of the clot starts earlier than in a saliva-free blood clot (Schulte 1970). A practical consequence of these findings for oral wounds healing by organization is that in the initial stages, saliva should be prevented from entering the wound. If saliva enters such wounds, the solidity of the clot is reduced and subsequent clot breakdown is likely.

2:2:6 Comparison with skin

It is of interest and value to compare the conditions occurring on the surface of the skin with those which have been described for the oral mucosa. The skin surface is covered by a thin film of fluid which is derived from the secretions of the apocrine and eccrine sweat glands, the sebaceous glands and from transepidermal permeation from the deeper tissues. The thin film of fluid is composed of the following substances; water, amino acids, urea, uric acid, ammonia, sodium, chloride, potassium, iron, calcium, lactate and lactic acid, glucose, free fatty acids, squalene cholesterol, and various vitamins (Marples 1965a).

The most important single function of the human skin is to act as a two-way barrier, preventing the loss of water, electrolytes, and other body constituents, and barring the entry of noxious or unwanted molecules from the external environment. In addition, contaminating micro-organisms are constantly removed from the surface by desquamation.

The efficiency of the mechanical barrier effect of the skin depends on water, since it is the only known plasticizer of horny material (Blank 1953). If the water content of the corneum drops below 10% the layer becomes brittle, cracks easily and allows potential irritants to penetrate it in increased amounts. Water is supplied to the skin surface by two main routes; by sweat-gland activity and transepidermal permeation from the deeper tissues. The mechanisms concerned with the water content and water loss from the skin tend to produce conditions such that the skin is maintained in a moist condition: that is, neither too dry nor visibly wet. Excessive moisture on the skin is a feature of a number of microbial skin conditions, for example candidosis, and Pillsbury & Kligman (1954) have stressed the importance of dryness in the prevention of secondary infection in dermatological conditions.

The most important function of sweat is thermo-regulation; evaporation of sweat causing heat loss from the body. Sweat also supplies large amounts of lactic acid and lactate to the skin surface. Although fundamentally similar to plasma from which it is derived, sweat is hypotonic and possesses a lower concentration of electrolytes and very little glucose. Sodium and chloride are the main ions of sweat. The electrolytes may have an antibacterial effect, depending on whether the particular micro-organism is inhibited by the concentration of the electrolytes present on the skin surface or not.

There is a wide variation in the pH of the skin surface not only with age and sex but in different areas of one individual (Marples 1965b). On average a pH value of 5·00 is regarded as normal. The low pH value of skin is mainly due to the lactic acid concentration of sweat. In the past some workers attached considerable importance to the destructive effect of skin acidity on various micro-organisms, the so-called 'acid mantle' (Burtenshaw 1945), although later workers have tended to discount this theory.

Several functions have been attributed to sebum but they are by no means undisputed. It has been suggested that a lipid film controls moisture less from the surface of the epidermis, but it is disputable if this film is derived from sebum, or whether the lipid is supplied by the surface epidermal cells themselves (Ebling 1970). It is widely believed that free fatty acids on the skin surface inhibit the growth of pathogenic bacteria and fungi. Sebum contains saturated fatty acids that have antifungal and antibacterial properties, but their practical importance is still uncertain, since Kligman (1963) claims that they are inactivated in the presence of keratin. At the present time desiccation of the skin surface and the antibacterial action of various fatty acids, particularly oleic acid, are believed to be the two main factors concerned in protection of the skin from pathogens (Ricketts *et al* 1951; Naylor 1970).

2:3 Reduced Secretion

2:3:1 Clinical implications

It is generally accepted that the three main ecological components of the mouth are the oral tissues, saliva and the oral microbial flora. Normally, the interactions of these components leads to a clinical state which we describe as health. When one of the components is greatly altered, however, for example virtual cessation of salivary secretion, an abnormal clinical state often results which we call disease. A severe reduction in salivary flow occurs in two main groups of patients, those in whom salivary gland function has been severely reduced by irradiation for carcinoma of the salivary glands, and those with severe Sjögren's syndrome. Frank et al (1965) reported that in the former group the saliva was reduced in volume, viscid with a low pH and an increased total nitrogen content. Many of the patients developed a superficial type of dental caries on areas normally caries-resistant. Patients with severe Sjögren's syndrome also have an increased incidence of dental caries (Bloch et al 1965). The oral mucosa in this condition may also show various abnormalities. The tongue is most commonly involved and clinically may present with a combination of redness, loss of papillae, fissuring and lobulation (Bertram 1967). In some cases, these appearances are accompanied by a painful sensation. Atrophy of other areas of the oral mucosa is also found in patients with xerostomia due to Sjögren's syndrome. Adams (1973) has shown that the salivary component of the mucus barrier protecting the surface of the oral mucosa is missing in patients with Sjögren's syndrome, with the result that the cell-derived component of the mucus barrier is exposed to the oral environment. This abnormality may result not only in areas of stagnation on the oral mucosal surface, but also facilitate proliferation and invasion of the epithelial surface by micro-organisms, especially yeasts. It is interesting to note that patients with Sjögren's syndrome have significantly greater numbers of yeasts, *Staph. aureus* and coliform bacilli compared with normal, healthy controls (MacFarlane & Mason 1973). In addition 70% of patients in the Sjögren's group had a history of candidosis. The clinical implication of these findings is that patients with xerostomia due to Sjögren's syndrome should be kept under regular clinical and microbiological surveillance for recurrence of candidosis. More obvious changes in patients with xerostomia are due to loss of the lubricant properties of saliva. Moistening of food for bolus formation and subsequent swallowing becomes very difficult and clarity of speech is also affected. In addition, the sensation of taste may be greatly reduced.

There is no doubt that saliva is necessary for the health of the oral mucosa. Some of the protective mechanisms are self-evident, e.g. lubrication and mechanical washing action, while others, especially those concerned with the epithelial salivary interface, appear more complex.

2:3:2 Tests for functional activity

Salivary flow rate estimation refers to the quantitative measurement of salivary secretion. Whole or mixed saliva can be measured, but removal of saliva from the mouth to a measuring tube or vessel involves suction (Bertram 1967), drainage or spitting (Kerr 1961), and the reproducibility of these methods is doubtful. Most workers have measured the flow of separated gland secretions. For the major salivary glands the technique employs a modified Carlson Crittenden cup which is held in place over the main duct orifice by air suction. Collecting devices are available for both parotid and submandibular secretions. Saliva is collected into graduated measuring tubes and the most reliable results are obtained under conditions of stimulation using a sialagogue such as 5% citric acid solution or pilocarpine. Various tests and normal ranges for salivary flow rates have been described by different workers (Curry & Patey 1964; Bloch et al 1965; Mason 1966; Bertram 1967; Ericson 1969; Chisholm 1970). Many factors, however, including the time of day, age and sex of the subject, the effects of various commonly prescribed drugs and local or systemic disease, influence salivary flow rates and the values obtained must be interpreted against this background.

Sialography refers to the introduction of a radio-opaque contrast medium to the salivary duct system. The medium is allowed to flow or is injected into the duct and a radiograph—the filling phase film—is taken. The subject is then given a piece of lemon to suck in order to stimulate salivary secretion, and this should rapidly expel the medium from the duct system. A second radiograph—the secretory phase film—is then taken and normally no retention of medium will be observed.

Biopsy is a valuable diagnostic procedure which often gives an indication of the nature of a disease process affecting the glands as well as some information about salivary gland function in a small area. With regard to the major salivary glands care must be taken to avoid damage to important neurovascular anatomical structures and minimize the risk of fistula formation. For these reasons, biopsy of the major glands is limited generally to the situation where neoplasia is suspected. However, in a number of disease processes where the salivary glands are affected generally, e.g. Sjögren's syndrome or sarcoidosis, then biopsy of the intra-oral minor salivary glands may be of great value (Chapter 10).

Scintiscanning and scintigraphy of the salivary glands are promising new investigative techniques. They require to be more fully evaluated, however, as tests of salivary gland function in disease states. However, they have the great advantage of examining the major salivary glands at the same time. The technique takes advantage of the fact that the major and minor salivary glands, like the thyroid gland, concentrate iodide to many times the plasma level. An artificial isotope such as ^{99m}Te pertechnetate, which has similar properties to iodide but gives a very low radiation dosage to the patient, is injected intravenously. The detecting head of the scanner (scintiscanner), or the gamma camera (scintigraphy), picks up the radioactive emissions from the head and neck region of the subject and translates them to a colour print-out or photograph of the salivary glands.

Variations in concentration of salivary constituents in disease states such as fibrocystic disease (Saggers *et al* 1967), disorders of adrenal and thyroid glands (Mason *et al* 1966; Mandel 1967; Chisholm *et al* 1973), have also been reported and it is probable that collection of saliva for analysis will become more common in clinical diagnosis in the future.

2:4 References

ADAMS D. (1973) Saliva, the mucus barrier and the health of the oral mucosa. PhD. Thesis, University of Wales.

ADINOLFI M., GLYNN A.A., LINDSAY M. & MILNE C.M. (1966) Serological properties of gamma A antibodies to *E. coli* present in human colostrum. *Immunol.*, **10,** 515.

AFONSKY D. (1961) *Saliva and its Relation to Oral Health*. University of Alabama Press, Birmingham.

BARRETT A. J. (1971). The biochemistry and function of mucosubstances. *Histochem. J.*, **3,** 213.

BECKETT A.H., BOYES R.N. & TRIGGS E.J. (1968) Kinetics of buccal absorption of amphetamines. *J. Pharm. Pharmacol.*, **20,** 92.

BERTRAM U. (1967) Xerostomia. *Acta odont. Scand.*, **25,** Suppl. 49.

BETTLEY F.R. (1970) The epidermal barrier and percutaneous absorption. In CHAMPION R.H., GILLMAN T., ROOK A.J. & SIMS R.T. *An Introduction to the Biology of the Skin*, 342–354. Blackwell Scientific Publication, Oxford.

BIBBY B.G., HINE M.K. & CLOUGH O.W. (1938) The antibacterial action of human saliva. *J. Am. dent. Ass.*, **25,** 1290.

BLAIR-WEST J.R., COGHAM J.P., DENTON D.A. & WRIGHT R.D. (1967) Effect of endocrines on salivary glands. In CODE C.F. *Handbook of Physiology*, Section 6, Alimentary Canal, Vol. II, *Secretion*, 639–640. American Physiology Society, Washington D.C.

BLANK I.H. (1953) Further observations on factors which influence the water content of the stratum corneum. *J. invest. Derm.*, **21,** 259.

BLOCH K.J., BUCHANAN W.W., WOHL M.J. & BUNIM J.J. (1965) Sjögren's syndrome. *Medicine (Baltimore)*, **44,** 187.

BLOOMFIELD A.L. (1921) Dissemination of bacteria in the upper air passages. 1. The circulation of foreign particles in the mouth. *Am. Rev. Tuberc.*, **5**, 903.
BLOOMFIELD A.L. (1922) Dissemination of bacteria in the upper air passages. II. The circulation of bacteria in the mouth. *Johns Hopk. Hosp. Bull.*, **33**, 145.
BRANDTZAEG P. & MANN W.V. (1964) A comparative study of the lysozyme activity of human gingival pocket fluid, serum and saliva. *Acta odont. Scand.*, **22**, 441.
BRILL N. (1962) The gingival pocket fluid. *Acta odont. Scand.*, **20**, Suppl. 32.
BURGEN A.S.V. & EMMELIN N.G. (1961) *Physiology of the Salivary Glands*, 140–194. Edward Arnold, London.
BURNETT G.W. & SCHERP H.W. (1968) *Oral Microbiology and Infectious Disease*, 3rd edition, 309–324. Williams & Wilkins Co., Baltimore.
BURTENSHAW J.M.L. (1945) Self-disinfection of the skin: a short review and some original observations. *Brit. med. Bull.*, **3**, 731.
CALDWELL R.C. & PIGMAN W. (1966) Changes in protein and glycoprotein concentrations in human submaxillary saliva under various stimulatory conditions. *Archs. oral Biol.*, **11**, 437.
CATALANOTTO F.A. & SWEENEY E.A. (1972) The effects of surgical desalivation of the rat upon taste acuity. *Archs. oral Biol.*, **17**, 1455.
CHAUNCEY H.H., SHANNON I.L. & FELLOW R.P. (1967) Effect of oral and nasal chemoreception on parotid gland secretions. In SCHNEYER L.H. & SCHNEYER C.A. *Secretory Mechanisms of the Salivary Glands*, 351. Academic Press, New York.
CHISHOLM D.M. (1970) The salivary glands in connective tissue disease. Ph.D. Thesis, University of Glasgow.
CHISHOLM D.M., BEELEY J.A. & MASON D.K. (1973) Salivary proteins in Sjögren's syndrome: separation by isoelectric focusing in acrylamide gels. *Oral Surg.*, **35**, 620.
CHISHOLM D.M., BLAIR G.S., LOW P.S. & WHALEY K. (1971) Hydrostatic sialography as an index of salivary gland disease in Sjögren's syndrome. *Acta radiol. (Stockh.)*, **11**, 577.
COHEN B., LOGOTHETOPOULOS J.H. & MYANT N.B. (1955) Autoradiographic localisation of iodine-131 in the salivary glands of the hamster. *Nature, Lond.*, **176**, 1268.
CROOKS J. (1964) Ergotamine tartarate in migraine. *Practitioner*, **193**, 228.
CURRY R.C. & PATEY D.H. (1964) A clinical test for parotid function. *Brit. J. Surg.*, **51**, 891.
DAWES C. (1965) Some characteristics of parotid and submandibular salivary proteins. *Archs. oral. Biol.*, **10**, 269.
DAWES C. (1966) The composition of human saliva secreted in response to a gustatory stimulus and to pilocarpine. *J. Physiol. (Lond.)*, **183**, 360.
DAWES C. (1969) The effects of flow rate and duration of stimulation on the concentration of protein and the main electrolytes in human parotid saliva. *Archs. oral Biol.*, **14**, 277.
DAWES C. (1970a) Effect of diet on salivary secretion and composition. *J. dent. Res.*, **49**, 1263.
DAWES C. (1970b) The approach to plasma levels of the chloride concentration in human parotid saliva at high flow rates. *Archs. oral. Biol.*, **15**, 97.

DAWES C. (1970c) Effects of different stimuli on the protein content of human parotid saliva. *I.A.D.R. Abstracts* (North American Division), No. 498.

DAWES C. (1972) Circadian rhythms in human salivary flowrate and composition. *J. Physiol. (Lond.)*, **220**, 529.

DAWES C. & WOOD C.M. (1973) The composition of human lip mucous gland secretions. *Archs. oral Biol.*, **18**, 343.

DE WARDENER H.E. & HERXHEIMER A. (1957) The effect of a high water intake on salt consumption, taste thresholds and salivary secretion in man. *J. Physiol. (Lond.)*, **139**, 53.

DISCHE Z., PALLAVICINI C., KAVASAKI H., SMIRNOW N., CIZAK L.J. & CHIEN S. (1962) Influence of the nature of the secretory stimulus on the composition of the carbohydrate moiety of glycoproteins of the submaxillary saliva. *Arch. Biochem.*, **97**, 459.

DOGON I.L. & AMDUR B.H. (1965) Further characterization of an antibacterial factor in human parotid secretions active against *Lactobacillus casei*. *Archs. oral Biol.*, **10**, 605.

DOGON I.L. & AMDUR B.H. (1970) Evidence for the presence of two thiocyanate-dependent antibacterial systems in human saliva. *Archs. oral Biol.*, **15**, 987.

EBLING F.J.B. (1970) Sebaceous glands. In CHAMPION R.H., GILLMAN T., ROOK A.J. & SIMS R.T. *An Introduction to the Biology of the Skin*, 187. Blackwell Scientific Publications, Oxford.

EGELBERG J. (1967) The topography and permeability of vessels at the dento-gingival junction in dogs. *J. periodont. Res.*, Suppl. 1.

ELLISON S.A. (1967) Proteins and glycoproteins of saliva. In CODE C.F. *Handbook of Physiology*, Section 6, *Alimentary Canal*, Vol. II, *Secretion*, 531–559. American Physiology Society, Washington D.C.

ERICSON S. (1969) An investigation of human parotid saliva secretion rate in response to different types of stimulation. *Archs. oral Biol.*, **14**, 591.

ERICSON S. (1971) The variability of the human parotid flow rate on stimulation with citric acid, with special reference to taste. *Archs. oral Biol.*, **16**, 9.

FARBMAN A.I. & ALLGOOD J.P. (1971) Inervation sensory receptors and sensitivity of the oral mucosa. In SQUIER C.A. & MEYER J. *Current Concepts of the Histology of Oral Mucosa*, 250–273. Charles C. Thomas, Springfield, Illinois.

FELLER R.P. & SHANNON I.L. (1970) Taste, tactile stimulation and parotid flow in the human. *J. oral Med.*, **25**, 87.

FLEMING A. (1922) On a remarkable bacteriolytic element found in the tissues and secretions. *Proc. R. Soc. (B)*, **93**, 306.

FRANK R.M., HERDLEY J. & PHILIPPE E. (1965) Acquired dental defects and salivary gland lesions after irradiation for carcinoma. *J. Am. dent. Ass.*, **70**, 868.

GEDDES D.A. (1972) Failure to demonstrate the antibacterial factor of Green in caries-free parotid saliva. In MACPHEE T. *Host Resistance to Commensal Bacteria*, 84–89. Churchill Livingstone, Edinburgh and London.

GIBALDI M. & KANIG J.L. (1965) Absorption of drugs through the oral mucosa. *J. oral Ther. & Pharma.*, **1**, 440.

GIBBONS R.J., DE STOPPELLAR J.D. & HARDEN L. (1966) Lysozyme insensitivity of bacteria indigenous to the oral cavity of man. *J. dent. Res.*, **45**, 877.

GREEN G.E. (1959) A bacteriolytic agent in salivary globulin of caries-immune human beings. *J. dent. Res.*, **38**, 262.
GREEN G.E. (1966) Properties of a salivary bacteriolysin and comparison with serum Beta lysin. *J. dent. Res.*, **45**, 882.
HARDEN R.McG., HILDITCH T.E., KENNEDY I., MASON D.K., PAPADOPOULOS S. & ALEXANDER W.D. (1967) Uptake and scanning of the salivary glands in man using pertechnetate ^{99m}Tc. *Clin. Sci.*, **32**, 49.
HENKIN R.I., GRAZIADEI P.P. & BRADLEY B.F. (1969) The molecular basis of taste and its disorders. *Ann. intern. Med.*, **71**, 791.
HENRIQUES B.L. (1961) Acinar duct transport in dogs submaxillary salivary gland. Abstract. *J. dent. Res.*, **40**, 719.
HENRIQUES B.L. (1962) A technique of studying salivary gland function. *Am. J. Physiol.*, **203**, 1086.
HOERMAN K.C., ENGLANDER H.R. & SHKLAIR I.L. (1956) Lysozyme—its characteristics in human parotid and submaxillo-lingual saliva. *Proc. Soc. exp. Biol. (N.Y.)*, **92**, 875.
JENKINS G.N. (1966a) *The Physiology of the Mouth*, 3rd edition, 305–316. Blackwell Scientific Publications, Oxford.
JENKINS G.N. (1966b) *The Physiology of the Mouth*, 3rd edition (revised reprint), 444–451. Blackwell Scientific Publications, Oxford.
JOLLES P. (1967) Relationship between chemical structure and biological activity of hen egg-white lysozyme and lysozymes of different species. *Proc. R. Soc. (B)*, **167**, 350.
JUNQUEIRA L.C.U. (1964) Studies on the physiology of rat and mouse salivary glands. III. On the function of the striated ducts of mammalian salivary glands. In SCREDONY L.M. & MEYER J. *Salivary Glands and their Secretions*, 123. Pergamon Press, Oxford.
KAABER S. (1971a) Studies on the permeability of human oral mucosa. I. Gravimetric determination of biological fluids at microgram levels. *Acta odont. Scand.*, **29**, 653.
KAABER S. (1971b) Studies on the permeability of human oral mucosa. II. The permeability of dry palatal mucosa to water, sodium and potassium. *Acta odont. Scand.*, **29**, 663.
KAABER S. (1971c) Studies on the permeability of human oral mucosa. III. The permeability of dry buccal mucosa to water, sodium and potassium. *Acta odont. Scand.*, **29**, 683.
KELLUM R.E. (1967) Human sebaceous gland lipids. *Archs. Derm.*, **95**, 218.
KERR A.C. (1961) The physiological regulation of salivary secretion in man. *Int. Ser. of Monographs on Oral Biology*, 9. Pergamon Press, Oxford.
KERR A.C. & WEDDERBURN D.L. (1958) Antibacterial factors in the secretions of human parotid and submaxillary glands. *Brit. dent. J.*, **105**, 321.
KLEBANOFF S.J., CLEM W.H. & LUEBKE R.G. (1966) The peroxidase–thiocyanate–hydrogen peroxide antimicrobial system. *Biochem. biophys. Acta (Amst.)*, **117**, 63.
KLEBANOFF S.J. & LUEBKE R.G. (1965) The antilactobacillus system of saliva. Role of salivary peroxidase. *Proc. Soc. exp. Biol. (N.Y.)*, **118**, 483.

KLIGMAN A.M. (1963) The uses of sebum. In MONTAGNA W., ELLIS R.A. & SILVER A.F. *Advances in Biology of Skin*, Vol. 4, 110. Pergamon Press, Oxford.

KLINKHAMMER J.M. (1968) Quantitative evaluation of gingivitis and periodontal disease. *Periodontics*, **6**, 207.

LILIENTHAL B. (1955) An analysis of the buffer system in saliva. *J. dent. Res.*, **34**, 516.

MCBURNEY D.H. & PFAFFMAN C. (1963) Gustatory adaptation to saliva and sodium chloride. *J. exp. Psychol.*, **65**, 523.

MACFARLANE T.W. & MASON D.K. (1972) Local environmental factors in the host resistance to commensal microflora of the mouth. In MACPHEE T. *Host Resistance to Commensal Bacteria*, 64–75. Churchill Livingstone, Edinburgh.

MACFARLANE T.W. & MASON D.K. (1973) Changes in the oral flora in Sjögren's syndrome. *J. clin. Path.*, **27**, 416.

MANDEL I.D. (1967) Diagnostic clues in saliva. *Diagnostica*, **4**, 11.

MANDEL I.D., KATZ R., ZENGO A., KUTSCHER A.H., GREENBERG R.A., KATZ S., SHARF R. & PINTOFF A. (1968) The effect of pharmacologic agents on salivary secretion and composition in man. Pilocarpine, atropine and anticholinesterases. *J. oral Ther.*, **4**, 192.

MARPLES M.J. (1965a) *The Ecology of the Human Skin*, 103. Charles C. Thomas, Springfield, Illinois.

MARPLES M.J. (1965b) *The Ecology of the Human Skin*, 130. Charles C. Thomas, Springfield, Illinois.

MASON D.K. (1966) Studies in salivary glands and their secretions in health and disease. M.D. Thesis, University of Glasgow.

MASON D.K., HARDEN R.McG. & ALEXANDER W.D. (1966) Problems of interpretation in studies of salivary constituents. *J. oral Med.*, **21**, 66.

MASSON P.L., HEREMANS J.F. & DIVE C.H. (1966a) An iron-binding protein common to many external secretions. *Clin. chim. Acta*, **14**, 735.

MASSON P.L., HEREMANS J.F., PRIGNOT J.J. & WAUTERS G. (1966b) Immunohistochemical localization and bacteriostatic properties of an iron-binding protein and bronchial mucus. *Thorax*, **21**, 538.

MILES A.E.W. (1958) Sebaceous glands in the lip and cheek mucosa of man. *Brit. dent. J.*, **105**, 235.

MISTRETTA C.M. (1971) Permeability of tongue epithelium and its relation to taste. *Am. J. Physiol.*, **220**, 1162.

NAYLOR G.R.E. (1970) Bacteria and the skin. In CHAMPION R.H., GILLMAN T., ROOK A.J. & SIMS R.T. *An Introduction to the Biology of the Skin*, 203. Blackwell Scientific Publications. Oxford.

NOUR-ELDIN F. & WILKINSON J.H. (1957) The blood clotting factors in human saliva. *J. Physiol. (Lond.)*, **136**, 324.

Orban's Oral Histology and Embryology (1972) SICHER H. & BHASKAR S.R. (eds), 7th edition, 269–297. C.V. Mosby Co., St Louis.

PARK W.M. & MASON D.K. (1966) Hydrostatic sialography. *Radiol.*, **86**, 116.

PETERSEN O.H. (1972) Electrolyte transports involved in the formation of saliva. In EMMELIN N. & ZOTTERMAN Y. *Oral Physiology*, 21–31. Pergamon Press, Oxford and New York.

PILLSBURY D.M. & KLIGMAN A.M. (1954) Some current problems in cutaneous bacteriology. In MACKENNA R.M.B. *Modern Trends in Dermatology*, 2nd Series, 187. Butterworth & Co., London.
PUSKULIAN L. (1972) Salivary electrolyte changes during the normal menstrual cycle. *J. dent. Res.*, **51**, 1212.
RICKETTS C.R., SQUIRE J.R. & TOPLEY E. (1951) Human skin lipids with particular reference to the self sterilizing power of the skin. *Clin. Sci.*, **10**, 89.
SAGGERS B.A., LAWSON D., STERN J. & EDGSON A.C. (1967) Rapid method for the detection of cystic fibrosis of the pancreas in children. *Arch. Dis. Childh.*, **42**, 187.
SCHNEYER L.H. & SCHNEYER C.A. (1967) Inorganic composition of saliva. In CODE C.F. *Handbook of Physiology*, Section 6, *Alimentary Canal*, Vol. II, *Secretion*, 497–530. American Physiology Society, Washington D.C.
SCHULTE W. (1970) Saliva and blood coagulation. In WALKER R.V. *Oral Surgery*, 494–495. E. & S. Livingstone, Edinburgh.
SHANNON I.L. & PRIGMORE J.R. (1960) Parotid fluid flow rate. Its relationship to pH and chemical composition. *Oral Surg.*, **13**, 1488.
SHANNON I.L., TERRY J.M. & CHAUNCEY H.H. (1969). Effect of a maxillary mouth-guard on the parotid flow rate response to flavoured solutions. *Proc. Soc. exp. Biol. (N.Y.)*, **130**, 1052.
SIEGEL I.A., HALL S.H. & STAMBAUGH R. (1971) Permeability of the oral mucosa. In SQUIER C.A. & MEYER J. *Current Concepts of the Histology of Oral Mucosa*, 274–286. Charles C. Thomas, Springfield, Illinois.
SPEIRS R.L. (1971) The effects of interactions between gustatory stimuli on the reflex flow-rate of human parotid saliva. *Archs. oral Biol.*, **16**, 351.
STEPHEN K.W., CHISHOLM D.M., HARDEN R.McG., ROBERTSON J.W.K., WHALEY K. & STUART A. (1971) Diagnostic value of quantitative scintiscanning of the salivary glands in Sjögren's syndrome and rheumatoid arthritis. *Clin. Sci.*, **41**, 555.
STEPHEN K.W., ROBERTSON J.W.K., HARDEN R.McG. & CHISHOLM D.M. (1973) Concentration of iodide, pertechnetate, thiocyanate and bromide in saliva from parotid, submandibular and minor salivary glands in man. *J. Lab. clin. Med.*, **81**, 219.
TANDLER B. (1963) Ultrastructure of human submaxillary gland. II. The base of the striated duct cells. *J. Ultrastruct. Res.*, **9**, 65.
TOLO K. (1971) Transport across stratified non-keratinized epithelium. *J. periodont. Res.*, **6**, 237.
TREFZ B. (1972) Histochemical investigations of the modal specificity of taste. *J. dent. Res.*, **51**, 1203.
TREGAER R.T. (1966) *Physical Function of the Skin*, 6–13. Academic Press Inc., New York.
VAN KESTERN M., BIBBY B.G. & BERRY G.P. (1942) Studies on the antibacterial factors of human saliva. *J. Bact.*, **43**, 573.
YOUNG G., RESCA H.G. & SULLIVAN M.T. (1951) The yeasts of the normal mouth and their relation to salivary acidity. *J. dent. Res.*, **30**, 426.
ZELDOW B.J. (1961) Studies on the antibacterial action of human saliva. *J. dent. Res.*, **40**, 446.

CHAPTER 3
IMMUNOGLOBULIN SYSTEMS OF ORAL MUCOSA AND SALIVA*

PER BRANDTZAEG†

3:0 Introduction

Immunoglobulins (Igs) are the antibody proteins produced by the host in response to foreign or antigenic material; they are the effector substances which alone or by means of various biological amplification systems exert so-called humoral immunity. The specificity of the underlying immune reaction is determined by the antibody activity exhibited by the Igs, whereas the biological consequences depend in addition on other structural characteristics of these unique molecules. The rapid expansion of the science of immunology during recent years can to a considerable extent be ascribed to increased knowledge about the structure of Igs and improved characterization of the cells producing them.

It is now well recognized that an *immune reaction* may be either beneficial or harmful to the host. Thus, protective immunity and immunopathology represent two faces of the same coin. This is schematically depicted in Fig. 3.1. The chief effect of the *primary immune response* against an antigen is to recruit cells which subsequently are responsible for an altered reactivity of the host. These immunological memory cells are the basis for a rapid and prolonged *secondary immune response* when the

---

* The author's investigations have been supported by grants from the Norwegian Research Council for Science and the Humanities; Grosserer N.A. Stangs Legat; and Anders Jahres Fond. Patient material for the studies has to a great extent been provided by Professor P. Berdal, Department of Oto-Rhino-Laryngology, Rikshospitalet.

† Research Fellow of the Norwegian Cancer Society, and Director of the Immunohistochemical Laboratory, Institute of Pathology, Rikshospitalet, Oslo, Norway.

same antigen is encountered again. The products of this anamnestic, intensified response are a large number of lymphocytes and a high concentration of antibodies readily made available to react with the antigen. Now the host is allergic to the antigen if the term is used as originally stated by von Pirquet (1906): 'The vaccinated person behaves . . . in a different manner from him who has not previously been in contact with such an agent.' Depending on the specific biological circumstances, this changed reactivity of the sensitized host will mediate protection (immunity) or damage (hypersensitivity). Today, however, the term *allergy* is commonly used to denote only the latter situation, while the manifestation of heightened responsiveness to antigens in general is called *immunity* regardless of the biological effect.

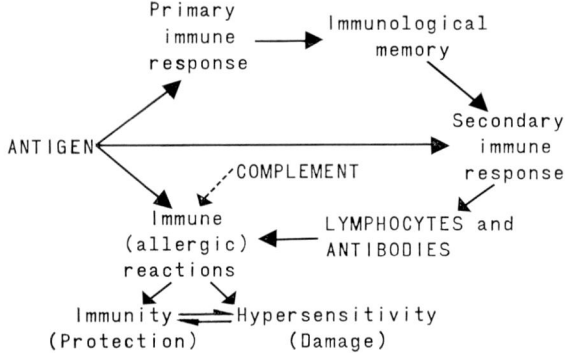

Fig. 3.1. Antigen-induced biological events leading to protective immunity or hypersensitivity.

In most immune reactions both protective and damaging processes are going on at the same time. On clinical and morphological grounds the outcome of this interplay will be called *protective immunity* or *hypersensitivity* according to the dominating facet. Several more or less well-characterized factors contribute to the result: e.g. the type of responding lymphocyte and the class of executive Ig; the participation of biological amplification systems, especially serum complement; the nature and supply of antigenic material; and, finally, the tissue site where the antigen is encountered by the immunocompetent cells and the specific antibodies. The immune reaction aims principally at antigenic elimination. In most cases following a secondary immune response this is successful, and the effects of pathogenic bacteria, viruses, fungi, and other exogenous antigens are readily neutralized to the benefit of the host. When antigen elimination is unsuccessful, however, the immune reaction may contribute to undue tissue damage because of a continuous triggering of biological amplification systems leading to inflammation; this is bound to occur when there is a persistent supply of stimulating antigen from an endogenous (*autoantigens*) or exogenous source. Adverse consequences similarly ensue a too violent reaction because of an unbalanced immune response; this may have a genetic basis or be due to irregularities during the development of the immune system.

This chapter deals with protective and deleterious aspects of the immunoglobulin systems operating in the human oral mucosa, adjacent tissues, and saliva. Since oral immunology is a young science, some of the presented ideas lack solid evidence and are rather derived at by extrapolation of information obtained in other sites of the organism. This especially applies to the actual antibody functions of locally produced Igs for which only scanty data are available when it comes to the oral cavity. The immunoglobulin systems of human skin are briefly taken into consideration since several dermatological diseases with features of immune reactions present symptoms in the oral mucosa.

3:1 T and B Cells

The specific immune mechanisms in man and several other species seem in the main to depend on two functionally different types of lymphocytes called T and B cells (Roitt *et al* 1969; Parrott & deSousa 1971) which develop from bone-marrow-derived lymphoid stem cells (Fig. 3.2). The T-cell precursors migrate to the *thymus* where they mature and proliferate, and subsequently become seeded to the blood. In birds the B-cell precursors migrate to the *bursa of Fabricius*, which is a sac-like lymphoepithelial structure arising as a dorsal diverticulum from the cloaca. The bursa equivalent has as yet not been defined in mammals. Some evidence indicates that in these species the B cells mature and proliferate in gut-associated lymphoepithelial tissues, whereas according to another widely held view the bone marrow serves not only as a source of lymphoid stem cells but also as a micro-environment for the differentiation of mammalian B cells.

The diversity of immunological responsiveness subsequently exhibited by circulating B cells is generated during this first developmental stage (Cooper *et al* 1972; Ritzmann *et al* 1973). Exactly how this comes about is not known; but a thymic and, respectively, a 'bursal' hormone may be responsible for a very high rate of cell proliferation. It is therefore quite possible that the primary lymphoid organs are mutant-breeding microenvironments where a large number of different immunologically competent cell lines emerge. The specificities of these clones are expressed through cell surface *'antigen receptors'* or *'recognition molecules'*. These

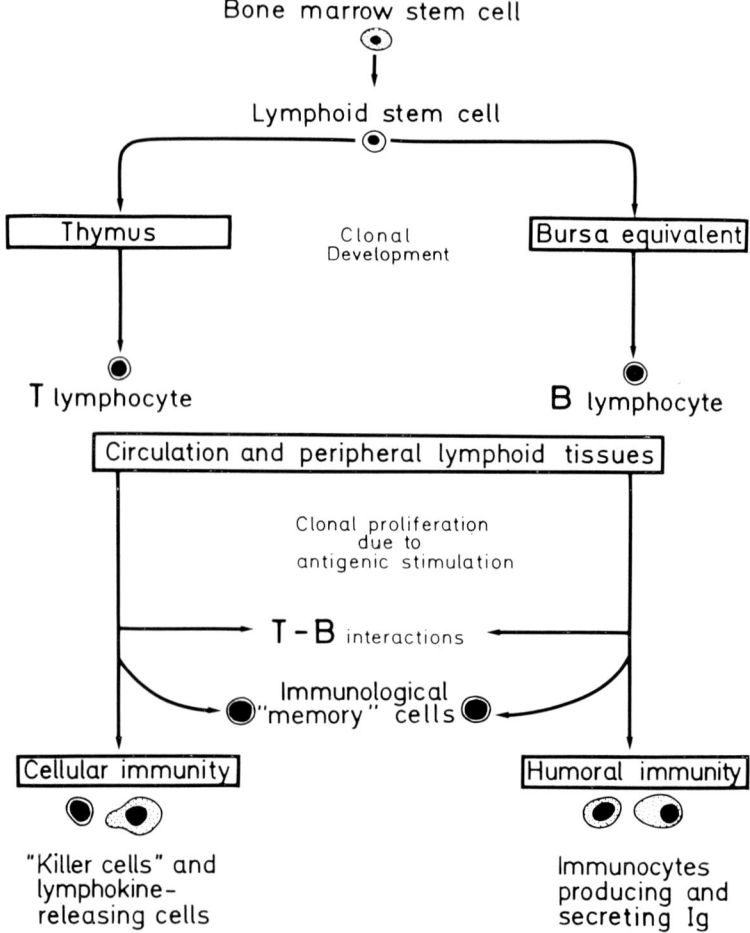

Fig. 3.2. Schematic representation of the two major functional limbs of the immune apparatus.

must necessarily exhibit a great variability among the different cell lines, and the genes coding for their structures have hence been termed '*V genes*'. According to a recent hypothesis (Jerne 1971) the V genes originally code exclusively for histocompatibility antigens. However, clones with autospecificity will survive only as mutants during the proliferation period in the primary immunological organs. Thus, while *tolerance* to the host's own tissue antigens develops, random somatic mutation generates a diverse population of cell lines sensitive to an immense variety of heterologous antigens. A relatively large number of clones directed against the histocompatibility antigens of other individuals of the same species will on the other hand survive; these subsequently form the basis for the 'allo-aggression' which causes the difficulties with graft rejection in transplantation surgery.

When the T and B lymphocytes appear in the blood they may be regarded as sensitive 'scout' cells which will explore every sector of the body actively seeking out antigenic substances. From the blood they migrate into the spleen and lymph nodes and, to a much smaller extent, into interstitial spaces within many non-lymphoid tissues. From these peripheral routes of migration the lymphocytes will eventually return via the lymphatics to the blood (Ford & Gowans 1969). Although both T and B cells participate in this continuously recirculating pool of lymphocytes, their contributions and migration patterns are significantly different (Ford & Marchesi 1971). Thus, T cells become concentrated in the mid-cortex of lymph nodes and in the periarteriolar regions of the spleen, whereas B cells are found preferentially in germinal centres and in the medullary cords of the nodes and the red pulp of the spleen. The biological value of the peripheral distribution of lymphocytes is not only to facilitate the induction of primary immune responses by enabling contact between antigens and the corresponding antigen-sensitive cells; lymphocyte recirculation is also important in disseminating surviving descendants of the cells stimulated in the primary response (*'immunological memory cells'*) so that an augmented secondary response can take place throughout the body wherever the same antigen reappears. Altogether, outside the primary lymphoid organs lymphopoiesis is based on antigen-dependent clonal proliferation (Fig. 3.2); and the peripheral or secondary lymphoid organs play an increasingly important immunological role as the individual matures and ages.

Circulating B cells can be distinguished from T cells as they contain membrane-associated Ig molecules in concentrations high enough to be detected by the direct immunofluorescence technique (Fig. 3.3). It is generally held that these molecules are synthesized by the same cells and represent their antigen receptors. Normally about 10% of human peripheral blood lymphocytes contain surface Ig and hence should represent B lymphocytes (Fröland & Natvig 1972). The proportion of T lymphocytes has not been definitely determined in man, but some evidence indicates that they constitute the majority of the remaining 90% (Williams et al 1973). However, there is as yet no well-defined marker for human T cells, and there is moreover disagreement with regard to the nature of their antigen receptors. Some investigators claim that the receptors are Ig molecules which cannot be detected by immunofluorescence partly because they are buried in the cell membrane, and partly because they are rapidly liberated. The released T-cell receptors have been found to be highly cytophilic for macrophages (Marchalonis & Cone 1973). This property may explain at least one facet of the *T–B cell interactions* (Fig. 3.2) which are a prerequisite for a successful humoral immune response to

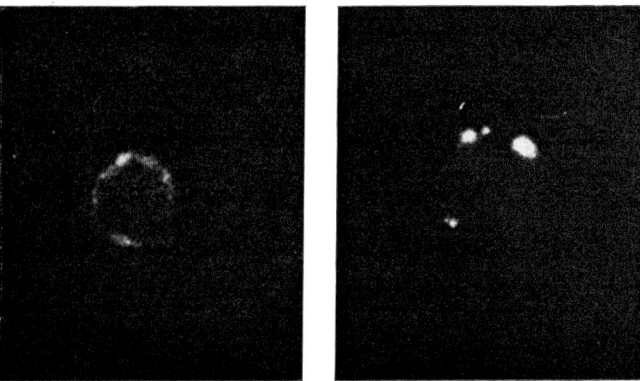

Fig. 3.3. B cells from peripheral blood. Viable lymphocytes from a normal individual were reacted with rhodamine-labelled antibodies to human immunoglobulin-light chains. Surface immunoglobulin is revealed as a diffuse, uneven fluorescent rim (left) or as larger granules (right). Magnification: 1000 ×. From: Brandtzaeg 1973d.

many antigens. When receptor–antigen complexes are released from the T-cell surface they may adhere to macrophages or dendritic reticulum cells; the antigens will consequently be presented to the recirculating B lymphocytes as a concentrated or 'polymeric' material which stimulates these cells more briskly. In addition to the antigen-specific cooperation between T and B cells there is evidence for non-specific helper functions. An experimentally induced T-cell response can thus promote a superimposed B-cell response directed towards a different antigen (Flax et al 1969); this may be due to blastogenic or mitogenic factors released from the activated T cells (David 1971).

Antigenically stimulated T lymphocytes develop into effector cells of *cellular immunity* (Fig. 3.2). It is generally held that they do not exert their

Table 3.1 Some properties of the major classes of human serum immunoglobulins

	IgG	IgM	IgD	IgE	IgA
WHO designation					
Sedimentation coefficient	7S	19S	7S	8S	7S (10–13S)*
Molecular weight	150,000	900,000	185,000	200,000	160,000
Concentration in serum (mg/100 ml)	800–1,600	50–200	<15	<0.07	140–400
Relative concentration in tissue fluid	High	Low	Very low	Very low	Intermediate
Active transfer through secretory epithelia	−	+	−	−	+†
Active transfer through placental membrane	+	−	−	−	−
Complement activation	+	+	−	−	−
Adherence to surface receptors of:					
Macrophages	+	?	?	?	?
Polymorphonuclear leukocytes	+	−	−	−	−
Monocytes and some lymphocytes	+	−	−	−	−
Mast cells and basophils	?	−	−	+	−

* 10–15% of polymers in normal serum.
† Does not apply to 7S IgA.

The L chains are common to all Ig classes, and each molecule contains either the κ or the λ type. An Ig unit theoretically contains two antigen-binding sites located at structurally variable regions (black areas in Fig. 3.4)

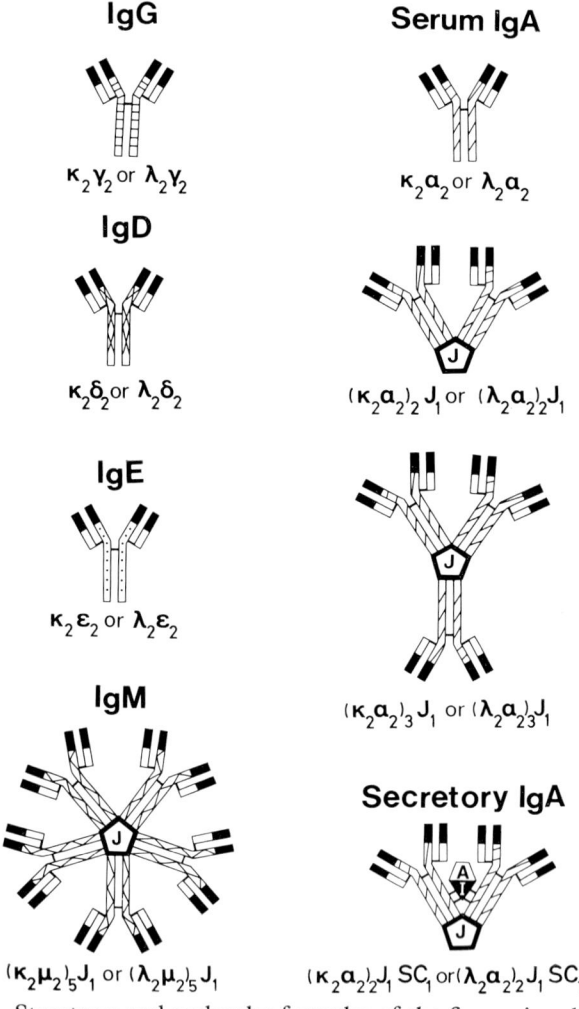

Fig. 3.4. Structures and molecular formulas of the five major classes of human immunoglobulins. κ and λ, light polypeptide chains; γ, δ, ε, μ and α, heavy polypeptide chains; J, J chain; and SC, secretory component indicated by its two major antigenic determinants A and I.

of the N-terminal part of the L and H chains. The amino acid sequence of these regions is coded by the V genes (cf. previous section), and this explains the diversity of antibody specificities exhibited by the Ig molecules. The remaining constant polypeptide sequence determines the than initially believed. Thus, it has recently been shown that Ig-synthesizing cell lines can release the migration inhibition factor (MIF) which has been regarded as a lymphokine produced only by T cells (Tsuchimoto et al 1972).

The immune systems of mucous membranes have up till now been studied mainly with respect to humoral immunity. Antibodies in the external secretions have been recognized as important resistance factors since the early studies of Besredka (1927) and Burrows & Havens (1948) on antibacterial immune responses in the gastrointestinal tract. However, despite our lacking knowledge about T-lymphocyte functions in mucosal tissues it can be deduced from the information cited above that these cells must be of significance locally at least by augmenting B-cell responses. There is evidence that such a helper function is particularly conducive to IgA responses (Clough et al 1971) which are responsible for most antibodies appearing in the secretions. In addition it has recently been shown that topical application of antigen in the respiratory tract of guinea-pigs can induce a T-cell response which may be more or less confined to the local tissue site (Waldman & Henney 1971; Nash & Holle 1973).

An attempt at defining a local immune response as 'cellular' or 'humoral' will probably hardly give the full truth whether it is based on conventional morphological and serological evaluation, or on refined studies of peripheral lymphocytes. It should be clear from the above discussion that in most if not all situations the host's response to foreign material includes components of both cellular and humoral immunity. Moreover, the possibilities of studying human T lymphocytes from a local lesion are at present very limited. Despite these difficulties it is important to try to characterize disease processes of mucous membranes and skin as mainly involving T- or B-cell reactions; understanding of the major effector mechanism may aid in diagnosis and treatment.

3:2 Immunoglobulins: Classes and Characteristics

The human immunoglobulins comprise five major structural classes: IgG, IgD, IgE, IgM and IgA (Fig. 3.4). They are all composed of at least one basic Ig unit containing two identical heavy (H) and two identical light (L) polypeptide chains which are joined by disulphide bonds and non-covalent interactions. The molecular weight (MW) of this unit is 150,000–160,000, and it exhibits a sedimentation coefficient of approximately 7S. The various Ig classes can be distinguished chiefly because their H chains are structurally different, as indicated by differently drawn patterns in Fig. 3.4.

effects by means of Ig molecules but rather by cell-interaction with the antigenic target ('*killer cells*') and by production and release of so-called '*lymphokines*'. *In vitro* such substances have been found to exhibit a variety of pharmacological activities such as promotion of vascular permeability, chemotaxis, cytotoxicity, accumulation and activation of macrophages, and stimulation of osteoclasts (David 1971; Horton *et al* 1972). Cellular immunity is believed to be of importance in: (*1*) delayed hypersensitivity reactions of skin and mucous membranes; (*2*) protection against viruses, fungi, and intracellular bacterial pathogens; (*3*) immunological surveillance against oncogenesis; (*4*) some so-called autoimmune diseases; and (*5*) transplantation immunity.

After antigen recognition and interaction through the surface receptors, B lymphocytes become activated to produce and secrete Ig molecules of the corresponding antibody specificity. *Humoral immunity* (Fig. 3.2) is thus ultimately expressed by the activity of these effector proteins which are released by apocrine secretion from immunocytes with varying morphology, the plasma cell being the end stage (Avrameas *et al* 1971). The concept of phenotypic restriction has been firmly established for B cells; members of an immunocyte clone are thus so highly specialized that they can produce antibody molecules of only one specificity (Osoba 1969; Petersen & Ingraham 1969; Benjamin & Weigle 1970, Thursh 1970). Each cell moreover releases only one class of Ig molecules, at least at a given time (Cebra & Bernier 1967). A switch in the synthesis of Ig class may occur in antigenically stimulated B cells, but only at a very low frequence since less than 1·5% of double-producers are found in sensitive test systems (Cosenza & Nordin 1970; Nossal *et al* 1971). During the first stage of clonal development, however, there may be a high frequency of switch in the genetic commitment (Cooper *et al* 1972). Each clone thus appears to be represented in the circulation by cells programmed to make antibodies of a single specificity, but of several Ig classes.

A classification of lymphocytes as T and B cells is probably an oversimplification. Several attempts at subgrouping have already appeared in the literature. Recent evidence indicates that there is at least one population of circulating human lymphocytes which cannot be satisfactorily classified as either T or B cells (Fröland & Natvig 1973). These lymphocytes are characterized by surface receptors with affinity for the Fc portion of IgG (cf. subsequent section). They can hence interact with antibody molecules and may play a role in so-called antibody-dependent, cell-mediated cytotoxic reactions (Wislöff & Fröland 1973). The effector mechanisms of activated T and B cells may moreover be less distinguished characteristic that allows classification into κ and λ for the L chains, and into γ, δ, ϵ, μ and α for the H chains (Fig. 3.4). Important functions (e.g. complement activation, affinity for various cell types, placental transfer) can be ascribed to the C-terminal parts of the H chains, and will hence differ between the classes (Table 3.1). These properties mediate the participation of biological amplification systems in immune reactions; the outcome is thus highly dependent on the Ig class to which the executive antibodies belong. The enzyme papain splits those parts of the Ig unit which exhibit antibody activity (*Fab fragments*) from the C-terminal parts of the H chains (*Fc fragment*) which are responsible for other biological functions. When the enzyme pepsin is used, the Fc portion is degraded whereas the portions with antibody activity are obtained as a single, divalent $F(ab')_2$ *fragment*. Techniques for fragmentation have been particularly well established for IgG.

In addition to differences in the primary structure, the various Ig classes exhibit pronounced physicochemical heterogeneity. IgG, IgD and IgE generally occur as monomeric 7S units only, whereas IgM and IgA regularly occur as polymers (Fig. 3.4). The tendency to polymerize may depend on the presence of a polypeptide called J chain which is common to IgM and IgA polymers, but cannot be detected in monomeric IgA, IgG and IgD (Halpern & Koshland 1970; Mestecky *et al* 1971). In normal human serum almost all of the IgM molecules are 19S pentamers, whereas only 10–15% of the IgA molecules are polymerized as 10–13S dimers or trimers. In external secretions, on the other hand, about 90% of the IgA molecules are 11S dimers (MW = 390,000) and larger polymers which in addition to L, H and J chains contain an epithelial glycoprotein called 'secretory component' (SC). In Fig. 3.3 SC is designated by its two major antigenic determinants, I and A (Brandtzaeg 1971b). The secretory IgA molecule has a closely packed quaternary structure where the J chain (Kobayashi *et al* 1973) and part of the SC (the I determinant) are inaccessible (Brandtzaeg 1971b); this may explain its relatively high resistance to proteolytic degradation (Brown *et al* 1970; Shuster 1971; Tax & Korngold 1971; Parkin *et al* 1973). Such a property serves to protect the molecular integrity of antibodies functioning in external secretions since these belong mainly to the secretory IgA class. Normal external secretions in addition contain small amounts of 19S IgM (Brandtzaeg *et al* 1970). SC is also associated with these molecules but not in such a stabilized quaternary structure. Thus, the I determinant is partially accessible, and after purification only 60–70% of the molecules have retained their SC (Brandtzaeg 1975).

IgG is the major Ig class in normal human serum (Table 3.1); this apparently reflects that peripheral lymphoid organs such as spleen and lymph nodes during secondary immune responses are chiefly synthesizing IgG. More than 50% is distributed extravascularly (Waldmann & Strober 1969); IgG is therefore also the major Ig class of tissue fluids in general, but is not actively transported to the external secretions. It is considered the most important antibacterial and virus-neutralizing antibody of the internal milieu. Its Fc portion has affinity for macrophages and neutrophilic granulocytes; phagocytosis of IgG–antigen complexes may hence be enhanced since they can adhere to the phagocytic cells. Through its Fc portion antigen-complexed IgG is also a potent activator of the series of enzymes comprised by the term serum complement (see Chapter 9). A number of biological consequences may ensue complement activation. Some of these may be beneficial, such as enhanced phagocytosis, bacteriolysis, chemotaxis of polymorphonuclear leukocytes, and stimulation of inflammation. However, complement activation may also produce detrimental effects through cytolysis and persistent, Arthus-type inflammatory reactions. Antibodies of the IgG class are therefore important in hypersensitivity reactions of type II and III (see Chapter 9) according to the classification of Coombs & Gell (1968). It is moreover possible that IgG antibodies play a role in cell-mediated cytotoxic reactions, since a population of lymphocytes have surface receptors with affinity for the Fc portion of this immunoglobulin.

IgM is usually produced early in the immune response; it is largely confined to the blood stream, only about 25% being distributed extravascularly (Waldmann & Strober 1969). Its chief function may therefore be in the blood, for example in cases of bacteriaemia. However, it has recently been shown that IgM is actively transported into external secretions (Brandtzaeg 1971a), and that some mucosal sites may have a significant supply of this immunoglobulin due to local synthesis (Brandtzaeg 1975). IgM antibodies are extremely efficient agglutinating and cytolytic agents. Complement activation by IgM in combination with the enzymatic action of lysozyme can produce efficient lysis of Gram negative bacteria (Glynn 1969). Many of the so-called 'natural' antimicrobial antibodies are IgM; among these should be included the isoagglutinins (anti-A, anti-B), whose synthesis most likely is stimulated by cross-reacting microbial antigens (Springer 1967). Antibodies to endotoxins also tend to appear in this class.

IgD is a mysterious protein to which no definite function as yet has been ascribed. A very high frequency of circulating B lymphocytes with membrane-associated IgD has recently been reported for newborns (Rowe et al 1973); this may in the future provide a clue to its biological value. Perhaps IgD is an important B-cell antigen receptor.

IgE exhibits affinity for the surface of mast cells and basophils; this explains its major contribution to immediate (atopic) hypersensitivity of type I (see Chapter 9). When antigen combines with the corresponding IgE antibody on the cell surface, the membrane is altered so that degranulation and release of vasoactive amines and certain enzymes ensues. Although this is commonly visualized as an immediate hypersensitivity reaction, IgE probably also has a physiological role by increasing vascular permeability and stimulating inflammation. It has been speculated that this may be important to the defence against certain parasites, since the level of IgE often is considerably raised during such infections. The action of IgE may on the other hand trigger local anaphylactic reactions (Type III hypersensitivity) by augmenting the deposition of IgG-antigen complexes at the reaction site (Benveniste 1973).

IgA has probably a function both in the internal (blood and tissue fluid) and external milieus (exocrine secretions). Lack of conventional complement-activating properties is firmly established for this immunoglobulin (Adinolfi et al 1966b; Ishizaka et al 1966; Vaerman & Heremans 1968). Nevertheless, IgA has recently been shown to be able to activate a proactivator for the third complement factor (Müller-Eberhard 1971); but this alternate pathway has very low cytolytic capacity and its biological significance is doubtful. Most likely, therefore, IgA antibodies present in the internal milieu may exert a blocking effect in competition with comparable antibodies of other classes; this may serve to moderate possible deleterious reactions produced by IgG and IgM, for example in type II and III hypersensitivity conditions. The host may similarly be protected against a too rapid antibody-mediated release of endotoxins from bacteria because of the blocking properties of IgA antibodies (Hall et al 1971). Adverse consequences of immune reactions have so far not been ascribed to this Ig class. The unexplored possibility exists, however, that IgA antibodies to tumour antigens may coat malignant cells and thus protect them against elimination by T lymphocytes.

The chief function of IgA probably takes place in the external milieu where it normally is the predominant antibody protein and occurs as a highly stabilized polymeric immunoglobulin (Fig. 3.4). The notion that secretory IgA antibodies may inhibit mucosal penetration and thereby act in a 'first line of defence' against deleterious agents is increasingly gaining acceptance; but most of the supporting evidence comes from studies of viral infections (Hanson & Brandtzaeg 1973). Despite the fact that secretory IgA has been shown to be effective as a virus-neutralizing antibody, very little information is available about its potential antibacterial functions. Since IgA does not mediate conventional complement activation, a bacteriolytic effect would not be expected for antibodies of this class. Nevertheless, Adinolfi et al (1966a) reported that human colostral IgA combined with complement plus lysozyme was able to lyse E. coli. This is an interesting observation as lysozyme is ubiquitously present in exocrine secretions. Complement factors, on the other hand, are not available in pure glandular fluids, but may appear in the external milieu as a result of exudation (Brandtzaeg 1966; Larsson et al 1973). However, a recent study indicates that the bactericidal effect of IgA plus lysozyme may rather depend on serum factors which do not belong to the complement system (Burdon 1973); it is not known whether these factors are present in the secretions in adequate concentrations. Reports on the phagocytosis-promoting (opsonizing) activity of secretory IgA are directly contradictory. Knop et al (1971) found that IgA from colostrum of sows was much more efficient than IgG and IgM in augmenting engulfment and intracellular killing of E. coli by phagocytes. Girard & Kalbermatten (1970) reported that the same microbe could be opsonized by human secretory IgA antibodies, and that this effect was enhanced by lysozyme but not by complement. Kaplan et al (1972), on the other hand, found the opsonization of incompatible erythrocytes by human colostral IgA to be complement dependent. Others (Eddie et al 1971; Wilson 1972; Zipursky et al 1973) have been unable to demonstrate any convincing opsonizing activity of secretory IgA, suggesting that some of the above results may be due to traces of IgM in the test preparations.

 Coating and agglutination of microorganisms seems to be the only well-established antibacterial activity of secretory IgA (Brandtzaeg et al 1968a; McClelland et al 1972; Williams & Gibbons 1972). The biological consequences may none the less be very important, as simple combination with IgA may inhibit a bacterium from sticking to epithelial cells and hence reduce its ability to colonize on the mucosa (Williams & Gibbons 1972). Studies of patients with selective lack of IgA have demonstrated that their mucous membranes are relatively permeable to a variety of extraneous antigens such as food and milk proteins (Buckley & Dees 1969; Ammann & Hong 1970; Kaufman & Hobbs 1970; Huntley et al 1971; Schwartz & Buckley 1971); and potentially allergen-blocking antibodies have been detected in nasal secretory IgA of some atopic patients (Dolovich et al 1970; Turk et al 1970). Simple complexing with antigens may thus explain the capacity of secretory IgA antibodies to constitute a general immunological trapping mechanism protecting mucous membranes.

3:3 Immunoglobulins of Oral Fluids

3:3:1 Quantitation of Ig

The various Ig classes are identified and quantitated in human body fluids by means of immunological techniques. Proper results generally depend on the use of animal sera monospecific to the Fc portion of each class. Cross-reactivity with the Fab portion can lead to false interpretation of findings obtained with techniques such as immunoelectrophoresis and double-diffusion in gel. Quantitation in addition depends on similar antigenic properties of the employed standard protein and the measured Ig. Homogeneity in the size of the compared molecules is, moreover, a prerequisite for reliability with the most commonly used quantitative method, *single-radial immunodiffusion* (SRID), since the result is a function of antigen diffusion into an antibody-containing gel (Mancini *et al* 1965). Up till now standards of variable quality have been used in different laboratories, and most published results are hardly comparable. In 1971 the WHO proposed that serum quantitations of IgG, IgM and IgA should be made with reference to an international standard; this is a lyophilized pooled human serum which is available for distribution (Anderson *et al* 1971). It is recommended that concentrations be reported as international units (I.U.) on the basis of the reference preparation rather than as mg/ml on the basis of a local protein standard. Similar reference preparations are now available for IgD and IgE.

In order to avoid difficulties of interpretation, however, levels of serum Ig should be given both as weight and as I.U., at least for a transitional period. Moreover, since an international reference standard is not available for secretory IgA the quantitation of this immunoglobulin has at present to be based on weight. Each laboratory dealing with these problems should, therefore, have its own working standard of pooled normal human serum (NHS) which is used for all concentration measurements of IgG, IgM, serum IgA and secretory IgA. This standard must be calibrated against the WHO reference preparation and against purified serum Igs and secretory IgA. Factors can then be calculated for conversion from the results obtained as per cent of NHS values to I.U. and mg/ml (Brandtzaeg *et al* 1970). Although the diffusion properties of IgA in serum and secretions are very different, a linear relationship can be obtained for a conversion of the SRID results obtained with the NHS standard to secretory IgA levels as mg/ml (Brandtzaeg et al 1970). Nevertheless, as secretions often contain a mixture of 7S IgA, 11S IgA and larger polymers, accurate quantitation of the total IgA level is rarely possible. Some attempts have been made to quantitate selectively secretory IgA by means of an antiserum specific for SC; this is bound to give an erroneous result, since most secretions contain appreciable quantities of free SC which will participate in the precipitation (Brandtzaeg 1971c). A sophisticated method has recently been developed in which different molecular species of IgA are separated by thin layer chromatography prior to immunological quantitation (Hanson et al 1971).

Conventional SRID detects Ig levels down to about 0·5 mg/100 ml, but the accuracy of the method is not satisfactory below 2 mg/100 ml. The sensitivity can be increased about twenty times by introducing a radioactively labelled 'anti-antibody' layer (Rowe 1969) and developing the precipitin rings by autoradiography (*radioimmunodiffusion*). Very low levels, particularly those of IgE, still have to be quantitated by *solid phase radioimmunoassay* which has a sensitivity of about 0·5 μg/100 ml. In this procedure a specific antiserum to IgE is coupled to an insoluble dextran carrier; the IgE level in the test sample is obtained by comparing its capacity to inhibit the antibody binding of radioactively labelled IgE with the inhibition produced by standard solutions of the same immunoglobulin. However, low Ig levels are prone to be overestimated by this method for two reasons. Firstly, Ig fragments containing parts of the H chains can participate in the competition for antibody sites; and, secondly, the test samples may contain factors that block antibody sites non-specifically. These pitfalls should be kept in mind, especially when external secretions are tested (Stokes et al 1973).

3:3:2 Salivary secretions

A survey of the Ig levels reported for human salivary secretions presents a diversity of results (Brandtzaeg et al 1970). This can mainly be ascribed to lack of standardization with regard to the method of fluid collection, concentration and storage, the quantitation technique, and the type of standard protein. With reference to an isolated parotid IgA preparation, Brandtzaeg et al (1970) reported that stimulated parotid secretions from nine healthy subjects on the average contained 3·95 mg IgA/100 ml (Table 3.2.) The observed range was 1·70–6·29. In a subsequent study of

Table 3.2 Immunoglobulin levels of human parotid secretions and whole saliva*

Samples	Concentrations (mg/100 ml ± S.D.)			Secretion rate of IgA (μg/min/gland ± S.D.)	Conc. ratios	
	IgG	IgM	IgA		IgG:IgM	IgG:IgA
Stimulated parotid secretion (9)†	0·036 ± 0·030	0·043 ± 0·036	3·95 ± 1·37	27·2 ± 8·7	0·84	0·009
'Unstimulated' parotid secretion (5)	N.D.‡	N.D.	11·96 ± 4·83	10·0 ± 6·6	N.D.	N.D.
'Unstimulated' whole saliva from:						
Normal individuals (8)	1·44 ± 0·90	0·21 ± 0·19	19·40 ± 5·37	N.D.	6·86	0·07
Periodontitis patients (13)	6·97 ± 3·36	0·76 ± 0·54	37·14 ± 22·47	N.D.	9·17	0·19

* Data from Brandtzaeg *et al* (1970) and Brandtzaeg (1971e).
† Number of individuals in parentheses.
‡ Not determined.

44 healthy adults, Oon & Lee (1973) found a normal distribution of the parotid IgA levels, and there was no significant difference between males and females. At least 90% of the parotid IgA normally consists of SC-containing 11S dimers and larger polymers (Brandtzaeg et al 1970). In agar-gel immunoelectrophoresis it migrates like amylase and definitely more slowly than serum IgA (Fig. 3.5A). In conventional disc electrophoresis (7% polyacrylamide) it is separated into three fractions as a result of size heterogeneity (Fig. 3.5B); the major band represents 11S molecules while the two minor bands close to the cathode represent larger polymers (Brandtzaeg et al 1970).

Although IgA accounts for less than 3% of the total protein of parotid

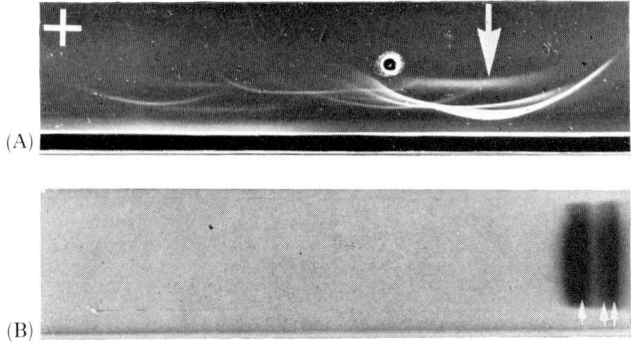

Fig. 3.5. A, immunoelectrophoresis of human parotid secretion developed with a corresponding rabbit antiserum; arrow indicates the IgA line. B, disc electrophoresis of purified parotid IgA; size heterogeneity is indicated by banding (arrows). Modified from: Brandtzaeg et al 1970.

secretions (Brandtzaeg 1971e), its concentration normally is at least 100 times that of IgG (Table 3.2). The parotid IgA : IgG ratio is thus on the average more than 400 times increased compared with the same ratio in serum. A smaller but distinct increase is also observed for the IgM : IgG ratio, indicating that both IgA and IgM are selectively transmitted through glandular epithelium. IgD has so far not been detected in parotid secretions, whereas the level of IgE has been reported to be 0·1–1·0 μg/100 ml, suggesting a selective external transfer (Bennich & Johansson 1971). However, recent studies have indicated that these data are based on artificial overestimation (Stokes et al 1973). The same applies to the surprisingly high levels of whole saliva IgE estimated by solid phase radioimmunoassay (Özkaragöz et al 1972). Subsequent measurements based on radioimmunodiffusion (Waldman et al 1973) have substantiated that the mechanism underlying the transmission of small amounts of IgE into saliva is by no means comparable with the active glandular transfer of IgA and IgM.

The Ig content of saliva is highly dependent on the flow of fluid; 'unstimulated' parotid secretions thus contain about three times more IgA than stimulated (Table 3.2). It is, therefore, of little value to quantitate salivary IgA levels without taking the flow rate into consideration. Some investigators have tried to avoid this problem by reporting parotid IgA in mg/100 mg of total protein; but this is very misleading as the secretory responses of the various parotid components are quite different. Upon gustatory stimulation the average secretion rate (μg/min/gland) increases about 16 times for amylase, about 5 times for lactoferrin and free SC, and only about 2·5 times for IgA (Brandtzaeg 1971e). The profile of total protein is largely influenced by the concentration of amylase which is a major constituent of the fluid. Relating the level of parotid IgA to the level of total protein is hence no compensation for the influence of flow rate, but rather adds to the confusion. It would be advantageous to report the output of all parotid proteins in secretion rates (μg/min/gland). Stimulated fluid is probably preferable as a test sample since it is more easily collected and less adversely affected by storage than unstimulated. With continuous gustatory stimulation the parotid IgA level remains fairly constant for more than 1 hour; when the stimulus is removed the concentration will generally, after a few minutes, reach the original 'unstimulated' level, but the secretion rate remains relatively high at least for 15 minutes of rest (Brandtzaeg 1971e).

Quantitation of Ig in whole saliva poses additional problems. Firstly, the contributions to this fluid from the minor, submandibular and parotid glands vary greatly according to the rate of flow (Kerr 1961). Secondly, the flow rate of whole saliva cannot be so accurately measured as that of the parotid secretion. Thirdly, the fluid has to be cleared by centrifugation before quantitation, and this may introduce a variable loss of Ig. Despite these disadvantages, whole saliva is commonly used as a 'representative' external secretion because it is easily obtained. To increase its volume chewing of paraffin has commonly been chosen for secretory stimulation. This should definitely be avoided, however, since the wax adsorbs organic material, and the chewing enhances leakage of plasma proteins into the oral cavity. While the 7S fraction of parotid IgA has been estimated to be about 10%, it is 13–17% in unstimulated whole saliva, depending on the state of the mucosa (Brandtzaeg et al 1970). The relative concentration of IgG is also significantly increased in whole saliva (Table 3.2), and this is a function of the degree and extent of gingival inflammation (Brandtzaeg et al 1970). Hence, the extraglandular contribution of Ig can in the main be ascribed to the admixture of crevicular fluid. Gingival health, therefore, must be

Table 3.3 Antimicrobial activities associated with salivary IgA

Antigens	Antibody determinations*	References
Blood-group substances†	N+(1)‡	1. Tomasi et al 1965
Diphtheria toxoid	P−(2,3)	2. Newcomb et al 1969
Enterobacter	N±(4)	3. Sirisinha &
Enterococcus	N+(5)	Charupatana 1970
Escherichia coli	N+(4,5,6)	4. McClelland et al 1972
Klebsiella	N+(4)	5. Sirisinha &
Pneumococcus	N+(7)	Charupatana 1971
Proteus	N±(4)	6. Tourville et al 1968
Providencia	N±(4)	7. Mouton et al 1970
Pseudomonas aeruginosa	N±(4)	8. Williams &
Salmonella typhosa	N+(3)	Gibbons 1972
Salmonella paratyphosa	P+(3)	9. Waldman et al 1968
Serratia marcescence	N−(4)	10. Mann et al 1968
Streptococcus	N+(5,8)	11. Nakao et al 1970,
Tetanus toxoid	P−(3)	Chiba & Nakao 1972
Veillonella	N+(5)	12. Berger et al 1967
Vibrio cholerae	P−(3)	13. Douglas et al 1967
Influenza virus	N±(9)	14. Chilgren et al 1967
Influenza virus inactivated	P±(10)	
Mumps virus	I+(11)	
Poliovirus	N+(12)	
Poliovirus inactivated	P±(3)	
Rhinovirus	I+(13)	
Candida albicans	I+(14)	

* N = in normal subjects
  P = after parenteral vaccination
  I = after infectious disease
  + = definite antibody titre
  ± = antibody detected in some samples
  − = no detectable antibody titre
† Included because of cross-reactions with microbial antigens
‡ References 1–14

considered when whole saliva levels of different Ig classes are determined. There is also some evidence of Ig fragmentation in this fluid, which may additionally interfere with immunological quantitation (Brandtzaeg et al

1970). Moreover, storage of whole saliva for 1 year at −20°C severely reduces measurable Ig concentrations (Brandtzaeg et al 1970). In the light of all these pitfalls the utmost caution should be exercised in the interpretation of quantitative data based on samples of whole saliva.

It is difficult to evaluate the numerous early reports on antibodies present in whole saliva; the responsible Igs could have been derived from gland-associated immunocytes, gingival immunocytes, or the blood. Recently antibodies to a great variety of microbial antigens have been reported to be carried specifically by salivary IgA (Table 3.3), although in most studies a definite identification as secretory IgA has not been accomplished. It appears from the table that antibody titres normally are found chiefly to antigens expected to be represented in the oral microbiota; and that parenteral immunization is an inefficient way of inducing a salivary IgA response. This is in agreement with findings from other mucosal sites demonstrating that topical application of antigen is the most potent stimulus for glandular IgA synthesis (Hanson & Brandtzaeg 1973). It is not known, however, how an antigen present on the oral mucosa can reach the rather remote major salivary glands and induce an immune response there. Much work hence remains to be done before manipulation of the salivary immune system can be visualized. It is possible that synthesis of IgA antibodies in the major salivary glands depends on dissemination of pre-stimulated immunocytes from other tissue sites, mainly the gut and the tonsils. That this indeed can occur is indicated by the presence in human colostrum of secretory IgA antibodies whose glandular synthesis is hardly a result of local antigen stimulation.

No reported attempt has been made to relate specific antibacterial IgA titres in saliva to the severity of *dental caries* or *periodontal inflammation*. Quantitations of total salivary IgA in relation to these diseases have provided contradictory results (Table 3.4), which probably reflects the technical difficulties discussed above. Accumulation of dental plaque, especially when combined with enhanced antigen absorption through inflamed gingivae, may conceivably lead to an intensified glandular immune response and a raised level of salivary IgA in periodontal disease. There is, on the other hand, some evidence to indicate that a lowered level of salivary IgA may be associated with decreased resistance to infection (Brasher & Deiterman 1972). Some of the findings in Table 3.4 are based on technically better investigations than others, yet it is impossible to claim that the observed negative association between salivary IgA output and caries susceptibility represents a true cause–effect relationship.

There are few reports on salivary Ig levels and antibody titres in relation to other oral diseases. In *Sjögren's syndrome* the minute quantities of parotid fluid that can be collected have been found to contain relatively more IgG than whole saliva from control subjects (Bluestone et al 1972); and an apparent correlation between the serum and parotid IgG levels indicated that this immunoglobulin had entered the secretion by passive diffusion through damaged secretory structures. An increased albumin content of the parotid fluid may be a still better indicator of protein leakage. In *cystic fibrosis*, a disease that can affect the salivary glands, the

Table 3.4 Quantitation of salivary IgA levels in relation to dental caries and periodontitis

Condition	Secretion*	IgA level	References
Caries	PS	Normal	Shklair et al 1969
Caries	PS	Normal	Zengo et al 1971
Caries	PS	Normal	Serre et al 1972
Caries	PS	Lowered	Örstavik & Brandtzaeg 1975
Caries	SMS	Lowered	Zengo et al 1971
Caries	WS	Lowered	Lehner et al 1967
Caries	WS	Lowered†	Everhart et al 1972
Caries	WS	Normal	Shklair et al 1969
Caries	WS	Normal	Sims 1972
Caries	WS	Raised‡	Everhart et al 1972
Caries	WS	Raised	Serre et al 1972
Periodontitis	PS	Normal	Lindstrom & Folke 1968
Periodontitis	PS	Raised	Chandler et al 1972
Periodontitis	PS	Raised	Örstavik & Brandtzaeg 1975
Periodontitis	WS	Raised	Lindstrom & Folke 1968
Periodontitis	WS	Raised	Brandtzaeg et al 1970

* PS, parotid secretion; SMS, submandibular gland secretion; and WS, whole saliva
† Younger age group
‡ Older age group

IgA concentration of submandibular secretions has been reported to be two to three times increased (Gugler et al 1968), whereas the parotid concentration apparently is normal (South et al 1967). Neither of the studies included determinations of secretion rates, but it was noted that the average flow of submandibular fluid was decreased in the patients. Whether the raised submandibular IgA level should be ascribed to the reduced flow rate, a high serum level of IgA, or intensified immunoglobulin synthesis in the affected glands, remains to be evaluated. During natural *mumps* with *parotitis* there is a rise of the virus-neutralizing antibody titre in the saliva of most patients (Nakao *et al* 1970). The titre usually reaches a maximum when inflammation subsides; the antibodies are chiefly of the IgA class although some may belong to IgG, at least in whole saliva (Chiba & Nakao 1972). It has not been possible to detect a general defect in the local synthesis of IgA in patients with *mucocutaneous candidosis*; but the parotid IgA of some patients may be specifically deficient in antibodies to *C. albicans* (Chilgren *et al* 1967). There is some evidence to indicate that a low capacity to produce IgA antibodies may predispose to complications and recurrence of *herpes simplex infection* (Tokumaru 1966), and especially for the development of intraoral lesions (Greenberg & Brightman 1969). However, these studies were based on quantitation of serum rather than of salivary IgA.

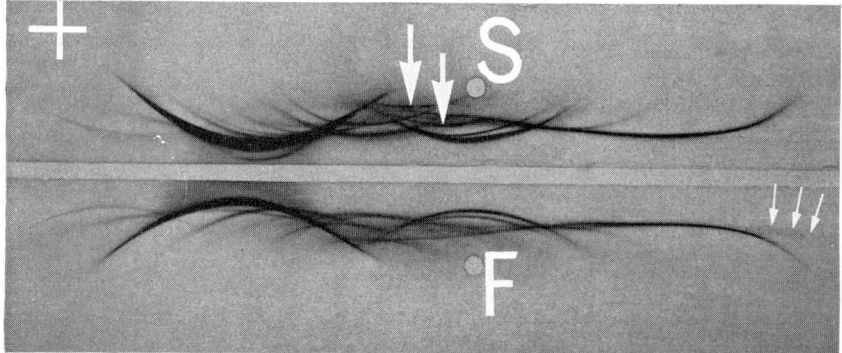

Fig. 3.6. Immunoelectrophoresis of serum (S) and a crevicular fluid sample (F) from the same patient developed with an antiserum to human serum. Only a few serum components are absent from the fluid (large arrows). The crevicular IgG exhibits fragmentation (small arrows).

3:3:3 Gingival crevicular fluid

The requirement for sample volume has limited Ig studies of crevicular fluid to cases with overt gingival inflammation. Both semiquantitative (Brandtzaeg 1965a) and quantitative (Holmberg & Killander 1971) determinations of IgG, IgA and IgM have indicated that these proteins are present in the fluid in about the same proportions and concentrations as in serum. This also applies to IgE (cited from Bennich & Johansson 1971), whereas IgD has not been examined. These findings along with a reported level of total protein similar to that of serum (Bang & Cimasoni 1971) strongly suggest that crevicular fluid should be considered an exudate;

and with the exception of some components, its immunoelectrophoretic protein pattern does indeed mimic that of serum (Fig. 3.6).

It may be argued that vascular and epithelial trauma during sample collection enhance extravasation thereby altering the composition of the crevicular fluid. However, Ig quantitation of unstimulated whole saliva substantiates that the 'resting' gingival crevice may transmit significant amounts of IgG. Table 3.5 demonstrates that the level of this immunoglobulin in saliva is best correlated with the sum of the periodontal index scores multiplied by the serum IgG concentration. This means that the transfer of IgG into the oral cavity takes place chiefly through the gingival crevice as a function of the degree and extent of periodontal inflammation with a superimposed influence of the serum IgG level. Also whole-saliva IgM is significantly correlated with similar factors (Table 3.5) as only minute amounts are derived from the salivary glands. The correlation coefficients listed for whole-saliva IgA, on the other hand, are not statistically significant. This is not surprising since merely 7% of the latter

Table 3.5 Influence of the immunoglobulin level in serum and the degree of gingival inflammation on the concentrations of IgG, IgM and IgA in whole saliva

Variables	Serum Ig	$\overline{PI}$	Σ PI	Serum Ig X $\overline{PI}$	Serum Ig X Σ PI
Salivary IgG	−0·013*	0·805	0·810	0·816	0·845
Salivary IgM	0·559	0·762	0·799	0·796	0·893
Salivary IgA	0·377	0·324	0·305	0·329	0·391

Ig, Immunoglobulins
$\overline{PI}$, average periodontal index score in a patient
Σ PI, sum of periodontal index scores in a patient
* Coefficient of correlation
Modified from Brandtzaeg *et al* 1970

immunoglobulin can be accounted for by extraglandular transmission, even in patients with periodontal inflammation (Brandtzaeg *et al* 1970). The estimate of this fraction is valid only if IgA contributed by the crevicular fluid is of the 7S monomeric type, an assumption that is supported by several findings. Firstly, SC can neither be detected in the fluid (Brandtzaeg *et al* 1970; Holmberg & Killander 1971) nor in the crevicular epithelium (Brandtzaeg 1972b); crevicular IgA, therefore, is not a secretory immunoglobulin. Secondly, the majority of the IgA immunocytes present in the inflamed gingivae have by a recently developed technique been shown to be monomer producers (Brandtzaeg 1973c, 1974d). Thirdly, about 90% of the serum IgA is monomeric, and this probably is the chief source of crevicular IgA.

Subsequent quantitations of a limited number of samples with a very sensitive SRID technique have indicated that there is some selectivity according to molecular size in the transfer of Igs into the crevicular fluid (Brandtzaeg 1972b). Thus, careful comparison with the serum of each patient demonstrated that the fluid is relatively deficient in IgA and especially in IgM. Furthermore, for one sample it could be estimated that 17% IgG and 7–8% IgA were contributed by local synthesis in the gingiva. Such distinctions between serum and the fluid are obviously prone to be masked because of trauma to the vascular bed adjacent to the crevicular epithelium. It is in full agreement with recent studies of other inflammatory fluids (Kushner & Sommerville 1971), however, that molecular sieving and local synthesis may change the protein composition in favour of IgG. In direct contrast with this view, Shillitoe & Lehner (1972) reported that the level of IgG in crevicular fluid is relatively more lowered than those of IgA and IgM. There is at present no explanation for this discrepancy; but it should be pointed out that several difficulties are involved in such studies. The proteolytic activity of crevicular fluid may produce Ig fragments (Fig. 3.6) which in different ways may invalidate immunological quantitation. An enzyme inhibitor, such as ϵ-amino-caproic acid, should therefore be added to the samples, and a check for Ig fragmentation should be done before quantitative analyses are performed. A possible sample contamination of salivary IgA must be excluded by tests with antiserum to SC.

Antibody activities have as yet not been reported for the crevicular fluid. Some bacteria from dental plaque are coated with IgA (Brandtzaeg et al 1968b), and IgG, IgA and IgM have been detected in sections of dental plaque (Schwartz & Gibson 1973); but the Igs may well be passively adsorbed and are, apparently, also incorporated in the enamel pellicle (Örstavik et al 1973). The detection of complement factors in the fluid (Brandtzaeg 1966; Shillitoe & Lehner 1972; Larsson et al 1973) along with IgG and IgM indicates a potential for biological amplification of antigen-antibody reactions which may occur in the gingival crevice. There is also some experimental suggestion that certain salivary substances may interact directly with the complement factors (Boackle & Pruitt 1973).

3:3:4 Jaw cyst fluid

Igs of cysts were first studied by Toller & Holborow (1969), who emphasized the predominance of IgA both in the fluid and in the plasma cells detected in the walls. However, if one unusual case is excluded, recalculation of their data for the remaining 18 gives mean cyst : serum ratios of 2·3 : 1, 2·1 : 1 and 1·8 : 1 for IgG, IgA and IgM respectively. Thus, the Igs generally occur in the fluid in about the same proportions as in serum (with a slight change disfavouring IgA and especially IgM); but their concentrations are on the average raised about 100%. In addition to

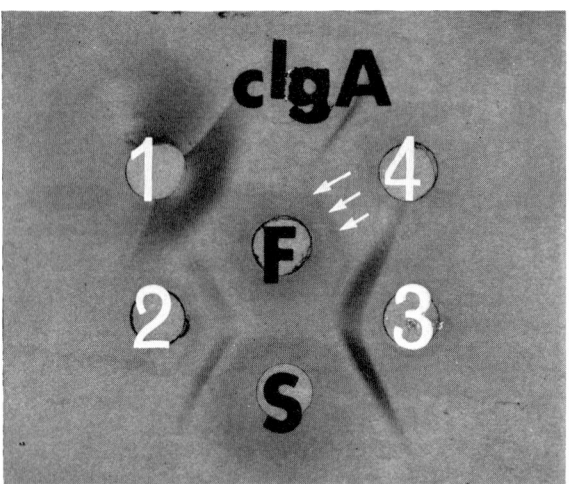

Fig. 3.7. Double-diffusion analyses of serum (S) and maxillary cyst fluid (F) from the same patient. Antisera: 1, anti-IgG; 2, anti-IgM; 3, anti-IgA; and 4, anti-SC. Traces of secretory IgA are present in the fluid as indicated by a faint precipitin line (arrows) fusing with that formed by colostral IgA (cIgA).

filtration from serum, therefore, Igs are most likely contributed by local synthesis, as supported by the finding that the Ig level may be relatively more raised than the albumin level (Brandtzaeg, unpublished). Most of the IgA appears to be monomeric, but traces of secretory IgA may be present, at least in some maxillary cysts (Fig. 3.7). This may either be ascribed to contamination by respiratory secretions, or a part of the wall may have secretory epithelial lining and contain a small population of dimer-producing IgA immunocytes. However, immunofluorescence examination of a limited number of cyst walls has indicated that the local immunocyte population in most areas is dominated by IgG cells (Brandtzaeg, unpublished). This agrees with the relatively high concentration of IgG in most cyst fluids. It is possible that the technical difficulties inherent in a proper enumeration of IgG cells (Brandtzaeg 1974a; Lai A Fat *et al* 1974) may have led Toller & Holborow (1969) to overestimate the proportion of IgA cells.

The stimulus for the local production of Igs in cyst walls is obscure, since the investigations cited above were carried out on apparently uninfected material. The recent observation (Skaug 1973) that IgG present in some cyst fluids may exhibit a 'monoclonal' electrophoretic pattern strongly suggests that a local antigenic stimulus is involved. Toller (1971) has speculated that there may be a local immune response against the occult epithelium, or against its breakdown products. This could explain the fact that small cysts may disappear spontaneously when infection is eliminated.

3:4 Immunoglobulins of Oral Tissues

3:4:1 Methods of detection

The simplest way to examine the content of Igs in a tissue is by *extraction*. The extract can be analysed either directly with techniques such as immunoelectrophoresis, double diffusion and SRID; or antisera produced against it will in similar tests reflect its antigenic composition. This is exemplified in Fig. 3.8, which shows immunoelectrophoretic analyses of a gingival extract and of the corresponding rabbit antiserum (Brandtzaeg & Fjellanger 1965). Two major precipitin arcs representing albumin and IgG appear when the extract reacts with an antiserum to human serum (Fig. 3.8A). The IgG line is distinctly split, however, indicating that proteolytic activity has produced Fab fragments which migrate more slowly than the intact immunoglobulin. The anti-extract reagent forms several precipitin lines with human plasma, those of albumin and IgG still dominating (Fig. 3.8B). This proves that these two components are the major serum proteins present in the gingiva. At least four tissue-specific antigens are demonstrated by the same reagent when its antibodies to plasma have been removed by absorption (Fig. 3.8C).

Although useful information may be obtained from analyses of tissue extracts, the results with regard to Igs are difficult to interpret. It is not possible to differentiate between Ig components derived from contaminating blood, from the extravascular compartment, or from local immunocytes. Moreover, antigenicity and size of the molecules may be severely altered because of enzymatic activities. Another approach is to identify immunologically radioactive proteins of the supernatant fluid from *tissue cultures* grown in a medium containing radioactively labelled amino acids, e.g. ^{14}C L-lysine and ^{14}C L-isoleucine. The results give an impression of the tissue's capacity for protein synthesis. Thus, in autoradiographs the densities of

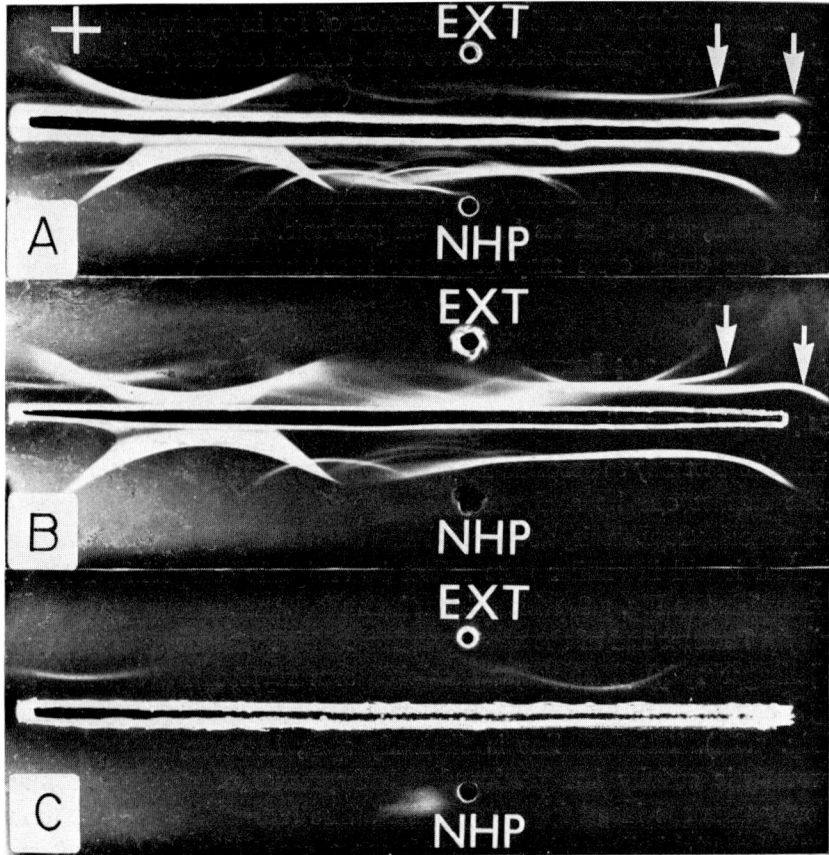

Fig. 3.8. Immunoelectrophoresis of an extract of human gingival tissue (EXT) and normal human plasma (NHP) developed with A, antiserum to human serum; B, antiserum to gingival homogenate; and C, antiserum to gingival homogenate absorbed with human plasma. Note fragmentation of IgG present in the extract (arrows).

precipitin lines representing the various Ig classes reflect the local population of Ig-producing immunocytes. The distribution of these cells within the tissue remains unknown, however, and a possible contamination by products of blood-borne immunocytes cannot be excluded. Examination of tissue sections by *immunofluorescence technique*, therefore, is often the method of choice. Firstly, the extravascular distribution of diffusible serum-derived or locally formed Igs can be studied on a semiquantitative basis (Brandtzaeg 1974a). Secondly, Ig-containing immunocytes can be counted and their distribution correlated with morphological features. The number of Ig-positive cells appears to be a valid expression of the local synthesis since such results are in good agreement with those obtained by tissue culture technique (Lai A Fat *et al* 1974). Immunofluorescence is hence a powerful tool by which various aspects of the local Ig supply can be studied; and most of the information given in the following sections has been obtained with this method. Although simple in principle, it is in practice a difficult technique, however, which presents many pitfalls, especially when used on tissue sections. It seems justified, therefore, to consider the major technical points in some detail.

The *direct method* is outlined to the left in Fig. 3.9; a particular antigen is traced in a tissue section by means of the corresponding antibody preparation conjugated with a fluorescent dye (*fluorochrome*). The name

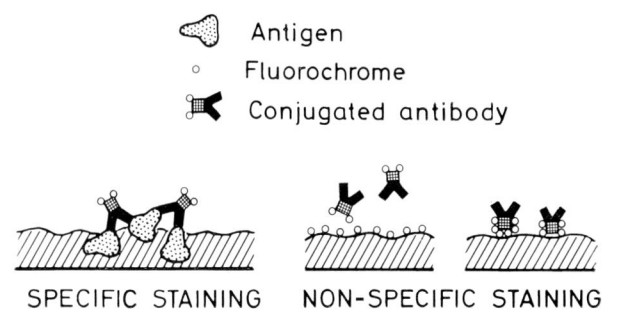

Fig. 3.9. Schematic representation of specific immunofluorescence staining (to the left), and non-specific staining due to free fluorochrome molecules (centre) or over-coupled protein (to the right).

'*fluorescent antibody technique*' has hence been commonly used. In the *indirect method* an unlabelled antiserum is first applied, and thereafter a labelled 'anti-antibody'. A similar principle ('*sandwich technique*') can also be used to visualize the antibody activity of cells; the section is first incubated with the relevant antigen and next with the corresponding conjugated antibody preparation. Antibody activity of sera or secretions can likewise be detected and titrated by the indirect method; a relevant substrate (e.g. a bacterial smear) is first incubated with serial dilutions of the body fluid, and then a fluorescent anti-Ig ('*antiglobulin*') reagent is applied. In all these situations the micro-precipitate, formed at sites of antigen–antibody combination, will act as a minute 'lamp' since the fluorochrome emits light of a longer wavelength than the excitation light to which it is exposed in the microscope. The two commonly used fluorochromes are *fluorescein isothiocyanate* (*FITC*), which emits green light upon excitation with blue or ultraviolet, and *tetramethylrhodamine isothiocyanate* (*MRITC*), which emits red light upon excitation with green. The use of interference filters in fluorescence microscopy (Faulk & Hijmans 1972) makes it possible to reveal selectively the reaction sites of 'green' and 'red' conjugates with different antibody specificities (Fig. 3.13); two antigenic components can hence be demonstrated simultaneously in a tissue section ('*double tracing*' or '*paired staining*'). The same principle can be applied for combinations of the direct and the indirect method; thus the Ig class of an immunocyte can be directly visualized by one colour

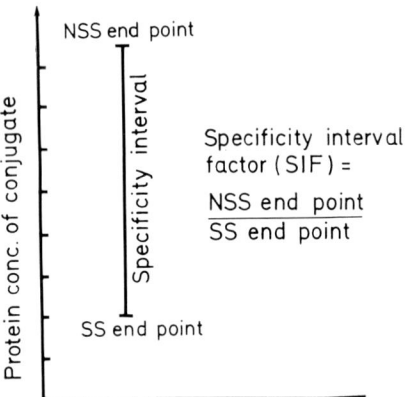

Fig. 3.10. The specific binding properties of a fluorescent conjugate depend on the magnitude of its specificity interval factor (SIF). The specificity interval represents the range of concentrations that can be expected to produce only immunological binding with the substrate. NSS, non-specific staining; SS, specific staining.

while its antibody activity is indirectly signified by the other (Brandtzaeg 1974a).

It is now generally accepted that the *immunological specificity* of a conjugate must be ascertained by immunofluorescence performance tests on appropriate substrates (Brandtzaeg 1972a, 1973b). Immunoelectrophoresis and double-diffusion are not sufficiently sensitive to reveal contaminating antibodies. Moreover, only immunofluorescence can truly disclose unwanted reactions due to non-precipitating antibodies or soluble immune complexes present in the conjugate. Another major source of error is lack of *binding specificity*. Since the fluorochromes are negatively charged, a high degree of labelling may reduce the isoelectric point of the conjugate proteins to such an extent that they combine with positive tissue elements because of electrostatic interactions (Fig. 3.9, to the right). Free fluorochrome remaining in the reagent may similarly result in non-specific staining (Fig. 3.9, in the centre). Leukocytes, particularly the eosinophilic granulocytes, as well as squamous epithelium are especially prone to become stained by 'over-coupled' proteins and free dye molecules (Brandtzaeg 1973b).

A fluorescent antibody preparation of good quality gives rise to non-specific staining (NSS) only at high protein concentrations, but still produces specific staining (SS) at low concentrations; such a conjugate has a wide '*specificity interval*' (Fig. 3.10) and consequently a high '*specificity interval factor*' (Brandtzaeg 1973b). This factor (SIF) can be increased in

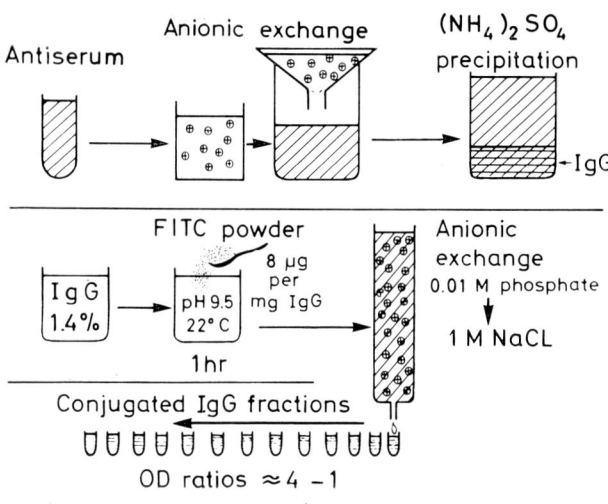

Fig. 3.11. Procedure for fluorochrome (FITC) conjugation of IgG purified from rabbit antiserum. Defined conjugate fractions can be obtained by anionic-exchange chromatography. Details are discussed in the text.

two ways: firstly, by using high-titred antisera; and, secondly, by removing 'over-coupled' and 'under-coupled' protein as well as free and loosely bound dye molecules. Conjugate fractions with molar fluorochrome to protein (F/P) ratios of 1–3 may be selected by anionic-exchange chromatography; if the antibody titre allows them to be used at a protein concentration ('*working dilution*') below 1 mg/ml non-specific phenomena due to electrostatic interactions pose no problem (Brandtzaeg 1973b).

A simple procedure for the production of optimum conjugate fractions is outlined in Fig. 3.11 (Brandtzaeg 1973a). The IgG of the antiserum is first isolated by batch adsorption with DEAE-Sephadex A-50, and further purified and concentrated by precipitation with ammonium sulphate. It is important to obtain IgG which appears pure in immunoelectrophoresis, since other serum proteins contaminating the preparation easily become over-coupled. The IgG concentration is adjusted to 1·2–1.6% and a small amount of fluorochrome powder is added. Optimum conjugation is usually attained with about 8 µg FITC or 35–40 µg MRITC per mg IgG. The coupling reaction should proceed for 1 hour at room temperature with continuous stirring and control of pH. The latter must be held between 9·45 and 9·55 by adjustments with 0·1 N NaOH. After subsequent equilibration against 0·01 M phosphate buffer by dialysis overnight, the conjugate can be fractionated by anionic-exchange chromatography. (MRITC conjugates must first be filtered through Sephadex G-50 to remove certain dye molecules which are not retained by the anionic exchanger.) The fractions eluted with 0·04–0·1 M NaCl added to the phosphate buffer usually have the best staining properties.

The requirements with regard to sensitivity level and specificity interval should be kept in mind when conjugates are produced and the chromatographic fractions selected. The highest dilution giving satisfactory fluorescence intensity, as well as the immunological specificity of each preparation, has to be established by performance testing on appropriate substrates. The binding specificity of the selected conjugate at its working dilution must be ascertained by antiserum blocking or, preferably, by antigen absorption in excess. Lack of fluorescence in such controls is no proof of immunological specificity, however, since the blocking and absorbing reagents may contain the same unwanted activities as the conjugate. Suggestive information about the immunofluorescence properties of the conjugate can be obtained in advance by measuring its *precipitating activity* and determining spectrophotometrically its *protein concentration* and *optical density (OD) ratio* (Brandtzaeg 1973a). This ratio is calculated by dividing the OD measured at 280 nm by the OD measured at the absorption maximum for the conjugated fluorochrome; it is recommended as a reproducible index of the conjugation degree. The above characteristics of the employed reagents should be stated when immunofluorescence observations are communicated. Details about the conjugates presently used in the author's laboratory can be found in recent publications (Brandtzaeg 1973b, 1974a).

3:4:2 Major salivary glands

IgG is normally the predominant Ig component of interstitial fluid in the salivary glands. This can be demonstrated by immunofluorescence of specimens in which the total protein content has been precipitated by alcohol fixation (Brandtzaeg 1974a). The brightest staining is related to vessel walls and basement membrane zones of epithelial structures (Fig. 3.12A). Similar distributions are found for IgA (Fig. 3.12B) and IgM (Fig. 3.12C), but signified by less intense staining. Most IgG contained in the extravascular pool is probably derived from serum, since cultures of

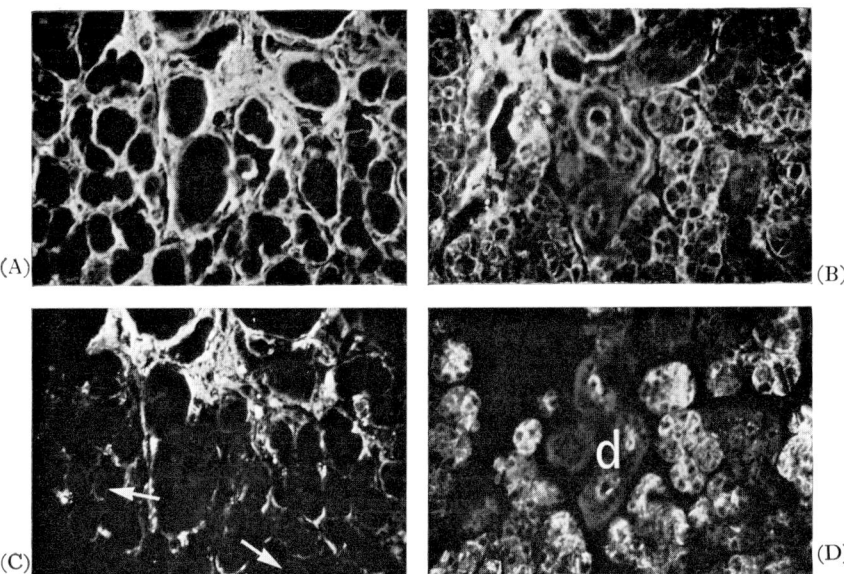

Fig. 3.12. Immunohistochemical demonstration of IgG (*A*), IgA (*B*), IgM (*C*) and SC (*D*), comparable fields in neighbouring sections of directly alcohol-fixed normal submandibular gland tissue. IgG dominates in the connective tissue ground substance and basement membranes, but is undetectable in most acini and ducts. IgA is present in several immunocytes which generally are masked by the background staining. Acini contains IgA, and traces of IgM (arrows), particularly concentrated intercellularly. SC is present in acini but absent from striated ducts (d) excepting a luminal rim. Magnification: 140 ×.

salivary glands produce only trace amounts of this immunoglobulin (Hurlimann & Zuber 1968). The same applies to IgM, whereas active IgA synthesis can be detected (Hurlimann 1971). The immunocytes responsible for the local Ig formation are generally quite masked by the diffuse background staining in directly alcohol-fixed tissue. When the diffusible proteins have been removed by washing the specimen prior to fixation (Brandtzaeg 1974a), however, the Ig-containing cells are clearly revealed against a dark background in a scattered distribution between the acini, and in groups adjacent to the striated ducts (Fig. 3.13A). As expected they are chiefly of the IgA class, with a dominance of 97% calculated for the human parotid gland (Brandtzaeg et al 1968b). IgM cells on the average slightly outnumber those containing IgG. Double tracing substantiates the phenotypic restriction of the local immunocytes; each cell contains only one Ig class (Fig. 3.13B).

Despite the distinct preponderance of IgG in the interstitial fluid, the epithelial structures are virtually devoid of this immunoglobulin in normal glands (Fig. 3.12A); but faint cytoplasmic and distinct intercellular fluorescence is commonly present for IgA, especially in acini and intercalary ducts (Fig. 3.13C, left part). Acinar staining may be more readily revealed in submandibular glands, always confined to the serous cells (Fig. 3.12D). IgM can hardly be detected in the epithelium, although occasional traces exhibit a pattern similar to that of IgA (Fig. 3.12C); this is more distinct in patients selectively lacking IgA, who have enhanced local synthesis and secretion of IgM (Brandtzaeg et al 1968b; Brandtzaeg 1971a). A very striking feature is the retention of IgA along the epithelial cell membranes after the tissue washing procedure (Fig. 3.13A); this is by contrast with the complete removal of the large amounts of extracellular IgG (Fig. 3.13B). The same observation has been made for other glands, indicating that IgA generally is bound to the membranes of secretory epithelial cells (Brandtzaeg 1974b).

Synthesis of SC has been demonstrated in cultures of human salivary glands (Hurlimann & Zuber 1968); but there are several conflicting reports with regard to its cellular origin. Tomasi et al (1965) first detected SC in parotid acinar cells by means of immunofluorescence. In a subsequent study Tourville et al (1969) found it as well in duct cells and especially in submandibular mucous-type acinar cells. Rossen et al (1968), on the other hand, reported the mucous acini to be negative whereas scattered interstitial cells in the parotid and submandibular glands were judged to contain both IgA and SC. Recently Kraus & Mestecky (1971) were unable to reveal SC in parotid acini but felt that it might be present in some duct cells. In our laboratory SC can definitely be detected only in secretory epithelial cells of the serous type; and the intensity of the specific fluorescence in specimens of salivary glands cannot be compared with that obtained for nasal and intestinal glands (Brandtzaeg 1974a,b). There is, moreover, pronounced variation between salivary glands from different individuals; this may be related to the rate of secretion at the time of biopsy. The most intense SC fluorescence seen till now for salivary glands was obtained with

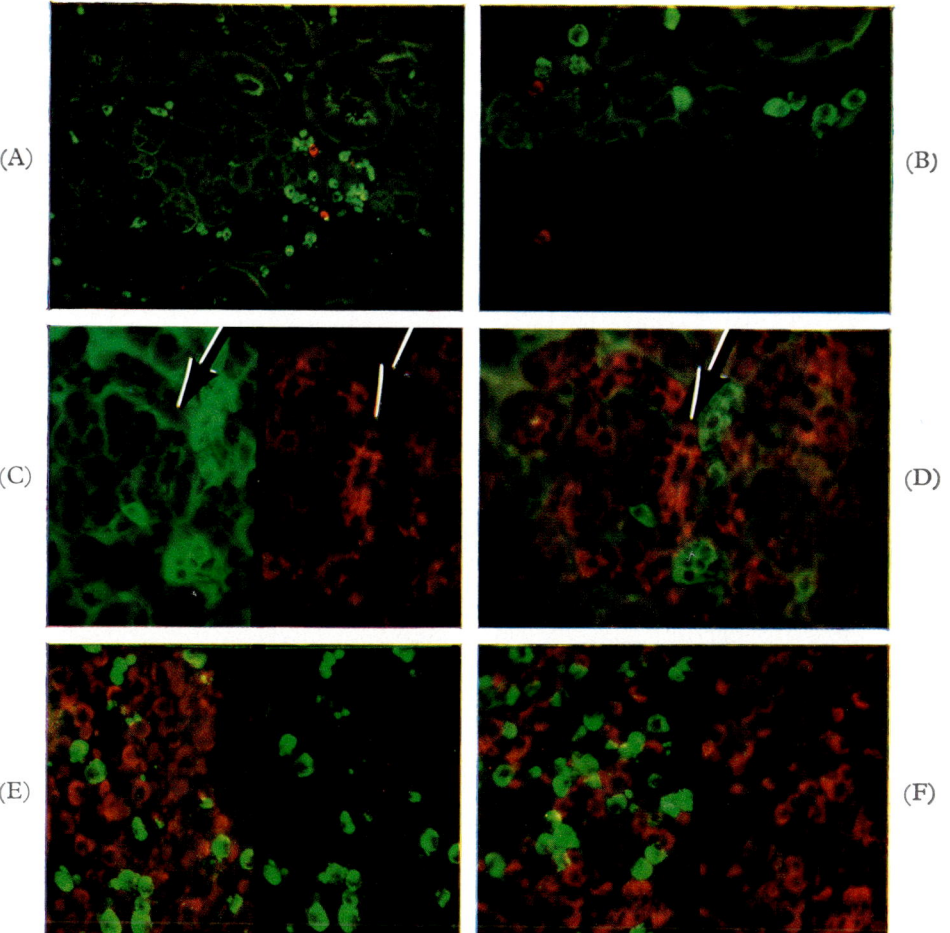

Fig. 3.13. *A*, paired staining for IgA (green) and IgM (red) in a section of washed normal submandibular tissue; note dominance of IgA immunocytes and retention of IgA along the membranes of acinar cells. *B*, paired staining for IgA (green) and IgG (red) in a section adjacent to that in *A*; note dominance of IgA immunocytes and virtually complete removal of IgG from the acinar cell membranes as demonstrated by selective red filtration of the same field (bottom). *C*, paired staining for IgA (green) and SC (red) in a section of directly alcohol-fixed normal parotid tissue; selective green filtration (left part) reveals IgA in immunocytes and diffusely in the connective tissue; acini and an intercalary duct (arrow) also contain IgA, especially related to the cell membranes; selective red filtration (right part) reveals SC exclusively in the epithelium and especially in the intercalary duct. *D*, double exposure of the same field as in *C* demonstrates that both SC and IgA (mixed colour) are present in the cell membranes and in the apical part of the secretory epithelial cells, whereas SC alone (red granules) is present in the Golgi region. *E*, paired staining for IgG (red) and IgA (green) in a section of washed gingival tissue from a patient with periodontitis; note in double exposure (left part) the dominance of IgG immunocytes adjacent to negative epithelium (upper right corner); selective green filtration of the same field (right part) substantiates absence of IgA in the IgG immunocytes. *F*, preparation like that in *E*, but from another patient with relatively more IgA immunocytes in his gingiva; selective red filtration of the same field (right part) substantiates absence of IgG in the IgA immunocytes. Original magnifications: 70× (*A*) 180× (*B–F*).

a parotid specimen from a small baby who received little gustatory or mechanical flow stimulation, since he was nourished intravenously. Variations are also noted for the different secretory elements. The intercalary duct cells generally fluoresce distinctly, whereas the parotid acinar cells may be almost negative (Fig. 3.13C, right part). In the submandibular gland serous-type acinar cells commonly are relatively more bright, with accentuation of the membranes (Fig. 3.12D). Striated duct cells are negative or at least very faintly stained; but their luminal borders are lined by a rim of fluorescent material positive for both SC and IgA (Fig. 3.12B, D). It is not possible to decide whether this is extra- or intra-cellularly. Major duct cells may or may not exhibit cytoplasmic fluorescence for SC. By paired tracing it can be shown that some SC-positive acinar cells may at the same time contain lactoferrin and amylase, while other cells may contain only one or two of these components (Brandtzaeg, unpublished).

According to our findings the overall epithelial distributions of IgA and SC hence appear quite similar, and this can be substantiated by double tracing (Fig. 3.13D). Thus, there is mixed fluorescence related to the cell membranes and in the apical part of the cytoplasm of secretory epithelial cells. However, in the Golgi region adjacent to the nuclei SC occurs alone in a granular pattern. Such differential intracellular distribution for these two components is much more readily revealed in nasal and intestinal glands (Brandtzaeg 1974a,b). It has moreover been shown that while only free SC is present in the Golgi region, the apical part of the secretory cells as well as their membranes contain SC covalently bound to dimeric IgA (Brandtzaeg 1974b). On the basis of these observations a model for the external transfer of IgA through secretory epithelia has been proposed (Fig. 3.14). It is postulated that the immunoglobulin is selectively received and bound in the cell membranes because of non-covalent affinity between SC and dimeric IgA (Brandtzaeg 1974a,b); the complexes then become mobilized and covalently stabilized and reach the cytoplasm outside the Golgi region by pinocytosis or facilitated diffusion; thereafter they are extruded into the gland lumen along general secretory pathways. Epithelial transmission of 19S IgM is probably mediated by a similar mechanism, but the formed complexes are not so stable as those of SC and dimeric IgA (Brandtzaeg 1975). An excess of free SC, as revealed both in the epithelial cells (Brandtzaeg 1974b) and in the secretions (Brandtzaeg 1971c), is probably important not only for the initial formation of the SC–Ig complexes but also for their subsequent stabilization (Brandtzaeg 1974c). The suggested receptor function of membrane-associated SC is strongly supported by *in vitro* experiments. When dimeric IgA is mixed with SC spontaneous complexing occurs (March 1970); and this also holds true for 19S IgM (Brandtzaeg 1974c). The J chain, common to dimeric IgA and 19S IgM, probably determines the affinity of these molecules for SC (Eskeland & Brandtzaeg 1974). Finally, most gland-associated IgA

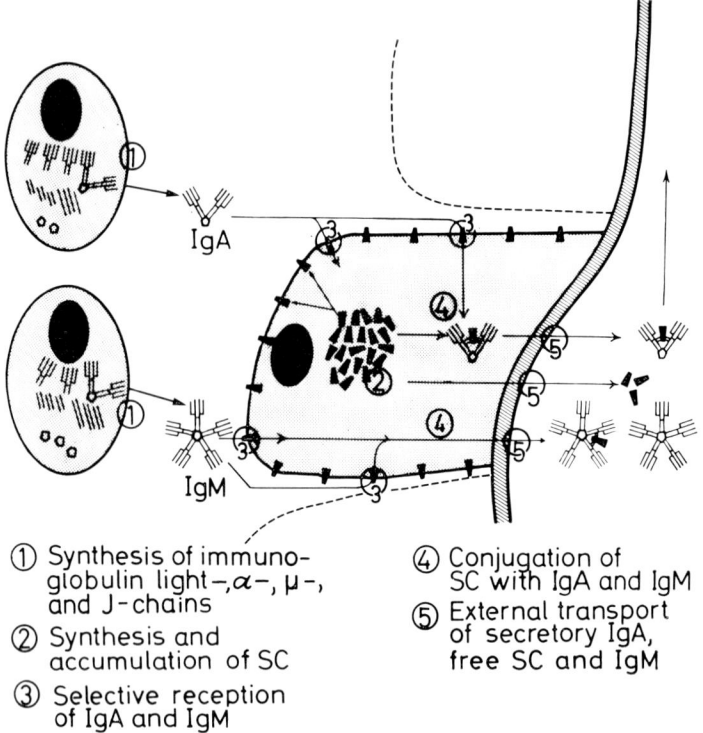

① Synthesis of immuno-globulin light–, α–, μ–, and J-chains
② Synthesis and accumulation of SC
③ Selective reception of IgA and IgM
④ Conjugation of SC with IgA and IgM
⑤ External transport of secretory IgA, free SC and IgM

Fig. 3.14. Schematic representation of gland-associated synthesis and selective external transfer of dimeric IgA and 19S IgM. It is proposed that SC acts as a specific receptor for these two immunoglobulins, and that SC–Ig complexes are formed and become mobilized and partially stabilized in the membrane of secretory epithelial cells. The completed secretory immunoglobulins finally reach the gland lumen (to the right) via the cytoplasm outside the Golgi region. While the combination of IgA with SC is efficient and gives rise to very stable complexes, this is so for only 60–70% of the IgM; the rest of the secreted IgM contains SC in a loose association which depends on an excess of free SC. From: Brandtzaeg 1974a,b.

immunocytes do indeed produce dimeric molecules which hence are readily available for external transmission by the proposed mechanism (Brandtzaeg 1973c, 1974d).

Despite the many reports on antibodies associated with salivary IgA

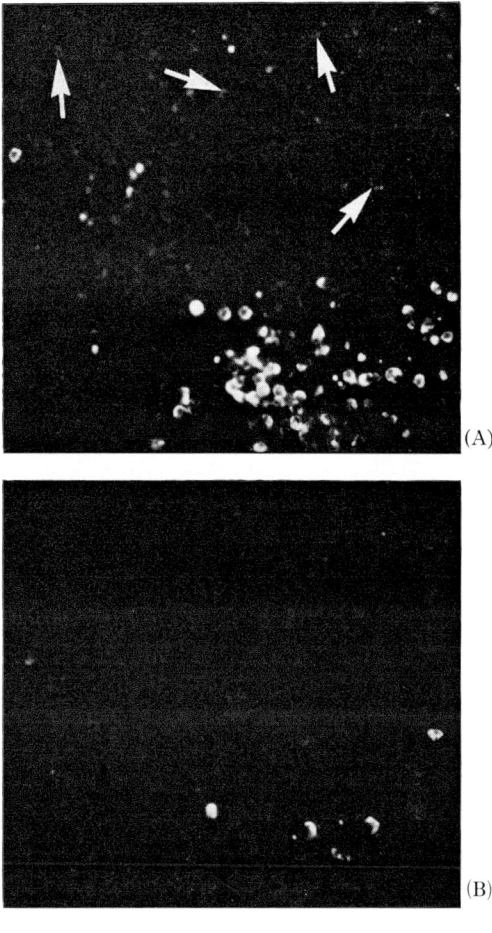

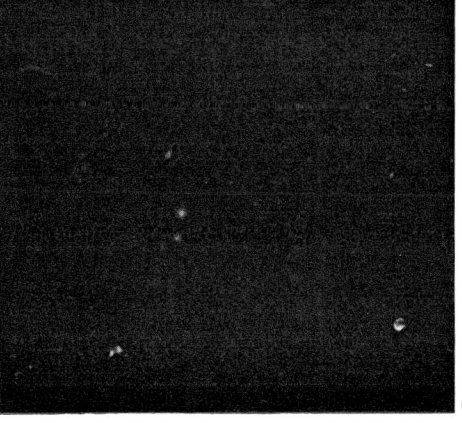

Fig. 3.15. Immunohistochemical demonstration of IgG (*A*), IgA (*B*) and IgM (*C*), comparable fields in neighbouring sections of a washed parotid specimen from a patient with Sjögren's syndrome. Note dominance of IgG immunocytes and that traces of IgG have been retained (arrows) around many of the numerous infiltrating lymphocytes. Magnification: 180 ×.

(Table 3.3), such activities have as yet not been identified in human glandular IgA immunocytes. This definitely has to be done in order to substantiate the postulated biological significance of the local immune system. Emmings & Genco (1972) were able to detect local IgA cells containing antibody to bovine albumin in rabbits whose submandibular glands had been injected with this antigen. However, when the antigen was deposited along with an adjuvant, the majority of the local antibody-containing cells were of the IgG class. We have observed the same response when insoluble antigens have been injected into the rabbit salivary glands (Brandtzaeg, unpublished). Hence, it seems to be a rule that when relatively large amounts of antigens are retained in the glandular tissue, thus representing a powerful and persistent stimulus, an IgG response associated with chronic inflammation will ensue.

It is of interest in this connection that a marked glandular synthesis of IgG regularly takes place in *Sjögren's syndrome*. This is illustrated in Fig. 3.15 for an advanced case with destruction of epithelial elements and dense lymphoid cell infiltration in the parotid gland. Although most cells are lymphocytes, considerable groups of Ig-containing immunocytes, clearly dominated by the IgG class, are also present. This agrees with observations on labial salivary glands which in cultures produce IgG, and to a lesser extent IgM, apparently as a function of the disease severity (Talal *et al* 1970). By indirect immunofluorescence technique it has been shown that about 50% of sera from patients with Sjögren's syndrome exhibit activity to salivary duct cells, and these antibodies are chiefly of the IgG class (Feltkamp & Rossum 1968). It is tempting to speculate that they are synthesized locally in the affected glands because of a persistent stimulus from autoantigens; whether this humoral immune response leads to intensified or retarded gland destruction is not known (Anderson *et al* 1973). About the same percentage of the patients have circulating antibodies to altered human IgG (*'rheumatoid factors'*); and there is evidence to indicate that these are indeed locally produced (Anderson *et al* 1972), perhaps in a response to IgG antibodies complexed with a tissue antigen or with some unidentified infectious agent. Cellular immunity to salivary gland antigens is apparently also involved in Sjögren's syndrome (Berry *et al* 1972); and most likely both humoral and cellular mechanisms play a role in the pathogenesis. Many of the lymphocytes infiltrating the diseased glands are 'coated' with IgG which is not easily removed by washing (Fig. 3.15A); the possibility exists that these cells have Fc receptors and mediate cytotoxic processes upon interaction with IgG–antigen complexes.

Although IgA cells normally represent the predominant lymphoid component of salivary glands, the above findings clearly demonstrate that this is not necessarily so during disease. The origin of the IgG cells

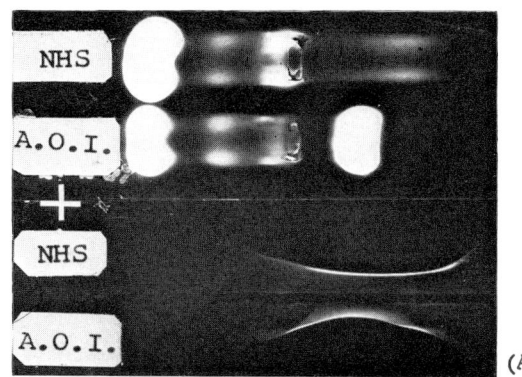

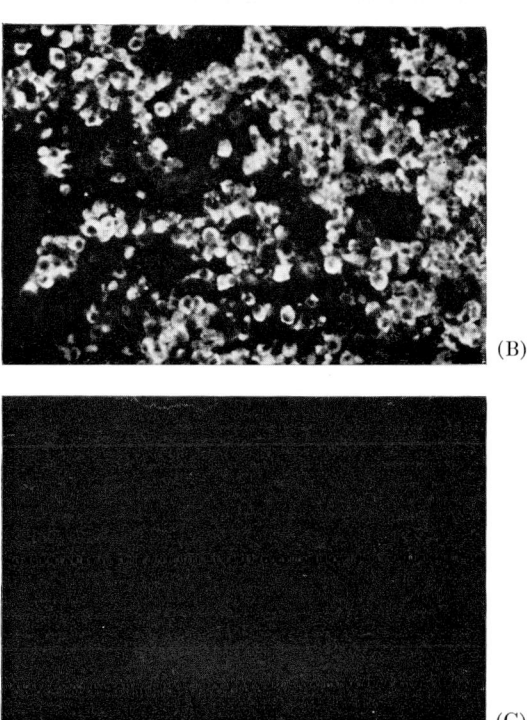

Fig. 3.16. Analyses of serum and biopsy specimen from a patient with a tumour in the parotid region. *A*, agar electrophoresis (top) of the patient's serum (A.O.I.) demonstrates a 'monoclonal' protein band contrasting the heterogeneous pattern of IgG in normal human serum (NHS); immunoelectrophoresis (bottom) developed with an antiserum to γ-chain substantiates that the monoclonal protein is IgG. *B–C*, paired immunohistochemical staining for IgG (red) and IgA (green) of a washed specimen from the tumour; red filtration (*B*) reveals numerous IgG immunocytes whereas green filtration of the same field (*C*) demonstrates complete lack of IgA immunocytes. Magnification: 210 ×.

dominating the local B-cell response in Sjögren's syndrome is not known; but most likely their precursors are seeded into the affected glands from the recirculating lymphocyte pool. As discussed in a following section this process may at least in part take place at random. Thus, in patients with co-existing Sjögren's syndrome and *Waldenström's macroglobulinaemia*, members of the malignant cell clone may appear in the salivary glands and synthesize monoclonal IgM there (Anderson *et al* 1972). It should be stressed that even for patients with monoclonal IgG in their sera, a salivary gland tumour should not be disregarded as a possible source. This is exemplified in Fig. 3.16, which shows analyses of serum and a parotid biopsy specimen from a patient who had a swelling adjacent to his left ear. Although patients with *multiple myeloma* generally have symptoms from bone-marrow lesions or kidneys, they may present with extraosseous tumours as the first signs of the disease. It is important to be able to distinguish these from the benign, so-called *primary plasmacytoma* which may occur in the oral mucosa (Martinelli & Rulli 1968), probably as a result of some chronic irritant. The malignant tumour contains virtually only one class of immunocytes (Fig. 3.16B,C), whereas more than one class is found in the benign. If a monoclonal protein can be detected in the serum, its Ig class should conform with that of the plasma cells in a malignant lesion. *Burkitt's lymphoma* is a malignant tumour that has a predilection for the jaws and commonly appears as a parotid swelling. The lymphoid cells from these tumours can in most cases be shown to carry IgM (κ) on their surface, but are apparently not secreting the immunoglobulin (Klein *et al* 1971). The clonal proliferation seems to be induced by a herpes-type virus. Although most prevalent in children of restricted areas in Africa, the disease has also been reported to occur in other parts of the world. It may be related to infectious mononucleosis, and tends to respond to chemotherapy.

3:4:3 Buccal and labial mucosa—comparison with skin

In harmony with the description for the major salivary glands, IgG is normally the predominant Ig component of the connective tissue ground substance throughout the oral mucosa. This observation is based on an immunohistochemical method that apparently preserves the total content of diffusible proteins in the specimens (Brandtzaeg 1974a). Judged from immunofluorescence intensities, the relative concentrations of IgG, IgA and IgM in the tissue fluid are high, intermediate and low respectively. Washing prior to fixation generally removes these extracellular components (Fig. 3.17A). Diffusible Igs are also present in the dermis of normal skin (Allansmith & Buell 1965), but apparently in lower concentrations than in oral mucosa and salivary gland stroma (compare fluorescence intensity of dermis in Fig. 3.18A with that of stroma in Fig. 3.12A). This may depend

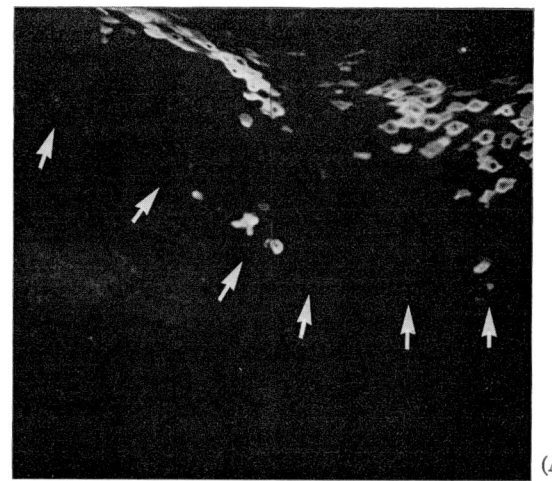

(A)

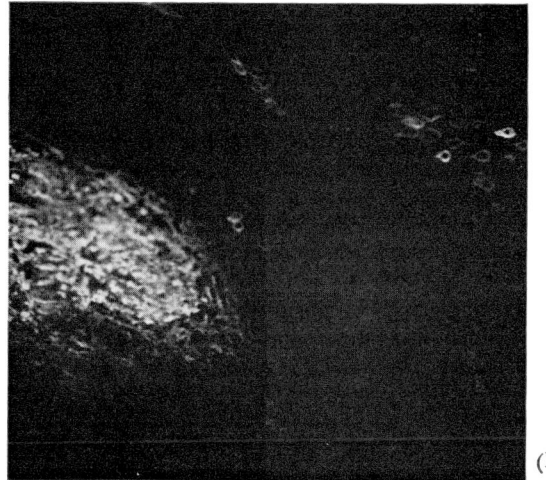

(B)

Fig. 3.17. Immunohistochemical demonstration of IgG (A), IgA (B) and SC (C), comparable fields in neighbouring sections of a washed specimen from the transition zone between normal labial mucosa (to the right) and a tumour (to the left) on the inside of the lower lip of a patient. The squamous epithelium contains cells with cytoplasmic IgG and, in lower concentrations, IgA. The connective tissue beneath the basement membrane (arrows) is devoid of Igs except for an accumulation of IgA (and SC) in the area of the mucosal swelling. Magnification: 70 ×.

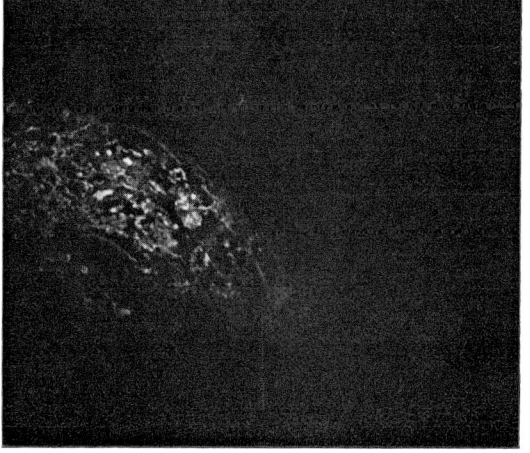

(C)

on differences in vascularity, since the Igs of these tissues, with the exception of secretory IgA, normally must be derived almost exclusively from the blood. It has been calculated that while most serum IgM (76%) is remains in the intravascular space, the majority of IgG and IgA (52–58%) is distributed extravascularly (Waldmann & Strober 1969). This dynamic equilibrium is determined by serum concentration and by molecular size (Nakamura et al 1968); but experimental evidence substantiates that there are differences among the various extravascular compartments (Mancini 1963). Moreover, no synthesis of Igs can be detected in cultures of normal skin (Lai A Fat et al 1973, 1974); and outside the glands, the buccal and labial mucosae are normally devoid of Ig-containing immunocytes (Fig. 3.17A,B).

A striking finding for both the oral mucosa and the skin is the presence of Igs in epithelial cells; the molecules appear to be 'bound' in the cytoplasm, since they are not removed by the washing procedure (Fig. 3.17A,B). Fennell & Vazquez (1962), in an immunohistochemical study of the female genital tract, first noted that plasma proteins may occur in squamous epithelia. Allansmith et al (1964), in their study of normal human skin, observed Ig-containing epidermal cells appearing singly or in clusters beneath the stratum corneum. We have confirmed this as illustrated in Fig. 3.18A. The positive cells mainly contain IgG, some IgA, and virtually no detectable IgM. This agrees with the distribution of plasma proteins in human gingival epithelium as first described by Brandtzaeg & Kraus (1965). Since also albumin and small amounts of fibrinogen were found in the positive cells these authors, as well as Fennell & Vazquez (1962), concluded that the cytoplasmic occurrence of Igs in squamous epithelia is a non-specific phenomenon depending on protein diffusion from the tissue fluid. Lehner (1969), on the other hand, subsequently placed great emphasis on his finding of Igs in the epithelial cells of oral mucosal specimens from patients with aphthous ulcers and Behçet's syndrome; he suggested that the Igs might represent autoantibodies bound to epithelial antigens. This cannot be generally true, since similar observations are made for normal skin and oral mucosa without ulcerative disease (Fig. 3.17). SC is not found in the Ig-positive cells (Fig. 3.17C), so the phenomenon should not be considered comparable with the transport of Igs through secretory epithelia. It may be of biological significance, though, by transferring protective serum antibodies to the surface. The Igs apparently diffuse outwards from cell to cell, and may also be passively transported as the renewal process of the epithelium goes on. The keratotic layer seems to act as a diffusion barrier, forcing the proteins sideways; this is suggested by the commonly observed superficial bands of positive cells (Fig. 3.18A). Most likely some sort of trauma to the epithelium explains its uptake of Igs. Thus, Kent (1967, 1969) has shown that plasma proteins readily diffuse into injured cells, and that they subsequently cannot easily be

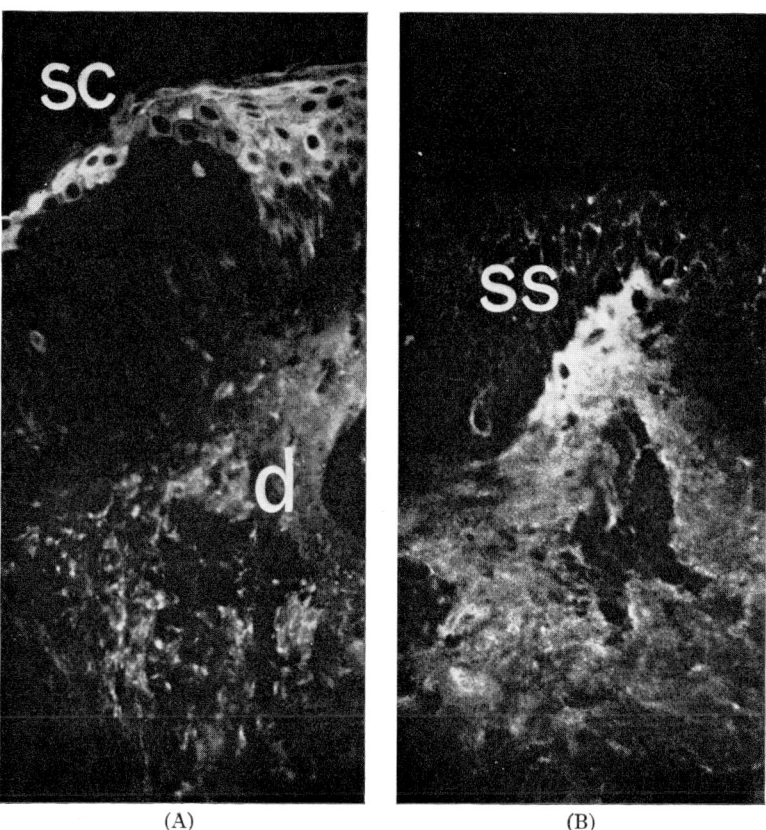

Fig. 3.18. Immunohistochemical demonstration of IgG in directly alcohol-fixed specimens of human skin from a patient with pyoderma gangraenosum migrans. *A*, specimen removed from apparently normal skin peripheral to the lesions. *B*, specimen from the margin of an ulcer. IgG is distributed diffusely in the dermis (d), in a band of epithelial cells beneath the stratum corneum (sc), and between the cells of the stratum spinosum (ss). Magnification: 200 ×.

removed from the cytoplasm by washing. It does indeed remain to be proved that the intracellular diffusion of proteins in squamous epithelia takes place *in vivo*, rather than being a result of biopsy trauma or autolytic processes.

The immune system of the mixed salivary glands, scattered in the buccal and labial mucosa, has not been studied in detail. These glands apparently contribute just less than 10% of the volume of whole saliva (Dawes & Wood 1973). Since they are situated relatively near the surface, however, they probably receive a considerable antigenic stimulation from the oral microbiota and extraneous substances; they may hence contribute significantly to the antibody activities of whole saliva. In a study of buccal and labial glands in monkey (*Macaca irus*) we have found a moderate number of IgA immunocytes distributed between the acini (Brandtzaeg & Tolo,

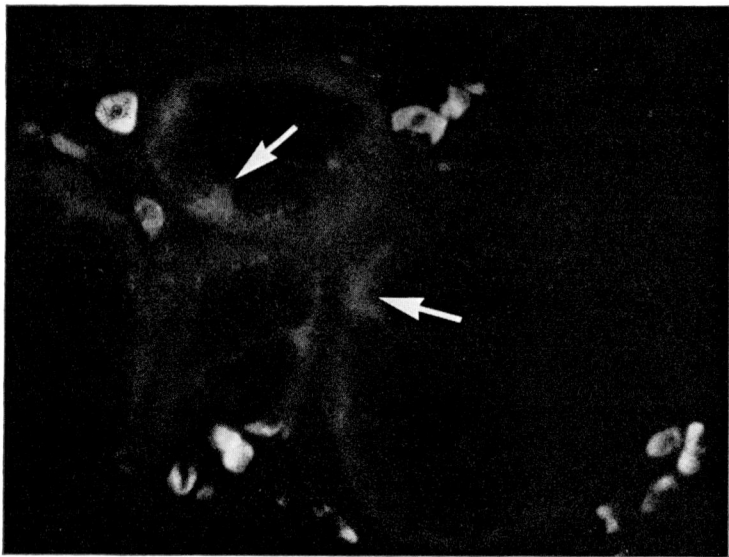

Fig. 3.19. Double exposure of paired immunohistochemical staining for IgA (red) and SC (green) in a section of directly alcohol-fixed monkey labial glands. Scattered IgA immunocytes are present between the acini, and SC plus traces of IgA (mixed colour) appear in the serous demilunes (arrows). Mucous acinar cells are completely negative. Magnification: 570 ×.

unpublished); SC could as expected (cf. previous section) be detected only in the serous demilunes along with occasional traces of IgA (Fig. 3.19). That the human minor glands likewise produce IgA and SC is exemplified in Fig. 3.17; this illustration should also demonstrate that these secretory proteins may aid in the diagnosis of oral lesions. The specimen was excised from a patient who presented with a small tumour on the inside of her lower lip. Neither the surgeon nor the pathologist felt that the diagnosis *mucocele* was justified. Nevertheless, immunohistochemistry of the washed biopsy specimen revealed selective retention of IgA (Fig. 3.17B) along with SC (Fig. 3.17C) beneath the elevated surface epithelium. Human sweat, on the contrary, contains more IgG than IgA (Page & Remington 1967), indicating that passive diffusion from the tissue fluid contributes to its composition. Tourville et al (1969) were unable to reveal IgA-producing cells in the dermis; but they reported marked immunofluorescence for SC in the sweat glands. The lack of Ig-containing immunocytes adjacent to these glands has been confirmed in our laboratory; we moreover obtained negligible or no fluorescence for SC in their epithelial elements (Brandtzaeg, unpublished). To us this is a reasonable result, since the level of free SC in sweat appears to be less than 5% of that in parotid secretion (Brandtzaeg 1971c); and only a fraction of the small amounts of sweat IgA is of the secretory type (Brandtzaeg et al 1970). It is quite clear, therefore, that the protection of the skin surface cannot depend on an active supply of Igs.

In *Sjögren's syndrome* the production of IgA by labial glands is inversely correlated with the degree of lymphoid cell infiltration (Talal et al 1970); and, as described for the major salivary glands, the synthesis of IgM and especially IgG increases as a function of the disease severity. This feature is of diagnostic importance if labial biopsy specimens can be examined immunohistochemically. Local B-cell responses associated with chronic inflammation in the oral mucosa are also outside the glands dominated by IgG immunocytes. This is well established for the gingivae (see subsequent section); and in the buccal mucosa adjacent to *aphthous ulcers* we have found ratios of about 18 : 2 : 1 for the numbers of IgG : IgA : IgM immunocytes respectively (Brandtzaeg, unpublished). Recently, definite IgG synthesis was likewise demonstrated quite regularly in lesions of human skin, whereas local production was detected only occasionally for IgA and very rarely for IgM, IgD and IgE (Lai A Fat et al 1973, 1974); this applies to both *bullous pemphigoid* and *pemphigus* as well to a variety of other skin diseases. The antibody activities of the locally produced Igs in lesions of oral mucosa and skin are unknown. As discussed for Sjögren's syndrome (see previous section) it is tempting to speculate that they are in part the products of an autoimmune response. In most of these diseases circulating antibodies to various epithelial elements have been detected: in Sjögren's syndrome reacting with the duct cells (Feltkamp & Rossum 1968); in aphthous stomatitis reacting with the cytoplasm of oral spinal epithelial cells (Donatsky & Dabelsteen 1973); in pemphigus reacting with the intercellular areas of squamous epithelia (Beutner et al 1970); and in bullous pemphigoid reacting with the basement membrane zone (Beutner et al 1970).

No attempt has been made to trace the origin of the antibodies to epithelial elements. Neither is there any conclusive information about their role in the pathogenesis. Those produced in pemphigus and bullous pemphigoid are not species specific. This, along with their clear-cut differential reaction pattern (Fig. 3.20), is of significant help in the diagnosis (Beutner *et al* 1970); but one should be aware of certain pitfalls both when the indirect and the direct immunofluorescence method is used. The pemphigus antigen has a distribution in squamous epithelia mimicking that of blood group substances (Fig. 3.20A,B). Depending on the substrate used for the indirect method, and the isoagglutinin titres of the sera tested,

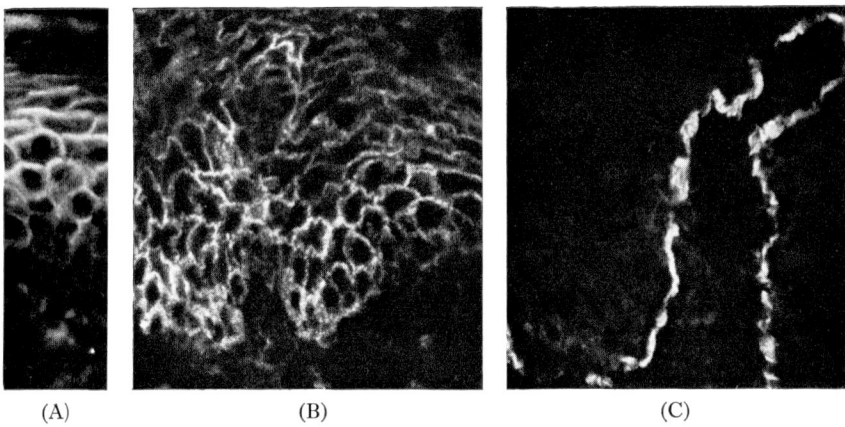

(A) (B) (C)

Fig. 3.20. Indirect immunohistochemical demonstration of *A*, blood group substance in a section of human gingiva (modified from: Brandtzaeg 1965b); *B*, pemphigus antigen in a section of guinea-pig labial mucosa; and *C*, bullous pemphigoid (basement membrane) antigen in a section of guinea-pig labial mucosa. The sections in *B* and *C* were incubated with the respective patient sera diluted 1 : 4, and thereafter with a conjugated rabbit anti-human Ig reagent. Magnification: 430 ×.

there is the possibility of false, positive reactions. Oral lesions may be the first sign of pemphigus (Eversole *et al* 1972); and about 75% of all cases will eventually have oral manifestations (Hardy *et al* 1971). When circulating antibodies are undetectable the oral lesions may pose a great diagnostic problem (Hasler 1972). In such cases has it been recommended that biopsy specimens should be examined by the direct immunofluorescence method in order to reveal the epithelial distribution of IgG (Jordon *et al* 1971). A pattern similar to that obtained with the indirect method may indicate that autoantibodies have become bound to the intercellular areas *in vivo*, and the diagnosis may thus be confirmed (Bean *et al* 1971). Such an approach can easily lead to erroneous interpretations, however, since IgG generally occurs intercellularly in squamous epithelia adjacent to inflammatory lesions (Figs. 3.18B and 3.23). This is solely a result of exudation combined with a widening of the intercellular spaces in the affected epithelium. The localization of complement factors to the same areas is no proof of a local antigen–antibody reaction, since these proteins also are contained in the exudate. Similar reservations apply to the direct test used in the diagnosis of bullous pemphigoid. Deposition of IgG and complement factors along the epithelial basement membrane may indeed be a non-specific phenomenon, and may moreover be produced by immune complexes in other diseases, especially in lupus erythematosus (Kay & Tuffanelli 1969; Beutner *et al* 1970).

3:4:4 Palatine and pharyngeal tonsils

The role of the tonsils in the immune system is still undefined. They have been considered a candidate in the search for the mammalian 'bursa equivalent', while other studies indicate that they should be regarded exclusively as secondary, peripheral lymphoid organs. They are situated in a region that is bound to be constantly bombarded by antigens from microbes and extraneous substances. Beneath the lining epithelium numerous *lymphoid follicles* are embedded in a mass of dense lymphatic tissue. Most of the follicles are of the secondary (stimulated) type with prominent *germinal centres* which are particularly rich in B lymphocytes (cf. Introduction). The follicles contain a web of *reticular cells* (also called '*dendritic macrophages*'); these apparently exert an important antigen-retaining function (Nossal 1969). Contrary to the macrophages distributed elsewhere in the tissues, the reticular cells do not engulf the antigen but keep it on the surface, perhaps complexed with released T-cell receptor or cytophilic antibody. By means of immunofluorescence IgG and IgM can readily be detected in the germinal centres, where they to some extent persist even after thorough washing (Brandtzaeg, unpublished). These Igs may represent immune complexes bound to the surface of the dendritic reticulum cells. When the antigen in this way is presented to the recirculating B cells it probably acts as a concentrated, potentiated stimulus. Unlike the lymph nodes, the tonsils do not have afferent lymphatics and sinuses; antigen supply is therefore not based on filtration of lymph from other areas, but rather on local access. The surface of the tonsils is indeed well suited for antigen trapping with numerous invaginations (*tonsillar crypts*) or folds; and electron microscopic observations indicate that antigens readily reach the subepithelial areas (Oláh *et al* 1972).

A large number of Ig-containing cells are present in the tonsils, focally distributed between the epithelium and the periphery of the lymphoid follicles, and scattered throughout the lymphatic tissue (Crabbé & Heremans 1967). IgG immunocytes predominate (Fig. 3.21), especially after the age of about 4 years (Ishikawa et al 1972). Only a small number of IgM, IgD and IgE cells can be found, whereas IgA immunocytes commonly are quite numerous, chiefly adjacent to the epithelium. In some areas most of them are monomer-producers, whereas other areas contain a

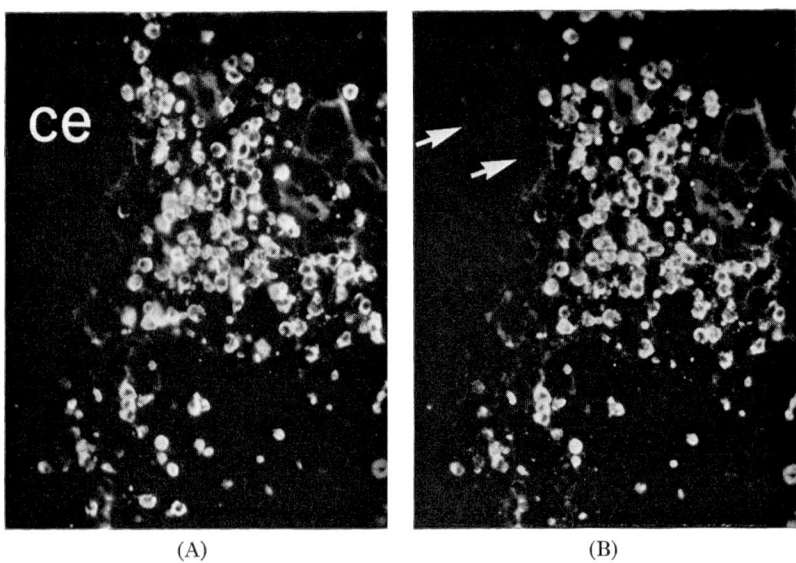

Fig. 3.21. Paired immunohistochemical staining for IgG (red) and IgA (green) in a washed specimen from human palatine tonsil. *A*, double exposure demonstrates a dense immunocyte population adjacent to crypt epithelium (ce). *B*, selective red filtration shows that most of the cells contain IgG and that traces of this immunoglobulin are present intercellularly (arrows) in the crypt epithelium. Magnification: 170 ×.

predominance of dimer-producing IgA immunocytes (Brandtzaeg 1974d). These are particularly concentrated adjacent to SC-containing epithelial cells. Secretory, columnar-type epithelium commonly covers the pharyngeal but rarely the palatine tonsils. The surface and crypts of the latter are generally lined by a squamous epithelium which is devoid of SC and does not transport IgA (Brandtzaeg 1973c); passive intercellular transmission of IgG is often seen, however (Fig. 3.21). Occasionally, Ig-positive groups of epithelial cells may be encountered as described for other squamous epithelia.

It is apparent that the tonsils cannot be considered as structures with a typical secretory immune system; neither do they exhibit a typical inflammatory immune response similar to the gingival one which includes very few dimer-producing IgA immunocytes (Brandtzaeg 1974d). Most likely, therefore, the humoral immunological competency of the tonsils represents a composite of (1) a secondary immune apparatus specialized for antigen trapping; (2) an inflammatory immune response; and (3) a secretory IgA system. The first component may chiefly play a protective role by distributing antigenically stimulated immature B cells to mucosal glands of the nasopharyngeal region and perhaps to the salivary glands; the tonsillar lymphoid follicles do contain 'blasts' with potency for J chain synthesis which is a characteristic of gland-associated immunocytes (Brandtzaeg 1974d). It remains to be clarified whether the tonsils should in addition be regarded as primary lymphoid organs which generate B-cell clones prior to antigenic stimulation.

Several early reports suggested that the tonsils are potent antibody-producing organs. In a more recent study Ogra (1971) demonstrated a marked reduction of the poliovirus antibody levels in nasopharyngeal secretions from children whose palatine and pharyngeal tonsils were removed after previous vaccination with live, attenuated virus. This finding is of great interest in view of epidemiological observations indicating that tonsillectomy and adenoidectomy is an important predisposing factor in the pathogenesis of poliomyelitis. Most likely the tonsils play a similar role in the protection against many other infectious agents, although this remains to be verified. If their chief role is the generation and dissemination of B-cell clones, their function may be of greatest significance in early childhood.

3:4:5 Gingiva

The connective tissue ground substance of gingiva is permeated by serum-derived Igs just as described above for the labial and buccal mucosa. This holds true even for specimens with little or no signs of inflammation, but may be more pronounced when overt gingivitis is present (Brandtzaeg & Kraus 1965). Diffuse immunofluorescence for IgG is so intense that cells containing this protein are almost completely obscured (Figs. 3.22A and 3.23A,B). IgA immunocytes, on the other hand, can generally be readily seen against a less bright background (Fig. 3.22B). The interstitial fluid normally contains very little IgM, and the fluorescence for this immunoglobulin is chiefly related to vessel walls and basement membrane zones. Ig-positive epithelial cells are found scattered or in groups and bands as

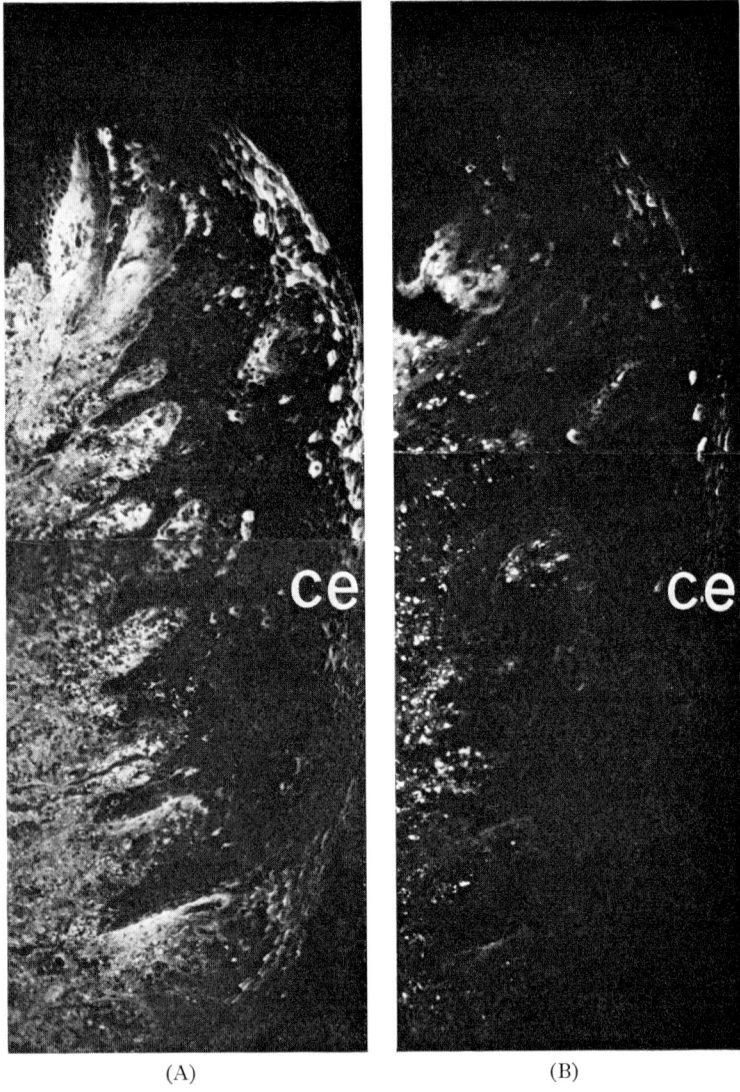

Fig. 3.22. Immunohistochemical demonstration of IgG (*A*) and IgA (*B*) in neighbouring sections of directly alcohol-fixed human gingiva from a patient with periodontitis. IgG is present diffusely in the connective tissue, obscuring a large number of IgG immunocytes. IgG is also present intracellularly in epithelial cells at the gingival margin and intercellularly in the crevicular epithelium (ce). The distribution of IgA mimics that of IgG, but is signified by less intense staining. IgA immunocytes are readily revealed against the relatively dark background. Magnification: 80×.

described above for other squamous epithelia. In the gingiva they have a predilection for the sulcus area close to the margin (Fig. 3.22). It is possible that trauma to this region or the age of these cells makes their membranes unduly permeable, thus allowing uptake of plasma proteins from the crevicular fluid. When inflammation is present Igs are readily detectable intercellularly in the crevicular epithelium and more rarely in the oral surface epithelium (Brandtzaeg & Kraus 1965; Brandtzaeg 1966). The epithelial fluorescence for IgG is always dominant; but with the increased sensitivity of present immunofluorescence techniques even traces of IgM can be revealed intra- as well as inter-cellularly.

Specimens of monkey gingivae fixed in correct relation to the tooth permit a detailed immunohistochemical study of the Ig distribution in the crevicular epithelium (Fig. 3.23A). The most prominent intercellular fluorescence is found adjacent to the sulcus, extending both apically and marginally from the area of transition between the oral epithelium and that directly facing the tooth. The most apical part of the latter may be fairly devoid of fluorescence, but a superficial bright rim indicates that Igs have been present all the way between the epithelium and the tooth (Fig. 3.23A). The extension of intercellular staining is clearly correlated with the extension of inflammatory infiltration. This morphological association is probably explained by the widening of intercellular spaces that has been revealed electron-microscopically in connection with inflammation (Freedman *et al* 1968; Gavin 1970). Double tracing substantiates that IgG and IgA follow exactly the same route through the crevicular epithelium (Fig. 3.23B,C). Since moreover no SC is detectable in gingival epithelium, Ig transmission into the crevice must be regarded as a passive diffusion phenomenon. There is thus good agreement between the relative fluorescence intensities of the various Igs intercellularly and their measurable concentrations in the crevicular fluid.

A slight inflammatory infiltration is commonly present in the gingiva even in the absence of clinical gingivitis. It is generally accepted that this can be ascribed to an influence on the host by the bacteria present in small accumulations of dental plaque adjacent to the gingival margin. When these accumulations grow because of neglected oral hygiene, the average degree of gingival inflammation increases proportionally although the response is subjected to great individual differences. In the early stages the cellular picture is dominated by mononuclear cells, mostly medium-large and small lymphocytes (Zachrisson 1968). In an established chronic gingivitis, however, the majority of the inflammatory cells can be characterized morphologically as belonging to the plasma-cell line

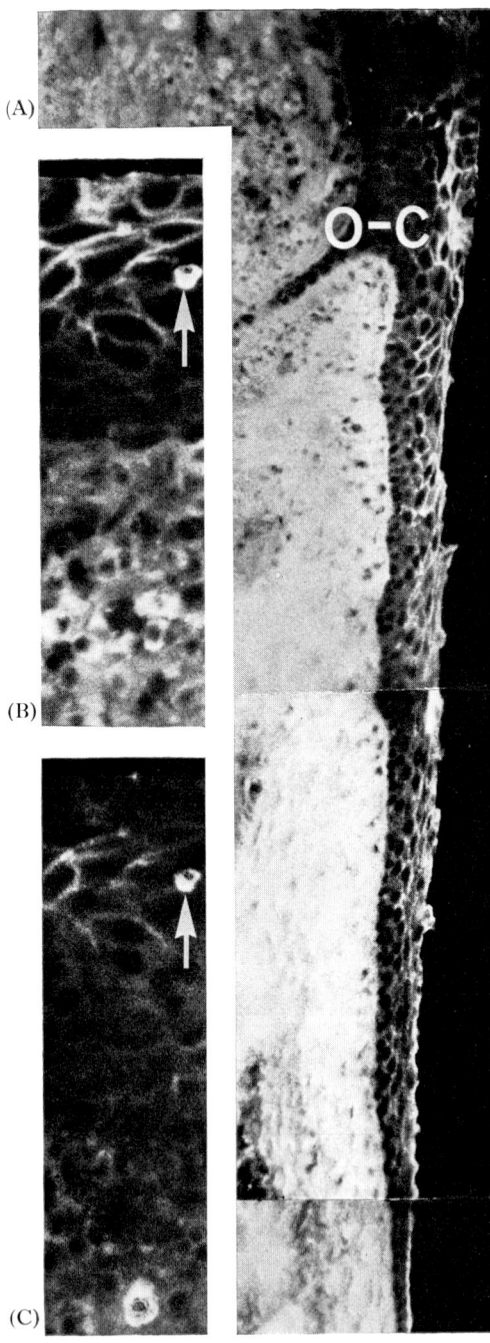

Fig. 3.23. *A*, immunohistochemical demonstration of IgG in monkey crevicular epithelium and adjacent connective tissue; the approximate transition zone between the oral epithelium and that directly facing the tooth is labelled o–c; adjacent to this zone numerous IgG immunocytes are partially masked in the connective tissue. *B–C*, a field from the same crevicular epithelium (at the top) after paired staining for IgG (green) and IgA (red); selective green (*B*) and red (*C*) filtration reveal that the two Igs are both present intercellularly, but there is a clear dominance of IgG; a fluorescent body (arrow), probably a phagocytic cell, contains both IgG and IgA. Magnification: 200 × (*A*) and 440 × (*B*, *C*).

(Freedman et al 1968; Gavin 1970). This is substantiated by immunofluorescence studies of washed biopsy specimens (Brandtzaeg & Kraus 1965; Brandtzaeg 1966); double tracing reveals that IgG and IgA immunocytes are so densely packed, especially in the marginal areas, that little space is left for other cells to be present (Fig. 3.13E,F). The morphology of the Ig-containing immunocytes is highly variable, many of them resembling blast cells with a relatively scanty cytoplasm. Their phenotypic restriction is well established by paired staining with selective colour filtration (Fig. 3.13E,F), which also excludes the possibility that some cells are positive due to inward diffusion of plasma proteins through injured membranes.

In monkeys (Macaca irus) with experimentally induced gingivitis we have tried to find out where the Ig-containing cells first appear in the gingiva (Brandtzaeg & Tolo, unpublished). There seems to be no consistent pattern; in some specimens the first clusters of immunocytes are found adjacent to the sulcus, whereas in others they appear near the blood vessels more centrally in the connective tissue. In contrast to the report of MacDonald & Cowley (1972), we observed a distinct dominance of IgG cells even in the early inflammatory infiltrates. The average ratio of IgG : IgA immunocytes in human specimens with moderate gingivitis has been estimated to be 4·3 : 1; in densely infiltrated specimens it was 7·2 : 1 (Brandtzaeg 1972b). There is marked variation between different individuals and between different specimens from the same patient, however; and in some areas the number of IgA cells may approach that of IgG cells (Fig. 3.13F). The average number of IgM immunocytes, on the contrary, is usually less than 1% of those containing IgG.

Local production of Igs in connection with the development of gingivitis therefore seems to follow the pattern of a classic secondary, systemic immune response which in man is characterized by a progressive dominance of IgG over IgA synthesis (Bandilla et al 1969). Primary immune responses are rather characterized by preferential appearance of IgM and IgA antibodies. The gingival immunocyte pattern moreover differs markedly from gland-associated immune responses in several ways: (*1*) the predominant IgG synthesis; (*2*) the pronounced excess of monomer producers in the local IgA-cell population (Brandtzaeg 1974d); and (*3*) the lack of replacement of IgA immunocytes by IgM cells in patients with selective IgA deficiency (Brandtzaeg, unpublished). If it is generally true that the rate of Ig-production per immunocyte is decreased in the order IgA : IgM : IgG by the proportions 5·6 : 3·7 : 1 (Gitlin & Sasaki 1969), then the gingival synthesis of IgA and IgM would be higher than indicated by the cell counts referred to above. However, recent tissue culture experiments have confirmed the predominant IgG synthesis of human gingival tissue, and that IgM is a negligible product (Lai A Fat et al 1973, 1974). This response pattern moreover agrees with that resulting from persistent antigen stimulation in the rabbit gingiva (Brandtzaeg 1972b; Kraus et al 1972). The findings do not harmonize with the immunofluorescence observations of Thonard et al (1966), Platt et al (1970) and MacDonald & Cowley (1972), but the discrepancy can most likely be explained by differences in technique. Special precautions must be taken to detect all of the IgG immunocytes in an immunohistochemical preparation, partly because these cells often exhibit a relatively faint fluorescence, and partly because they are easily masked by diffuse background staining (Brandtzaeg 1974a). IgD and IgE synthesis cannot be revealed in cultures of gingiva (Lai A Fat et al 1973, 1974,) and cells of these classes are extremely rare in chronically inflamed specimens (Nisengard et al 1971, Brandtzaeg, unpublished).

Several attempts have been made to define the antibody specificities of the immunocytes appearing in the inflamed gingivae. The test antigens have mainly been selected from plaque bacteria, and as yet most experiments have turned out to be negative. In a recent publication Mayron & Loiselle (1973) reported that FITC-conjugated bacteria stained gingival sections, particularly the epithelium; and they felt that this was evidence for antibacterial activities. It is very hard to accept that their result is due to specific binding, since the epithelium does not contain diffusely distributed Igs. The concentration of a specific antibody is after cellular release much less than that of total interstitial Igs; immunofluorescence localization would hence be expected to be confined almost exclusively to the cytoplasm of immunocytes (Brandtzaeg 1974a). Squamous epithelium is moreover particularly prone to become non-specifically stained (Brandtzaeg 1973b). Until immunohistochemical evidence for the presence of antibodies in gingiva has been based on properly characterized reagents, the available data have to be interpreted with the utmost caution. Berglund (1971), on the other hand, used tissue culture technique and definitely showed that B cells capable of responding to crude antigen from *Fusobacterium* are present in the gingiva; but direct proof of local antibody synthesis to plaque components is still lacking. Affinity for altered IgG has recently been demonstrated in gingival sections by a very sensitive mixed agglutination technique (Kristoffersen & Tönder 1973). It is not known whether these 'rheumatoid factor'-like activities can be ascribed to local antibody synthesis, or are due to the accumulation of serum-derived Igs or complement factors in the lesion.

It is well established that gingivitis and periodontitis may develop in patients with various types of Ig deficiency (Brandtzaeg 1966, 1972b; Barrickman *et al* 1973). Studies of such cases may help in the evaluation of the possible protective or deleterious role of antibodies in periodontal disease. Interpretation of the results is more difficult than originally believed, however, since the co-operation of lymphocytes and antibodies in immune reactions is very complex. It has been found that patients with general hypo-γ-globulinaemia have numerous cells with surface-associated IgG in their inflamed nasal mucosae (Brandtzaeg 1974a). Most of these are probably derived from the circulating pool of lymphocytes with Fc

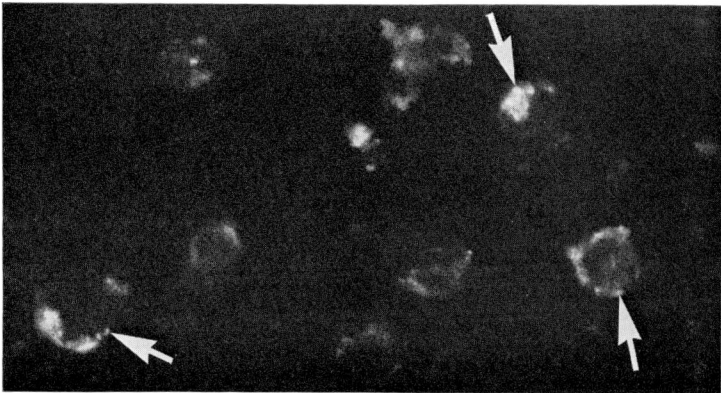

Fig. 3.24. Immunohistochemical demonstration of IgG in a washed specimen of gingiva from a hypo-γ-globulinaemic patient (1·7 mg IgG/100 ml serum) with gingivitis. Mononuclear cells with specifically fluorescing, apparently membrane-associated granules (arrows) are clearly disclosed against a dark background. Magnification: 1000×.

receptors, which cannot be convincingly classified as B or T cells (Fröland & Natvig 1973). It seems that members of this third population are able to concentrate IgG on their surface even when it is present in only minute amounts in blood and tissue fluid. This is exemplified in Fig. 3.24 for the chronically inflamed gingiva of a patient with only 1·7 mg IgG/100 ml serum. Hence, by co-operation with lymphocytes trace amounts of Igs may play a role in local immune reactions if the surface-bound molecules exhibit antibody activities specific for available antigens. There is evidence to indicate that lymphocytes with Fc receptors can mediate cytotoxic reactions (Wislöff & Fröland 1973).

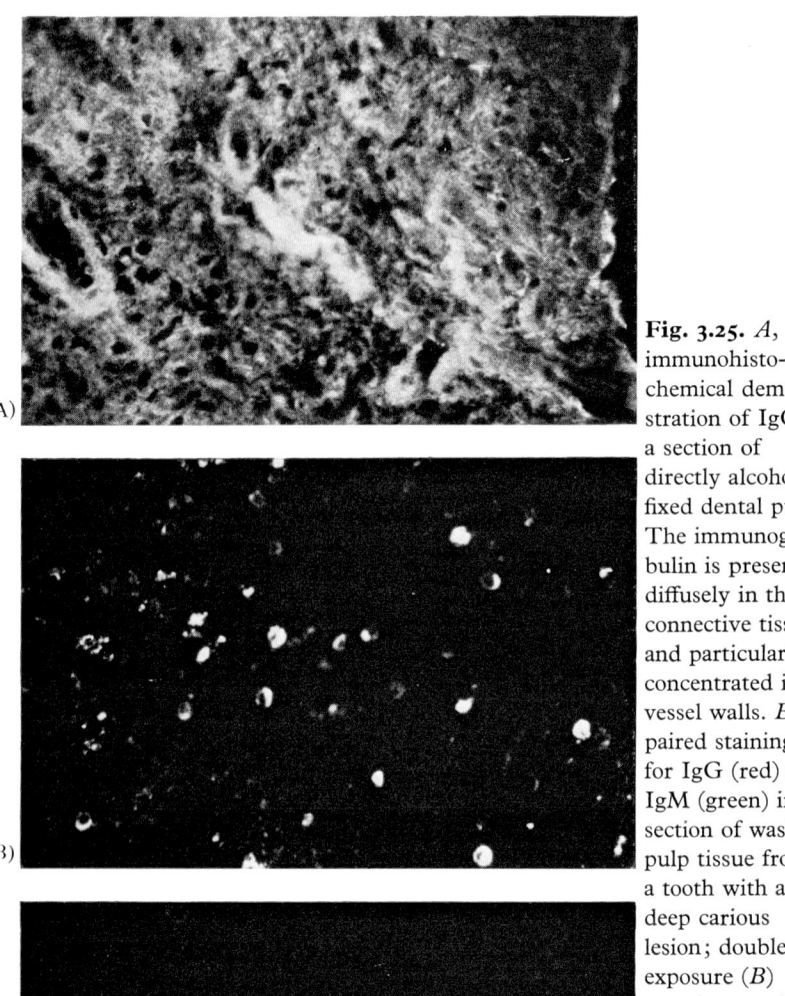

Fig. 3.25. *A*, immunohistochemical demonstration of IgG in a section of directly alcohol-fixed dental pulp. The immunoglobulin is present diffusely in the connective tissue and particularly concentrated in vessel walls. *B–C*, paired staining for IgG (red) and IgM (green) in a section of washed pulp tissue from a tooth with a deep carious lesion; double exposure (*B*) reveals a small number of immunocytes scattered throughout the section; selective green filtration (*C*) shows that only 3–4 of the cells contain IgM. Magnification: 220×.

3:4:6 Dental pulp

Very little attention seems to have been paid to the immunological aspects of pulpitis. Several investigators have by conventional histological techniques detected plasma cells in inflamed dental pulps, but only a brief report (Honjo *et al* 1970) has classified the cells with regard to cytoplasmic Igs. These workers found a preponderance of IgG immunocytes, and suggested that local antibody formation is an aspect of pulpitis. We have confirmed that the dental pulp is apparently no different from the oral mucosa with regard to the supply of serum-derived Igs (Fig. 3.25A) as well as when it comes to the local immune response associated with chronic inflammation (Fig. 3.25B,C). The ratios of IgG : IgA : IgM immunocytes in a limited material from teeth with deep carious lesions have been estimated to be about 5 : 2·5 : 1 (Brandtzaeg & Örstavik, unpublished). The dental pulp should be well suited for the investigation of locally induced antibody synthesis; and information in this field is certainly needed to understand more about the mechanisms of pulpitis and other inflammatory diseases.

3:5 The Role of Immunoglobulins in the Physiology and Pathology of the Oral Cavity—Concluding Remarks

Studies on the normal distribution of Igs in mucous membranes and skin have clearly revealed that one important aspect of local immunity is the supply of serum-derived antibodies. The connective tissue ground substance is generally permeated by IgG, and to a lesser extent by IgA and IgM. Antibodies present in serum must consequently also be represented in a local tissue site. This has recently been verified for the human gingiva with regard to antimicrobial activities (Berglund 1971; Hartzer *et al* 1971). Accumulation of serum antibodies should be particularly pronounced in inflamed areas. Enhanced respiratory immunity has thus been found in systemically immunized experimental animals after irritant-induced extravasation of circulating antibodies into the mucosa (Fazekas de St Groth 1951; Fazekas de St Groth *et al* 1951). This has been termed '*pathotopic potentiation*' of local immunity, and may likewise play a role in the protection of skin and oral mucosa. It is possible that the crevicular fluid can be regarded as an aspect of pathotopic potentiation of gingival protection, although there is no direct evidence to support this view. Moreover, Hand *et al* (1971) in a study of chronically inflamed urinary bladders questioned the importance of serum-type antibodies in mucosal surface protection; they may not be sufficiently stable for an effective external function (Haneberg 1974). Recent animal experiments have, on the other hand, indicated that antibodies present intercellularly in gingival epithelium restrict the penetration of antigens into the subepithelial compartment (McDougall 1974). In the connective tissue the serum-derived antibodies may mediate beneficial or adverse reactions. The latter situation is likely to occur when antigen elimination is unsuccessful. Auer pointed out in 1920 that a mild inflammation can be severely aggravated by local accumulation of serum antibodies combined with a systemic supply of the corresponding antigen; subsequent studies have demonstrated that this holds true also when the antigen is topically applied (Kraft et al 1963; Ford & Kirsner 1964). Theoretically, the initial gingival lesion should be an ideal situation for the development of a so-called 'Auer-phenomenon' due to continuous contribution of dental plaque and food antigens. Similar mechanisms may be involved in the propagation of autoimmune disease when the generation or release of autoantigens has started.

In addition to the local aspects of systemic immunity, two distinct humoral effector systems of potential protective value have been delineated for the oral mucosa and the salivary glands. As previously suggested for the respiratory and intestinal tract (Brandtzaeg 1973e), a *'first line of mucosal defence'* depends on gland-associated immune responses providing dimeric IgA and, to a smaller extent, polymeric IgM. These Igs are selectively transmitted through secretory epithelia. During this process they become stabilized by combination with an epithelial glycoprotein (SC), and are subsequently well suited for a function in the external milieu. Local IgG-cell responses probably constitute a *'second line of mucosal defence'* directed against antigens which are not efficiently handled by the secretory Ig system. This may pertain to extraneous agents penetrating the epithelial lining as well as to endogenous components rendered immunogenic during an inflammatory process or by other obscure mechanisms. It is for example quite possible that products from reactions between serum-derived antibodies and continuously supplied antigens eventually stimulate local formation of IgG 'anti-antibodies'. Several recent reports have suggested an association between transient or permanent lack of IgA and a variety of diseases such as respiratory tract infections, atopic allergy, coeliac disease and rheumatoid arthritis, as well as other conditions with autoimmune aspects. It has also been noted that patients with IgA deficiency have a relatively high incidence of circulating antibodies to food and milk proteins, indicating that their mucosal penetrability is increased (for review, see Hanson & Brandtzaeg 1973). This may explain not only low resistance to bacterial and viral infections, but also undue absorption of extraneous antigens potentially cross-reacting with host components and thereby inducing self-destructing, autoimmune phenomena. Hence, it seems very likely that the surface of mucous membranes is normally protected by secretory IgA antibodies. The deleterious effects of a selective lack of this immunoglobulin may, however, to some extent be masked by enhanced local synthesis and secretion of IgM (Brandtzaeg et al 1968b; Brandtzaeg 1971a). In the skin a 'first line of defence' is not mediated by a secretory Ig system, but rather depends on an intact physical barrier.

The secretory Ig system matures relatively rapidly, and IgA may be detected at an earlier age in saliva than in serum. Almost 'adult' salivary IgA levels have been reported to develop within 6 weeks for most infants (Selner et al 1968); such quantitations, therefore, are of great diagnostic importance when an immunological defect is suspected. The origin of the local IgA-dimer-producing cells is unknown. They are most likely generated in a 'bursa equivalent' organ. It is interesting in this connection that some areas of the tonsils contain many such cells although apparently having a very limited capacity for external transfer of dimeric IgA. The impressive selective homing of IgA-dimer immunocytes to tissues containing secretory epithelium is perhaps determined by cell affinity for SC which is released into the interstitial fluid and serum in small amounts (Brandtzaeg 1971d, 1973c). The homing of IgM cells to glandular areas may be similarly influenced by a concentration gradient of SC; this is especially important when the maturation of IgA cells is defective. There is moreover some evidence to indicate that the secretory IgM system plays a role in newborns before the secretory IgA system has developed. Experiments in animals have clearly demonstrated that the local proliferation and maturation of immunocytes is stimulated to a great extent by the normal microbial flora living on the mucosa (Crabbé et al 1970). This indirectly suggests that one important function of the secretory Ig system is to regulate the relationship between the host and the commensal bacteria.

As outlined in Fig. 3.14 the supply of protective secretory antibodies on the mucosal surface depends on five critical steps: (*1*) local Ig synthesis; (*2*) SC formation; (*3*) epithelial reception of dimeric IgA and 19S IgM; (*4*) stabilization of the SC–Ig complexes; and (*5*) the final external transport of the secretory Igs. A defect in one of these steps may conceivably lead to inadequate host resistance. Until now, however, studies on local immunity have revealed only an association between defective Ig synthesis and disease. Much therefore remains to be learned about other aspects of the secretory immune system. When it comes to oral diseases, moreover, there is a complete lack of conclusive information both with regard to the importance of local IgA synthesis and methods for its stimulation in the salivary glands. Preliminary reports have indicated that a combination of parenteral vaccination and oral inoculation of live streptococci have led to inhibition of dental caries development in experimental animals (Wagner 1967; Bowen 1969); but these studies certainly need confirmation by more extensive investigations which include evaluation of antibodies belonging to the secretory Igs.

A local immune response dominated by IgG cells seems to develop in association with chronic inflammation regardless of the tissue site and the initiating antigenic stimulus. This has been clearly shown both for the oral mucosa and the skin, as well as for synovia (Smiley *et al* 1968; Sliwinski & Zvaifler 1970; Herman *et al* 1971), kidneys (Lehmann *et al* 1968) and urinary bladder (Hand *et al* 1970). An IgG response may moreover become superimposed on the normal gland-associated IgA–immunocyte system as demonstrated for the salivary glands in Sjögren's syndrome, as well as for inflamed nasal (Brandtzaeg *et al* 1967), gastric (Fjellanger *et al* 1968) and intestinal mucosae (Brandtzaeg *et al* 1974). The predominant synthesis of IgG in inflammatory lesions is probably explained by two mechanisms. Firstly, the tissue site continuously receives lymphocytes from the recirculating pool and will hence exhibit immunological competency 'mirroring' that of spleen and lymph nodes; it has been shown that the transformation of B lymphocytes to Ig-secreting immunocytes takes place after their migration into the inflamed tissue (Moore & Schoenberg 1964; Loewi *et al* 1971). Secondly, the chronicity of the lesion is related to the local persistence or continuous supply of some obvious or obscure antigenic material; due to unsuccessful elimination this will provide the long-lasting stimulus required for an IgG response (Hanna & Peters 1971).

Lymphocyte homing from the blood into inflammatory lesions is only partly understood. Determinations indicate that the flux of lymphocytes through a chronically inflamed tissue equals the flux through a lymph node of the same mass (Smith *et al* 1970). The seeding into the inflammatory focus has been assumed to be a random process (Jasin & Ziff 1969; Williamson *et al* 1969; Koster & McGregor 1971; Werdelin & McCluskey 1971), but recent experiments suggest that antigen can specifically select a very small sub-fraction of cells from the recirculating pool (Lance & Cooper 1972; Rowley *et al* 1972). In addition, newly formed descendants from immune responses apparently exhibit affinity for inflamed tissue regardless of specificity (Koster *et al* 1971; Asherson & Allwood 1972). Around a depot of antigen in the rabbit gingiva 30–40% of the Ig-containing cells were found to be relevant antibody producers, while 60% were engaged in synthesis of what might appear to be 'non-reactive' immunoglobulin (Brandtzaeg 1972b). Similar results have been obtained with other techniques for systemic (Urbain-Vansanten 1970; Vos-Cloetens *et al* 1971) as well as for local immune responses (Cooke & Jasin 1972; Graham & Shannon 1972). In hyperimmunized animals a fraction of the local immunocytes containing so-called 'non-reactive' Ig can indeed be shown to express the systemic immune competency of the host (Jasin & Ziff 1969; Herman *et al* 1971; Brandtzaeg 1973d). The proliferation and maturation of these cells in the lesion may be explained by accumulation of circulating corresponding antigen, or by blastogenic factors released from other locally activated T or B cells (Schimpl & Wecker 1973). As summarized in Table

Table 3.6 Potential stimuli for local immunoglobulin synthesis in chronic inflammation

1. Antigens from local collections of micro-organisms
2. Circulating antigens accumulating in the inflammatory focus
3. Blastogenic factors released from locally activated T or B cells
4. Altered IgG (immune complexes)
5. Altered endogenous tissue components
6. Microbial mitogens (e.g. lipopolysaccharides, dextram, levam)

3.6, additional stimuli for local Ig formation associated with chronic inflammation may be altered autologous IgG in circulating or locally produced immune complexes (Bokisch *et al* 1972), altered endogenous tissue components revealed during the inflammatory process (Willoughby & Ryan 1970), and microbial mitogens (Andersson *et al* 1972). This should serve to point out some of the complexity of inflammatory B-cell responses.

The biological significance of the Igs synthesized in an inflammatory focus remains speculative. Like serum-derived antibodies, they probably exert their chief functions in the tissue itself with beneficial or deleterious effects. In addition to direct antimicrobial activities IgG present in the inflamed tissue may be converted to a factor chemotactic for neutrophilic granulocytes (Yoshinaga *et al* 1970). The importance of these cells in the local defence has been stressed in several studies. Chemotaxis may also be mediated indirectly via complement activation when local IgG antibodies react with antigens. Since neutrophils moreover contain surface receptors for IgG (Messner & Jelinek 1971) antibodies of this class may promote phagocytosis by being cytophilic in addition to being directly opsonizing. On the other hand, antigen–antibody reactions taking place on the surface of neutrophils probably contribute to the lysis of these cells and to the release of inflammatory mediators. Collagen fibres likewise seem to have affinity for immune complexes (Cooke *et al* 1972; Straus 1972); and since lymphocytes with Fc receptors apparently occur in inflammatory lesions, IgG antibodies may direct such cells with their cytotoxic capacity to the fibrous elements. It is of interest in this connection that lymphocytes can be observed in intimate contact with degenerating fibroblasts in inflamed gingivae (Schroeder & Page 1972).

Several recent studies have emphasized the possibility that immunological mechanisms may be important in destructive gingival inflammation (Rizzo & Mitchell 1966; Ranney 1970; Ranney & Zander 1970; Kraus *et al* 1972; McDougall 1972). It has been shown that molecules with a size like albumin can diffuse across apparently normal crevicular epithelium (Tolo 1971), and that antigen penetration is enhanced when the epithelium is exposed to irritants (Dick & Trott 1971). Thus, antibodies to bacterial products, to irrelevant antigens, to altered IgG, and to newly exposed tissue antigens may all contribute to a continuous supply of immune complexes which in turn give rise to an Arthus-type reaction (Cochrane 1967) perhaps combined with cytotoxic phenomena. By such mechanisms immune reactions may be responsible for the perpetuation of inflammation and explain chronicity (Lachmann 1967). It has also been proposed that gingivitis contains a component of immediate, reagin-mediated hypersensitivity because a few IgE immunocytes have been detected in the chronic infiltrates (Nisengard *et al* 1971). This immunoglobulin exhibits selective affinity for mast cells (Tomioka & Ishizaka 1971), which are abundant in the gingiva (Zachrisson 1967) and whose potent inflammatory mediators are released after degranulation. However, the presence of IgE immunocytes does not necessarily indicate that Type I immediate hypersensitivity is a major contributor to the inflammatory reaction. Studies of respiratory mucosa have revealed no increase in the number of IgE immunocytes in connection with asthma, but rather suggested that IgE is a normal participant in chronic inflammatory lesions (Callerame *et al* 1971; Gerber *et al* 1971), where it perhaps augments the accumulation of IgG-antigen complexes (Benveniste 1973).

The postulated protective and deleterious effects of the two major components of local immune responses are summarized in Table 3.7. Adverse effects of IgA have not as yet been demonstrated. In the tissue such antibodies probably exert a blocking effect since they lack conventional complement-activating properties; if the antibody specificity is directed towards malignant cells, cancer enhancement may ensue due to protection against elimination by T cells. The blocking effect of IgA antibodies may, nevertheless, generally be conducive to health by slowing down deleterious consequences of antibody reactions involving IgG (and IgM). Thus, it seems likely that a beneficial outcome of local immune

Table 3.7 Postulated protective and deleterious consequences of local immune responses

The secretory IgA response	The inflammatory IgG response
Protective	*Protective*
Antigen trapping in mucous coat	Virus and toxin neutralization
Allergen blocking	Enzyme inhibition
Virus neutralization	Allergen blocking
Coating and aggregation of bacteria, and inhibition of bacterial colonization on epithelial cells (and teeth?)	Bacteriolysis
	Chemotaxis and opsonization
	Inflammation due to immune complexes
Opsonization (?)	
Bacteriolysis (?)	
Deleterious	*Deleterious*
Enhancement of cancer (?)	Rapid release of pharmacologically active substances from bacteria and host cells
	Persistent inflammation due to immune complexes (Arthus-type reaction)

responses is dependent not only on an efficient 'first line of defence', but also on a balance in the synthesis of IgG and IgA antibodies in the 'second line of defence'; a shift of the latter response in favour of IgG may in several ways disturb the local immune homeostasis with aggravation and perpetuation of the inflammatory process as a result. It must be concluded, however, that much remains to be learned about protective and destructive aspects of chronic inflammation with regard to the relative importance of humoral and cellular factors as well as interactions between T and B cells.

3:6 References

ADINOLFI M., GLYNN A.A., LINDSAY M. & MILNE C.M. (1966a) Serological properties of γA antibodies to *Escherichia coli* present in human colostrum. *Immunology*, **10**, 517–526.

ADINOLFI M., MOLLISON P.L., POLLEY M.J. & ROSE J.M. (1966b) γA-Blood group antibodies. *J. exp. Med.*, **123**, 951–967.

ALLANSMITH M. & BUELL D. (1965) Immunoglobulins in the skin of allergic and nonallergic individuals. *J. Immunol.*, **95**, 951–958.

ALLANSMITH M., GOIHMAN-YAHR M. & BUELL D.N. (1964) Demonstration of gamma-2 globulin in human skin. *J. Allergy*, **35**, 313–321.

AMMANN A.J. & HONG R. (1970) Selective IgA deficiency and autoimmunity. *Clin. exp. Immunol.*, **7**, 833–838.

ANDERSON L.G., CUMMINGS N.A., ASOFSKY R., HYLTON M.B., TARPLEY T.M., TOMASI T.B., WOLF R.O., SCHALL G.L. & TALAL N. (1972) Salivary gland immunoglobulin and rheumatoid factor synthesis in Sjögren's syndrome. Natural history and response to treatment. *Am. J. Med.*, **53**, 456–463.

ANDERSON L.G., TARPLEY T.M., TALAL N., CUMMINGS N.A., WOLF R.O. & SCHALL G.L. (1973) Cellular-versus-humoral autoimmune responses to salivary gland in Sjögren's syndrome. *Clin. exp. Immunol.*, **13**, 335–342.

ANDERSON S.G., BANGHAM D.R., BATTY I., BECKER W. & OTHERS (1971) Measurements of concentrations of human serum immunoglobulins. *Eur. J. Immunol.*, **1**, 223–225.

ANDERSSON J., SJÖBERG O. & MÖLLER G. (1972) Induction of immunoglobulin and antibody synthesis *in vitro* by lipopolysaccharides. *Eur. J. Immunol.*, **2**, 349–353.

ASHERSON G.L. & ALLWOOD G.G. (1972) Inflammatory lymphoid cells. Cells in immunized lymph nodes that move to sites of inflammation. *Immunology*, **22**, 493–502.

AUER J. (1920) Local autoinoculation of the sensitized organism with foreign protein as a cause of abnormal reactions. *J. exp. Med.*, **32**, 427–444.

AVRAMEAS S., KUHLMANN W., MILLER H.R.P. & LEDUC E. (1971) Two antibody-producing cell types in four species. *Immunology*, **20**, 85–89.

BANDILLA K.K., MCDUFFIE F.C. & GLEICH G.J. (1969) Immunoglobulin classes of antibodies produced in the primary and secondary responses in man. *Clin. exp. Immunol.*, **5**, 627–641.

BANG J.-S. & CIMASONI G. (1971) Total protein in human crevicular fluid. *J. dent. Res.*, **50**, 1683 (only).

BARRICKMAN R.W., CALLERAME M.L. & CONDEMI J.J. (1973) Gingivitis in hypogammaglobulinemia. *J. Periodont.*, **44**, 171–174.

BEAN S.F., ALT T.H. & KATZ H.I. (1971) Oral pemphigus and bullous pemphigoid. Immunofluorescent studies of two patients. *J. Am. med. Ass.*, **216**, 673-674.

BENJAMIN D.C. & WEIGLE W.O. (1970) Frequency of single spleen cells from hyperimmune rabbits producing antibody of two different specificities. *J. Immunol.*, **105**, 537–540.

BENNICH H. & JOHANSSON S.G.O. (1971) Structure and function of human immunoglobulin E. *Advances in Immunology*, **13**, 1–55.

BENVENISTE J. (1973) Définition expérimentale d'un role nouveau pour l'IgE. Déclenchement immunologique de la déposition des immune complexes. *Nouv. Presse Méd.*, **2**, 703–706.
BERGER R., AINBENDER E., HODES H.L., ZEPP H.D. & HEVIZY M.M. (1967). Demonstration of IgA polio-antibody in saliva, duodenal fluid and urine. *Nature, Lond.*, **214**, 420–422.
BERGLUND S.E. (1971) Immunoglobulins in human gingiva with specificity for oral bacteria. *J. Periodont.*, **42**, 546–551.
BERRY H., BACON P.A. & DAVIS J.D. (1972) Cell-mediated immunity in Sjögren's syndrome. *Ann. Rheum. Dis.*, **31**, 298–302.
BESREDKA A. (1927) *Local Immunization*. Williams & Wilkins, Baltimore.
BEUTNER E.H., CHORZELSKI T.P. & JORDON R.E. (1970) *Autosensitization in Pemphigus and Bullous Pemphigoid*, 194. Charles C. Thomas, Springfield, Illinois.
BLUESTONE R., GUMPEL, J.M., GOLDBERG L.S. & HOLBOROW E.J. (1972) Salivary immunoglobulins in Sjögren's syndrome. *Int. Arch. Allergy*, **42**, 686–692.
BOACKLE R.J. & PRUITT K.M. (1973) The interaction of human salivary secretions with the complement system. *I.A.D.R. Abstracts*, No. 330.
BOKISCH V.A., BERNSTEIN D. & KRAUSE R.M. (1972) Occurrence of 19S and 7S anti-IgGs during hyperimmunization of rabbits with streptococci. *J. exp. Med.*, **136**, 799–815.
BOWEN W.H. (1969) A vaccine against dental caries: A pilot experiment in monkeys (*Macaca irus*). *Brit. dent. J.*, **126**, 159–160.
BRANDTZAEG P. (1965a) Immunochemical comparison of proteins in human gingival pocket fluid, serum and saliva. *Archs. oral Biol.*, **10**, 795–803.
BRANDTZAEG P. (1965b) Localization of blood-group substances A and B in alcohol-fixed human gingivae by indirect immunofluorescence technique. *Acta odont. Scand.*, **23**, 335–345.
BRANDTZAEG P. (1966) Local factors of resistance in the gingival area. *J. periodont. Res.*, **1**, 19–42.
BRANDTZAEG P. (1971a) Human secretory immunoglobulins. II. Salivary secretions from individuals with selectively excessive or defective synthesis of serum immunoglobulins. *Clin. exp. Immunol.*, **8**, 69–85.
BRANDTZAEG P. (1971b) Human secretory immunoglobulins. III. Immunochemical and physicochemical studies of secretory IgA and free secretory piece. *Acta Path Microbiol Scand.*, Section B, **79**, 165–188.
BRANDTZAEG P. (1971c) Human secretory immunoglobulins. IV. Quantitation of free secretory piece. *Acta Path. Microbiol. Scand.*, Section B, **79**, 189–203.
BRANDTZAEG P. (1971d) Human secretory immunoglobulins. V. Occurrence of secretory piece in human serum. *J. Immunol.*, **106**, 318–323.
BRANDTZAEG P. (1971e) Human secretory immunoglobulins. VII. Concentrations of parotid IgA and other secretory proteins in relation to the rate of flow and duration of secretory stimulus. *Archs. oral Biol.*, **16**, 1295–1310.
BRANDTZAEG P. (1972a) Evaluation of immunofluorescence with artificial sections of selected antigenicity. *Immunology*, **22**, 177–183.
BRANDTZAEG P. (1972b) Local formation and transport of immunoglobulins related to the oral cavity. In MACPHEE I.T. *Host Resistance to Commensal Bacteria*, 116–150. Churchill Livingstone, London.

BRANDTZAEG P. (1973a) Conjugates of immunoglobulin G with different fluorochromes. I. Characterization by anionic-exchange chromatography. *Scand. J. Immunol.*, **2**, 273-290.
BRANDTZAEG P. (1973b) Conjugates of immunoglobulin G with different fluorochromes. II. Specific and non-specific binding properties. *Scand. J. Immunol.*, **2**, 333-348.
BRANDTZAEG P. (1973c) Two types of IgA immunocytes in man. *Nature, New Biology*, **243**, 142-143.
BRANDTZAEG P. (1973d) Immunology of inflammatory periodontal lesions. *Int. dent. J.*, **23**, 438-454.
BRANDTZAEG P. (1973e) Structure, synthesis and external transfer of mucosal immunoglobulins. *Ann. Immunol. (Inst. Pasteur)*, **124C**, 417-438.
BRANDTZAEG P. (1974a) Mucosal and glandular distribution of immunoglobulin components. Immunohistochemistry with a cold ethanol-fixation technique. *Immunology*, **26**, 1101-1114.
BRANDTZAEG P. (1974b) Mucosal and glandular distribution of immunoglobulin components. Differential localization of free and bound SC in secretory epithelial cells. *J. Immunol.*, **112**, 1553-1559.
BRANDTZAEG P. (1974c). Characteristics of SC–Ig complexes formed *in vitro*. *Advanc. exp. med. Biol.*, **45**, 87-97.
BRANDTZAEG P. (1974d). Presence of J chain in human immunocytes containing various immunoglobulin classes. *Nature*, **252**, 418-420.
BRANDTZAEG P. (1975) Human secretory immunoglobulin M. *Immunology* (in press).
BRANDTZAEG P., BAKLIEN K., FAUSA O. & HOEL P.S. (1974) Immunohistochemical characterization of local immunoglobulin formation in ulcerative colitis. *Gastroenterology*, **66**, 1123-1136.
BRANDTZAEG P. & FJELLANGER I. (1965) Immunological studies on tissue components of human gingiva. *Odont. Tidskr. (Scand. J. dent. Res.)*, **73**, 621 (Abstract).
BRANDTZAEG P., FJELLANGER I. & GJERULDSEN S.T. (1967) Localization of immunoglobulins in human nasal mucosa. *Immunochemistry*, **4**, 57-60.
BRANDTZAEG P., FJELLANGER I. & GJERULDSEN S.T. (1968a) Adsorption of immunoglobulin A onto oral bacteria *in vivo*. *J. Bacteriol.*, **96**, 242-249.
BRANDTZAEG P., FJELLANGER I. & Gjeruldsen S.T. (1968b) Immunoglobulin M: Local synthesis and selective secretion in patients with immunoglobulin A deficiency. *Science*, **160**, 789-791.
BRANDTZAEG P., FJELLANGER I. & GJERULDSEN S.T. (1970) Human secretory immunoglobulins. I. Salivary secretions from individuals with normal or low levels of serum immunoglobulins. *Scand. J. Haematol.*, Suppl. 12, 1-83.
BRANDTZAEG P. & KRAUS F.W. (1965) Autoimmunity and periodontal disease. *Odont. Tidskr. (Scand. J. dent. Res.)*, **73**, 281-393.
BRASHER G.W. & DEITERMAN L.H. (1972) Salivary IgA and infection in children with atopy. *Ann. Allergy*, **30**, 241-244.
BROWN W.R., NEWCOMB R.W. & ISHIZAKA K. (1970) Proteolytic degradation of exocrine and serum immunoglobulins. *J. clin. Invest.*, **49**, 1374-1380.
BUCKLEY R.H. & DEES S.C. (1969) Correlation of milk precipitins with IgA deficiency. *New Engl. J. Med.*, **281**, 465-468.

BURDON D.W. (1973) The bactericidal action of immunoglobulin A. *J. Med. Microbiol.*, **6**, 131–139.
BURROWS W. & HAVENS I. (1948) Studies on immunity to asiatic cholera. V. The absorption of immune globulin from the bowel and its excretion in the urine and feces of experimental animals and human volunteers. *J. Infectious Dis.*, **82**, 231–250.
CALLERAME M.L., CONDEMI J.J., ISHIZAKA K., JOHANSSON S.G.O. & VAUGHAN J.H. (1971) Immunoglobulins in bronchial tissues from patients with asthma, with special reference to immunoglobulin E. *J. Allergy*, **47**, 187–197.
CEBRA J. & BERNIER G.M. (1967) Quantitative relationships among lymphoid cells differentiated with respect to class of heavy chain, type of light chain, and allotypic markers. In SMITH R.T., GOOD R.A. & MIESCHER P.A. *Ontogeny of Immunity*, 65–77. University of Florida Press, Gainsville.
CHANDLER D.C., LUNDBLAD R.L. & SILVERMAN M.S. (1972) Salivary IgA and periodontal disease—a quantitative and differential study. *I.A.D.R. Abstracts*, No. 371.
CHIBA Y. & NAKAO T. (1972) Mumps virus neutralizing antibody in saliva following natural infection. *Tohoku J. exp. Med.*, **106**, 75–81.
CHILGREN R.A., QUIE P.G., MEUWISSEN H.J. & HONG R. (1967) Chronic mucocutaneous candidiasis, deficiency of delayed hypersensitivity and selective local antibody defect. *Lancet*, **2**, 688–693.
CLOUGH J.D., MIMS L.H. & STROBER W. (1971) Deficient IgA antibody responses to arsanilic acid bovine serum albumin (BSA) in neonatally thymectomized rabbits. *J. Immunol.*, **106**, 1624–1629.
COCHRANE C.G. (1967) Mediators of the Arthus and related reactions. *Prog. Allergy*, **11**, 1–35.
COOKE T.D., HURD E.R., ZIFF M. & JASIN H.E. (1972) The pathogenesis of chronic inflammation in experimental antigen-induced arthritis. II. Preferential localization of antigen–antibody complexes to collagenous tissues. *J. exp. Med.*, **135**, 323–339.
COOKE T.D. & JASIN H.E. (1972) The pathogenesis of chronic inflammation in experimental antigen–induced arthritis. I. The role of antigen in the local immune response. *Arthritis and Rheumatism*, **15**, 327–337.
COOMBS R.R.A. & GELL P.G.H. (1968) Classification of allergic reactions responsible for clinical hypersensitivity and disease. In GELL P.G.H. & COOMBS R.R.A. *Clinical Aspects of Immunology*, 2nd edition, 575–596, Blackwell Scientific Publications, Edinburgh.
COOPER M.D., LAWTON A.R. & KINCADE P.W. (1972) A two-stage model for development of antibody-producing cells. *Clin exp. Immunol.*, **11**, 143–149.
COSENZA H. & NORDIN A.A. (1970) Immunoglobulin classes of antibody-forming cells in mice. *J. Immunol.*, **104**, 976–983.
CRABBÉ P.A. & HEREMANS J.F. (1967) Distribution in human nasopharyngeal tonsils of plasma cells containing different types of immunoglobulin polypeptide chains. *Lab. Invest.*, **16**, 112–123.
CRABBÉ P.A., NASH D.R., BAZIN H., EYSSEN H. & HEREMANS J.F. (1970) Immunohistochemical observations on lymphoid tissues from conventional and germfree mice. *Lab. Invest.*, **22**, 448–457.

DAVID J.R. (1971) Migration inhibitory factor and mediators of cellular hypersensitivity *in vitro*. In AMOS B. *Progress in Immunology*, 399–412. Academic Press, New York.

DAWES C. & WOOD C.M. (1973) The contribution of oral minor mucous gland secretions to the volume of whole saliva in man. *Archs. oral Biol.*, **18,** 337–342.

DICK H.M. & TROTT J.R. (1971) The role of inflammation and sensitization on antigen penetration in rabbit gingiva. *J. Periodont.*, **42,** 796–803.

DOLOVICH J., TOMASI T.B. & ARBESMAN C.E. (1970) Antibodies of nasal and parotid secretions of ragweed-allergic subjects. *J. Allergy*, **45,** 286–294.

DONATSKY O. & DABELSTEEN E. (1973) Recurrent aphthous stomatitis. An immunological study. *I.A.D.R. Abstracts* (Scandinavian Division), No. 25.

DOUGLAS R.G., ROSSEN R.D., BUTLER W.T. & COUCH R.B. (1967) Rhinovirus neutralizing antibody in tears, parotid saliva, nasal secretions and serum. *J. Immunol.*, **99,** 297–303.

EDDIE D.S., SCHULKIND M.L. & ROBBINS J.B. (1971) The isolation and biologic activities of purified secretory IgA and IgG anti-*Salmonella typhimurium* 'O' antibodies from rabbit intestinal fluid and colostrum. *J. Immunol.*, **106,** 181–190.

EMMINGS F. & GENCO R. (1972) IgA antibody-forming cells in rabbit submandibular glands. *I.A.D.R. Abstracts*, No. 876.

ESKELAND T. & BRANDTZAEG P. (1974) Does J chain mediate the combination of 19S IgM and dimeric IgA with the secretory component rather than being necessary for their polymerization? *Immunochemistry*, **11,** 161–163.

EVERHART D.L., GRIGSBY W.R. & CARTER W.H. (1972) Evaluation of dental caries experience and salivary immunoglobulins in whole saliva. *J. dent. Res.*, **51,** 1487–1491.

EVERSOLE L.R., KENNEY E.B. & SABES W.R. (1972) Oral lesions as the initial sign in pemphigus vulgaris. *Oral Surg. Oral Med. & Oral Path.*, **33,** 354–361.

FAULK W.P. & HIJMANS W. (1972) Recent developments in immunofluorescence. *Progr. Allergy*, **16,** 9–39.

FAZEKAS DE ST GROTH S. (1951) Studies in experimental immunology of influenza. IX. The mode of action of pathotopic adjuvants. *Austral. J. exp. Biol. med. Sci.*, **29,** 339–352.

FAZEKAS DE ST GROTH S., DONNELLEY M. & GRAHAM D.M. (1951) Studies in experimental immunology of influenza. VIII. Pathotopic adjuvants. *Austral. J. exp. Biol. med. Sci.*, **29,** 323–337.

FELTKAMP T.E.W. & VAN ROSSUM A.L. (1968) Antibodies to salivary duct cells, and other autoantibodies, in patients with Sjögren's syndrome and other idiopathic autoimmune diseases. *Clin. exp. Immunol.*, **3,** 1–16.

FENNELL R.H. & VAZQUEZ J.J. (1962) Immunochemical study of plasma proteins of female genital tract. *Acta Cytol.*, **6,** 340–342.

FJELLANGER I., BRANDTZAEG P. & GJERULDSEN S.T. (1968) Immunohistochemical localization of gamma-globulins in human gastric mucosa. In SEMB L.S. & MYREN J. *The Physiology of Gastric Secretion*, 110–117. Universitetsforlaget, Oslo.

FLAX M.H., ELLIOTT J.H., DALY J.J., WILLMS-KRETSCHMER K., MCCARTHY J.S. & LESKOWITZ S. (1969) Local plasmacytopoiesis in delayed hypersensitivity reactions. *J. Immunol.*, **102,** 1214–1219.

FORD H. & KIRSNER J.B. (1964) 'Auer colitis' in rabbits induced by intrarectal antigen. *Proc. Soc. exp. Biol. Med.*, **116**, 745–748.
FORD W.L. & GOWANS J.L. (1969) The traffic of lymphocytes. *Seminars in Hematology*, **6**, 67–83.
FORD W.L. & MARCHESI V.T. (1971) Lymphocyte recirculation and its immunological significance. Workshop 5. In AMOS B. *Progress in Immunology*, 1159–1164. Academic Press, New York.
FREEDMAN H.L., LISTGARTEN M.A. & TAICHMAN N.S. (1968) Electron microscopic features of chronically inflamed human gingiva. *J. periodont. Res.*, **3**, 313–327.
FRÖLAND S.S. & NATVIG J.B. (1972) Surface-bound immunoglobulin on lymphocytes from normal and immunodeficient humans. *Scand. J. Immunol.*, **1**, 1–12.
FRÖLAND S.S. & NATVIG J.B. (1973) Identification of three different human lymphocyte populations by surface markers. *Transplant. Rev.*, **16**, 114–162.
GAVIN J.B. (1970) Ultrastructural features of chronic marginal gingivitis. *J. periodont. Res.*, **5**, 19–29.
GERBER M.A., PARONETTO F. & KOCHWA S. (1971) Immunohistochemical localization of IgE in asthmatic lungs. *Am. J. Path.*, **62**, 339–350.
GIRARD J.P. & DE KALBERMATTEN A. (1970) Antibody activity in human duodenal fluid. *Eur. J. clin. Invest.*, **1**, 188–195.
GITLIN D. & SASAKI T. (1969) Immunoglobulins G, A, and M determined in single cells from human tonsils. *Science*, **164**, 1532–1534.
GLYNN A.A. (1969) The complement lysozyme sequence in immune bacteriolysis. *Immunology*, **16**, 463–471.
GRAHAM R.C. & SHANNON S.L. (1972) Peroxidase arthritis. I. An immunologically mediated inflammatory response with ultrastructural cytochemical localization of antigen and specific antibody. *Am. J. Path.*, **67**, 69–94.
GREENBERG M.S. & BRIGHTMAN V.J. (1969) Immunoglobulin levels in patients with recurrent intraoral herpes simplex infections. *I.A.D.R. Abstracts*, No. 9.
GUGLER E., PALLAVICINI J.C., SWERDLOW H., ZIPKIN I. & SANT' AGNESE P.A. di (1968) Immunological studies of submaxillary saliva from patients with cystic fibrosis and from normal children. *J. Pediat.*, **73**, 548–559.
HALL W.H., MANION R.E. & ZINNEMAN H.H. (1971) Blocking serum lysis of *Brucella abortus* by hyperimmune rabbit immunoglobulin A. *J. Immunol.*, **107**, 41–46.
HALPERN M.S. & KOSHLAND M.R. (1970) Novel subunit in secretory IgA. *Nature, Lond.*, **228**, 1276–1278.
HAND W.L., SMITH J.W., MILLER T.E., BARNETT J.A. & SANFORD J.P. (1970) Immunoglobulin synthesis in lower urinary tract infection. *J. Lab. clin. Med.*, **75**, 19–29.
HAND W.L., SMITH J.W. & SANFORD J.P. (1971) The antibacterial effect of normal and infected urinary bladder. *J. Lab. clin. Med.*, **77**, 605–615.
HANEBERG B. (1974) Human fecal agglutinins to rabbit erythrocytes. *Scand. J. Immunol.*, **3**, 71–76.
HANNA M.G. & PETERS L.C. (1971) Requirement for continuous antigenic stimulation in the development and differentiation of antibody-forming cells: Effect of antigen dose. *Immunology*, **20**, 707–718.

HANSON L.Å. & BRANDTZAEG P. (1973) Secretory antibody systems. In STIEHM E.R. & FULGINITI V.A. *Immunologic Disorders in Infants and Children*, 107–126. W.B. Saunders, Philadelphia.

HANSON L.Å., HOLMGREN J. & WADSWORTH C. (1971) A radial immuno-gel filtration method for characterization and quantitation of macromolecules. *Int. Arch. Allergy*, **40**, 806–819.

HARDY K.M., PERRY H.O., PINGREE G.C. & KIRBY T.J. (1971) Benign mucous membrane pemphigoid. *Archs. Derm.*, **104**, 467–475.

HARTZER R.C., TOTO P.D. & GARGIULO A.W. (1971) Immune reactions in the gingiva of the pregnant and nonpregnant human female. *J. Periodont.*, **42**, 239–245.

HASLER J.F. (1972) The role of immunofluorescence in the diagnosis of oral vesiculobullous disorders. *Oral Surg. Oral Med. & Oral Path.*, **33**, 362–374.

HERMAN J.H., BRADLEY J., ZIFF M. & SMILEY J.D. (1971) Response of the rheumatoid synovial membrane to exogenous immunization. *J. Clin. Invest.*, **50**, 266–273.

HOLMBERG K. & KILLANDER J. (1971) Quantitative determination of immuno-globulins (IgG, IgA and IgM) and identification of IgA-type in the gingival fluid. *J. periodont. Res.*, **6**, 1–8.

HONJO H., TSUBAKIMOTO K., UTSUMI N. & TSUTSUI M. (1970) Localization of plasma proteins in the human dental pulp. *J. dent. Res.*, **49**, 880 (only).

HORTON J.E., RAISZ L.G., SIMMONS H.A., OPPENHEIM J.J. & MERGENHAGEN S.E. (1972) Bone resorbing activity in supernatant fluid from cultured human peripheral blood leukocytes. *Science*, **177**, 793–795.

HUNTLEY C.C., ROBBINS J.B., LYERLY A.D. & BUCKLEY R.H. (1971) Characterization of precipitating antibodies to ruminant serum and milk proteins in humans with selective IgA deficiency. *New Engl. J. Med.*, **284**, 7–10.

HURLIMANN J. (1971) Immunoglobulin synthesis and transport by human salivary glands. Immunological mechanisms of the mucous membranes. *Current Topics in Pathology*, **55**, 69–108.

HURLIMANN J. & ZUBER C. (1968) *In vitro* protein synthesis by human salivary glands. I. Synthesis of salivary IgA and serum proteins. *Immunology*, **14**, 809–817.

ISHIKAWA T., WICHER K. & ARBESMAN C.E. (1972) Distribution of immunoglobulins in palatine and pharyngeal tonsils. *Int. Arch. Allergy*, **43**, 801–812.

ISHIZAKA T., ISHIZAKA K., BORSOS T. & RAPP H. (1966) C'1 fixation by human isoagglutinins: Fixation of C'1 by γG and γM but not by γA antibody. *J. Immunol.*, **97**, 716–726.

JASIN H.E. & ZIFF M. (1969) Immunoglobulin and specific antibody synthesis in a chronic inflammatory focus: Antigen-induced synovitis. *J. Immunol.*, **102**, 355–369.

JERNE N.K. (1971) The somatic generation of immune recognition. *Eur. J. Immunol.*, **1**, 1–9.

JORDON R.E., TRIFTSHAUSER C.T. & SCHROETER A.L. (1971) Direct immuno-fluorescent studies of pemphigus and bullous pemphigoid. *Archs. Derm.*, **103**, 486–491.

KAPLAN M.E., DALMASSO A.P. & WOODSON M. (1972) Complement-dependent opsonization of incompatible erythrocytes by human secretory IgA. *J. Immunol.*, **108**, 275–278.

KAUFMAN H.S. & HOBBS J.R. (1970) Immunoglobulin deficiencies in an atopic population. *Lancet*, **2**, 1061–1063.
KAY D.M. & TUFFANELLI D.L. (1969) Immunofluorescent techniques in clinical diagnosis of cutaneous disease. *Ann. intern. Med.*, **71**, 753–762.
KENT S.P. (1967) Diffusion of plasma proteins into cells: A manifestation of cell injury in human myocardial ischemia. *Am. J. Path.*, **50**, 623–637.
KENT S.P. (1969) Diffusion of plasma proteins into cells. A manifestation of cell injury in rabbit skeletal muscle exposed to lecithinase C. *Arch. Path.*, **8**, 407–412.
KERR A.C. (1961) The physiological regulation of salivary secretions in man. GREULICH R.C., MACDONALD J.B. & RUSHTON M.A. In *International Series of Monographs on Oral Biology*, Vol. I. Pergamon Press, Oxford.
KLEIN E., ESKELAND T., INOUE M. & STROM R. (1971) Surface immunoglobulin-moieties on lymphoid cells. *Ann. N.Y. Acad. Sci.*, **177**, 306–325.
KNOP J., BREU H., WERNET P. & ROWLEY D. (1971) The relative antibacterial efficiency of IgM, IgG and IgA from pig colostrum. *Austral. J. exp. Biol. med. Sci.*, **49**, 405–413.
KOBAYASHI K., VAERMAN J.P. & HEREMANS J.F. (1973) J-chain determinants in polymeric immunoglobulins. *Eur. J. Immunol.*, **3**, 185–191.
KOSTER F.T. & MCGREGOR D.D. (1971) The mediator of cellular immunity. III. Lymphocyte traffic from the blood into the inflamed peritoneal cavity. *J. exp. Med.*, **133**, 864–876.
KOSTER F.T., MCGREGOR D.D. & MACKANESS G.B. (1971) The mediator of cellular immunity. II. Migration of immunologically committed lymphocytes into inflammatory exudates. *J. exp. Med.*, **133**, 400–409.
KRAFT S.C., FITCH F.W. & KIRSNER J.B. (1963) Histologic and immunohisto-chemical features of the Auer 'colitis' in rabbits. *Ann. J. Path.*, **43**, 913–926.
KRAUS F.W. & MESTECKY J. (1971) Immunohistochemical localization of amylase, lysozyme and immunoglobulins in the human parotid gland. *Archs. oral Biol.*, **16**, 781–789.
KRAUS F.W., MESTECKY J. & GRUPE H.E. (1972) Immune response to clostridial collagenase in gingiva and other tissues of the rabbit. *J. dent. Res.*, **51**, 293–301.
KRISTOFFERSEN T. & TÖNDER O. (1973) Anti-immunoglobulin activity in inflamed human gingiva. *I.A.D.R. Abstracts* (Scandinavian Division), No. 83.
KUSHNER I. & SOMMERVILLE J.A. (1971) Permeability of human synovial membrane to plasma proteins. Relationship to molecular size and inflammation. *Arthritis and Rheumatism*, **14**, 560–570.
LACHMANN P.J. (1967) Allergic reactions, connective tissue, and disease. In *Scientific Basis of Medicine Annual Reviews*, 36–58.
LAI A FAT R.F.M., CORMANE R.H. & VAN FURTH R. (1974) An immunohisto-pathological study on the synthesis of immunoglobulins and complement in normal and pathological skin and the adjacent mucous membranes *Brit. J. Dermatol.* **90**, 123–135.
LAI A FAT R.F.M., SUURMOND D. & VAN FURTH R. (1973) *In vitro* synthesis of immunoglobulins, secretory component, and complement in normal and pathological skin and the adjacent mucous membranes. *Clin. exp. Immunol.*, **14**, 377–395.
LANCE E.M. & COOPER S. (1972) Homing of specifically sensitized lymphocytes to allografts of skin. *Cellular Immunol.*, **5**, 66–73.

LARSSON U., ATTSTRÖM R. & LAURELL A.-B. (1973) Complement factors in gingival crevice material and in saliva. *I.A.D.R. Abstracts* (Scandinavian Division), No. 86.
LEHMANN J.D., SMITH J.W., MILLER T.E., BARNETT J.A. & SANFORD J.P. (1968) Local immune response in experimental pyelonephritis. *J. clin. Invest.*, **47**, 2541–2550.
LEHNER T. (1969) Pathology of recurrent oral ulceration and oral ulceration in Behçet's syndrome: Light, electron and fluorescence microscopy. *J. Pathol.*, **97**, 481–494.
LEHNER T., CARDWELL J.E. & CLARRY E.D. (1967) Immunoglobulins in saliva and serum in dental caries. *Lancet*, **1**, 1294–1297.
LINDSTROM F.D. & FOLKE L.E.A. (1968) Salivary IgA in periodontal disease. *I.A.D.R. Abstracts*, No. 410.
LOEWI G., DORLING J. & GLYNN L.E. (1971) The origin of antibody-producing cells in experimental synovitis. *Internat. Arch. Allergy Applied Immunol.*, **41**, 132–137.
MACDONALD D.G. & COWLEY G.C. (1972) Local formation of immunoglobulins in gingivae. In MACPHEE T. *Host Resistance to Commensal Bacteria*, 151–157. Livingstone, Edinburgh.
MACH J.-P. (1970) *In vitro* combination of human and bovine free secretory component with IgA of various species. *Nature, Lond.*, **228**, 1278–1282.
MANCINI G., CARBONARA A.O. & HEREMANS J.F. (1965) Immunochemical quantitation of antigens by single radial immunodiffusion. *Immunochemistry*, **2**, 235–254.
MANCINI R.E. (1963) Connective tissue and serum proteins. *Int. Rev. Cytol.*, **14**, 193–222.
MANN J.J., WALDMAN R.H., TOGO Y., HEIMER G.G., DAWKINS A.T. & KASEL J.A. (1968) Antibody response in respiratory secretions of volunteers given live and dead influenza virus. *J. Immunol.*, **100**, 726–735.
MARCHALONIS J.J. & CONE R.E. (1973) Biochemical and biological characteristics of lymphocyte surface immunoglobulin. *Transplant. Rev.*, **14**, 3–49.
MARTINELLI C. & RULLI M.A. (1968) Primary plasmacytoma of soft tissue (gingiva). *Oral Surg. Oral Med. & Oral Path.*, **25**, 607–609.
MAYRON L.W. & LOISELLE R.J. (1973) Bacterial antigens and antibodies in human periodontal tissue. *J. Periodont.*, **44**, 164–166.
MCCLELLAND D.B.L., SAMSON R.R., PARKIN D.M. & SHEARMAN D.J.C. (1972) Bacterial agglutination studies with secretory IgA prepared from human gastrointestinal secretions and colostrum. *Gut*, **13**, 450–458.
MCDOUGALL W.A. (1972) Ultrastructural localization of antibody to an antigen applied topically to rabbit gingiva. *J. periodont. Res.*, **7**, 304–314.
MCDOUGALL W.A. (1974) The effect of topical antigen on the gingiva of sensitized rabbits. *J. Periodont. Res.*, **9**, 153–164.
MESSNER R.P. & JELINEK J. (1971) Receptors for human γG globulin on human neutrophils. *J. clin. Invest.*, **49**, 2165–2171.
MESTECKY J., ZIKAN J. & BUTLER W.T. (1971) Immunoglobulin M and secretory IgA: Presence of a common polypeptide chain different from light chains. *Science*, **171**, 1163–1165.

MOORE R.D. & SCHOENBERG M.D. (1964) Origin of plasma cells in sites of inflammation. *Nature, Lond.*, **203**, 1293-1294.
MOUTON R.P., STOOP J.W., BALLIEUX R.E. & MUL N.A.H. (1970) Pneumococcal antibodies in IgA of serum and external secretions. *Clin. exp. Immunol.*, **7**, 201-210.
MÜLLER-EBERHARD H.J. (1971) Biochemistry of complement. In AMOS B. *Progress in Immunology*, 553-565. Academic Press, New York.
NAKAMURA R.M., SPIEGELBERG H.L., LEE S. & WEIGLE W.O. (1968) Relationship between molecular size and intra- and extravascular distribution of protein antigens. *J. Immunol.*, **100**, 376-383.
NAKAO T., CHIBA Y. & CHIBA S. (1970) Hemagglutination inhibition activity for mumps virus in saliva. *Tohoku J. exp. Med.*, **100**, 369-373.
NASH D.R. & HOLLE B. (1973) Local and systemic cellular immune responses in guinea-pigs given antigen parenterally or directly into the lower respiratory tract. *Clin. exp. Immunol.*, **13**, 573-583.
NEWCOMB R.W., ISHIZAKA K. & DEVALD B.L. (1969) Human IgG and IgA diphtheria antitoxins in serum, nasal fluids and saliva. *J. Immunol.*, **103**, 215-224.
NISENGARD R.J., BEUTNER E.H. & GAUTO M. (1971) Immunofluorescence studies of IgE in periodontal disease. *Ann. N.Y. Acad. Sci.*, **177**, 39-47.
NOSSAL G.J.V. (1969) *Antibodies and Immunity*, 238. Basic Books, Inc., London.
NOSSAL G.J.V., WARNER N.L. & LEWIS H. (1971) Incidence of cells simultaneously secreting IgM and IgG antibody to sheep erythrocytes. *Cellular Immunol.*, **2**, 41-53.
OGRA P.L. (1971) Effect of tonsillectomy and adenoidectomy on nasopharyngeal antibody response to poliovirus. *New Engl. J. Med.*, **284**, 59-64.
OLÁH I., SURJÁN L. & TÖRO I. (1972) Electronmicroscopic observations on the antigen reception in the tonsillar tissue. *Acta Biol. Acad. Sci. Hung.*, **23**, 61-73.
OON C.H. & LEE J. (1972) A controlled quantitative study of parotid salivary secretory IgA-globulin in normal adults. *J. Immunological Methods*, **2**, 45-48.
ÖRSTAVIK D. & BRANDTZAEG P. (1975). Secretion of parotid IgA in relation to gingival inflammation and dental caries experience in man. *Archs. oral Biol.* (in press).
ÖRSTAVIK D., KRAUS F.W. & COOK C.H. (1973) Immunohistochemical analysis of proteins in the acquired enamel pellicle. *I.A.D.R. Abstracts*, No. 538.
OSOBA D. (1969) Restriction of the capacity to respond to two antigens by single precursors of antibody-producing cells in culture. *J. exp. Med.*, **129**, 141-152.
ÖZKARAGÖZ K., SMITH H.J. & GÖKCEN H. (1972) IgE levels in serum, saliva and urine of normal individuals. *Acta Allergologica*, **27**, 392-396.
PAGE C.O. & REMINGTON J.S. (1967) Immunologic studies in normal human sweat. *J. Lab. clin. Med.*, **69**, 634-650.
PARKIN D.M., MCCLELLAND D.B.L., SAMSON R.R., MCA LEES M. & SHEARMAN D.J.C. (1973) The effect of acid, pepsin and trypsin on human colostral IgA agglutinins. *Eur. J. clin. Invest.*, **3**, 66-71.
PARROTT D.M.V. & DESOUSA M. (1971) Thymus-dependent and thymus-independent populations: origin, migratory patterns and lifespan. *Clin. exp. Immunol.*, **8**, 663-684.

PETERSEN B.H. & INGRAHAM J.S. (1969) The limitation of individual cells to the production of a single specificity of antibody in response to a coupled hapten–antigen complex. *Immunochemistry*, **6**, 379–390.
PIRQUET C. VON (1906) Quoted from COOMBS R.R.A. & GELL P.G.H. (1968) p. 576.
PLATT D., CROSBY R.G. & DALBOW M.H. (1970) Evidence for the presence of immunoglobulins and antibodies in inflamed periodontal tissues. *J. Periodont.*, **41**, 215–222.
RANNEY R.R. (1970) Specific antibody in gingiva and submandibular nodes of monkeys with allergic periodontal disease. *J. periodont. Res.*, **5**, 1–7.
RANNEY R.R. & ZANDER H.A. (1970). Allergic periodontal disease in sensitized squirrel monkeys. *J. Periodont.*, **41**, 12–21.
RITZMANN S.E., DANIELS J.C., SAKAI H. & BEATHARD G.A. (1973) The lymphocyte in immunobiology. *Ann. Allergy*, **31**, 109–125.
RIZZO A.A. & MITCHELL C.T. (1966) Chronic allergic inflammation induced by repeated deposition of antigen in rabbit gingival pockets. *Periodontics*, **4**, 5–10.
ROITT I.M., TORRIGIANI G., GREAVES M.F., BROSTOFF J. & PLAYFAIR J.H.L. (1969). The cellular basis of immunological responses. *Lancet*, **2**, 367–371.
ROSSEN R.D., MORGAN C., HSU K.C., BUTLER W.T. & ROSE H.M. (1968) Localization of 11S external secretory IgA by immunofluorescence in tissues lining the oral and respiratory passages in man. *J. Immunol.*, **100**, 706–717.
ROWE D.S. (1969) Radioactive single radial diffusion: a method for increasing the sensitivity of immunochemical quantification of proteins in agar gel. *Bull. Wld. Hlth. Org.*, **40**, 613–616.
ROWE D.S., HUG K., FAULK W.P., MCCORMICK J.N. & GERBER H. (1973) IgD on the surface of peripheral blood lymphocytes of the human newborn. *Nature New Biol.*, **118**, 155–157.
ROWLEY D.A., GOWANS J.L., ATKINS R.C., FORD W.L. & SMITH M.E. (1972) The specific selection of recirculating lymphocytes by antigen in normal and preimmunized rats. *J. exp. Med.*, **136**, 499–513.
SCHIMPL A. & WECKER E. (1973) Stimulation of IgG antibody response *in vitro* by T cell-replacing factor. *J. exp. Med.*, **137**, 547–552.
SCHROEDER H.E. & PAGE R. (1972) Lymphocyte–fibroblast interaction in the pathogenesis of inflammatory gingival disease. *Experientia*, **28**, 1228–1230.
SCHWARTZ D.P. & BUCKLEY R.H. (1971) Serum IgE concentrations and skin reactivity to anti-IgE antibody in IgA-deficient patients. *New Engl. J. Med.*, **284**, 513–517.
SCHWARTZ H.A. & GIBSON W.A. (1973) Immunofluorescent demonstration of IgG, IgM and IgA in human dental plaque. *I.A.D.R. Abstracts*, No. 324.
SELNER J.C., MERRILL D.A. & CLAMAN H.N. (1968) Salivary immunoglobulin and albumin: Development during the newborn period. *J. Pediat.*, **72**, 685–689.
SERRE A., BENFREDJ G. & LEVY D. (1972) Les immunoglobulines A salivoires. Étude des corrélationes avec les indices de carie et de quelques facteurs de variabilité des résultats. *Rev. Immunol. (Paris)*, **36**, 47–54.
SHILLITOE E.J. & LEHNER T. (1972) Immunoglobulins and complement in crevicular fluid, serum and saliva in man. *Archs. oral Biol.*, **17**, 241–247.

SHKLAIR I.L., ROVELSTAD G.H. & LAMBERTS B.L. (1969) A study of some factors influencing phagocytosis of cariogenic streptococci by caries-free and caries-active individuals. *J. dent. Res.*, **48**, 842–845.

SHUSTER J. (1971) Pepsin hydrolysis of IgA—delineation of two populations of molecules. *Immunochemistry*, **8**, 405–411.

SIMS W. (1972) The concept of immunity in dental caries. II. Specific immune responses. *Oral Surg.*, **34**, 69–86.

SIRISINHA S. & CHARUPATANA C. (1970) Antibody responses in serum, secretions, and urine of man after parenteral administration of vaccines. *Infection and Immunity*, **2**, 29–37.

SIRISINHA S. & CHARUPATANA C. (1971) Antibodies to indigenous bacteria in human serum, secretions, and urine. *Canad. J. Microbiol.*, **17**, 1471–1473.

SKAUG N. (1973) Immunoglobulins in fluid from non-keratinizing jaw cysts. *I.A.D.R. Abstracts* (Scandinavian Division), No. 26.

SLIWINSKI A.J. & ZVAIFLER N.J. (1970) *In vivo* synthesis of IgG by rheumatoid synovium. *J. Lab. clin. Med.*, **76**, 304–310.

SMILEY J.D., SACHS C. & ZIFF M. (1968) *In vitro* synthesis of immunoglobulin by rheumatoid synovial membrane. *J. clin. Invest.*, **47**, 624–632.

SMITH J.B., MCINTOSH G.H. & MORRIS B. (1970) The migration of cells through chronically inflamed tissues. *J. Pathol.*, **100**, 21–29.

SOUTH M.A., WARWICK W.J., WOLLHEIM F.A. & GOOD R.A. (1967) The IgA system. III. IgA levels in the serum and saliva of pediatric patients—evidence for a local immunological system. *J. Pediat.*, **71**, 645–653.

SPRINGER G.F. (1967) The relation of microbes to blood-group-active substances. In TRENTIN J.J. *Cross-reacting Antigens and Neoantigens*, 29–47. Williams & Wilkins, Baltimore.

STOKES C.R., HOSKING C.S., TURNER M.W. & JOHANSSON S.G.O. (1973) Urinary IgE: a reappraisal. *Eur. J. Immunol.*, **3**, 241–242.

STRAUS W. (1972) Location of the antigen, antibody and antigen–antibody complexes in delayed-type hypersensitivity skin reactions to horseradish peroxidase. *J. Histoch. Cytochem.*, **20**, 604–620.

TALAL N., ASOFSKY R. & LIGHTBODY P. (1970) Immunoglobulin synthesis by salivary gland lymphoid cells in Sjögren's syndrome. *J. clin. Invest.*, **49**, 49–54.

TAX A. & KORNGOLD L. (1971) Comparison of the effect of elastase on human secretory IgA and serum IgA. *J. Immunol.*, **107**, 1189–1191.

THONARD J.C., CROSBY R.C. & DALBOW M.H. (1966) Detection of IgM and IgA immunoglobulins in diseased human periodontal tissue. Abstract No. 328. *I.A.D.R. 44th General Meeting*.

THURSH D.R. (1970) The immune response to (3-amino, 5-succinylaminobenzoyl)-p-aminophenylarsenic acid. Immunofluorescent studies of cells making anti-arsanilic acid antibody or anti-m-aminosuccinanilic acid antibody. *Immunology*, **18**, 807–819.

TOKUMARU T. (1966) A possible role of γA-immunoglobulin in herpes simplex virus infection in man. *J. Immunol.*, **97**, 248–259.

TOLLER P.A. (1971) Immunological factors in cysts of the jaws. *Roy. Soc. Med.*, **64**, 555–559.

TOLLER P.A. & HOLBOROW E.J. (1969) Immunoglobulins and immunoglobulin-containing cells in cysts of the jaws. *Lancet*, **2**, 178–181.

TOLO K.J. (1971) A study of permeability of gingival pocket epithelium to albumin in guinea pigs and Norwegian pigs. *Archs. oral. Biol.*, **16**, 881–888.

TOMASI T.B., TAN E.M., SOLOMON A. & PRENDERGAST R.A. (1965) Characteristics of an immune system common to certain external secretions. *J. exp. Med.*, **121**, 101–124.

TOMIOKA H. & ISHIZAKA K. (1971) Mechanisms of passive sensitization. II. Presence of receptors for IgE on monkey mast cells. *J. Immunol.*, **107**, 971–978.

TOURVILLE D.R., ADLER R.H., BIENENSTOCK J. & TOMASI T.B. (1969) The human secretory immunoglobulin system: Immunohistological localization of γA, secretory 'piece', and lactoferrin in normal human tissues, *J. exp. Med.*, **129**, 411–429.

TOURVILLE D., BIENENSTOCK J. & TOMASI T.B. (1968) Natural antibodies of human serum, saliva, and urine reactive with *Escherichia coli*. *Proc. Soc. exp. Biol. Med.*, **128**, 722–727.

TSUCHIMOTO T., TUBERGEN D.G. & BLOOM A.D. (1972) Synthesis of macrophage migration inhibition factor (MIF) by immunoglobulin-producing lymphocyte lines and their clones. *J. Immunol.*, **109**, 884–885.

TURK A., LICHTENSTEIN L.M. & NORMAN P.S. (1970) Nasal secretory antibody to inhalant allergens in allergic and non-allergic patients. *Immunology*, **19**, 85–95.

URBAIN-VANSANTEN G. (1970) Concomitant synthesis, in separate cells, of non-reactive immunoglobulins and specific antibodies after immunization with tobacco mosaic virus. *Immunology*, **19**, 783–797.

VAERMAN J.-P. & HEREMANS J.F. (1968) Effect of neuraminidase and acidification on complement-fixing properties of human IgA and IgG. *Internat. Arch. Allergy Applied Immunol.*, **34**, 49–52.

VOS-CLOETENS C. DE, MINSART-BALERIAUX V. & URBAIN-VANSANTEN G. (1971) Possible relationships between antibodies and non-specific immunoglobulins simultaneously induced after antigenic stimulation. *Immunology*, **20**, 955–962.

WAGNER M. (1967) Specific immunization against Streptococcus faecalis induced dental caries in the gnotobiotic rat. *Bacteriological Proceedings*, **67**, 99 (Abstract).

WALDMAN R.H. & HENNEY C.S. (1971) Cell-mediated immunity and antibody responses in the respiratory tract after local and systemic immunization. *J. exp. Med.*, **134**, 482–494.

WALDMAN R.H., MANN J.J. & KASEL J.A. (1968) Influenza virus neutralizing antibody in human respiratory secretions. *J. Immunol.*, **100**, 80–85.

WALDMAN R.H., VIRCHOW C. & ROWE D.S. (1973) IgE levels in external secretions. *Int. Arch. Allergy*, **44**, 242–248.

WALDMANN T.A. & STROBER W. (1969) Metabolism of immunoglobulins. *Progr. Allergy*, **13**, 1–110.

WERDELIN O. & MCCLUSKEY R.T. (1971) The nature and the specificity of mononuclear cells in experimental autoimmune inflammations and the mechanisms leading to their accumulation. *J. exp. Med.*, **133**, 1242–1263.

WILLIAMS R.C., DE BOARD J.R., MELLBYE O.J., MESSNER R.P. & LINDSTROM F.D. (1973) Studies of T- and B-lymphocytes in patients with connective tissue diseases. *J. clin. Invest.*, **52**, 283–295.

WILLIAMS R.C. & GIBBONS R.J. (1972) Inhibition of bacterial adherence by

secretory immunoglobulin A: A mechanism of antigen disposal. *Science*, **177,** 697–699.
WILLIAMSON J.J., DOLBY A.E. & ADAMS D. (1969) Studies of the origin of mononuclear cells in delayed hypersensitivity reaction of oral mucosa. *J. dent. Res.*, **48,** 689–695.
WILLOUGHBY D.A. & RYAN G.B. (1970) Evidence for a possible endogenous antigen in chronic inflammation. *J. Pathol.*, **101,** 233–239.
WILSON I.D. (1972) Studies on the opsonic activity of human secretory IgA using an *in vitro* phagocytosis system. *J. Immunol.*, **108,** 726–730.
WISLÖFF F. & FRÖLAND S.S. (1973) Antibody-dependent lymphocyte-mediated cytotoxicity in man: No requirement for lymphocytes with membrane-bound immunoglobulin. *Scand. J. Immunol.*, **2,** 151–157.
YOSHINAGA M., MAYUMI M., YAMAMOTO S. & HAYASHI H. (1970) Immunoglobulin G as possible precursor of chemotactic factor. *Nature, Lond.*, **225,** 1138–1139.
ZACHRISSON B.U. (1967) Mast cells in the human gingiva. II. Metachromatic cells at low pH in healthy and inflamed tissues. *J. periodont. Res.*, **2,** 87–105.
ZACHRISSON B.U. (1968) A histological study of experimental gingivitis in man. *J. periodont. Res.*, **3,** 11–20.
ZENGO A.N., MANDEL I.D., GOLDMAN R. & KHURANA H.S. (1971) Salivary studies in human caries resistance. *Archs. oral Biol.*, **16,** 557–560.
ZIPURSKY A., BROWN E.J. & BIENENSTOCK J. (1973) Lack of opsonization potential of 11S human secretory γA. *Proc. Soc. exp. Biol. Med.*, **142,** 181–184.

CHAPTER 4
ORAL MUCOUS MEMBRANE MARKERS OF INTERNAL DISEASE: PART I

J. HAROLD JONES

4:0 Introduction

Many diseases which involve the whole body produce at some stage in their development oral changes, albeit often slight and overshadowed by the major manifestations of these diseases. The oral changes may be part of the primary disease process or they may be a complication of it. They are often distinctive because of the unique structure and function of the mouth and because of the peculiarities of its milieu, microbial, biochemical and otherwise.

This chapter seeks to survey in a general way oral mucous membrane manifestations distinctive or dominant in certain systemic diseases and to compare some of these with the skin changes seen in the same diseases. It is not intended to give a comprehensive account of the oral changes in all systemic diseases, particularly when these are minor or non-specific in character. The chapter omits reference to diseases detailed elsewhere in this book. In general Chapter 5 deals with systemic abnormalities which are well understood and whose oral manifestations have been recognized for many years, while this chapter refers to systemic abnormalities ill understood or with oral manifestations about which little has been written. The chapter may serve to highlight areas of potential growth of knowledge.

4:1 Diseases of the Gastrointestinal Tract

The idea that the same spectrum of disease may occur in the mouth as in other parts of the gastrointestinal tract is an attractive one which is not wholly supported by experience. Nevertheless, there are complex interrelationships between oral and gastric or intestinal diseases which involve the diverse results of genetic defects, the oral complications of abnormalities lower in the alimentary canal, suppositions of a common aetiology for certain oral and alimentary canal diseases, and oral manifestation of disorders which are predominantly intestinal.

4:1:1 The Peutz–Jegher's syndrome

Circumoral melanic pigmentation may result from a defect inherited through a Mendelian dominant gene of high penetrance which is not sex linked and point to the presence of one form of intestinal polyposis as a second expression of the same defect; the two comprising the Peutz–Jegher's syndrome. The pigmentation is macular and occurs intraorally as well as on the facial skin. The cutaneous pigmentation may fade after 25 years but the oral pigmentation persists. Cases with melanic pigmentation only occur and may later develop the intestinal features of the syndrome (Lin 1967). The intestinal polyps in the Peutz–Jegher's syndrome are hamartomatous and do not predispose to malignancy, although intestinal malignancy and hamartomatous polyposis may co-exist rarely in one person (Dozois *et al* 1969).

4:1:2 Oesophageal reflux

Some patients with glossopyrosis or glossodynia also complain of symptoms suggestive of oesophageal reflux such as heartburn, regurgitation and discomfort on swallowing. In such patients it is difficult to prove an association between the oral symptoms and oesophageal malfunction, and the former often fail to respond to topical remedies. The idea that oesophageal reflux is at fault is similar to the suggestion that reflux of acid contents of the oesophagus into the pharynx may cause laryngeal disease (Delahunty 1972), which is supported by acid barium swallow studies (Donner *et al* 1966). Although the suggestion remains unproven (*Brit. med. J.* 1972), the matter requires further investigation. There is also the possibility that hiatus hernia may be associated with sideropaenia and, in consequence, indirectly produce effects in the mouth and pharynx (Smiley *et al* 1963).

4:1:3 Peptic ulceration

It has been suggested that oral aphthous ulceration and peptic ulceration in the stomach or duodenum have a common aetiology. A history of dyspepsia is given by about 30% of oral ulcer patients but peptic ulceration is found in only 9%. It has been concluded that the stomach is not unusually vulnerable in oral ulcer subjects by virtue of a single aetiology (Sircus *et al* 1957).

4:1:4 Malabsorption

Intestinal malabsorption, primary or secondary to other disease, may result in nutritional deficiency and in the oral signs of this deficiency. Oral ulceration and glossitis occur frequently in idiopathic steatorrhoea (Badenoch 1960; Cooke 1953) and may be associated with the defective absorption of vitamin B_{12}, folic acid and iron which occurs in that condition (Shear & Kramer 1964).

4:1:5 Acrodermatitis enteropathica

Acrodermatitis enteropathica (Gorlin 1969) is an uncommon condition which affects children and which often has a familial incidence. Pustular eruptions occur on the lips and perioral skin and there may be a stomatitis or glossitis which is often candidal in origin. Diarrhoea, of a type indicating malabsorption, is usual and there is hair loss and alteration in the nails.

4:1:6 Crohn's disease and ulcerative colitis

Oral manifestations of Crohn's disease and ulcerative colitis are well recognized. Chronic oral ulcers, swellings of the lip, hypertrophic lesions of the buccal mucosa with a corrugated or cobble-stone appearance may show the typical histology of Crohn's disease and be associated with more extensive involvement elsewhere in the gut (Stankler *et al* 1972; Verbov 1973). In some cases the diagnosis of Crohn's disease has been made on the basis of the oral lesions (Issa 1971; Varley 1972). The specific lesions of Crohn's disease in the mouth, which are uncommon, should not be confused with aphthous ulceration, which occurs in 20% of patients with Crohn's disease (Kyle 1972).

About 5% of patients with ulcerative colitis have skin disease thought to be associated with the colitis (Johnson & Wilson 1969). Several forms of skin disease are recognized in this context and the oral and ocular mucosae may be involved in pyodermatitis vegetans. The oral lesions, referred to as pyostomatitis vegetans (McCarthy & Shklar 1963), consist of purulent vegetating eruptions.

4:2 Internal Malignancy

4:2:1 Metastases

Metastases occur less frequently in the oral soft tissues than in the jaw bones, but malignant tumours of the kidney, breast, bronchus, colon, eye, testis, liver, oesophagus and stomach have produced secondary deposits in the oral soft tissues (Lucas 1972). Such deposits in the tongue have been variously described as ulcerated, pedunculated, polypoid, crater-like, haemorrhagic and pigmented (Zegarelli *et al* 1973).

4:2:2 Non-metastatic markers

Non-metastatic markers of internal malignancy are well recognized and include endocrine, neurological and skin manifestations. The skin markers are acanthosis nigricans, dermatomyositis, gyrate erythemata, Bowen's disease and certain blistering eruptions (Sneddon 1963). Oral involvement in acanthosis nigricans associated with carcinoma of the stomach has been reported (Bang 1970; Navaratnam & Hodgson 1973), and in another case acanthosis with oral lesions occurred in a 56-year-old man with polyposis of the colon (Cohenour & Gamble 1971). Oral pigmentation without papillomata has been reported in association with bronchogenic carcinoma in a 58-year-old woman (Merchant 1973).

It has been suggested that the subepidermal blistering eruptions which occur in patients with carcinoma are more likely to affect the mucosa than the usual variety of senile pemphigoid (Sneddon 1963). One paper has related oral pemphigoid with unspecified uterine disease (Cahn 1969), and another, oral bullae with distant malignancy in six cases (Stern 1970). It is not clear at the present time whether bullous changes in the mouth, in general or of a particular type, should be regarded as likely pointers to hidden malignancy.

4:2:3 Herpes zoster

Herpes zoster may be secondary to systemic disease; or to ganglionic or nerve involvement in other infections, or by chemicals, tumours or trauma. An instance in which facial herpes zoster was the primary manifestation of previously undiagnosed lymphatic leukaemia has been reported (Chaconas 1960) and, in contrast, the suggestion that malignancy may occur in association with herpes zoster scar tissue has been considered in respect of oral lesions (Nally & Ross 1971).

4:2:4 Multiple mucosal neuromas

The presence of multiple mucosal neuromas should encourage the clinician to search for an associated endocrine tumour such as medullary thyroid carcinoma or phaeochromocytoma (Williams & Pollock 1966). The appearance of the neuromas can precede the carcinoma by as much as ten years and several members of one family may be afflicted, indicating the necessity for investigation of the relatives of an affected individual and proper genetic counselling (Walker 1973). It is postulated that the oral mucosal neuroma–medullary thyroid carcinoma syndrome is caused by a generalized disorder of neural crest development (Schimke et al 1968).

4:2:5 Mycosis fungoides

Mycosis fungoides has been described as the 'reticulosis *par excellence* of the dermatologist' (Samman 1972) and involvement of the oral mucous membrane is uncommon in it. Where oral involvement does occur it is often late in the course of the disease and overshadowed by other evidences of it (Schimpf 1964; Calhoun & Johnson 1966; Cohn et al 1971). The oral lesions manifest the typical histology and have been described as erythematous and ulcerated on the buccal mucosa and gums. Patients with the disease may have a red, shiny and smooth tongue.

4:3 Diseases of the Connective Tissue

The connective tissue diseases are generally taken to include rheumatoid arthritis, systemic lupus erythematosus, progressive systemic sclerosis, dermatomyositis and polyarteritis nodosa (Boyle & Buchanan 1971). Apart from temporomandibular joint involvement, xerostomia may be an outstanding oral feature in rheumatoid arthritis (see Chapter 10) (Bloch et al 1965).

4:3:1 Systemic lupus erythematosus

Oral or nasopharyngeal ulceration is one of fourteen manifestations of systemic lupus erythematosus, and a person is said to have the disease if four or more of these are present serially or simultaneously during any period of observation (Cohen & Canoso 1972). Patients may present with atypical migratory gingivitis in which the attached gingiva show small separate triangular and linear lesions consisting of depressed deep red areas bordered by radiating white striae and minute blood vessels, suggesting a diagnosis of lichen planus (Edwards & Gayford 1971). The ulcers may be deep and ragged and some patients complain of glossopyrosis (Herschfus 1972).

There may be considerable difficulty in differentiating the oral lesions in lichen planus from those of lupus erythematosus but the differentiation is important, since the latter may be the first evidence of a systemic disease which ultimately may hazard the patient's life. Oral ulceration in systemic lupus erythematosus may be due to herpetic infection and oral candidosis may occur (Jones 1973). It is not surprising that microbial agents dormant in the mouth produce infections in this disease because of the disordered immunity which occurs as part of it or as an effect of its treatment. Such infections must be differentiated from the primary effects of the disease since they may respond to appropriate antimicrobial therapy, or be aggravated by topical remedies given under the impression that they represent a primary manifestation of systemic lupus erythematosus.

A desquamative form of gingivitis has been reported in lupoid hepatitis (Berdon & Girasole 1972); showing hyperkeratosis, acanthosis, dyskeratosis, a lymphocytic infiltrate and degenerative changes in the basal layer and underlying collagen on histology. In the instance referred to, recovery was aided by the patient relinquishing her habit of chewing two to three packs of mint-flavoured chewing gum per day, and it is not clear how important a factor this was in producing the patient's oral lesions.

4:3:2 Progressive systemic sclerosis (scleroderma)

Oral lesions may be seen in this diffuse form of scleroderma. The patient has a mask-like face and difficulty in opening the mouth due to the rigidity of the facial soft tissue. Intraorally, livid discoloration and oedema of the mucosa occurs in the early stages of the disease, followed sometimes by shortening and induration of the lingual fraenum (Strassburg & Knolle 1972). Later the white-yellowish mucous membrane is fixed to unyielding underlying tissue and there is interference in mastication, swallowing and speech. Widening of the periodontal membrane as visualized radiographically, sometimes referred to as Blackburn's sign, may occur (Stafne & Austin 1944), but this inconstant feature may not affect all the teeth (Munroe & Knauer 1962), and may disappear in the late stages of the disease (Krogh 1950).

4:3:3 Dermatomyositis

The polymyositis which is part of this disease may affect the tongue and extreme tenderness and weakness may be found (McCarthy & Shklar 1964). Focal haemorrhage and necrosis of the oral mucous membrane occurs in about 20% of patients and the possible association of dermatomyositis with internal malignancy should be borne in mind by the clinician.

4:3:4 Polyarteritis nodosa, variants and similar diseases

4:3:4a CLASSICAL POLYARTERITIS

In classical polyarteritis there is widespread necrotizing arteritis affecting all layers of the walls of small and medium-sized vessels in a patchy fashion and producing a systemic illness with protean focal symptoms and signs. The arterial lesions may occur in the oral tissues and produce signs such as unilateral sagging of the soft palate during life, or they may be demonstrated at necropsy (Gottsegen & Gorlin 1949). Oral ulceration, sometimes linear in form or beginning in a painless papule, is also found in this disease (Plumpton 1965).

4:3:4b CUTANEOUS POLYARTERITIS NODOSA

Ten per cent of all cases of polyarteritis nodosa are of a benign type best described as 'cutaneous polyarteritis nodosa' (Borrie 1973). The only tissues affected are the skin, muscles and peripheral nerves and this variety of polyarteritis has distinctive features which allow its recognition. The mucous membranes are not affected, and those cutaneous lesions which are associated with ulcerative or granulomatous lesions in the nose or mouth are particular causes for concern to the clinician (Winkelmann & Ditto 1964).

4:3:4c WEGENER'S GRANULOMATOSIS

Wegener's granulomatosis is a rare disease in which destructive ulcerative lesions of the upper and lower respiratory tract are often the precursors of a generalized necrotizing arteritis and glomerulitis. The disease occasionally presents as a characteristic gingivitis, the recognition of which permits early diagnosis in those cases in which it occurs. The gingivitis appears as multiple, proliferative, raised and friable granulomatous papillary lesions which may be limited to the facial surfaces of the gums, and involve the interproximal free and attached gingiva as well as the adjacent alveolar mucosa. These lesions are often painful and have the consistency of wet, soft, spongy rubber. The histology of the gingival lesions may not permit certain diagnosis and vascular changes may be lacking (Cawson 1965; Kakehashi *et al* 1965). The histological features in the various case reports have tended to be less distinctive than the clinical features (Scott & Finch 1972b), but the gingival histology does resemble that seen elsewhere in this disease with collections of Langhan's and foreign body giant cells involved in an intense granulomatous inflammation. Epithelial hyperplasia may be striking.

4:3:4d GIANT CELL ARTERITIS

The outstanding symptom in giant cell arteritis is pain which may occur in the tongue particularly during eating or on talking (Henderson 1967). Episodic blanching of the tongue has been reported in this disease (Grahame *et al* 1968) and gangrene of the anterior part of the tongue may also occur (Davis & Davis 1966).

4:4 Granulomatous Diseases of Unknown Aetiology

4:4:1 Boeck's sarcoid (sarcoidosis)

Boeck's sarcoid is a systemic granulomatous disease of unknown aetiology, often widespread in the body and with depression of certain immunological reactions. Involvement of the nose and mouth occurs in approximately 3% of patients with the disease but the lesions are often small and easily overlooked (Mayock *et al* 1963).

Asymptomatic enlargement of the major salivary glands (Heerfordt's syndrome) may occur, preceded by a mild febrile illness of one week to several months' duration. Parotid gland involvement, often bilateral and with enlargement of the submandibular glands, is usual. Uveitis and other ocular lesions may occur in association with the salivary gland enlargement, and facial nerve paralysis is present in about half the cases (Epker 1972).

Analysis of twenty-five cases of intraoral involvement in sarcoidosis gleaned from the world literature (Tarpley *et al* 1972) has shown that the buccal mucous membrane, lips, gums, palate, tongue, tonsil and the floor of the mouth may be affected in the disease. Biopsy of apparently normal tissues in patients with sarcoidosis has yielded evidence of the disease in the palate (Cahn et al 1964), gingival tissue (Tillman 1964), and in labial minor salivary glands (Chisholm et al 1971; Tarpley et al 1972). Intraoral swellings in sarcoidosis are usually plaque-like or irregular, often tender, on the alveolar mucous membrane (Hobkirk 1969), floor of the mouth (Orlean & O'Brien 1966), tongue (Tillman et al 1966), or multiple (Kolas & Roche 1960), and sometimes producing gingival enlargement (Dawson Watts 1968). Diffuse granulomatous lesions with superficial desquamation and the appearance of bleb-like structures may occur (Covel 1954) and there may be chronic inflammation of the mandible with sequestration and alveolar bone loss (Macdonald et al 1969). More striking in sarcoidosis than the intraoral change is cervical lymphadenopathy.

4:4:2 Melkersson–Rosenthal syndrome

In this syndrome there is a diffuse and often brawny red swelling of the upper or lower lips or cheeks. The swelling has a rapid onset and may be accompanied by mild constitutional upset. It subsides but recurs at irregular intervals until the affected part is rubbery in consistency. Facial or other cranial nerve palsy and fissuring of the tongue, which is sometimes enlarged, occur in about one-third of the cases. Histology may reveal granulomatous inflammation which is indistinguishable from that found in sarcoidosis. Genetic factors and infective agents have been implicated in the aetiology of the condition (Nally, 1970). Reference to the Melkersson–Rosenthal syndrome is included, since its aetiology is little understood and it is possible that it can occur in several distinct diseases some of which are more widespread in their involvement.

4:5 Oral Manifestations of the Accumulation of Metabolic Products

A variety of metabolic products are deposited in the tissues. The skin and the oral mucous membranes may be affected and examples of the oral manifestations of this will be considered in the present section (Table 4.1).

4:5:1 Amyloidosis

Amyloidosis occurs in a heredofamilial form, as a complication of other diseases, and primary. Heredofamilial amyloidosis is sometimes associated with severe gastrointestinal complaints such as constipation alternating with diarrhoea and malabsorption, and there is widespread deposition of amyloid in the body (Cohen 1967). A case report (Hornová & Dluhošová 1968) of primary amyloidosis of gingiva and conjunctiva and mental disorder in a brother and sister probably represents an example of heredofamilial amyloidosis with oral manifestations. Of note was the icing-like coating on the hyperplastic gingiva.

Table 4.1 The oral manifestations of the accumulation of metabolic products

Disease	Mucosal manifestations	Particular clinical aspects
Amyloidosis	Macroglossia, petechiae, blood blisters, dryness	Diagnosis possible by gingival or lingual biopsy
Cystinosis	Stomatitis	Stomatitis occurs in latent phase
Haemochromatosis	Pigmentation, advanced periodontitis	Exclude other causes of intraoral pigmentation
Hurler's syndrome	Macroglossia, gingival hyperplasia	Difficulty in oral surgery
Lipoid proteinosis	Yellow-coloured plaques	Possible misdiagnosis as 'leukoplakia'
Erythropoietic porphyria	Atrophic cheilitis, advanced periodontitis	—
Hepatic porphyria	Blisters, later painful ulcers	Blisters may follow dental treatment. Exacerbations induced by certain drugs
Xanthomatosis	Yellow-coloured nodules	Possible misdiagnosis as 'squamous carcinoma'
Phenylketonuria	Macroglossia, ptyalism	—

Amyloid may be deposited in many organs as a complication of chronic infections, connective tissue diseases, regional enteritis, ulcerative colitis, neoplasms and diabetes. In the past tuberculosis was dominant among the possible aetiologies of secondary amyloidosis but is now less important in this respect. There does not seem to be any pattern of gastrointestinal amyloidosis unique to either primary or secondary form of the disease but gross depositions in the mouth are more usually associated with the former (Cohen 1967).

Macroglossia occurs in 10–12% of patients with primary amyloidosis as a diffuse symmetrical enlargement which interferes with oral function and may prevent mouth closure. The enlarged and relatively immobile tongue often has lateral indentations due to pressure against the teeth, and it is usually described as firm, with a thickened fraenum. Petechiae occur on the oral mucosa and 'blood blisters' on the tongue or gums which rupture to leave 'aphthae'-like ulcers (Keith 1972). Localized deposits appear as papules or as verruca-like or tumour-like masses (Stanback & Peagler 1968). The mouth is often dry and sore and this contributes to the difficulty in swallowing (Aach & Kissane 1972). Skin lesions also occur in primary amyloidosis.

Amyloid deposition has been reported in the oral submucosa as an effect of prolonged snuff taking (Lyon et al 1964) and in association with some odontogenic tumours (Vickers et al 1965).

The diagnosis of amyloidosis may be confirmed by biopsy. The tongue is suggested by some to be a better site for biopsy than the gum (Keith 1972). 'The key to the successful diagnostic biopsy is proper staining of the tissues and examination with the appropriate optical equipment', and tissue properly stained with Congo red and viewed with the polarizing microscope offers a high degree of sensitivity and specificity for amyloid (Cohen 1967).

4:5:2 Cystinosis

Cystinosis is a genetically based metabolic disorder, characterized by the deposition of cystine crystals in several tissues with photophobia, growth retardation and vitamin D-resistant rickets as the outstanding clinical signs of it. Stomatitis occurs during the latent stage of the disease causing difficulty in feeding. Smears from the oral lesions do not contain cystine crystals or *Candida* but coagulase-positive staphylococci may be present (Nazif & Osman 1973).

4:5:3 Haemochromatosis

Skin pigmentation, due to melanin and haemosiderin accumulation, is common in haemochromatosis. Gingival or mucosal pigmentation occurs in 15–25% of cases as an Addisonian melanosis of the attached gingiva or a bluish-grey haemosiderosis of the hard palate. The latter is said to be a characteristic feature of haemochromatosis, and rapid periodontal destruction also occurs in spite of appropriate therapy (Frantzis et al 1972).

4:5:4 Hurler's syndrome

Hurler's syndrome is one of the mucopolysaccharidoses and the oral manifestations of it have been comprehensively reviewed recently (Gardner 1971).

Gingival hyperplasia is an inconsistent finding in Hurler's syndrome. Enlargement of the gums in this disease may be due to enlargement of the alveolar processes, hyperplastic gingivitis associated with mouth breathing or poor oral hygiene, or to the basic connective tissue defect. Sometimes the palate is involved in the fibromatosis (Fay 1972). The tongue is usually thickened and enlarged, as are the lips, and these changes, together with generalized relative inelasticity of the soft tissues, may present difficulty in surgery (Hopkins *et al* 1973).

4:5:5 Lipoid proteinosis (hyalinosis cutis et mucosae)

Oral lesions are to be expected in the primary or Urbach-Wiethe type of this disease but not in the light-sensitive type—more correctly termed erythropoietic protoporphyria (Cairns 1972). Yellow-coloured firm plaques occur on the lips, palate and elsewhere, and the tongue may be thickened with relative immobility. The oral lesions are occasionally misdiagnosed as 'leukoplakia', but the presence of skin lesions and hoarseness dating from early childhood should suggest the diagnosis which may be substantiated by biopsy (Williams 1971; Simpson 1972).

4:5:6 Porphyria

Porphyrins are found in haemoglobins, chlorophyll, catalyse and cytochromes, and are produced mainly in the haematopoietic bone marrow and eliminated in the liver. Increased synthesis or reduced degradation results in their accumulation in the body and in the disease porphyria. Porphyria (Gilhuus-Moe & Koppang 1972) may be the result of increased synthesis (erythropoietic porphyria) or of reduced elimination (hepatic porphyria). The latter may occur as a genetically determined disorder and without skin lesions (acute intermittent porphyria), as a genetically determined disorder with skin lesions (porphyria cutanea tarda hereditaria), or as a complication of other liver disease (porphyria cutanea tarda symptomatica).

Erythropoietic porphyria is associated with skin photosensitivity and the formation of bullae and scars. Reddish-brown discolouration of the deciduous and permanent teeth (erythrodontia) occurs, and erythrodontia, atrophic cheilitis and advanced localized periodontitis are considered pathognomic of the disease (Rayne 1967).

Hepatic porphyria occurs more frequently in Swedes and in South Africans than in other races. Acute intermittent porphyria is characterized by pronounced abdominal, psychic and neuromuscular symptoms, and exacerbations of it may be initiated by sulphonamides, barbiturates and occasionally alcohol. In porphyria cutanea tarda hereditaria, subepithelial bullous skin lesions occur on exposure to sunlight and the skin is excessively vulnerable to minor traumas. In hepatic porphyria painful bullous lesions may appear in the mouth after dental treatment, and histology will reveal features similar to those seen in the cutaneous lesions (Gilhuus-Moe & Koppang 1972).

4:5:7 Xanthomatosis

In recent years there has been a considerable expansion in our knowledge of hyperlipidaemia and of xanthomatosis, but for the purpose of this chapter xanthomatosis may be defined as the widespread occurrence of collections of lipid-containing cells in the dermis and can be present in primary or secondary forms. The former is due to a biochemical defect often associated with abnormality of the serum lipids and the latter is secondary to some other disease resulting in overloading of the lipid transport mechanisms. Oral lesions have been reported in the primary form of the disease as yellowish nodules on the skin and oral mucosa, tongue and hard palate (Raffle & Hall 1968). These nodules may be indurated and ulcerated so as to mimic the clinical appearance of a squamous carcinoma.

The mucous membranes are involved in at least one-third of cases of xanthoma disseminatum; a rare disease characterized by widespread skin xanthomata and often diabetes insipidus but usually without disturbance of lipid metabolism (Beare 1971). Oral lesions may also occur in juvenile xanthoma which affects the skin and eyes in very young children and usually disappears spontaneously (Crocker 1951).

4:5:8 Miscellaneous deposits

Macroglossia and salivary excess may occur in phenylketonuria (Myers et al 1968). Sulphatides are found within myelinated nerves in the dental pulp, lip and elsewhere in the oral region in metachromatic leukodystrophy

(Gardner & Zeman 1970), but oral signs of this disease are not recognized clinically.

4:6 Oral Manifestations of Systemic Reticulohistiocytic Proliferation

4:6:1 Histiocytosis X

Stomatitis, intraoral haemorrhage, ulceration of the gingiva and mucous membranes may be found in the rapidly progressing, acute, disseminated phase of histiocytosis X, Letterer–Siwe disease, which occurs in children and in which there is sometimes a familial pattern of involvement (Johnson & Mohnac 1967).

Hand–Schüller-Christian disease describes the more chronic phase of histiocytosis X, which is slowly progressive and systemic in its involvement. More than 60% of patients with this disease present with oral symptoms or signs (Sleeper 1951), which include infiltrating masses, delayed healing after tooth extraction, necrotizing gingivitis, and bone loss simulating periodontal disease (Johnson & Mohnac 1967; Boggs & McMahon 1968; Scott & Finch 1972a). The disease runs a prolonged course, so that several years may elapse between the initial oral lesions and evidence of systematization (Whitehead 1972).

The eosionophilic granuloma phase of histiocytosis X is usually solitary and within bone, but the disease may involve soft tissues, including the oral mucosa where the lesions are evident as necrotic, friable and painful ulcerated areas.

Because of the overlap in clinical and histopathologic aspects of the diseases referred to above, the traditional concept of three separate entities is untenable (Blevins *et al* 1959) and thus the emergence of the unifying term 'histiocytosis X'. The difficulty in precise categorization of the disease in an individual patient is illustrated in some reports which also emphasize that the oral manifestations of histiocytosis X are different from those occurring in other locations, probably because of the unique structural and microbial environment of the mouth which predisposes to secondary infection (Winther *et al* 1972).

4:7 Conclusions

There are similarities between the oral and the cutaneous manifestations of many of the diseases described above. Occasionally the oral manifestations are distinctive and sometimes this is because systemic imbalance permits full rein to the potential pathogenicity of oral microbia. In some diseases the oral and the cutaneous manifestations appear dissimilar, but it may be that future work will provide evidence of an underlying unity in these manifestations. Some internal diseases with skin manifestations do not have a recognized oral counterpart but such an oral manifestation may exist, to be uncovered in the future.

4:8 References

AACH R. & KISSANE J. (1972) Amyloidosis. *Am. J. Med.*, **53**, 495.
BADENOCH J. (1960) Steatorrhoea in the adult. *Brit. med. J.*, **2**, 963.
BANG G. (1970) Acanthosis nigricans maligna. *Oral Surg.*, **29**, 370.
BEARE J.M. (1968). In ROOK A., WILKINSON D.S. & EBLING F.J.G. *Textbook of Dermatology*, 1229. Blackwell Scientific Publications, Oxford.
BERDON J.K. & GIRASOLE R.V. (1972) Oral manifestations of lupoid hepatitis. *Oral Surg.*, **33**, 900.
BLEVINS C., DAHLIN D.C., LOVESTEDT S.A. & KENNEDY R.L.J. (1959) Oral and dental manifestations of histiocytosis X. *Oral Surg.*, **12**, 473.
BLOCH K.J., BUCHANAN W.W., WOHL M.J. & BUNIM J.J. (1965) Sjögren's syndrome. *Medicine*, **44**, 187.
BOGGS D.C. & MCMAHON L.J. (1968) Hand–Schüller–Christian disease presenting as gingivitis. *Oral Surg.*, **26**, 261.
BORRIE P. (1973) Cutaneous polyarteritis nodosa. *Brit. J. Derm.*, **87**, 87.
BOYLE J.A. & BUCHANAN W.W. (1971) *Clinical Rheumatology*. Blackwell Scientific Publications, Oxford and Edinburgh.
Brit. med. J. (1972) Acid and the larynx. **3**, 193.
CAHN L.R. (1969) The oral mucous membrane markers of malignancy. *Oral Surg.*, **27**, 431.
CAHN L.R., EIZENBUD L., BLAKE M.N. & STERN D. (1964) Biopsies of normal appearing palates of patients with known sarcoidosis. *Oral Surg.*, **18**, 342.
CAIRNS R.J. (1972) In ROOK A., WILKINSON D.S. & EBLING F.J.G. *Textbook of Dermatology*, Vol. 2, 1858. Blackwell Scientific Publications, Oxford.
CALHOUN N.R. & JOHNSON C.C. (1966) Oral manifestation of mycosis fungoides. *Oral Surg.*, **22**, 261.
CAWSON R.A. (1965) Gingival changes in Wegener's granulomatosis. *Brit. dent. J.*, **118**, 30.
CHACONAS C.P. (1960) Herpes zoster—a primary manifestation of chronic lymphatic leukaemia. *Oral Surg.*, **13**, 1429.
CHISHOLM D.M., LYELL A., HAROON T.S., MASON D.K. & BEELEY J.A. (1971) Salivary gland function in sarcoidosis. *Oral Surg.*, **37**, 766.
COHEN A.S. (1967) Amyloidosis. *New Engl. J. Med.*, **277**, 522, 574, 628.

COHEN A.S. & CANOSO J.J. (1972) Criteria for the classification of systemic lupus erythematosus—status 1972. *Arthritis and Rheumatism*, **15,** 540.
COHENOUR W. & GAMBLE J.W. (1971) Acanthosis nigricans. *J. Oral Surg.*, **29,** 48.
COHN A.M., PARK J.K. & RAPPAPORT H. (1971) Mycosis fungoides with involvement of the oral cavity. *Arch. Otolaryngol.*, **93,** 330.
COOKE W.T. (1953) Personal communication quoted by Sircus *et al* (1957).
COVEL E. (1954) Boeck's sarcoid of mucous membrane. *Oral Surg.*, **7,** 1242.
CROCKER A.C. (1951) Skin xanthomas in childhood. *Pediatrics, Springfield*, **8,** 573.
DAVIS A.E. & DAVIS T.P. (1966) Gangrene of the tongue caused by temporal arteritis. *Med. J. Aust.*, **2,** 459.
DAWSON WATTS K. (1968) Sarcoidosis. *Brit. J. oral Surg.*, **6,** 108.
DELAHUNTY J.E. (1972) Acid laryngitis. *J. Laryngol.*, **86,** 335.
DONNER M.W., SILBIGER M.L., HOOKMAN P. & HENDRIX (1966) Acid-barium swallows in the radiographic evaluation of clinical esophagitis. *Radiology*, **87,** 220.
DOZOIS R.R., JUDD E.S., DAHLIN D.C. & BARTHOLOMEW L.G. (1969) The Peutz–Jegher's syndrome. *Arch. Surg.*, **98,** 509.
EDWARDS M.B. & GAYFORD J.J. (1971) Oral lupus erythematosus. *Oral Surg.*, **31,** 332.
EPKER B.N. (1972) Obstructive and inflammatory diseases of the major salivary glands. *Oral Surg.*, **33,** 2.
FAY J.T. (1972) An early case of Hurler's syndrome. *J. oral Med.*, **27,** 64.
FRANTZIS T.G., SHERIDAN P.J., REEVE C.M. & YOUNG L.L. (1972) Oral manifestations of hemochromatosis. *Oral Surg.*, **33,** 186.
GARDNER D.G. (1971) The oral manifestations of Hurler's syndrome. *Oral Surg.*, **32,** 46.
GARDNER D.G. & ZEMAN W. (1970) Oral findings in metachromatic leukodystrophy. *Oral Surg.*, **29,** 431.
GILHUUS-MOE O. & KOPPANG H.S. (1972) Oral manifestations of porphyria. *Oral Surg.*, **33,** 926.
GORLIN R.J. (1969) Genetic disorders affecting mucous membranes. *Oral Surg.*, **28,** 512.
GOTTSEGEN R. & GORLIN R.J. (1949) Periarteritis nodosa. *Oral Surg.*, **2,** 1250.
GRAHAME R., BLUESTONE R. & HOLT P.J.L. (1968) Recurrent blanching of the tongue due to giant cell arteritis. *Ann. intern. Med.*, **69,** 781.
HENDERSON A.H. (1967) Tongue pain with giant cell arteritis. *Brit. med. J.*, **4,** 337.
HERSCHFUS L. (1972) Lupus erythematosus. *J. oral Med.*, **27,** 12.
HOBKIRK J.A. (1969) Sarcoidosis with oral lesions. *J. oral Surg.*, **27,** 891.
HOPKINS R., WATSON J.A., JONES J.H. & WALKER M. (1973) Two cases of Hunter's syndrome. *Brit. J. oral Surg.*, **10,** 286.
HORNOVÁ J. & DLUHOŠOVÁ O. (1968) Primary amyloidosis of gingiva and conjunctiva and mental disorder in a brother and sister. *Oral Surg.*, **25,** 457.
ISSA M.A. (1971) Crohn's disease of the mouth. *Brit. dent. J.*, **130,** 247.
JOHNSON M.L. & WILSON H.T.H. (1969) Skin lesions in ulcerative colitis. *Gut*, **10,** 255.
JOHNSON R.P. & MOHNAC A.M. (1967) Histiocytosis X. *J. oral Surg.*, **25,** 7.
JONES J.H. (1973) Unpublished data.

KAKEHASHI S., HAMNER III J.E., BAER P.N. & MCINTYRE J.A. (1965) Wegener's granulomatosis. *Oral Surg.*, **19**, 120.
KEITH D.A. (1972) Oral features of primary amyloidosis. *Brit. J. oral Surg.*, **10**, 107.
KOLAS S. & ROCHE W.C. (1960) Sarcoidosis lesions primary in the oral cavity. *J. oral Surg.*, **18**, 169.
KROGH H.W. (1950) Dental manifestation of scleroderma. *J. oral Surg.*, **8**, 242.
KYLE J. (1972) *Crohn's Disease*, 78. Heinemann, London.
LIN T.Y. (1967) Peutz–Jegher's syndrome. A case report. *Brit. dent. J.*, **123**, 278.
LUCAS R.B. (1972) *Pathology of Tumours of the Oral Tissues*. Churchill Livingstone, Edinburgh.
LYON H., POULSEN H.E. & PINDBORG J.J. (1964) Studies in oral leukoplakias. *Acta path. microbiol. Scand.*, **60**, 305.
McCARTHY P. & SHKLAR G. (1963) A syndrome of pyostomatitis vegetans and ulcerative colitis. *Archs. Derm.*, **88**, 913.
McCARTHY P.L. & SHKLAR G. (1964) *Diseases of the Oral Mucosa*. McGraw-Hill Book Co., New York.
MACDONALD D.G., ROWAN R.M. & BLAIR G.S. (1969) Sarcoidosis involving the mandible. *Brit. dent. J.*, **126**, 168.
MAYOCK R.L., BERTRAND P., MORRISON C.E. & SCOTT J.H. (1963) Manifestations of sarcoidosis. *Am. J. Med.*, **35**, 67.
MERCHANT H.W. (1973) Oral pigmentation associated with bronchogenic carcinoma. *Oral Surg.*, **36**, 675.
MUNROE L.S. & KNAUER C.M. (1962) Gastrointestinal manifestations of systemic sclerosis. *Amer. Pract.*, **13**, 636.
MYERS H.M., DUMAS M. & BALLHORN H.B. (1968) Dental manifestations of phenylketonuria. *J. Am. dent. Ass.*, **77**, 587.
NALLY F.F. (1970) Melkersson–Rosenthal syndrome. *Oral Surg.*, **29**, 694.
NALLY F.F. & ROSS I.H. (1971) Herpes zoster of the oral and facial structures. *Oral Surg.*, **32**, 221.
NAVARATNAM A. & HODGSON G.A. (1973) Acanthosis nigricans with carcinoma of the stomach. *Brit. J. Derm.*, **89**, Suppl. 9, 46.
NAZIF M. & OSMAN M. (1973) Oral manifestations of cystinosis. *Oral Surg.*, **35**, 330.
ORLEAN S.L. & O'BRIEN J.J. (1966) Sarcoidosis manifesting a soft lesion in the floor of the mouth. *Oral Surg.*, **21**, 819.
PLUMPTON S. (1965) Polyarteritis nodosa. *Brit. dent. J.*, **118**, 249.
RAFFLE E.J. & HALL D.C. (1968) Xanthomatosis presenting with oral lesions. *Brit. dent. J.*, **125**, 62.
RAYNE J. (1967) Porphyria erythropoietica. *Brit. J. oral Surg.*, **5**, 68.
SAMMAN P.D. (1972) In ROOK A., WILKINSON D.S. & EBLING F.J.G. *Textbook of Dermatology*, 2nd edition, 1396. Blackwell Scientific Publications, Oxford.
SCHIMKE R.N., HARTMANN W.H., PROUT T.E. & RIMOIN L.D. (1968) Syndrome of bilateral pheochromocytoma, medullary thyroid carcinoma and multiple neuromas. *New Engl. J. Med.*, **279**, 1.
SCHIMPF A. VON (1964) Zur klinik und therapie der mycosis fungoides. *Arch. klin. exp. Derm.*, **221**, 97.

SCOTT J. & FINCH L.D. (1972a) Histiocytosis X with oral lesions. *J. oral Surg.*, **30,** 748.
SCOTT J. & FINCH L.D. (1972b) Wegener's granulomatosis presenting as gingivitis. *Oral Surg.*, **34,** 920.
SHEAR M. & KRAMER S. (1964) Atrophic glossitis and recurrent oral ulceration in idiopathic steatorrhoea. *J. dent. Ass. S.A.*, **19,** 324.
SIMPSON H.E. (1972) Oral manifestations in lipoid proteinosis. *Oral Surg.*, **33,** 528.
SIRCUS W., CHURCH R. & KELLEHER J. (1957) Recurrent aphthous ulceration of the mouth. *Quart. J. Med.*, **26,** 235.
SLEEPER E.L. (1951) Eosinophilic granuloma of bone. *Oral Surg.*, **4,** 896.
SMILEY T.B., MCDOWELL R.F.C. & COSTELLO W.T. (1963) Sideropenic dysphagia and hiatus hernia. *Lancet*, **2,** 7.
SNEDDON I.B. (1963) Skin markers of malignancy. *Brit. med. J.*, **2,** 405.
STAFNE E.C. & AUSTIN L.T. (1944) A characteristic dental finding in acrosclerosis and diffuse scleroderma. *Am. J. Orthodont. oral Surg.*, **30,** 25.
STANBACK III J.S. & PEAGLER F.D. (1968) Primary amyloidosis. *Oral Surg.*, **26,** 774.
STANKLER L., EWEN S.W.B. & KERR N.W. (1972) Crohn's disease of the mouth. *Brit. J. Derm.*, **87,** 501.
STERN D. (1970) Influence of systemic cancer on oral tissues. *Oral Surg.*, **29,** 229.
STRASSBURG M. & KNOLLE G. (1972) *Diseases of the Oral Mucosa*. Buch- and Zeitschriften-Verlag 'Die Quintessenz', Berlin.
TARPLEY T.M., ANDERSON L., LIGHTBODY P. & SHEAGREN J.N. (1972) Minor salivary gland involvement in sarcoidosis. *Oral Surg.*, **33,** 755.
TILLMAN H.H. (1964) Sarcoidosis with unsuspected oral manifestations. *Oral Surg.*, **18,** 130.
TILLMAN H.H., TAYLOR R.G. & CARCHIDI J.E. (1966) Sarcoidosis of the tongue. *Oral Surg.*, **21,** 190.
VARLEY E.W.B. (1972) Crohn's disease of the mouth. *Oral Surg.*, **33,** 570.
VERBOV J. (1973) Crohn's disease with lip and mouth involvement. *Brit. J. Derm.*, **88,** 517.
VICKERS R.A., DAHLIN D.C. & GORLIN R.J. (1965) Amyloid-containing odontogenic tumors. *Oral Surg.*, **20,** 476.
WALKER D.M. (1973) Oral mucosal neuroma—medullary thyroid carcinoma syndrome. *Brit. J. Derm.*, **88,** 599.
WHITEHEAD F.I.H. (1972) Histocytosis X. *Brit. J. oral Surg.*, **10,** 199.
WILLIAMS E.D. & POLLOCK D.J. (1966) Multiple mucosal neuromata with endocrine tumours: a syndrome allied to von Recklinghausen's disease. *J. Path. & Bact.*, **91,** 71.
WILLIAMS R.F. (1971) Lipoid proteinosis. *Oral Surg.*, **31,** 624.
WINKELMANN R.K. & DITTO W.B. (1964) Cutaneous and visceral syndromes of necrotizing or 'allergic' angiitis. *Medicine*, **43,** 59.
WINTHER J.E., FEJERSKOV O. & PHILIPSEN H.P. (1972) Oral manifestations of histocytosis X. *Acta Derm. Venereol. (Stockh.)*, **52,** 75.
ZEGARELLI D.J., TSUKADA Y., PICKREN J.W. & GREENE G.W. (1973) Metastatic tumour to the tongue. *Oral Surg.*, **35,** 202.

CHAPTER 5
ORAL MUCOUS MEMBRANE MARKERS OF INTERNAL DISEASE: PART II, DISORDERS OF THE ENDOCRINE SYSTEM, HAEMOPOIETIC SYSTEM AND NUTRITION

M. M. FERGUSON

5:0 Introduction

Cellular metabolism is carefully regulated by hormones and adequacy of nutritional factors. When a single factor is disturbed sequential changes occur in many tissues: it is often difficult to decide exactly how a particular manifestation has arisen and one must consider possible actions on all systems of the body as well as directly upon the tissue being examined.

The purpose of this chapter is to discuss the effect of changes in the endocrine status, haemopoietic tissue and nutrition, on the oral mucosa. These systems frequently interact and an attempt has been made to differentiate those oral manifestations which occur as a primary event from those developing as a secondary consequence.

5:1 Endocrine Glands

The secretions of the ductless glands regulate metabolic pathways and in so doing facilitate the organism's adaptation to its fluctuating environment. Although many of the hormones have been ascribed specific actions it should be appreciated that there is often considerable interaction with the final outcome being accomplished under the control of several endocrine secretions. When a disorder occurs in one gland this can lead to compensating increases or to hypofunction in others.

5:1:1 Pituitary gland

The pituitary gland consists of three distinct lobes, each of which secretes a group of protein or polypeptide hormones. The established hormones together with their main actions are summarized in Table 5.1. Discussion in this section will be limited to those hormones which appear to have a direct effect upon oral mucosa in contrast to being mediated through another endocrine gland.

Table 5:1 Pituitary hormones

Lobe of pituitary	Hormone	Main action
Anterior lobe	Growth hormone	Generalized increase in growth
	ACTH	Stimulates adrenocortical secretion
	TSH	Stimulates thyroid secretion
	FSH	Stimulates ovarian follicle growth and probably also the secretion of oestrogen
		Promotes gametogenesis in males
	LH (ICSH)	Stimulates luteinization of ovarian follicles which results in progesterone secretion
		Stimulates Leydig interstitial cells in testis to produce androgens
	Prolactin	Stimulates mammary gland secretion of milk
		Has a luteinizing effect on ovarian follicles in rodents
Intermediate lobe (also anterior and posterior lobe in several species including human)	α-MSH β-MSH	Stimulate melanophores in certain species Unsure of role in humans
Posterior lobe	Vasopressin (ADH)	Water retention
	Oxytocin	Uterine contraction and milk ejection

5:1:1a GROWTH HORMONE

Growth hormone has an anabolic effect promoting growth in a wide variety of tissues. This is accomplished by influencing protein, carbohydrate and lipid metabolism. Excessive secretion of growth hormone is usually caused by acidophilic adenomata and is associated with gigantism in children and acromegaly in adults.

In acromegaly the lips and tongue become hypertrophic, with the lips enlarging and protruding. The enlarged tongue fills the oral cavity and sometimes may even exhibit scalloping around the margins due to pressure indentations from the teeth. The lingual papillae may also hypertrophy.

We are not aware of any changes in the oral mucosa itself due to over-stimulation with growth hormone although Bardik (1969) demonstrated an increase in the proliferation rate of oesophageal epithelium.

5:1:1b GONADOTROPHIC HORMONES

Post-menopausal women are more frequently troubled with atrophy and tenderness of the mucous membranes; the oral cavity often mirrors the vagina in such patients, although to a lesser degree. The obvious cause for this complaint would seem to be a simple decrease in circulating oestrogens and progestogens. However, substitution therapy is commonly disappointing and the conclusion is that other factors may be involved. A similar search towards the aetiology of osteoporosis is also being made.

One factor worth considering is that in post-menopausal women the levels of follicle stimulating hormone (FSH) and luteinizing hormone (LH) increase about fivefold (Riggs et al 1973) with the ovaries remaining unresponsive. No one has shown FSH or LH to have any direct effect upon any oral tissues or evidence of there being receptors for gonadotropins but it is interesting to note that human chorionic gonadotrophin (HCG) when given to oöphorectomized monkeys caused degenerative changes to occur in the buccal and gingival mucosae. The epithelium was reduced in thickness, keratinization decreased and inflammatory cells appeared in the underlying connective tissue (Ziskin et al 1936; Ziskin and Blackberg 1940). Similar changes occurred in the buccal and gingival mucosae of three women injected with HCG (Ziskin 1937). Lindhe & Branemark (1967b) reported that topical HCG caused a microcirculatory disturbance in hamster cheek pouch.

Older males do not appear to be troubled with oral problems associated with endocrine changes. This may be influenced by the fact that whereas oestrogen secretion drops considerably in post-menopausal females, it actually increases in males over 45 years of age to a level twice as high as in younger men and about three times as high as in post-menopausal females. There is a possibility that this increase in males may be to some extent attributed to adrenal secretion, as Ziskin & Blackberg (1940) showed that hypophysectomy and oöphorectomy in female monkeys resulted in degenerative changes occurring in gingivae which contrasts to males hypophysectomized and castrated: these animals remained healthy and even showed some similarities to females which had been treated with oestrogen. The increase in oestrogen secretion with age in males may also be a contributory factor to the increased mitotic rate in oral mucosa (Meyer et al 1956). However, an opposite trend is found in rats (Karring & Löe 1973).

5:1:1c NON-SPECIFIC ACTION FROM ANTERIOR PITUITARY

Sutton & Ashworth (1940) reported a series of male and female patients with glossitis, stomatitis and angular cheilitis. No nutritional factors were found to relieve the symptoms. The diagnosis of hypopituitarism was reached and all of the group responded very rapidly to injections of anterior pituitary extract. Either these subjects could have been affected by a lack of one of the hormones from the anterior lobe of the pituitary or their problem may have been a manifestation of hypofunction by another gland. Thyroid extract and insulin afforded no relief to one of the group.

5:1:2 Adrenal cortex

The adrenal cortex secretes glucocorticosteroids, mineralocorticosteroids, androgens, progestogens and oestrogens. ACTH is responsible for regulating the synthesis principally of glucocorticosteroids and the rate of secretion of ACTH is in turn partially governed by the levels of circulating glucocorticosteroids: a negative feedback system operates.

5:1:2a HYPOADRENOCORTICALISM

Hypofunction of the adrenal cortex may result either from a failure of the anterior pitiutary to secrete ACTH or from destruction of the adrenal cortical cells themselves. The commonest causes of adrenal cortical destruction are idiopathic (probably autoimmune) adrenal atrophy and tuberculous destruction of the adrenal cortex. The term Addison's disease is applied to the hypofunction resulting from both of these entities although Addison's initial description was only of tuberculous involvement.

Addison's disease is associated with cutaneous pigmentation and with pigmentation of the oral mucosa. The buccal mucosa is most commonly affected but patchy pigmentation may also be seen on the labial, gingival, palatal and lingual mucosae. This coloration is due to melanin and may appear brown, blue-black or black, depending on the vascularity of the

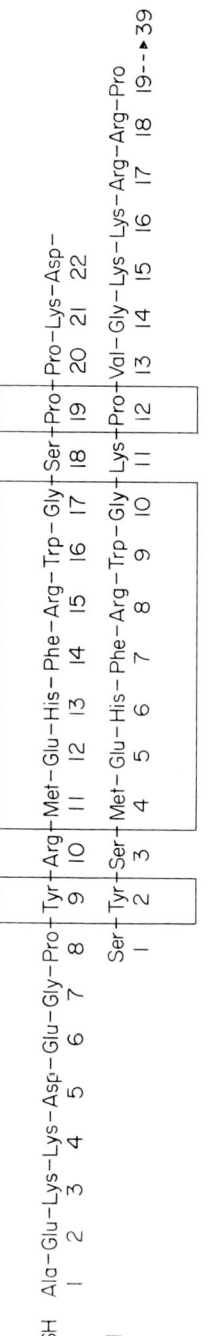

Fig. 5.1. Relationship between the amino-acid sequence of ACTH and human β-MSH.

tissues as well as of the epithelial character. The melanocytes are found in the basal layer of the epithelium and on stimulation will produce and deposit melanin granules.

The intermediate lobe of the pituitary gland secretes polypeptide hormones which will cause the dispersion of melanophore granules in lower vertebrates—these are melanocyte stimulation hormones (MSH). The structure of β-MSH varies from species to species but the amino acid sequences bear a similarity to ACTH (see Fig. 5.1). Pure ACTH has melanocyte-stimulating activity that is about 1/100 that of β-MSH, but MSH's have no physiologically significant ACTH activity. In lower vertebrates, MSH activity is confined to the intermediate lobe of pituitary, but in mammals MSH's have also been detected in the anterior and posterior lobes.

The role of MSH in mammals is unclear, as there are no melanophores in the skin. However, MSH does seem to influence the skin in disease states and has been shown to darken the skin of humans by accelerating melanin synthesis. The controversial point is whether MSH or ACTH causes the pigmentation in Addison's disease. In hypoadrenocorticalism due to a pituitary disorder no pigmentary changes take place; if anything there is an abnormal pallor. A considerable concentration of ACTH would be required to produce the pigmentation and doubt has been expressed as to whether or not the ACTH levels in the plasma are sufficiently high. In addition to this, β-MSC secretion increases as does ACTH secretion, and thus is elevated in cases of Addison's disease. The consensus of opinion at present favours MSH as being responsible for the production of the muco-cutaneous pigmentaion.

Chronic muco-cutaneous candidosis is another feature of hypoadrenocorticalism (Craig *et al* 1955) and represents part of the associated general immunological upset (Irvine *et al* 1967) (see Chapter 9).

5:1:2b HYPERADRENOCORTICALISM

Increased secretion of adrenocortical steroids may result from pituitary or adrenal tumours as well as from bilateral adrenal hyperplasia. Cushing's syndrome is the name given to this state and the pathological changes brought about are principally due to the glucocorticosteroids. Therapeutic doses of costicosteroids will produce essentially the same clinical picture.

Glucocorticosteroids affect the epithelium, fibroblasts and ground substance (Castor & Baker 1950; Sethi *et al* 1961; Castor 1965; Zachariae 1966; Torak & Banoczy 1972) and it is perhaps surprising that the oral mucosa is not altered significantly in Cushing's disease. Exfoliative cytology of the oral mucosa in patients receiving steroids has revealed cells with nuclear changes (Medak et al 1973). The intraoral use of topical steroids often leads to candidal infections.

5:1:3 Thyroid gland

The hormones secreted by the thyroid gland are thyroxine and tri-iodothyronine. This is under the control of TSH from the anterior pituitary, which is in turn regulated partially by a feedback system of thyroid hormones and by hypothalamic neural mechanisms. The action of thyroid hormones is basically to stimulate oxygen consumption and the basal metabolic rate. They also influence carbohydrate and lipid metabolism.

5:1:3a HYPOTHYROIDISM

Inadequate secretion of thyroid hormones occurs in children and adults for a wide variety of reasons. Congenital hypothyroidism leads to the state of cretinism and these children develop, amongst many manifestations, an enlarged tongue which protrudes from the mouth. The lips, palate and gingivae are also enlarged and spongy (Buckman 1957). Puffiness of the face and oral tissues is also a feature of hypothyroidism, or myxoedema, in adults. The enlarged tissues are spongy and histology reveals loose connective tissue with a considerable infiltration of mucopolysaccharides. Carotenaemia is frequently present and gives the skin a yellow tinge due to the diminished conversion of carotene to vitamin A.

Hypothyroidism does not seem to be associated with any changes in the human oral epithelium but Rosenberg et al (1961) reported hyperparakeratosis and keratosis in rabbits following thyroidectomy.

Hypothyroidism, whether it is present singly or co-existing with multiple endocrinopathies, may present with chronic muco-cutaneous candidosis due to impaired cellular immunity (Papazian & Koch 1960; Kenny & Holliday 1964; Wuepper & Fudenberg 1967; Chilgren et al 1969; Hermans et al 1969; Montes et al 1972). It is possible that in these cases the multiple endocrinopathy and poor immune response are indicative of a common aetiology, although administration of thyroxine to some of the individuals resulted in a complete cure of their candidal infection.

5:1:3b HYPERTHYROIDISM

Excessive secretion of thyroid hormones does not lead to any specific lesion of the oral mucosa. The only oral soft tissue manifestation is a tremor of the tongue.

5:1:4 Parathyroid glands

The parathyroid glands secrete a hormone, parathormone, which maintains a constant level of ionized calcium in the extracellular fluid. Parathormone is secreted in direct response to a lowering of ionizable calcium and its action is to raise the plasma calcium and mobilize calcium from bone.

Abnormal levels of parathormone do not affect the oral mucosa, although the skin may become dry and the nails ridged and brittle in hypoparathyroidism.

Chronic muco-cutaneous candidosis has been reported in hypoparathyroidism occurring alone (Greenberg *et al* 1969) as well as in association with other endocrinopathies, especially Addison's disease.

5:1:5 Pancreatic islets

Insulin is secreted by the β-cells of the pancreatic islets and its action is to induce an increase in the rates of glycogen, lipid and protein synthesis, and a diminution in the rates of glycogenolysis and lipolysis. The level of insulin maintains a balance between catabolic and anabolic processes.

Diabetes mellitus is a condition where there is a lack of available insulin for cells, hence there is a resultant decrease in anabolism and increase in catabolism. Blood glucose levels are consequentially elevated. The aetiology of diabetes remains obscure and discussion of the various theories is outside the scope of the present work.

Certain basic pathological features are characteristic of diabetes; these include widespread thickening of the basement membranes in small vessels due to the excessive deposition of mucoproteins and collagen, atherosclerosis and an increased predisposition to infections.

The cutaneous manifestations of diabetes are necrobiosis lipoidica diabeticorum, atrophic circumscribed lesions of the lower limb and mucocutaneous candidosis.

Diabetes mellitus has no pathognomonic lesion in the oral cavity, although certain changes do appear in inadequately controlled individuals. Thickening of small blood vessel walls is probably not related to hyperglycaemia *per se*, and vascular changes have been reported in the periodontal membrane and gingiva (Russell 1966 & 1967). There is considerable evidence to suggest that periodontal disease and gingivitis are more common only in diabetics who are poorly controlled (Rutledge 1940; Lovestedt & Austin 1943; Cheraskin & Ringsdorg 1965; Chinn *et al* 1966; Finestone & Boorujy 1967; Benveniste *et al* 1967; Cohen *et al* 1970; Hove & Stallard 1970) and both Shklar *et al* (1962) and Cohen *et al* (1963) found an increased incidence of periodontitis in diabetic hamsters.

Xerostomia is another common finding in diabetics (Sheppard 1942; Banks 1945; Barach 1949) and is presumably related to dehydration. This dryness will almost certainly be partially responsible for the frequent symptoms of burning, general tenderness and altered taste (Brody *et al* 1971). These authors found that up to 39% of patients with oral symptoms had an abnormal tolerance curve whereas no more than 7% of the general population would possess this diabetic tendency. Another factor leading to the oral discomfort is the neuropathy resulting from microangiopathy of the nutrient vessels.

Resistance to infection is lowered in diabetes and fungal infections, especially candidosis, are common. Wounds heal poorly and minor traumatic ulcers may take a considerable period to resolve.

5:1:6 Gonads

The ovaries secrete oestrogens and progestogens while the testes secrete androgens along with a small amount of oestrogen. Placental secretions may be conveniently considered along with the gonads. Gonadal steroid hormone synthesis is mediated by the anterior pituitary with FSH, LH and ICSH, and by the placenta with HCG (see Table 5.1). The release of gonadotropins is in turn controlled by hypothalamic centres, with a negative feedback system operating to a considerable extent.

Inadequate, excessive or imbalanced levels of sex hormones have been implicated in a number of oral disorders, especially in females. Therefore, we feel that it would be worth considering some biochemical and physiological effects of this group of steroids before passing on to the clinical disorders themselves.

The principal oestrogens in humans are oestroadiol, oestrone and oestriol. Like most physiological steroids, oestrogens have a vast range of actions: they influence cell membranes, DNA and RNA synthesis. Target tissues for oestrogens possess a system of specific receptors which carries the hormone through the cell. It is possible, although by no means proven, that in order to be influenced by oestrogens at all the tissue must have a receptor, and this has been advanced as the reason that rabbit gingival mucosa with no receptors fails to respond to oestrogens (Rubright et al 1971, 1973), which is in contrast to rodents (Nutlay et al 1954; Formicola et al 1970; Jonek et al 1970). Human and other primates have an oral mucosa which is influenced by and can metabolize oestrogens (Ziskin et al 1936; Ziskin 1937, 1938; Litwack et al 1970; Deasy et al 1972; El Attar & Hugoson 1974), although we are not aware of receptors having been demonstrated here.

In sensitive epithelium two actions of oestrogen are to increase the rate of cellular proliferation and to promote keratinization; such changes are best exemplified by vagina but oral mucosa does follow a similar trend. Keratinization of oral and vaginal mucosa probably undergoes comparable changes during the menstrual cycle and pregnancy (Main & Ritchie 1967; Hugoson et al 1971), although Silverman & Shous (1966) did not detect this.

Vascular permeability is also increased by oestrogens (Lindhe & Brånemark 1967a,b), although progesterone is more active in this respect. The mechanism whereby this alteration is affected remains obscure.

Collagen synthesis is decreased by oestrogens in many tissues (Smith & Allison 1966; Yang et al 1973).

Progestogens also bind to receptor sites on target tissues, and there influence DNA and RNA metabolism. There appears to be some sort of complicated partial antagonistic relationship between oestrogens and progestogens with regard to cellular proliferation and, probably, to keratinization. The issue is further clouded by trying to differentiate between therapeutic and physiological levels. It seems that progesterone will not only cause proliferation of an atrophic mucosa, but regressive changes when the epithelium is at a highly proliferative stage.

Progesterone is metabolized to a number of metabolites in gingiva and this conversion is significantly increased in the presence of inflammation (El Attar et al 1973).

Progesterone promotes a widespread increase in vascular permeability which includes oral mucosa (Linde & Brånemark 1967a,b; Mohamed 1972). Several theories have been advanced about the mechanism whereby progesterone brings about this alteration in permeability. One suggestion has been that progesterone affects the nature of a carbohydrate fraction associated with the vessel wall and ground substance (Gersh & Catchpole 1960; Wolff et al 1967), and another has been its action on the pores (Haim 1966). Further alternatives presumably exist.

Androgens, of which testosterone is the principal member, apparently, do not play a significant role in controlling the proliferation or morphology of oral mucosa. One interesting observation is that administration of testosterone to rats resulted in the appearance of taste buds in abnormal locations on the vallate papille (Allara 1952).

Oral disorders attributable to sex hormones may be subdivided: (a) Puberty, (b) Menstrual cycle, (c) Pregnancy, (d) Post-menopausal, and (e) Hormone-dependent aphthae.

5:1:6a PUBERTY

The incidence of gingivitis increases significantly at the time of puberty and occurs earlier and to a greater degree in girls (Massler et al 1950; Parfitt 1957; Sutcliffe 1972). This peak corresponds to the greater secretion of gonadotropins, oestrogens and progestogens. The reaction is hyperplastic and soft, erythematous gingiva bleeds readily. Histology shows a non-specific gingivitis with vascular dilation, endothelial proliferation and chronic inflammation. In some instances the inflammatory reaction proceeds to pyogenic granulomata. The gingivitis of puberty seems to represent an increased response to plaque and calculus and it is possible to completely control the problem with adequate oral hygiene.

5:1:6b MENSTRUAL CYCLE AND
ORAL CONTRACEPTIVES

As has been stated above, the oral mucosa of females undergoes a cyclical variation with the menstrual cycle. The fluctuating levels of hormones are sometimes reflected in the mouth, and during menstruation there may be a tendency towards hyperaemic, tender gingivae which bleed readily during toothbrushing (Klein 1934; Mühlemann 1948). Gingival exudation increases at the time of menstruation in females with pre-existing gingivitis (Holm-Pederson & Loe 1967; Lindhe & Åttstrom 1967).

Oral contraceptives consist of a mixture of an oestrogen and a progestogen. The rationale behind their use is that the oestrogen suppresses FSH secretion and hence development of the Graafian follicle, while the progestogen ensures that withdrawal bleeding is prompt and physiological. The effects of oral contraceptives on other endocrines is discussed by Lucis & Lucis (1972).

Gingivitis is more common in females taking oral contraceptives (Lindhe & Bjorn 1967; Lynn 1967; Lindhe et al 1968a,b,c,d,e; Kaufman

1969; Sperber 1969; Das *et al* 1971), although not all preparations appear to cause this (Heiss & Grasser 1968; Klinger & Klinger 1970). The development of the hyperaemic reaction is probably, as it is also in pregnancy, due to the level of progesterone.

5:1:6c PREGNANCY

Many investigators have noted that gingivitis is more marked during pregnancy and that this reaction is not due to any alteration in previous oral hygiene standards (Pinard & Pinard 1877; Arkovy 1915; Ziskin *et al* 1933; Ziskin & Nesse 1946; Maier & Orban 1949; Hilming 1952; Löe & Silness 1963; Löe 1965; Holm-Pederson & Löe 1967; Cohen *et al* 1969; Hugoson 1971).

The gingivitis is again marked by hyperaemia, and vasodilation with non-specific chronic inflammation. This tendency starts to develop by about the eighth week of gestation and resolves fairly promptly in the puerperium. Healthy parts of the gingiva remain unaffected and the disorder is one of greater inflammatory response to plaque and irritations. Pregnancy tumours, or pyogenic granulomata, merely represent a prolonged and severe inflammatory reaction. Therefore, it is a situation which is not only transient but will respond to improved oral hygiene.

The obvious aetiological factor in gingivitis of pregnancy is the elevated progesterone levels. No reports are available correlating gingivitis with progesterone *levels,* although additional progesterone given to such patients is inclined to aggravate the situation. Conversely, oestrogens alleviate symptoms. This suggests that the problem is not simply related to progestogen concentrations but instead to the balance between oestrogens and progestogens (see section 5:1:6e). Sex hormones have been found to decrease inflammation in a granuloma of hamster cheek pouch (Lindhe & Sonesson 1967) and this has been postulated to be a possible reason for the lack of striking histological changes even when the gingivae are red and tense.

5:1:6d MENOPAUSE AND POST-MENOPAUSE

The menopause marks the cessation of menstruation: the transition through this phase may be fairly innocuous and abrupt or can be spread over a period. The term menopause is used to describe that period during which the body is undergoing a series of changes, often stormy, and the post-menopausal phase refers to the stage when a state of equilibrium has been re-established. This is the stage when ovarian function ceases, oestrogen and progesterone levels decline sharply and both FSH and LH outputs can increase about fivefold.

Oral symptoms are very common, particularly during the menopause itself, and Barone (1965) gave a figure of 80% of menopausal and post-menopausal women having complained about oral symptoms. The usual symptoms are glossopyrosis, burning sensation of buccal mucosa and abnormal taste sensations (Massler 1951). Sometimes there is difficulty separating complaints with an organic basis from psychological problems. In addition to this, minor discomforts tend to be magnified in a psycho-neurotic state.

Oral lesions vary between desquamative gingivitis and atrophic stomatitis and glossitis. Such problems cause difficulty in tolerating dentures. In our experience of these patients with atrophic stomatitis, the vaginal mucosa has often undergone comparable changes, becoming tender and friable.

Desquamative gingivitis is characterized by stripping of the gingival epithelium leaving a raw, red, tender surface. Histologically, the epithelium is non-keratinized with a thin spinous cell layer. Hydropic degeneration occurs in the basal cells and acantholysis and subepithelial bulla formation may occur. The underlying lamina propria is infiltrated with lymphocytes, plasma cells, macrophages and a few neutrophils (Foss *et al* 1953; Glickman & Smulow 1964; Scopp 1964).

Similar changes can occur on the buccal, labial, palatal and lingual mucosae, with atrophy being succeeded by stripping of the epithelium. This leaves the exposed connective tissue bright red and extremely tender.

Oestrogens are of use in some patients (Richman & Abarbanel 1943) but their use should be restricted to severe cases. The problem with systemic oestrogen therapy is that it may induce withdrawal bleeding from the uterus and the dilemma is then to be sure that the bleeding can be attributed simply to the oestrogen therapy and not to a carcinoma. Topical oestrogens in atrophic stomatitis have been less satisfactory than in atrophic vaginitis, possibly because it is difficult to maintain the hormone in contact with oral mucosa for any length of time.

5:1:6e OESTROGEN-SENSITIVE APHTHAE

In a certain group of females there is a relationship between recurrent aphthae and the latter part of the menstrual cycle (Woodburne 1941; Strauss 1947; Collings & Dukes 1952; Sircus *et al* 1957; Driscoll *et al*

1959; Ship *et al* 1961; Dolby 1968). Pregnancy is frequently associated with freedom from these ulcers and Carruthers (1967a,b) found that, in this group, aphthae responded favourably to oral contraceptives. Subsequently it was found that oestrogen alone would alleviate the problem (Bishop *et al* 1967; Frietag *et al* 1971). We made the interesting observation in one patient with these aphthae that although oestrogen alone cleared the ulcers, the combination with progestogen in an oral contraceptive did not and a further increase in the dose of oestrogen was necessitated. Possibly this points to a critical balance rather than an absolute concentration of oestrogen alone. The issue has recently become further clouded by the fact that some patients do not apparently respond to oestrogens but to progestogens (Ferguson, Hart & Lindsay—unpublished observations).

5:2 Diseases of the Blood and Haematopoietic System

In this section it is not our intention to review the details of the many disorders of the haematopoietic system but instead to consider the oral manifestations of groups of conditions giving rise to similar changes. It is of the utmost importance that the dental surgeon is aware of these signs, as the mouth is so commonly the first site where evidence of blood dyscrasias appear.

5:2:1 Defective haemostasis

Following injury, haemostasis is effected by a sequel of three mechanisms. Initially there is a reflex vasoconstriction followed by the aggregation of platelets. Finally, secondary haemostasis is achieved with the build-up of fibrin strands in the platelet clump to form a robust plug until healing has occurred.

The effectiveness of intravascular haemostasis is further influenced by the adequacy of the perivascular support.

This section is restricted to intravascular haemostatic mechanisms, although defects in the extravascular factors can also lead to purpura.

Intravascular disorders may be subdivided into two groups: platelets and blood coagulation.

5:2:1a PLATELETS

Inadequate platelet function may be due to a quantitative or qualitative deficiency, i.e. thrombocytopaenia and thrombocytosthenia respectively.

The oral manifestations of inadequate platelet function are the same and may be the first evidence of this altered condition (Hirch & Dameshek 1951; Linenberg 1964). Petechiae and coarser ecchymoses are frequently seen on the floor of the mouth, soft palate, buccal and labial mucosae. Minor traumata leads to disportionate bleeding and multiple petechial haemorrhages are found in relation to ill-fitting dentures. Bleeding occurs from the gingivae and oozes out from the margins with the slightest provocation.

Dental extractions can be followed by a prolonged and severe haemorrhage.

Thrombocytosis refers to a state where there is an increase over the normal amount of platelets. It occurs in a number of conditions and may be the primary indication of leukaemia or polycythemia. Although the individual platelets themselves are thought to be normal the excessive amount apparently interferes with thromboplastin production. The oral manifestations are ecchymoses and prolonged (post-extraction) bleeding.

5:2:1b BLOOD COAGULATION

An haemorrhagic diasthesis consequential to defective blood coagulation with deficiency of factor VIII or IX is called haemophilia. Deficiency of factor VIII (antihaemophilic factor) is by far the most common and is termed haemophilia A. Haemophilia B is used for a deficiency of factor IX (Christmas factor).

Individuals with coagulation defects vary considerably in the degree to which they are affected. At one end of the spectrum the only oral manifestation may be a slight prolongation in post-extraction haemorrhage, and at the other end there are spontaneous haemorrhages, purpura and prolonged bleeding following dental extraction. Petechiae are not as prominent as in platelet disorders nor is gingival oozing.

5:2:2 Anaemia

Anaemia is a quantitative or qualitative reduction of red blood cells which results in an inadequate availability of circulating haemoglobin. Basically it is caused by impaired production, excessive destruction or abnormal loss of erythrocytes. There is no convincing evidence to suggest that anaemia *per se* has any oral mucosal manifestations other than producing a mucosal pallor when the haemoglobin level falls below approximately 8·5 G%. Icterus is sometimes seen in haemolytic anaemias and a yellow tinge is also associated with vitamin B_{12} deficiency.

Deficiencies of iron, folic acid, vitamin B_{12} and pyridoxine all may lead to anaemia as well as oral mucosal changes, and these are discussed under nutrition.

The alterations in the soft tissues of the mouth associated with aplastic anaemia, as with the anaemias of leukaemia, can in all probability be ascribed to the other concomitant changes in the blood.

5:2:3 Polycythaemia

Polycythaemia is an abnormal increase in the circulating erythrocyte mass and, therefore, in haemoglobin. It is divided into relative polycythaemia, as in haemoconcentration, primary polycythaemia (polycythaemia vera) and secondary polycythaemia. Primary polycythaemia is a disease of middle age and after a variable time may progress to myelofibrosis or leukaemia.

The oral mucosal features of polycythaemia are a generalized deep reddish coloration to the oral mucosa with a bluish tinge especially noticeable on the lips. An increased bleeding tendency is sometimes found and is possibly related to the concomitant thrombocytosis (see section 5:2:1). In addition the blood is more viscous and thrombotic episodes also occur.

5:2:4 Leukopaenia and agranulocytosis

Leukopaenia is said to exist when the leukocyte count falls below 4,000 cells per cubic mm (de Gruchy 1972). Although occasionally the differential count may remain balanced it is far more common to find a disproportionate reduction in the neutrophils, and the term neutropaenia is then applied. Agranulocytosis represents a more marked decrease in the circulating granulocyte series and may be considered as an extreme form of neutropaenia.

Infections, drugs and radiation may all precipitate neutropaenia as well as more specific diseases affecting the bone marrow, such as aplastic anaemia, aleukaemic anaemia, myelofibrosis and lymphosarcoma. Chronic hypoplastic neutropaenia is associated with defective granulocytic precursors and in primary splenic neutropaenia there is increased destruction of granulocytic leukocytes within the spleen.

The outcome of these states is essentially a lowered ability to cope with infections. Variation occurs between individuals as to at what level of neutrophils oral manifestations appear, but in general the lower the white count the greater the tendency until in agranulocytosis there is almost universal ulceration of the mucosal surfaces. Extensive ulceration and necrosis develops on the palatal, buccal, labial, ligual, gingival and pharyngeal mucosae. The ulcerated areas become infected and covered with a greyish slough. The gingivae become inflamed, ulcerate and bleed readily. The microscopic picture of these oral lesions exhibits the usual signs of inflammation but neutrophils are conspicuously absent.

Cyclic or periodic neutropaenia is a disorder where for some unknown reason there is a cyclic diminution of neutrophils. This occurs about every 21 days and persists for a week: the periodicity is unrelated to any other known cycles (Page & Good 1957). In this condition, at the phase of lowered neutrophils, ragged ulcers develop which are identical to those occurring in other forms of neutropaenia. Gingivitis, stomatitis and aphthae are also common (Gorlin & Chaudhry 1960; Telsey et al 1962; Wade & Stafford 1963; Morley 1966; Morley et al 1967. These changes heal in about two weeks, only to reappear again shortly thereafter.

5:2:5 Leukaemia

Leukaemia is characterized by the widespread abnormal proliferation of the leukocyte precursors in haemopoietic tissues. It is divided into acute and chronic forms and each group is further subdivided into lymphocytic, myelocytic and monocytic varieties. In addition to these there are some less common variants with eosinophils or basophils being involved.

Leukaemia is a disease of all age groups, although acute forms are more common under 20 years of age and acute lymphocytic leukaemia markedly predominates under 10 years. Chronic leukaemia is the more common disorder over 20 years of age.

Figures for oral manifestations in leukaemia show considerable variation between authors (13–87%), but certain trends have emerged. Acute leukaemia is associated with a greater incidence of oral changes than is chronic leukaemia; probably about threefold. Of the acute leukaemias the lymphocytic variant has fewer oral changes.

The oral signs of leukaemia are well recognized as mucosal pallor, petechial haemorrhages and ecchymoses, gingivitis and gingival bleeding, ulceration, infection and gingival hypertrophy (Love 1936; Resch 1940; Burkett 1944; McCarthy & Karcher 1946; Wentz et al 1949; Duffy & Driscoll 1958; Boggs et al 1962; Lynch & Ship 1967a,b; Bodey 1971a; Curtis 1971).

The pallor is attributable to anaemia which is in turn caused by a combination of decreased erythropoiesis together with haemorrhages and possibly also a haemolytic tendency. The bleeding tendency can be accounted for by the diminution in platelets and to a lesser extent disordered coagulation and more active fibrinolysis. Manifestations of this haemorrhagic disorder are probably the commonest oral change of leukaemia. Gingivitis is another common finding but is said to occur only in the presence of inadequate oral hygiene. Certainly, we have found a dramatic improvement, even in near terminal cases when intensive oral hygiene measures are instituted. Gingival hypertrophy, which can reach the proportions of virtually engulfing the teeth, is a feature of monocytic and myelocytic forms: only rarely is it seen in lymphocytic leukaemia. This gross enlargement is due to a dense infiltrate of the particular leucocytes which disrupts the normal connective tissue morphology. Dilated capillaries and oedema of the subepithelial papillary layers are also seen. Chaudry and Gorlin (1962) reported a similar infiltration on the palate of an edentulous patient and considered that denture irritation may have been the aetiological factor.

Mucosal ulceration probably has a multifactorial aetiology. Small blood vessels may be completely occluded with the leukaemic cells and thus cause the overlying mucosa to become gangrenous and slough off. Granulocytopaenia and hypogammaglobulinaemia are common occurrences in leukaemia (Herch et al 1965; Bodey 1971b) and the large ragged ulcers become readily infected and necrotic. Organisms most frequently associated with these oral infections are candida, *E. coli*, *Pseudomonas pyocyanea*, klebsiella, staphylococci and streptococci. In addition, the chemotherapeutic agents employed in the management of leukaemia can themselves induce ulcerative stomatitis; these include amethopterin (see section on folate deficiency and amethopterin, 5:3:3), daunorubidomycin, 6-mercaptopurine, cytosine arabinoside, chlorambucil, cyclophosphamide, and phenylalanine mustard. Corticosteroids, by further depressing the immune response, promote the development of secondary infections.

The oral changes in leukaemia may become so painful and distressing as to seriously interfere with the ingestion of nutrients and even fluids. This in turn predisposes to further complications and the vicious cycle must be stopped with active local therapy.

5:3 Nutrition and Oral Mucosa

Mammals require a diet containing amino acids, fatty acids, vitamins and minerals, including trace elements. Carbohydrate is used essentially to fulfil the calorie requirements, although it will have a sparing effect on protein by reducing the necessity for gluconeogenesis. The calorie intake *per se* appears to influence the epidermis (Bullough 1949; Keys *et al* 1950) but no similar findings have been reported in oral mucosa. Intestinal bacteria are capable of synthesizing certain vitamins in significant quantities and this flora is affected not only by the chemical composition of the diet but probably also by the physical consistency.

Interrelationships exist between many nutrients; an abnormal intake of one frequently influencing the metabolism of others.

The concept of a balanced diet is one wherein all the known essential nutrients are ingested in specified ranges. These quantities have both lower and upper limits for each individual substance. This leads to a state of morphological and biochemical equilibrium which is conceived of as normal for the species. If any single factor is taken in a quantity outwith that range for which the equilibrium can be established then it is feasible to accept that this will necessitate the required range for each of the remaining essential factors in the diet to undergo a compensatory alteration. Therefore, one may consider the absolute requirements for any particular nutrient to be dependent upon the overall dietary pattern.

Findings substantiating the conclusions reached in the preceding paragraph are discussed under the separate nutrients.

Nutritional deficiencies may arise in a number of ways. Each general heading includes numerous mechanisms but it is not within the scope of the present text to discuss these in any detail.

The main categories are as follows:
1 Inadequate intake: e.g. poverty, low intelligence and in the elderly.
2 Disordered digestion: e.g. achlorhydria, post-gastrectomy, pancreatic disease and hepatobiliary disease.
3 Defective absorption: e.g. coeliac disease, regional ileitis, ulcerative colitis, intestinal parasites and alimentary infections.
4 Alterations in metabolism: e.g. methotrexate, trimethoprim and desoxypyridone.
5 Increased demands: e.g. pregnancy and hyperthyroidism.
6 Loss of nutrient: e.g. menstrual loss, alimentary tract bleeding and renal disease.

Investigations describing the effect of nutritional deficiencies upon the oral mucosa fall into two broad categories. Firstly, accounts are presented of the clinical state of the mucosa in humans with diagnosed deficiencies; the proof being the patient's response to specific replacement therapy. The second group includes experimental human and animal studies where a diet lacking in a single factor is given and the oral changes are noted. Administration of the specific agent with resolution of abnormalities again confirms the particular deficiency picture.

Unfortunately the published results are variable and even, in some cases, conflicting. Cheilitis, glossitis and stomatitis are common manifestations of nutritional deficiencies and we are not convinced that it is possible to differentiate, with any great degree of confidence, between many deficiency states. The situation is aggravated further by the changing patterns of early and late deficiency. This prompts us to advocate a standard approach to the patient in which a nutritional disorder is suspected: if no directive information comes from the clinical history and systemic examination then it would seem logical to assess the body status of as many nutrients as is reasonable. In practice, it is probably more convenient to screen for the most commonly occurring deficiencies, as well as utilizing generally available facilities, in the first instance, e.g. iron, folic acid and vitamin B_{12}.

A further point to consider is that in dealing clinically with humans, in contrast to experimental animals, nutritional deficiencies not infrequently occur as groups rather than isolated events and patterns of these groups can vary between different communities as well as various aetiological disorders.

5:3:1 Proteins and amino acids

Ingested proteins are not absorbed as such by animals but are broken down in the alimentary canal to small peptides and amino acids.

In order to maintain the nitrogen balance the amino acid intake must be at least equal to the loss: this has been calculated to correspond to approximately 1 gram of protein daily per kilogram body weight for the standard adult man.

Eight amino acids are essential for man (isoleucine, leucine, lysine, methionine, phenylalanine, threonine, tryptophan and valine). Arginine and histidine, though not essential for life, are required to permit normal growth. The remaining amino acids can be synthesized *in vivo* from the essential amino acids at suitable rates (Rosen *et al* 1946; Geiger 1947).

Deficiency of protein, and therefore of the essential amino acids, leads to the condition known as kwashiorkor. Certainly, protein deficiency has been shown to alter the intestinal absorption of iron, lipids, vitamins and carbohydrate (Keys *et al* 1950—Chap. 26; Arroyave *et al* 1959; El-Shobaki *et al* 1972; Mayoral *et al* 1972). This disorder, as it appears in man, however, probably represents multiple deficiencies.

Amino acids are also influential in the metabolism of other nutrients, for example, an increase of leucine in the diet has been shown to precipitate nicotinic acid deficiency (Belavady et al 1967).

A decreased immune response is known to occur in protein deficiency (Rosen & Geifhuysin 1971; Mathur et al 1972) and consideration should be given to this point in interpreting clinical data.

In protein deficiency the tongue becomes reddened and smooth around the anterior margins. Scalloping of the edges of the tongue may develop due to oedema and its consequent pressure against the teeth. Angular cheilitis occasionally occurs and fissures may also appear on the lower lip. Loss of pigment along the buccal border of the lips is especially marked in dark-skinned races. This is probably due to an inadequacy of tyrosine (Trowell et al 1952; Van Wyck 1965; Gillman 1970).

Cutaneous effects of specific amino acid deficiencies have been demonstrated in experimental animals although we are unaware of any such reports in oral mucosa.

Deeley (1965) made the interesting observation that by increasing the protein intake of a group of edentulous patients there was a significant increase in denture tolerance. Whether this can be attributed directly to the effect on oral mucosa or indirectly to salivary gland function remains to be resolved (for review of protein deficiency and salivary gland see Rauch & Gorlin 1970, p. 994).

The protein status of an individual may be estimated in a number of ways: in addition to total serum proteins, serum albumin, serum amino acids and urinary creatinine it is also possible to assess the general body protein status by measuring the protein content of a hair root tip (Kelsay 1969; Bradfield et al 1972; Bollet & Owens 1973).

5:3:2 Fatty acids

Two polyunsaturated fatty acids, linoleic acid and linolenic acid, which the body is unable to synthesize, have long been known to be essential in the diet (Burr & Burr 1929). Arachidonic acid, which was at one time similarly considered to be essential, can be synthesized *in vivo* from linoleic acid (Mead & Howton 1958).

These fatty acids are now known to be precursors of prostaglandins (Bergstrom 1964; Van Dorp et al 1964; Ziboh & Hsia 1971; Coniglio 1972; Jonsson & Ånggård 1972; Samuelsson 1972; Sprecher 1972; Tan & Privett 1973) and it has recently been reported that certain other fatty acids might also be considered as essential for this purpose (Schlenk 1972).

Ziboh & Hsia (1972) confirmed the importance of essential fatty acids for prostaglandin production by clearing the cutaneous scaly lesions of essential fatty acid deficiency in rats, with topical applications of prostaglandin E_2. The skin of experimental animals deficient in essential fatty acids becomes thickened, dry and scaly, together with increased capillary fragility and cell permeability (Gross 1940; Hansen & Wiese 1943; White, Foy & Cerecedo 1943; Hansen & Bur 1946; Sinclair 1952; Kramer & Levine 1953; Deuel et al 1954; MacMillan & Sinclair 1958). Keratinization and number of epidermal layers in chick skin are influenced by prostaglandins (Kirscher 1973). Cutaneous changes have also been observed in humans with dry scaly lesions appearing (Hansen et al 1963; Caldwell et al 1972).

The oral mucosa might be expected to be similarly affected although no such account has yet been published.

Essential fatty acid deficiency can be confirmed by the determination of fatty acids in plasma, lecithin, triglyceride and cholesterol ester (Press et al 1972).

5:3:3 Vitamins

Vitamin A

Many metabolic pathways are influenced by vitamin A, including glycolysis, glycogenesis and phosphorylation. Mucoprotein synthesis in epithelium is altered and the changes in keratinization brought about by varying levels of vitamin A might be attributed to this process.

The effect of vitamin A on epithelial proliferation and maturation pattern is well established: mitotic activity is increased and keratinization suppressed (Fell & Mellanby 1953; Bern et al 1955; Moore 1957 & 1967; Lawrence et al 1960; Laschet 1961; Prutkin 1967; Rothberg 1967; Christophers & Braun-Falco 1970; Plewig et al 1971; Rietz 1971; Logan 1972; Lukacs et al 1972; Zil 1972). Vitamin A also increases permeability of the cell membranes, including the lysosomal membrane (Fell & Dingle 1963; Weissman & Thomas 1963; Dingle & Lucy 1965; Roels 1966; Iqbal & Wynn 1970; Franquin et al 1970; Mack et al 1972). This results in the release of hydrolytic enzymes into the cytoplasm, as well as extracellularly, and may account for the action upon connective tissues.

Much evidence has been presented indicating a complex interrelationship between vitamin A and the endocrine system. Deficiency of vitamin A leads to thyroid hypertrophy while hypervitaminosis A produces atrophy. Thyroxine, on the other hand, is required for the conversion of carotene to vitamin A and in cases of hypothyroidism there is an accumulation of carotene giving rise to the well-known cutaneous yellow tinge of myxoedema.

Steroid production is also dependent on vitamin A, and in vitamin A deficiency there is a reduction in the synthesis of adrenocortical and sex hormones.

Deficiency in vitamin A leads to the development of a dry scaly skin with follicular hyperkeratosis. The oral mucosa undergoes comparable changes with non-keratinized stratified squamous epithelium transforming into keratinized epitheliun (Reiss 1936; Wolbach & Bessey 1942; Schneider 1965; Jolly 1967; Cavalaris & Krikos 1967; Franquin et al 1969, 1970, 1971; Hicks 1969; Baume et al 1970).

Clinically, hyperkeratotic white patches may be found on the oral mucosa. Xerostomia may also be present due to concomitant changes occurring in the salivary gland ducts (Hayes et al 1970).

Hypervitaminosis A leads to thinning of the oral epithelium which is manifested as dry scaly lips and tender gingivae which bleed readily (Smith 1964). This property of vitamin A and of its acid (retinoic acid) has led to its use, topically and systemically, in hyperkeratotic lesions of skin (Beer 1962; Heiss & Gross 1970; Pedace & Stoughton 1971) and oral mucosa (Smith 1962; Silverman et al 1963a,b; Ryssel et al 1971; Gunther 1972 a, b).

Measurement of plasma levels of vitamin A and carotenoids does not reflect vitamin A deficiency until the tissue stores, principally in the liver, are depleted (Dowling & Wald 1958). Hepatic levels of vitamin A are an accurate indicator of its body status (McLaren 1966), but this is hardly a convenient routine procedure. Other techniques for assessing tissue saturation of vitamin A are based on measuring the rhodopsin concentration in the eye by electroretinography or reflectance spectrophotometry (Jacobson 1961; Rushton 1962).

Vitamin B_1 (thiamine)

Once absorbed, thiamine is phosphorylated to form thiamine pyrophosphate, which acts as a coenzyme for carboxylases. This enzyme system is responsible for the decarboxylation of α-keto acids such as pyruvic and α-ketoglutaric acids. Thus, a deficiency of thiamine leads to the accumulation of pyruvic and lactic acids in the serum and tissues. The disease syndrome of thiamine deficiency is beriberi, which is principally a degenerative process of the nervous system.

Little convincing evidence exists regarding cutaneous or mucosal lesions in thiamine deficiency. Mann et al (1941) stated that a generalized hypersensitivity of the oral tissues occurred and Weisberger (1941) attributed small vesicles on the oral mucosa to thiamine deficiency. Jensen et al (1965) described a single patient with atrophy to the lingual papillae: although this individual appeared to be of a low thiamine status we calculate from their data that the serum iron saturation was only 8% (normal $>$ 16%).

The lack of lesions in oral mucosa is compatible with the fact that stratified squamous epithelium is thought to obtain its energy mainly by anaerobic glycolysis (Iqbal & Gerson 1971) and therefore is not so dependent on the aerobic enzyme systems of the Krebs tricarboxylic acid cycle. A comparable situation obtains in the kidney of thiamine-deficient animals: adenosine triphosphate production is only diminished in regions dependent on the tricarboxylic acid cycle.

In order to estimate body thiamine status it is necessary to perform a loading test and measure urinary excretion. Direct measurement of blood or urine thiamine levels reflect recent intake only and are not a true parameter of tissue saturation. A more accurate representation of body status than measuring serum thiamine directly is to quantify its metabolic product, thiamine pyrophosphate, by its effect on transketolase activity. Either a 24-hour urinary collection must be made or else the thiamine pyrophosphate is expressed in relation to urinary creatinine.

Vitamin B_2 (riboflavin)

Riboflavin is required for the synthesis of flavoprotein enzymes whose function is the carriage of hydrogen from reduced pyridine nucleotides to the cytochrome system. Accordingly, levels of flavoproteins drop markedly in riboflavin deficiency. As riboflavin is necessary for such a basic enzymatic step, abnormal levels can be reflected in protein, carbohydrate and lipid metabolism.

The amount of riboflavin necessary in the diet is governed by the other dietary constituents. A carbohydrate diet requires least riboflavin and as more protein or fat is introduced then the requirement for riboflavin increases in a corresponding manner.

Riboflavin deficiency leads to a decrease in serum folate and an increase in vitamin B_{12} (Foy et al 1966; Bovina et al 1969). These alterations are reflected in the marrow and may account for the anaemia (Lane &

Alfrey 1965). The albumin-globulin ratio undergoes profound changes, which confirms the need for riboflavin in protein metabolism.

The endocrine system is also affected by riboflavin deficiency with a diminution of thyroxine secretion (Nolte *et al* 1972). This in turn decreases the basal metabolic rate.

The skin and mucous membranes are prominently affected by riboflavin deficiency. A greasy, scaling dermatitis develops in the nasolabial folds, on the nose, on the ears, on the medial and lateral canthi of the eyelids, on the scrotum and on the vulvae. The cornea shows similar changes with the development of a superficial interstitial keratitis.

The oral changes in riboflavin deficiency are essentially cheilitis and glossitis. A bluish-purple discoloration occurs in the buccal mucosa, the tongue and the lips (Youmans 1950). Sialorrhoea is a marked feature: Jones *et al* (1944), who, in a group of over 1,700 people with riboflavin deficiency, reported: 'Salivation was often troublesome, and sometimes so excessive that saliva dripped from the mouth when this was opened for examination.'

There is some variance in accounts of the stages of development of the cheilitis of riboflavin deficiency. Sebrell & Butler (1938) describe the initial lesion as a pallor of the labial mucosa at the angles which is followed by maceration and shortly thereafter by superficial transverse fissures. These fissures are usually bilateral and extend downwards from the angle. Some authors have attempted to use the upward or downward slope of these fissures as a diagnostic feature but we are not convinced of the validity of this test. On the other hand, Jones *et al* (1944) stated that the initial lesion was a 'tiny, painful raw red area at the commissure of the lips'. This red area spreads on to the buccal mucosa and lower labial mucosa and is soon covered by a boggy white epithelium. At this stage fissures develop. These authors also report that the lesion is frequently unilateral, or at least the two sides are at different stages in development. That fissures occur at the angle of the lips is agreed by all investigators (Weisberger 1941; Nippert & McGinty 1943; Brown 1949a; Pollack 1956; Dreizen *et al* 1958). These lesions subsequently are covered by crusts which can be scraped off without bleeding. The epithelial denudation spreads along the lips, particularly the lower lip, and causes the lips to appear abnormally red. Painful ulceration of labial mucosa is also described. A further feature reported by Jones *et al* (1944) is the appearance of small papular swellings near the gingival margin of the lower labial mucosa.

In dogs, riboflavin deficiency is associated with patchy atrophy of the lingual filiform and fungiform papillae on the anterior two-thirds of the tongue (Afonsky 1955). Histology reveals that there is degeneration of the basal epithelial cells together with rarefaction of the epithelium and adjacent connective tissues. Similar changes occur in humans (Jones *et al* 1944) with progressive atrophy of the lingual papillae. In the early stages of the condition the tongue is reddened but it gradually becomes smooth, shiny and pale. A central fissure, shallow ulcers or petechial haemorrhages may then appear. Finally, wasting can occur with the lingual margins becoming thin and sharp rather than rounded.

A small percentage of the individuals described by Jones *et al* (1944) developed raw, red areas with a serpiginous outline on the hard palate. The margins were surrounded by a rim of 'sodden white epithelium'.

The measurement of urinary riboflavin or of erythrocyte riboflavin has the same limitations as many other vitamins in that the values thus obtained are a reflection on recent dietary experience rather than on tissue saturation.

Nicotinic acid (niacin)

Nicotinic acid is converted into nicotinamide, which is then utilized for the synthesis of diphosphopyridine nucleotide (DPN or NAD) and triphosphopyridine nucleotide (TPN or NADP). Both of these coenzymes have a dual role: they function as hydrogen receptors from metabolites, passing hydrogen on to the flavoprotein and cytochrome systems, and they also act as hydrogen donors for hydroxylation and reduction.

Originally there was some confusion about the dietary requirement of nicotinic acid but it is now established that the amino acid, tryptophan, can be converted into nicotinic acid within the gut as well as systemically (Chick 1951; Dalgleish 1955). Therefore the amount of nicotinic acid required in the diet is inversely related to tryptophan intake. A 'Nicotinic Acid Equivalent' has been worked out for the tryptophan requirement; this varies between species and in man the figure is approximately—60 mg tryptophan equivalent to 1 mg nicotinic acid.

The nicotinic acid requirement is also influenced by the composition of the remainder of the diet. Not only do levels of protein and fat ingestion bring about these alterations but the amount and even the type of carbohydrate are also relevant.

The manifestations of nicotinic acid deficiency, or pellagra, have been termed as the three D's—Diarrhoea, Dermatitis and Dementia. Alimentary upset often heralds the onset of pellagra, with loss of appetite, nausea and severe diarrhoea. The gastric and colonic mucosa become atrophic and occasionally develop small ulcers. The endocrine system is severely affected in pellagra with degenerative changes occurring in the thyroid and adrenal cortex.

Cutaneous lesions develop in areas exposed to sunlight or minor trauma. Initially there is erythema, pruritis or a burning sensation, and bullae, scales or pustules may appear. In the later stages the skin becomes rough, brittle, fissured and brown.

The oral manifestations of pellagra are glossitis, stomatitis and, less frequently, cheilitis (Denton 1925, 1928; Rhoads & Miller 1933; Elvehjem 1940; Field *et al* 1940; Afonsky 1955; Goldsmith *et al* 1956; Belvady *et al* 1967). Reddening of the oral mucosa is the earliest sign and it is this deep red colour that has given rise to the descriptive term 'Black Tongue' in dogs. The entire dorsum of the tongue undergoes atrophic changes with the filiform papillae disappearing before the fungiform papillae. Eventually the epithelium becomes thin and parakeratotic with the cells showing impaired differentiation, hydropic degeneration, pleomorphism and pyknosis. No inflammatory changes are said to occur in the underlying connective tissue. The central surface of the tongue, however, may ulcerate and become covered by a pseudomembrane containing numerous organisms.

The entire oral mucosa becomes involved in advanced stages of pellagra. Initially the floor of the mouth, buccal and labial mucosae are involved, but as the disorder progresses the palate and pharynx are similarly affected. Following the phase of reddening the mucosa becomes ulcerated and is then covered extensively with a greyish-green pseudomembrane.

Histology reveals that the earliest alterations occur in the lamina propria. This becomes loosely arranged with many intercellular spaces, dilated blood vessels and a chronic inflammatory cell infiltrate. Subsequently the overlying epithelium grows thinner until only a single layer of cells is left. Ulceration takes place and the connective tissue becomes covered with a pseudomembrane of fibrin, cell debris and bacteria. Polymorphonuclear leukocytes appear once ulceration has developed.

Angular cheilitis was noted in several of the post-mortem cases reported by Denton (1925). This does not seem to be a prominent feature of pellagra and maybe this report should be viewed with some reservations: all their cases were terminal and there is the possibility of other concomitant deficiencies.

The principal, and most readily measured, urinary metabolite of nicotinic acid is N-methyl nicotinamide. This is expressed in relation, like thiamine and riboflavin, to urinary creatinine.

Vitamin B_6

Vitamin B_6 is the generic for a group of three compounds: pyridoxine, pyridoxal and pyridoxamine. In the body these compounds are phosphorylated and function as coenzymes. Pyridoxal phosphate participates in many enzyme systems including amino acid transamination, decarboxylation and deamination. It is also involved in fatty acid synthesis as well as in various steps of carbohydrate metabolism.

Iron metabolism is disturbed by vitamin B_6 deficiency and a microcytic, hypochromic anaemia develops. This is associated with high serum levels of iron and an increase of haemosiderin in the marrow, spleen and liver (Borson & Mettier 1940; Wintrobe *et al* 1943; Snyderman *et al* 1952; Reid *et al* 1945; Harris & Horrigan 1964).

One interpretation of these results would seem to be that pyridoxine is required for the synthesis of iron-containing proteins and in cases of vitamin B_6 deficiency the iron accumulates in serum and tissues.

Jacobs & Cavill (1968a), in a study of patients with iron deficiency, concluded that the oral abnormalities could probably be attributed to pyridoxine deficiency. However, the interaction between pyridoxine and iron in oral mucosa is not clear, and further work is required.

Vitamin B_6 deficiency causes changes in serum proteins together with a lymphopenia and neutrophilia. The immune response could well be altered in such circumstances and the interpretation of clinical manifestations is obscured by this issue.

Vitamin B_6 deficiency produces a dermatitis with yellowish, greasy scaling particularly of the face. This is accompanied by pruritis and a burning sensation.

The oral manifestations are stomatitis, glossitis and cheilitis (Smith & Martin 1940; Mueller & Vilter 1950; Vilter *et al* 1953, 1954; Afonsky 1955). The anterior two-thirds of the dorsum of the tongue becomes red and swollen with the filiform papillae atrophying and the fungiform papillae remaining as red knobs. In dogs (Afonsky 1955) this atrophy has a patchy distribution. Histology shows degenerative changes occurring in the epithelium including decreased keratinization, hydropic degeneration and parakeratosis. Nerve degeneration is also seen, and is part of a generalized peripheral neuritis associated with pyridoxine deficiency.

The remaining oral mucosa becomes red and has a burning sensation. Small ulcers may appear. Fissures develop along the lips and at the labial commissures.

Several techniques are available for the estimation of vitamin B_6 status.

In deficiency, erythrocyte glutamic pyruvic transaminase (GPT) is markedly depressed and erythrocyte glutamic oxalacetic transminase (GOT) is depressed to a lesser extent (Marsh et al 1955; Raica & Sauberlich 1964; Cheney et al 1965). Pyridoxal phosphate can be measured directly in the plasma and in the urine (Kelsay et al 1968). Finally, a tryptophan load test may be used and urinary levels of xanthurenic acid, kynurenine and quinolinic acid measured. These biochemical assessments of vitamin B_6 status are discussed by Sauberlich (1968) and Sauberlich et al (1972).

Pantothenic acid

Pantothenic acid is a component of coenzyme A, the function of which is acylation in many metabolic pathways, for example the tricarboxylic acid cycle, fatty acid and amino acid oxidation. The importance of coenzyme A in steroid hormone biosynthesis is reflected in the marked adrenal necrosis and gonadal atrophy of pantothenic acid deficiency (Fidanza 1971).

The requirements for pantothenic acid are uncertain and although convincing deficiency states have been produced in animals, the manifestations are not as clear in humans (Bean & Hodges 1954).

Pantothenic acid is produced by the intestinal bacteria, but it is dubious if this is of much benefit to the host as the main site of synthesis is thought to be the colon. Another fact obscuring clear interpretation is the effect of protein in the diet: within limits, the more protein ingested the less pantothenic acid is required.

In animals with pantothenic acid deficiency, a scaling erythematous dermatitis occurs with a histological picture of hyperkeratosis and acanthosis. Later, the epidermis is inclined to undergo atrophic changes and even ulcerate (Sullivan & Nicholls 1942a; Wintrobe et al 1943; Elvehjem 1944; McCall et al 1946). In rats, the entire oral mucosa, including gingivae, is involved (Wainwright & Nelson 1945). There is an initial reaction with epithelial hyperkeratosis, hyperplasia and 'proliferation' of the basal cells. Subsequently the epithelium undergoes degenerative changes leaving the connective tissue uncovered. The authors remarked on the unusual absence of any inflammatory changes in the lamina propria even in the presence of considerable tissue destruction.

Afonsky (1955) described a mild diffuse atrophy of the lingual filiform papillae in dogs with a transformation of the epithelium from orthokeratosis to parakeratosis. Again the lamina propria was unaffected.

One report exists wherein four patients with glossitis responded to pantothenic acid therapy (Brown 1949b, c).

We are not familiar with any standard laboratory procedure for measuring pantothenic acid status.

Biotin

Biotin is involved in carboxylation and deamination systems and as such participates in protein, lipid and carbohydrate metabolism. The role of biotin as the protector from egg-white injury is clear. Egg-white contains a protein, avidin, which has a very high resistance to digestion within the alimentary tract and is not absorbed. What egg-white in fact does is bind the ingested biotin and thus creates a biotin deficiency. Therefore biotin deficiency can be precipitated either by inadequate intake or by eating large quantities of raw eggs: cooking inactivates the binding capacity of avidin.

A dry, scaly dermatitis due to biotin deficiency has been shown to develop in several animals as well as in man (Boas 1927; Gyorgy 1931, 1941; Sydenstricker *et al* 1942; Lehrer *et al* 1952). The microscopic picture of the skin reveals hyperkeratosis, some parakeratosis and acanthosis (Findlay & Stern 1929; Gyorgy *et al* 1937; Sullivan & Nicholls 1942b; Sullivan *et al* 1942).

There is some variation in the oral manifestations of biotin deficiency in man. Sydenstricker *et al* (1942) reported tongue changes in four volunteers, although the pattern was variable. One showed patchy atrophy of the papillae, similar in appearance to geographic tongue, one had papillary atrophy confined to the lateral thirds, and two had diffuse atrophy of the papillae. A common factor was that the tongues of the four individuals remained pale unlike that found in deficiencies of other vitamins. In a report of a single case of probable biotin deficiency Williams (1943) noted that although the typical cutaneous lesions developed the tongue remained normal.

Boas (1927) found that sublingual ulcers were fairly common in biotin-deficient rats.

The body status of biotin can be assessed by measuring the urinary excretion of biotin or by performing a loading test.

Vitamin B_{12}

Vitamin B_{12} is the generic term for a group of cobalamins: deoxyadenosylcobalamin is the predominant cobalamin in the diet but smaller quantities of other analogues are also found, namely hydroxycobalamin and methylcobalamin. Cyanocobalamin is a semisynthetic form used in the therapy of deficient states.

Vitamin B_{12} is involved in several metabolic pathways including the synthesis of purines and pyrimidines. As such it plays a vital role in nucleic acid (DNA and RNA) production and is considered to interact with folate in this respect.

Larrabee *et al* (1963) proposed the sequence of events depicted in Fig. 5.2, showing the function of vitamin B_{12} in the regeneration of tetrahydrofolate.

Therefore, inadequate amounts of vitamin B_{12} or folate will have a similar effect on tetrahydrofolate-mediated purine and pyrimidine synthesis. Ascorbic acid is also involved in this scheme and maintains the folic acid reductases in their tetrahydro form. Another aspect of the involvement of vitamin B_{12} with folate metabolism is its effect on the cellular uptake of 5-methyltetrahydrofolate.

Deficiency of vitamin B_{12} may arise in a number of ways, as was indicated in the introductory remarks on nutrition. Vitamin B_{12} deficiency leads to a diminution in gastric secretion of intrinsic factor as well as impairing the absorption of vitamin B_{12} itself (as well as of folate). The requirement of vitamin B_{12} is influenced by the dietary pattern and it is elevated by increasing the intake of proteins and fat.

Pernicious anaemia is a disorder peculiar to humans and is a state wherein there is an inadequate amount of available intrinsic factor as a consequence of atrophic gastritis. This is just one cause of vitamin B_{12} deficiency. Addisonian (idiopathic) anaemia and Biecmer's pernicious anaemia are synonymous terms originally used to describe a fatal form of anaemia associated with gastrointestinal changes and not due to inadequate diet. Coupland (1881) first appreciated that the clinical picture of vitamin B_{12} deficiency could be caused both by pernicious anaemia as well as by other mechanisms. The aetiology of pernicious anaemia is obscure and opinions are divided. One possibility is that the original lesion is of the gastric mucosa with atrophy of the parietal and chief cells occurring. During this process cellular material passes into the deeper tissues and leads to the production of antibodies. Antibodies to parietal cells can be demonstrated in about 90% of individuals with pernicious anaemia and antibodies to intrinsic factor only in half that number. Supporting this theory is the appearance of pernicious anaemia in cases of agammaglobulinaemia, thus indicating that it is not the antibodies which precipitate the disorder. Some evidence has been presented which indicates that

T-lymphocytes are involved, but the role of the cellular immune response in pernicious anaemia still requires further elucidation.

Another theory is that pernicious anaemia is an autoimmune disease and the evidence substantiating this is the presence of other autoantibodies, mainly thyroid, in cases of pernicious anaemia. (For further discussion of pernicious anaemia see Chanarin (1969).)

Deficiency of vitamin B_{12} causes changes in a number of tissues and the mechanism whereby these are affected might be in a reduction of DNA and RNA synthesis. Chromosomal abnormalities (Lawler *et al* 1971) as well as the more obvious nuclear alterations are characteristic of vitamin B_{12} deficiency and this is well illustrated in the macrocytic anaemia with megaloblastic erythropoiesis.

It should be appreciated that the *anaemia* of vitamin B_{12} deficiency has no effect on the oral tissues other than to produce a pallor of the mucous membranes when the haemoglobin falls below a level of about 8·5 G (see section 5:2:2).

Vitamin B_{12} deficiency is not associated with striking cutaneous changes, although a form of dermatitis has been reported in pigs (Richardson *et al* 1951). However, mucous membranes are affected and abnormally large nuclei in epithelial cells have been reported in vagina, nose, stomach, bronchi and urinary tract in addition to the oral cavity (Graham & Rheault 1954; Massey & Klagman 1955; Boen 1957; Boen *et al* 1958; Farrant 1958, 1960; Boddington 1959; Boddington & Spriggs 1959; Rubin 1959; Lloyd & Gary 1963; Foroozan & Trier 1967). Although there is a considerable volume of work on cytology there are surprisingly few reports of histology being carried out on mucosae.

The oral manifestations of glossitis and stomatitis in vitamin B_{12} deficiency have long been recognized (Barclay 1851; Möller 1851; Muller 1877; Hunter 1900, 1909; Stern 1914; Dreifuss 1924; Starr 1928; Lewis 1930; Oatway & Middleton 1932; Miller & Rhoads 1935; Brown 1946; Reisner *et al* 1951; Johnson 1957; Taft *et al* 1958; Jacobs 1960, 1961a,b; Cox 1962; Jensen *et al* 1965, 1967).

The oral mucosa may appear pale, due to anaemia, or it may be tinged yellow as a consequence of elevated serum bilirubin arising from increased haemolysis. Baker *et al* (1963) reported the presence of buccal pigmentation as well as cutaneous pigmentation in a group of patients with vitamin B_{12} deficiency. The appearance of the mouth was similar to that in Addison's disease but the pattern of cutaneous pigmentation was very different. Adrenal function was shown to be normal in the group. Brown (1946) commented on pigmentation being a feature of vitamin B_{12} deficiency, but Wintrobe (1967) felt that it was more prevalent in folate deficiency. The mechanism for this altered pigmentation, either increased or decreased, has not been explained.

The tongue is a sensitive index of vitamin B_{12} deficiency and undergoes changes in approximately 60% of patients with pernicious anaemia. This is a more variable figure in other aetiological groups of vitamin B_{12} deficiency and this apparently depends on the degree of deficiency. The oral manifestations fluctuate between a relatively quiescent atrophic phase and a severely inflamed phase. As the deficiency continues untreated the severity of the lesions progressively increases.

The dorsum of the tongue is affected either diffusely or in a patchy manner. Initially the tip is reddened and tender and this process gradually spreads around the lateral margins until it eventually involves the entire dorsum. This becomes bright red, oedematous, raw and is exquisitely tender. Fissures or furrows may develop with the descriptive term of 'scrotal tongue' being applied. The epithelium thins, becoming parakeratinized or non-keratinized and finally disintegrates, leaving large, shallow, white ulcers which frequently become infected with bacteria and fungi. Smaller ulcers, similar to recurrent aphthae, have also been described in the tongue. Both acute and chronic inflammatory cells congregate in the subepithelial connective tissue and these may migrate into the epithelium. Numerous dilated capillaries are present and the fibrous tissue of the lamina propria appears oedematous.

This phase of the raw, red tongue is excruciatingly painful, interferes with eating, and the apt clinical description of 'beefy tongue' is used. Hunter (1900) gave the equally descriptive simile of looking like 'raw liver'. Some authors have also noted the presence of reddish vesicles containing clear fluid around the tip of the tongue.

After a few weeks the acute symptoms and signs tend to subside and the dorsum takes on a smooth appearance. The filiform, fungiform and circumvallate papillae undergo atrophy in that order and as the deficiency continues between inflammatory and atrophic phases the papillae all disappear, leaving the tongue looking flabby, smooth and glazed. Ulcers may also appear during the atrophic quiescent phases.

Hjørting-Hansen & Bertram (1968) found that two of their patients had a knobbly appearance to the tongue and suggested that this was related to their xerostomia: the tongue often takes on a similar knobbled pattern in Sjögren's syndrome. Brown (1946) and Allington (1950) also comment on xerostomia in vitamin B_{12} deficiency.

The remainder of the oral mucosa is not usually as severely affected in the earlier stages of vitamin B_{12} deficiency, although as the disorder progresses the entire oral mucosa may be involved. The ventral surface of the tongue as well as the buccal, labial, palatal, gingival and pharyngeal mucosae all become red and tender. Ulcers appear either in the form of shallow erosions or as small aphthae. The pharynx, in particular, becomes both inflamed and ulcerated and this together with the upper oesophageal lesions produce dysphagia.

Jacobs (1960) examined biopsies of buccal mucosa in patients with pernicious anaemia and found decreased epithelial thickness, increased mitoses in basal cells, prickle cell mitotic figures, binucleated prickle cells, the presence of keratohyalin granules and a subepithelial infiltration of acute and chronic inflammatory cells, especially lymphocytes. He also noted a decrease in melanin which is in contrast to the clinical finding of Baker et al (1963). As has been stated above, the mechanism altering pigmentation, in either direction, has still to be elucidated.

Angular cheilitis is not a regular feature of vitamin B_{12} deficiency and we would disagree with Dreizen (1971), who states that cheilitis and glossitis are equally prevalent. We have found a report of only one case having angular cheilitis (Laache 1883). Another report states that a deep fissure developed in the lower lip but not at the commissure (Spies et al 1955).

Cytological examination of oral epithelial cells obtained either by mouth rinsing or scraping has revealed cells with significantly enlarged nuclei (Boen 1957; Boen et al 1958; Farrant 1958, 1960; Boddington 1959; Boddington & Spriggs 1959). These nuclei exhibit polymorphism and contain chromatin in clumps or in a finely reticulated pattern. Multinucleated cells may also be present (Boen 1957; Boen et al 1958; Farrant 1958, 1960; Boddington 1959; Boddington & Spriggs 1959). The appearance of these epithelial cells with enlarged and altered nuclei are similar to those obtained from other mucosal sites and although the picture is not specific for vitamin B_{12} deficiency it is a further confirmatory sign.

In addition to the clinical examination several techniques are available to aid in the diagnosis of vitamin B_{12} deficiency.

1   Blood: low haemoglobin, low red cell count, raised mean cell volume (MCV), raised mean cell haemoglobin concentration (MCHC).
Blood film showing characteristic appearances of erythrocytes and leukocytes.
2   Marrow: megaloblastic erythropoiesis.
3   Serum B_{12} level low: measured by radioassay or by bioassay.

4 Increased urinary excretion of methylmalonic acid, especially following an oral dose of valine.
5 Optimal response to vitamin B_{12} injection.
6 Gastric biopsy showing atrophic changes.
7 Parietal cell or intrinsic factor antibodies in serum.
8 Faecal excretion of radioactive vitamin B_{12} after oral administration.
9 Schilling test: measuring urinary excretion of a small injected dose of radioactive vitamin B_{12} followed by a large oral dose.
10 Hepatic uptake of radioactive vitamin B_{12} following oral administration.
11 Serum uptake of radioactive vitamin B_{12} following oral administration.
12 Whole body counting following oral administration of vitamin B_{12}.

Tests (6) to (12) are particularly designed to diagnose pernicious anaemia and often show a response towards normal when intrinsic factor is administered concurrently. However, some caution must be exercised in analysing the results because vitamin B_{12} deficiency *per se* may alter gastric secretion of intrinsic factor and hydrochloric acid as well as decreasing intestinal absorption. Also, antibodies to intrinsic factor, secretory IgA in particular, may be present in the stomach and gut and can interfere with vitamin B_{12} binding and absorption.

Folic acid

Folic acid or folate are general terms describing a group of glutamic acid conjugates of pteroic acid. When one molecule of glutamic acid is conjugated with pteroic acid the resultant compound is named pteroylglutamic acid. If two molecules of glutamic acid are conjugated it is called pteroyldiglutamic acid, and so on. Other groups, such as methyl- or formyl-, may also be added on to the molecule.

The common forms of folic acid in the diet are pteroylheptaglutamic acid, pteroyltriglutamic acid and 10-formylpteroylglutamic acid. However, the polyglutamyl forms of folic acid are not as readily used by man and the monoglutamate, therefore, is preferred for therapy (Crosby 1960).

Once ingested, the above polyglutamyl members are subjected to folate conjugases and reductases with tetrahydrofolate being formed as the active form. As such, folic acid is involved as a coenzyme in a number of different metabolic pathways. These include purine synthesis, by transferring carbon numbers 2 and 8 in the production of inosinic acid; and pyrimidine synthesis, by effecting the methylation of uridylate in thymidilate production. Folic acid is also required for the interconversion of serine and glycine as well as for the methionine methyl group synthesis. The methylation of uridylate is particularly sensitive to the folic acid antagonists, e.g. aminoperin, amethopterin, pyrinethanine and trimethoprim. Similar oral manifestations to folic acid deficiency have been described in patients receiving amethopterin (Dreizen et al 1970; Hausemen 1970; Randazzo et al 1972) and primidone (Stein & Lewis 1973).

Therefore, like vitamin B_{12}, a deficiency of folic acid will interfere with both DNA and RNA production by a common mechanism. However,

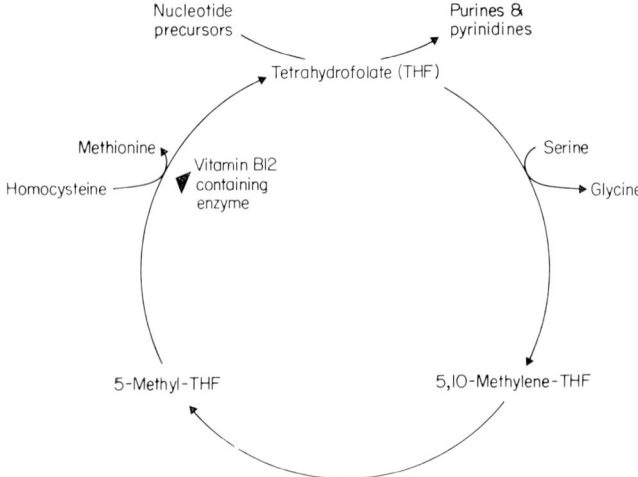

Fig. 5.2. Interconversions of functional forms of folic acid with metabolic roles indicated.

A vitamin-B_{12}-containing enzyme is required for the transmethylation reaction, in the formation of methionine.

the separate involvements of vitamin B_{12} and folic acid in other metabolic pathways are reflected in the different spectrum of manifestations of their respective deficiencies. (For a review of folic acid metabolism see Stokstad & Koch (1967).)

Deficiency of folic acid can lead to the development of a papular, scaly dermatitis, the histology of which reveals marked nuclear variability in size and form, diminution of the granular layer, hyperpigmentation and a leukocytic infiltration with the eosinophils being prominent (Rodriquez-Molina 1941, 1954; Stefanini 1948; Nagaraju et al 1971). Proctitis and vaginitis may also be troublesome.

The oral manifestations of folic acid deficiency are glossitis, ulcerative stomatitis and angular cheilitis (Low 1928; Manson-Bahr & Willoughby 1930; Day et al 1938; Wills & Evans 1938; Spies et al 1946; Stefanini 1948; Wills 1948; Rodriquez-Molina 1954; Afonsky 1955; Gardner 1958; Zalusky & Herbert 1961; Izak et al 1963; Dreizen & Levy 1969; Rose 1971). Although cutaneous pigmentation is a feature of folic acid deficiency, Stefanini (1948) found no intraoral pigmentation in over a thousand cases of tropical sprue.

As in other nutritional deficiencies predisposing to anaemia the mucosae may appear pale, although there is no good evidence that the lower haemoglobin with reduced oxygenation of the tissues leads to any abnormality of the mucosae *per se*.

The glossitis follows a similar course to that of vitamin B_{12} deficiency. Initially the dorsum becomes reddened, swollen and tender. This frequently commences around the lingual margins but eventually involves the dorsum of the anterior two-thirds. Ulcers appear, either in the form of superficial erosions or as small aphthae. The tongue at this stage is also described as 'beefy' and is most painful. Subsequently, the papillae atrophy, first the filiform and then the fungiform papillae. Finally the dorsum of the tongue becomes smooth and shiny.

Histology of the tongue in folate-deficient dogs (Afonsky 1955) shows areas both of epithelial proliferation and atrophy: keratinization is disturbed with disappearance of keratohyaline granules and a transformation to parakeratosis or even to non-keratinizing epithelium. The basal cells are abnormally large and the underlying connective tissue is infiltrated with leukocytes. Occasional nerve degeneration is also seen.

The buccal, gingival, labial, soft palatal and pharyngeal mucosae as well as the ventral surface of tongue develop a patchy stomatitis with aphthae commonly appearing. This widespread stomatitis is exceedingly painful and has been described as causing discomfort even when drinking water.

Dreizen et al (1970) examined the histology of oral mucosal tissues from folate-deficient marmosets and found widespread changes. The cells of the prickle and granular layers were enlarged and described as ballooning. The cytoplasm was lightly stained and the nuclei had a light lacy appearance with clumping of chromatin. Keratinization was decreased partially or completely. Extensive shallow ulceration was also reported.

There is little doubt that folic acid deficiency causes angular cheilitis, both in experimental animals and in man. The fissuring at the labial commissures is similar to that in other deficiency states and is frequently a site of secondary infection by bacteria and fungi. The predisposition to infection may be accentuated by leukopaenia.

Gingivitis and periodontitis is also reported to be more common in folic acid deficiency in humans, as compared to vitamin B_{12} (Day et al 1938), although Afonsky (1955) did not find this so in dogs. Doo (1971) recorded a number of histochemical changes in normal rat oral mucosa following the administration of relatively high doses of folic acid.

Cytology of epithelial cells from mucosal surfaces, including the mouth, shows cells with increased nuclear size which are indistinguishable from those found in vitamin B_{12} deficiency (Gardner 1956; Butterworth & Perez-Santiago 1957; Monto et al 1963; Staats et al 1965; Swanson & Thomassen 1965; van Niekerk 1966; Staats et al 1969).

The following parameters are used in diagnosing folic acid deficiency and it can be seen that part of the diagnosis lies in excluding vitamin B_{12} deficiency.

1 Blood: low haemoglobin, low red cell count, raised MCV.
2 Marrow-megaloblastic erythropoiesis.
3 Serum vitamin B_{12} level normal. (Note—folate deficiency can impair absorption of B_{12}.)
4 Normal B_{12} absorption and Schilling's test.
5 Normal urinary excretion of methylmalonic acid.
6 Elevated urinary excretion of formiminoglutamic acid (FIGLU) following oral histidine. (Note—vitamin B_{12} deficiency can elevate this up to 100 mg; folate deficiency often exceeds this figure.)
7 Serum folate is low—actual figure varies with technique used in assay.
8 Red cell folate is low. (Note—can also be low in vitamin B_{12} deficiency.)
9 Optimal haematological response following parenteral folate therapy.

Vitamin C (ascorbic acid)

Ascorbic acid is involved in a multitude of oxidation reduction reactions, and as such influences the metabolism of amino acids, lipids, carbohydrates and minerals. It is, therefore, not surprising that a deficiency of ascorbic acid (scurvy) leads to changes in many tissues. Mesenchymal tissue is particularly sensitive to ascorbic acid deficiency and considerable work has been carried out on the role of ascorbic acid in collagen synthesis. Increased capillary fragility also occurs in scurvy. The endocrine system undergoes significant alterations in the deficiency state and these may predispose to secondary manifestations.

The typical cutaneous changes seen in scurvy are a hyperkeratotic scaly dermatitis and petechiae. Several investigators have commented on the similarity of the epithelial changes in vitamin A and vitamin C deficiencies, although no clear relationship between the two has been shown. It is interesting to note that fatty acid metabolism is disturbed in scorbutic individuals (Ginter et al 1969) and that the clinical appearance of the skin in scurvy also is comparable to that found in essential fatty acid deficiency. Possibly ascorbic acid is required for prostaglandin synthesis.

The inflamed spongy gums of scurvy have been recognized since the time of Hippocrates. In dentulous subjects only, the gingivae become swollen, ulcerated and infected. They bleed readily and in advanced scurvy blood oozes spontaneously from the gingiva. Other than the periodontal changes few manifestations have been found elsewhere in the oral mucosa.

Machella (1942) recorded three cases of angular cheilitis which responded to vitamin C, and Ferguson & Dagg (1974) reported a single case in which aphthous stomatitis responded to vitamin C. Bartley et al (1953) also noted aphthae in a number of scorbutic people but could show no greater incidence than in a control group. Stafford (1965) strongly recommended the use of vitamin C in buccal ulceration, although he did not support this statement with any figures.

Salivary glands are affected by reduced levels of ascorbic acid and the sicca syndrome may develop (Hodges et al 1970; Hood et al 1970). The resultant xerostomia may predispose to a general tenderness of the oral mucosa (see Chapter 10).

Finally, petechiae, resulting from increased capillary fragility, may appear intraorally as well as over the skin.

Ascorbic acid deficiency can be diagnosed using the following procedures:
1 Test for increased capillary fragility, e.g. Hess's test.
2 Leukocyte ascorbic acid level (normal > 25 mg$/10^8$ WBC).
3 Urinary excretion of ascorbic acid after a saturation test.

Vitamin D

Vitamin D is the term used for two sterols, calciferol and cholecalciferol, which prevent rickets. The precise role of vitamin D at the cellular level remains obscure but the general effect is to elevate the serum calcium and phosphate.

Vitamin D deficiency does not appear to cause any clinical abnormalities of skin or oral mucosa, although Oliver et al (1972) reported that vitamin D deficiency depressed the rate of collagen synthesis in the oral mucosa.

In a group of patients receiving high doses of vitamin D for various reasons, Ziskin (1946) concluded that the gingival mucosa was 'improved', the epithelium 'thickened' and that the 'keratin seemed more mature'. No confirmatory studies have been presented.

Vitamin E (tocopherol)

Vitamin E is a potent reversible antioxidant which exerts a protective action on vitamin A, vitamin C and unsaturated fatty acids by inhibiting their oxidation.

Deficiency of vitamin E has not been associated with any specific cutaneous or mucosal changes, although it does affect the periodontium in rats (Schneider & Pose 1969).

Vitamin K

Vitamin K includes a group of fat-soluble derivatives of 1,4-naphthoquinone, the most potent member of which is menadione. Vitamin K is necessary for the synthesis of prothrombin, proconvertin, Stuart factor (factor X) and Christmas factor (factor IX). Therefore, a deficiency of this vitamin leads to a disorder of coagulation with a resultant haemorrhagic state (section 5:2:1).

5:3:4 Minerals and trace elements

Iron

Iron is involved both in oxygen transport, as in haemoglobin and myoglobin, and as a constituent of several tissue redox enzyme systems including cytochrome C, cytochrome oxidase, catalase, peroxidases, succinic dehydrogenase, xanthine oxidase, lipoamide oxidoreductase, flavoprotein dehydrogenases and oxidases. Iron is stored in tissues in the form of ferritin, a metalloprotein complex.

Iron, like copper, belongs to the group of elements known as the transition metals. These elements usually have more than one valence state and as such are able to undergo reversible valency changes and in so doing can be reduced by substrates and reoxidized by molecular oxygen.

Descriptions of the use of iron therapy are to be found dating back to 1500 B.C. in early Greek and Egyptian literature. The term chlorosis was introduced about the 17th century to describe the symptoms of severe iron deficiency anaemia, but it remained until the late 19th and early 20th century until the relationship of iron to erythropoiesis and its disorder was elucidated.

A controversial point which is still open to debate is whether symptoms of iron deficiency (sideropenia) may appear prior to the development of anaemia. The consensus of opinion is that the lowered haemoglobin *per se* is not responsible for the characteristic cutaneous and mucosal manifestations of sideropenia; that is, other than the pallor. The marrow is merely particularly sensitive to a diminution of available iron and probably is the first tissue wherein the effects of iron deficiency can be shown to produce clinical signs. Discussion continues about possible cases where epithelial lesions precede anaemia, and investigators have a tendency to become entangled in deciding exactly what level of haemoglobin constitutes anaemia. We do not think that this problem is of much concern and are prepared to accept that an occasional patient may present with oral manifestations of sideropenia without necessarily having anaemia. The minor fluctuations of haemoglobin through the day, as well as with technical variation, prompt us to suggest that there will be a host of individuals who would hover between being defined as 'sideropenic anaemia' and 'sideropenia sine anaemia' depending on their haemoglobin being 11·95 G and 12·05 G on two occasions.

There is no doubt that the activity of many iron-dependent enzymes in tissues are decreased in sideropenia (Cohen & Elvehjem 1934; Beutler 1957, 1959a,b,c; Gubler *et al* 1957; Beutler & Blaisdell 1958; Beutler *et al* 1960; Jacobs 1961, 1969; Dallman & Schwartz 1965; Srivastava *et al* 1965; Dallman *et al* 1967; Swarup *et al* 1967; Jaroshewsky *et al* 1970), although Dagg *et al* (1966) found no correlation between reduced cytochrome oxidase in buccal mucosa and the onset of symptoms. The initial stage of iron deficiency (latent deficiency) is represented by decreased tissue ferritin and then by a diminution of iron-containing enzymes. This process continues on to a reduction in serum iron with the iron saturation falling below 16% (sideropenia). Finally, clinical symptoms and signs become manifest.

Recently, an interesting issue has been raised suggesting that the oral manifestations found in patients with iron-deficiency anaemia should be attributed to a concurrent pyridoxine deficiency (Jacobs & Cavill 1968a). The pyridoxine status of the body, estimated as by erythrocyte glutamic pyruvate transaminase (i.e. an indicator of pyridoxine status), is often lowered in iron-deficiency anaemia (Cavill & Jacobs 1967; Jacobs & Cavill 1968b). The reason for this may be a poor diet lacking in pyridoxine as well as iron, or it may reflect an interference of intestinal absorption in sideropenia (Naiman *et al* 1964). However, we are not aware of any confirmation of these findings in oral mucosal lesions and *for the present purpose* we consider the oral changes occurring as due to iron deficiency. It should also be pointed out that the epithelial lesions of pyridoxine deficiency and iron deficiency though similar in some respects are not identical. This concept of a second deficiency having to occur concomitant with sideropenia before the muco-cutaneous manifestations appear may be an explanation for their variable occurrence. Other deficiencies which sometimes occur together with iron deficiency and which may produce similar tissue changes include zinc, cystine, folate, vitamin B_{12} and protein. Obviously, further work is required to answer the problem.

Cell-mediated immunity is significantly dimished in cases of sideropenia (Joyson *et al* 1972) and this may predispose to chronic infections. Higgs & Wells (1972) investigated the iron status of a group of patients with chronic muco-cutaneous candidiasis and showed that there was a decreased cell-mediated immune response which could be rectified by treating their iron deficiency. It is interesting to note that as long ago as 1928, Schmidt had demonstrated the need for iron in thymic function in mice: T-lymphocytes mediate the cellular immune response.

Iron deficiency precipitates a series of changes in a number of tissues including the muco-cutaneous integument. Koilonychia, maybe atrophy of the nasal mucosa (Bernat 1965; Barkve & Djupesland 1968) and pruritis vulvae (Wintrobe & Beebe 1933) occur. The skin may become pale and wrinkled once anaemia is present and pigmentary alterations may also be seen: the skin may become light brown in white races or depigmented in negroes (Wintrobe & Beebe 1933).

Changes in the oral mucosa are a fairly frequent feature of sideropenia, although not as common or as severe as in vitamin B_{12} deficiency. As has been stated above there is some confusion as to why the oral manifestations of iron deficiency do not appear more regularly or are more common in middle-aged or older people regardless of the degree of the deficiency.

Sideropenia causes a glossitis, angular cheilitis, stomatitis and ulceration of the mucosa (Witts 1931; Meulengracht 1932; Wintrobe & Beebe 1933; Waldenstrom 1938; Lundholm 1939; Darby 1946; Savilanti 1946; Cheli *et al* 1959; Baird *et al* 1961; Monto *et al* 1961; Beveridge *et al* 1965; Rose 1968; Jacobs 1969; Jaroshewsky *et al* 1970; Kalinin 1970).

The first change in the tongue is a burning sensation accompanied by a reddening at the tip and around the margins. The discomfort of iron deficiency does not approach the severity found in vitamin B_{12} or pyridoxine deficiencies. The dusky redness gradually spreads from the borders over the entire dorsum. Along with this the filiform papillae and then the fungiform papillae atrophy in a patchy or diffuse pattern leaving the anterior two-thirds of the dorsum fairly smooth. In more advanced cases the epithelium may lose the keratohyaline granules, become para-keratinized or non-keratinized, thin and eventually erode, leaving shallow ulcers which may become the seat of secondary fungal and bacterial infections. Small vesicles may also develop and on rupturing leave small ulcers similar to aphthae. Atrophic changes may also be seen in the underlying lingual musculature.

Less commonly the buccal mucosa undergoes comparable atrophic changes with a red eroded appearance. Vesicles have also been described on the buccal mucosa which similarly rupture and result in aphthae.

The histology of buccal mucosa in sideropenia is very similar to that found in vitamin B_{12} deficiency (Jacobs 1960), with the one main exception that in three cases of iron deficiency orthokeratosis was seen and in one of these there were also areas of parakeratosis. Savilanti (1946) described a case with leukoplakia on the buccal mucosa adjacent to the labial commissure. This increase in oral keratinization in sideropenia has also been seen in a cytological investigation (Jacobs 1959). Other than that, the buccal epithelium is often thinned, has a greater incidence of mitotic figures in prickle cells as well as binucleate prickle cells and a decrease in melanin, particularly where the pharynx was also involved. Lymphocytes and plasma cells were seen to be more frequent in the lamina propria. Histochemistry has shown alterations in the glycogen and sulphydryl content in oral mucosa of patients with iron deficiency (Jacobs 1961).

Angular cheilitis is another feature of sideropenia but is indistinguishable from that found in other deficiencies.

The pharyngeal and oesophageal mucosae are occasionally affected in iron deficiency and there is an increased incidence of carcinoma of oesophagus. This group with iron deficiency, dysphagia, a post-cricoid web and the increased tendency to develop carcinoma come under the classification of the Brown–Kelly–Patterson syndrome (Plummer–Vinson syndrome in U.S.A.) (see Chapter 7).

Exfoliative cytology of the oral cavity has revealed epithelial cells with a reduced cytoplasmic diameter and an increase in nuclear cytoplasmic ratio. No particular nuclear pattern was characteristic (Boddington

1959; Dabski 1960; Monto *et al* 1961). Jacobs (1959) found increased keratinization of buccal cells in Papanicolaou-stained smears.

The laboratory diagnosis of iron deficiency is based on the following measurements:

1 Decreased serum iron and increased transferrin, giving a saturation of less than 16% (Bainton & Finch 1964).
2 Increased erythrocyte protoporphyrins ($>$ 38 μg/100 ml RBC) (Dagg *et al* 1966).
3 Absence of stainable iron in the marrow.
4 Blood (as with vitamin B_{12} and folate deficiency these changes might follow the more direct estimations).
Low haemoglobin; MCV low.
Blood film—hypochromic microcytic erythrocytes.
5 Marrow: typical appearance of iron deficiency.

Zinc

Zinc is involved in many cellular metabolic activities both as an integral part of metallo-enzymes (e.g. alkaline phosphatase, carboxypeptidase, carbonic anhydrase, malate dehydrogenase, lactate dehydrogenase and glutamate dehydrogenase,) as well as functioning as a co-factor in a number of other enzyme systems (e.g. peptidases, enolase, arginase, carnosinase and oxalacetate decarboxylase). A number of these enzymes, as well as DNA polymerase and RNA polymerase, are decreased in zinc deficiency.

The presence of zinc in tissues was known of in the 19th century and was first ascribed a biochemical function in higher animals by Birckner (1919). Zinc deficiency has been shown to cause a scaly dermatitis, characterized by parakeratosis, in several agricultural animals (Tucker & Salmon 1955; Miller & Miller 1962; Ott *et al* 1964) and by hyperkeratosis along with foci of parakeratosis in rats (Follis *et al* 1941; Follis 1966). Although zinc deficiency has been reported to occur in humans (Prasad 1966) this does not appear to be associated with any mucosal disorders: Halsted *et al* (1972) noted flaking skin in a group of zinc-deficient individuals. Possibly this is due to the lesser degree of deficiency in humans compared to that produced in animals. However, morphological comparisons have been made between the cutaneous lesions of zinc deficiency in animals and psoriasis in humans. Zinc deficiency has also been shown to lead to defective collagen synthesis (Fernandez-Madrid *et al* 1971).

The oral mucosa in rats is sensitive to zinc deficiency, with the buccal mucosa in particular exhibiting the most striking changes (Follis *et al* 1941;

Alvares & Meyer 1968, 1973; Chen 1972; Alvares *et al* 1973). This was accompanied by a general thickening of the epithelium together with an increase in the rate of cell division. Changes reported in the upper cell layers of the buccal epithelium are increased cell dry weight, increased concentrations of ribosomes, mitochondria and endoplasmic reticulum (Osmanski & Meyer 1969). Chvapil *et al* (1972) demonstrated that zinc stabilized cellular membranes possibly by inhibiting peroxidation of membrane lipids.

Zinc deficiency has also been produced in monkeys (Macapinlac *et al* 1967a,b) and this was associated especially with changes in the tongue. The epithelium of the anterior of the dorsum was thickened, parakeratotic and exhibited nuclear hyperchromatism of the basal layer. The underlying muscle became atrophic.

Systematic therapy with zinc sulphate has been shown to promote wound healing in various sites (Pories *et al* 1966, 1967a,b; Husain 1969) including the gingivae of hamsters (Mesrobian and Shklar 1968). The reason for this apparently pharmacological effect in non-deficient subjects is obscure. Zinc is concentrated in healing tissues and this may indicate an increased demand for tissue production during healing. No studies appear to have been carried out on the use of zinc salts to accelerate healing of oral wounds in man.

The zinc status of the body may be estimated either by measuring plasma zinc of the zinc content of hair.

Magnesium

Magnesium functions as an activator for a number of enzymes and is necessary for oxidative phosphorylation.

Deficiency of magnesium has not been reported as a cause of mucocutaneous alterations in humans, but in dogs and rats an erythematous, desquamative dermatitis has been described (Kruse *et al* 1932; Orent *et al* 1932; Sullivan & Evans 1944). In a small group of magnesium-deficient rats Kruse *et al* (1932) noted that the gingivae became hypertrophic due to fibrous overgrowth: recession occurred and the molars became loose.

Copper

Copper, like iron, is a member of the transition group of elements and as such is involved in a number of redox enzyme systems. Copper metalloenzymes include cytochrome oxidase, dopamine-B-hydroxylase, monamine oxidase, tyrosinase and ascorbate oxidase.

Copper plays an important role in keratinization, probably aiding the formation of S—S cross-linkages. It is perhaps surprising that copper deficiency has not been associated with more muco-cutaneous disorders. Smith & Ellis (1947) reported depigmentation of the hair in copper-deficient rabbits together with an exfoliative dermatitis. No oral changes have been recorded.

Other trace elements

Many other trace elements are necessary for the general well-being of the animal but we are unaware of any literature discussing pathological changes of the oral mucosa in the deficient states. As with proteins, fats and vitamins, any change in one element is liable to precipitate a whole series of changes in serum and tissue concentrations of other elements and compounds. This in turn may confuse the exact mechanism whereby the deficiency is manifested clinically, and care must be exercised in separating primary from secondary effects.

5:4 References

AFONSKY D. (1955) Oral lesions in niacin, riboflavin, pyridoxine, pantothenic acid and folic acid deficient adult dogs. *Oral Surg.*, **8,** 206–212, 315–318, 438–440, 543–545, 656–658, 769–773 and 867–876.

ALLARA E. (1952) Sull influenza esercitata dagli ormoni sessauli sulla stuttura dell formazioni gustative di mus rattus albinus. *Riv. Biol.*, **44,** 209–229.

ALLINGTON H.V. (1950) Dryness of the mouth. *Arch. Derm. Syph.*, **62,** 829–850.

ALVARES O.F. & MEYER J. (1968) Regional differences in parakeratotic response to mild zinc deficiency. *Archs. Derm.* **98,** 191–201.

ALVARES O.F., MEYER J. & GERSON S.J. (1973) Activity and distribution of acid phosphatase in zinc-deficient parakeratotic rat buccal epithelium. *Scand. J. dent. Res.*, **81,** 481–488.

ALVARES O.F. & MEYER J. (1973) Thymidine uptake and cell migration in cheek epithelium of zinc-deficient rats. *J. oral Path.*, **2,** 86–94.

ARKÖVY J. (1915) Ueber Gingivitis gravidarum und Gingivitis periodica (dysmenorrhoica). *Öst.-ung. Vrtljschr. Zahnh.*, **31,** 197–203.

ARROYAVE G., VITERI F., BEHAR M. & SERUMSHAW N.S. (1959) Impairment of intestinal absorption of vitamin A palmitate in severe protein malnutrition (Kwashiorkor). *Am. J. Clin. Nutrit.*, **7,** 185–190.

BAINTON D.F. & FINCH C.A. (1964) The diagnosis of iron deficiency anaemia. *Am. J. Med.*, **37,** 62–70.

BAIRD I.McL., DODGE O.G., PALMER F.J. & WAWMAN R.J. (1961) The tongue and oesophagus in iron deficiency anaemia and the effect of iron therapy. *J. clin. Pathol.*, **14**, 603–609.

BAKER S.J., IGNATIUS M., JOHNSON S. & VAISH, S.K. (1963) Hyperpigmentation of skin. A sign of vitamin B_{12} deficiency. *Brit. med. J.*, **1**, 1713–1715.

BANKS S.O. (1945) Diabetes and its oral manifestations: a medico-dental problem. *Bull. Nat. Dent. Ass.*, **4**, 7–10.

BARACH J.H. (1949) Symposium on diabetes mellitus; arteriosclerosis and diabetes. *Am. J. Med.*, **7**, 617–624.

BARCLAY (no initials) (1851) Death from anaemia. *Med. Times Gaz.*, Vol. **23** (old series) or Vol. **2** (new series), 480–482.

BARDIK Y.V. (1969) Effect of growth hormone on duration of individual periods of the mitotic cycle in stratum basale cells of the rat esophageal epithelium. *Bull. exp. Biol., Med.*, **68**, 1290–1292.

BARKVE H. & DJUPESLAND G. (1968) Ozaena and iron deficiency. *Brit. med. J.*, **2**, 336–337.

BARONE J.V. (1965) Nutrition of edentulous patients. *J. Prosth. Dent.*, **15**, 804–809.

BARTLEY W., KREBS H.A. & O'BRIEN J.R.P. (1953) Vitamin C requirements of human adults. *Med. Res. Council Brit. Spec. Rept. Ser.* No. 280, 179 pp.

BAUME L.J., FRANQUIN J.C. & KÖRNER W.F. (1970) Some histological and histochemical observations in the oral epithelium of vitamin A deficient rats and rats receiving high doses of vitamin A. *Int. J. Vitamin Res.*, **40**, 471–482.

BEAN W.B. & HODGES R.E. (1954) Pantothenic acid deficiency induced in human subjects. *Proc. Soc. exp. Biol. Med.*, **86**, 693–698.

BEER P. (1962) Untersuchungen über die wirkung der Vitamin A-Säure. *Dermatologica*, **124**, 192–195.

BELAVADY B., MADHAVAN T.V. & GOPALAN C. (1967) Production of nicotinic acid deficiency (blacktongue) in pups fed diets supplemented with leucine. *Gastroenterology*, **53**, 749–753.

BENVENISTE R., BIXLER D. & CONNEALLY P.M. (1967) Periodontal disease in diabetics. *J. Periodont.*, **38**, 271–279.

BERGSTRÖM S. (1964) The enzymatic conversion of essential fatty acids into prostaglandins. *J. Biol. Chem.*, **239**, PC4006–4008.

BERN H.A., ELIAS J.J. & PICKETT P.B. (1955) The influence of vitamin A on the epidermis. *Am. J. Anat.*, **96**, 419–448.

BERNAT I. (1965) In *Ozaena: A Manifestation of Iron Deficiency*. Pergamon Press, Oxford.

BEUTLER E. (1957) Iron enzymes in iron deficiency. I. Cytochrome C. *Am. J. med. Sci.*, **234**, 517–527.

BEUTLER E. (1959a) Iron enzymes in iron deficiency states. *Illinois med. J.*, **116**, 16–19.

BEUTLER, E. (1959b) Iron enzymes in iron deficiency. IV. Cytochrome oxidase in rat kidney and heart. *Acta Haematol.*, **21**, 371–377.

BEUTLER E. (1959c) Iron enzymes in iron deficiency. VI. Aconitase activity and citrate metabolism. *J. clin. Invest.*, **38**, 1605–1616.

BEUTLER E. & BLAISDELL R.K. (1958) Iron enzymes in iron deficiency. III. Catalase in rat red cells and liver with some further observations on cytochrome C. *J. Lab.clin. Med.*, **52**, 694–699.

BEUTLER E., LARSH S. & TANZI F. (1960) Iron enzymes in iron deficiency. VII. Oxygen consumption measurements in iron deficient subjects. *Am. J. med. Sci.*, **239**, 759–765.

BEVERIDGE B.R., BANNERMAN R.M., EVANSON J.M. & WITTS L.B. (1965) Hypochromic anaemia. A retrospective study and follow-up of 378 in-patients. *Quart. J. Med.*, **34**, 145–161.

BIRCKNER V. (1919) The zinc content of some food products. *J. biol. Chem.*, **38**, 191–203.

BISHOP P.M.F., HARRIS P.W.R. & TRAFFORD J.A.P. (1967) Oestrogen treatment of recurrent aphthous mouth ulcers. *Lancet*, **1**, 1345–1347.

BOAS M.A. (1927) The effect of desiccation upon the nutritive properties of eggwhite. *Biochem. J.*, **21**, 712–724.

BODDINGTON M.M. (1959) Changes in buccal cells in the anaemias. *J. clin. Path.*, **12**, 222–227.

BODDINGTON M.M. & SPRIGGS A.I. (1959) The epithelial cells in megaloblastic anemias. *J. clin. Path.*, **12**, 228–234.

BODEY G.P. (1971a) Oral complications of the myeloproliferative diseases. *Postgrad. Med.*, **69**, 115–121.

BODEY G.P. (1971b) In *Oncology*, Vol. III, 446. Year Book Medical Publishers Inc., Chicago.

BOEN S.T. (1957) Changes in the nuclei of squamous epithelial cells in pernicious anaemia. *Acta med. Scand.*, **159**, 425–431.

BOEN S.T., MOLHUYSEN J.A. & STEENBERGEN J. (1958) Nuclear changes in oral epithelial cells in subacute combined degeneration of the spinal cord due to vitamin-B_{12} deficiency. *Lancet*, **2**, 294–296.

BOGGS D.R., WINTROBE M.M. & CARTWRIGHT G.E. (1962) The acute leukemias. *Medicine*, **41**, 163–225.

BOLLET A.J. & OWENS S. (1973) Evaluation of nutritional status of selected hospitalized patients. *Am. J. Clin. Nutrit.*, **26**, 931–938.

BORSON H.J. & METTIER S.R. (1940) Relief of hypochromic anemia in dogs with synthetic vitamin B_6: Influence of 'filtrate' factors. *Proc. Soc. exp. Biol. Med.*, **43**, 429–432.

BOVINA C., LANDI L., PASQUALI P. & MARCHETTI M. (1969) Biosynthesis of folate coenzymes in riboflavin deficient rats. *J. Nutrit.*, **99**, 320–324.

BRADFIELD R.B., JELLIFFE E.F.P. & JELLIFFE D.M. (1972) Assessment of marginal malnutrition. *Nature, Lond.*, **235**, 112.

BRODY H.A., PRENDERGAST J.J. & SILVERMAN S. (1971) The relationship between oral symptoms, insulin release, and glucose intolerance. *Oral Surg.*, **31**, 777–782.

BROWN A. (1946) Pernicious anaemia; a clinical study of 78 cases. *Glasgow med. J.*, **27**, 313–344.

BROWN A. (1949a) Glossitis in Addisonian pernicious anaemia. Effect of synthetic vitamins of the B group. *Brit. med. J.*, **1**, 704–706.

BROWN A. (1949b) Steatorrhoea and glossitis after ileocolostomy; effect of synthetic vitamins of B complex, autolysed yeast, and liver extracts. *Brit. med. J.*, **1**, 1073–1076.

BROWN A. (1949c) Steatorrhoea and glossitis after ileocolostomy; effect of synthetic vitamins of B complex, autolysed yeast and liver extract. *Brit. med. J.*, **1**, 197–215.
BUCKMAN N. (1957) Oral manifestations of cretinism. *Oral Surg.*, **10**, 938–947.
BULLOUGH W.S. (1949) Epidermal mitotic activity in the adult female mouse. *J. Endocrinol.*, **6**, 340–349.
BURKETT L.W. (1944) A histopathologic explanation for the oral lesions in acute leukemia. *Am. J. Orthodont.*, **30**, 516–523.
BURR G.O. & BURR M.M. (1929) A new deficiency disease produced by the rigid exclusion of fat from the diet. *J. biol. Chem.*, **82**, 345–367.
BUTTERWORTH C.E. & PEREZ-SANTIAGO E. (1957) Pathologic changes in jejunal biopsies from sprue patients. *Am. J. Diag. Dis.*, **2**, 659–662.
CALDWELL M.D., JONSSON H.T. & OTHERSEN H.B. (1972) Essential fatty acid deficiency in an infant receiving prolonged parenteral alimentation. *J. Pediat.*, **81**, 894–898.
CARRUTHERS R. (1967a) Oral ulcers. *Austr. dent. J.*, **12**, 279.
CARRUTHERS R. (1967b) Recurrent aphthous ulcers. *Lancet*, **2**, 259.
CASTOR C.W. (1965) The effects of chronic glucocorticoid excess on human connective tissue cells in vitro. *J. Lab. clin. Med.*, **65**, 490–499.
CASTOR C.W. & BAKER B.L. (1950) Local action of adrenocortical steroids on epidermis and connective tissue of skin. *Endocrinology*, **47**, 234–241.
CAVALARIS C.J. & KRIKOS G.A. (1967) Vitamin A produced mucous metaplasia. *J. Oral Therapeut. Pharmacol.*, **3**, 452–461.
CAVILL I.A.J. & JACOBS A. (1967) Erythrocyte transaminase activity in iron deficiency anaemia. *Scand. J. Haematol.*, **4**, 249–256.
CHANARIN I. (1969) In *The Megaloblastic Anaemias*. Blackwell Scientific Publications, Oxford.
CHAUDRY A.P. & GORLIN R.J. (1962) Unusual oral manifestations of chronic lymphatic leukemia. *Oral Surg.*, **15**, 446–449.
CHELI R., DODERO M., CELLE G. & VASSALOTTI M. (1959) Gastric biopsy and secretory findings in hypochomic anaemias. *Acta Haemat.*, **22**, 1–11.
CHEN, S-Y. (1972) Changes in fine structure and histochemical aspects of the nucleus in the buccal epithelium of the zinc deficient rat. Ph.D. Thesis, Univ. of Illinois, Chicago.
CHENEY M., SABRY Z.I. & BEATON G.H. (1965) Erythrocyte glutamic-pyruvic transaminase activity in man. *Am. J. Clin. Nutrit.*, **16**, 337–338.
CHERASKIN E. & RINGSDORF W.M. (1965) Gingival state and carbohydrate metabolism. *J. dent. Res.*, **44**, 480–486.
CHICK H. (1951) The causation of pellagra. *Nutrit. Abst. Rev.*, **20**, 523–535.
CHILGREN R.A., MEUWISSEN H.J., QUIE P.G. & HONG R. (1969) The cellular immune effect in chronic mucocutaneous candidiasis. *Lancet*, **1**, 1286–1288.
CHINN H., BRODY H., SILVERMAN S. & DI RAIMONDO V. (1966) Glucose tolerance in patients with oral symptoms. *J. Oral Therapeut. Pharmacol.*, **2**, 261–269.
CHRISTOPHERS E. & BRAUN-FALCO O. (1970) Mechanisms of parakeratosis. *Brit. J. Derm.*, **82**, 268–275.
CHVAPIL M. RYAN J.N, & ZUKOSKI C.F.. (1972) Effect of zinc on lipid peroxidation in liver microsomes. *Proc..Soc. exp. Biol. Med.*, **141**, 150–153.

COHEN D.W., FRIEDMAN L.A., SHAPIRO J., KYLE G.C. & FRANKLIN S. (1970) Diabetes mellitus and periodontal disease: two-year longitudinal observations. *J. Periodont.*, **41**, 49/709-52/712.
COHEN D.W., FRIEDMAN J., SHAPIRO J. & KYLE G.C. (1969) A longitudinal investigation of the periodontal changes during pregnancy. *J. Periodont.*, **40**, 563-570.
COHEN E. & ELVEHJEM C.A. (1934) The relation of iron and copper to the cytochrome oxidase content of animal tissues. *J. biol. Chem.*, **107**, 97-105.
COHEN M.M., SHKLAR G. & YERGANIAN G. (1963) Pulpal and periodontal disease in Chinese hamsters with hereditary diabetes mellitus. *Oral Surg.*, **16**, 104-112.
COLLINGS C.K. & DUKES C.D. (1952) Recurrent herpetic stomatitis treated by intradermal injections of influenza A and B virus vaccine. *J. Periodont.*, **23**, 48-52.
CONIGLIO J.G. (1972) Essential fatty acids. *Fed. Proc.*, **31**, 1429.
COUPLAND S. (1881) Gulstonian lectures on anaemia. *Lancet*, **1**, 445-447, 491-495, 531-535, 611-613, 689-692.
COX E.V. (1962) The clinical manifestations of vitamin B_{12} deficiency in Addisonian pernicious anaemia. In HEINRICH H.C. *Vitamin B_{12} and Intrinsic Factor*, 590. Ferdinand Enke Verlag, Stuttgart.
CRAIG J.M., SCHIFF L.H. & BOONE J.E. (1955) Chronic moniliasis associated with Addison's disease. *Am. J. Dis. Child.*, **89**, 669-684.
CROSBY W.H. (1960) The daily dose of folic acid. *J. Chron. Dis.*, **12**, 583-585.
CURTIS A.B. (1971) Childhood leukemias: initial oral manifestations. *J. Am. dent. Assoc.*, **83**, 159-164.
DABSKI H. (1960) Zmiany morfologiczne nablonka jamy ustnej w przebiegu niedokrwistosci Addisona-Biermera niedokrwistosc istotnej niedobarwliwej. *Polski tygodn. lek.*, **15**, 942-945 (abstracted in *Blood*, **16**, 1659).
DAGG J.H., GOLDBERG A., GIBBS N. & ANDERSON J.R. (1960) Detection of latent pernicious anaemia in iron-deficiency anaemia. *Brit. med. J.*, **2**, 619-621.
DAGG J.H., JACKSON J.M., CURRY B. & GOLDBERG A. (1966) Cytochrome oxidase in latent iron deficiency (sideropenia). *Brit. J. Haemat.*, **12**, 331-333.
DALGLEISH C.E. (1955) Metabolism of the aromatic amino acids. *Advances in Protein Chemistry*, **10**, 31-150.
DALLMAN P.R. & SCHWARTZ H.C. (1965) Myoglobin and cytochrome response during repair of iron deficiency in the rat. *J. clin. Invest.*, **44**, 1631-1638.
DALLMAN P.R., SUNSHINE P., & LEONARD Y. (1967) Intestinal cytochrome response with repair of iron deficiency. *Pediatrics*, **39**, 863-870.
DARBY W.J. (1946) Oral manifestations of iron deficiency. *J. Am. med. Ass.*, **130**, 830-835.
DAS A.K., BHOWMICK S. & DUTTA A. (1971) Oral contraceptives and periodontal disease. *J. Ind. dent. Ass.*, **47**-53, 61-66, 155-158.
DAY P.L., LANGSTON W.C. & DARBY W.J. (1938) Failure of nicotinic acid to prevent nutritional cytopenia in the monkey. *Proc. Soc. exp. Biol. Med.*, **38**, 860-863.
DEASY M.J., GROTA L.J. & KENNEDY J.E. (1972) The effect of estrogen, progesterone and cortisol on gingival inflammation. *J. periodont. Res.*, **7**, 111-124.
DEELEY R.A. (1965) The effect of protein versus placebo supplementation upon denture tolerance. *J. Prosth. Dent.*, **15**, 65-72.

DE GRUCHY G.C. (1973) In *Clinical Haematology in Medical Practice*, 3rd edition, 367. Blackwell Scientific Publications, Oxford.
DENTON J. (1925) The pathology of pellagra. *Am. J. trop. Med.*, **5,** 173-210.
DENTON J. (1928) A study of the tissue changes in experimental black tongue of dogs compared with similar changes in pellagra. *Am. J. Path.*, **4,** 341-351.
DEUEL H.J., MARTIN C.R. & ALFIN-SLATER R.B. (1954) The effect of fat level of the diet on general nutrition. *J. Nutrit.*, **54,** 193-199.
DINGLE J.T. & LUCY J.L. (1965) Vitamin A, carotenoids and cell function. *Biol. Rev.*, **40,** 422-461.
DOLBY A.E. (1968) Recurrent Mikulicz's oral aphthae. *Brit. dent. J.*, **124,** 359-360.
DOO B.S. (1971) Histochemical study on the oral mucosa of folic acid administered rats. *J. Korean dent. Ass.*, **9,** 235-239.
DOWLING J.E. & WALD G. (1958) Vitamin A deficiency and night blindness. *Proc. nat. Acad. Sci. U.S.*, **44,** 648-661.
DREIFUSS, W. (1924) Die pathologisch-histologischen Befunde im oberen Verdauungskanal bei pernizioser Anämie. *Virch. Arch. Path. Anal. Phys.*, **251,** 44-55.
DREIZEN S., STONE R.E. & SPIES T.D. (1958) Oral manifestations of nutritional disorders. *Dent. Clin. N. Am.*, 429-440.
DREIZEN S. & LEVY B.M. (1969) Histopathology of experimentally induced nutritional deficiency cheilosis in the marmoset (Callithrix Jacchus). *Archs. oral Biol.*, **14,** 577-582.
DREIZEN S., LEVY B.M. and BERNICK S. (1970) Studies on the biology of the periodontium of marmosets: VIII. The effect of folic acid deficiency on the marmoset oral mucosa. *J. dent. Res.*, **49,** 616-620.
DREIZEN S. (1971) Oral indications of the deficiency states. *Postgrad. Med.*, **49,** 97-102.
DRISCOLL E.J., SHIP I.I., BARON S., STANLEY H.R. & UTZ J.P. (1959) Chronic aphthous stomatitis, herpes labialis and related conditions. *Ann. intern. Med.*, **50,** 1474-1496.
DUFFY J.H. & DRISCOLL E.S. (1958) Oral manifestations of leukemia. *Oral Surg.*, **11,** 484-490.
EL ATTAR T.M.A. & HUGOSON A. (1974) The in vitro conversion of female sex steroid, estrone, in normal and inflamed gingiva. *Archs. oral Biol.*, **19,** 425-430.
EL ATTAR T.M.A., ROTH G.D. & HUGOSON A. (1973) Comparative metabolism of 4-^{14}C-progesterone in normal and chronically inflamed human gingival tissue. *J. periodont. Res.*, **8,** 79-85.
EL-SHOBAKI F.A., EL-HAWARY M.F.S., MORCOS S.R., ABDELKHALEK M.K., EL-ZAHWAHRY K. & SAKR R. (1972) Iron metabolism in Egyptian infants with protein-calorie deficiency. *Brit. J. Nutr.*, **28,** 81-89.
ELVEHJEM C.A. (1940) Relation of nicotinic acid to pellagra. *Physiol. Rev.*, **20,** 249-271.
ELVEHJEM C.A. (1944) Symposium on human vitamin requirements; introduction. *Fed. Proc.*, **3,** 158-159.
FARRANT P.C. (1958) Nuclear changes in oral epithelium in pernicious anaemia. *Lancet*, **1,** 830-831.
FARRANT P.C. (1960) Nuclear changes in squamous cells from buccal mucosa in pernicious anaemia. *Brit. med. J.*, **1,** 1694-1697.

FELL H.A. & MELLANBY E. (1953) Metaplasia produced in cultures of chick ectoderm by high vitamin A. *J. Physiol.*, **119**, 470–488.
FELL H.A. & DINGLE J.T. (1963) Studies on the mode of action of excess vitamin A. Lysosomal protease and the degradation of cartilage matrix. *Biochem. J.*, **87**, 403–408.
FERGUSON M.M. & DAGG J.H. (1974) Oral ulceration due to ascorbic acid deficiency. *Lancet*, **1**, 164.
FERNANDEX-MADRID F., PRASAD A.S. & OBERLEAS D. (1971) Effect of zinc deficiency on collagen metabolism. *J. Lab. clin. Med.*, **78**, 853.
FIDANZA A. (1971) Le azioni fisiologiche dell' acido pantotenico. *Acta Vitamin Enzymol.*, **25**, 135–144.
FIELD H., PARNALL C. & ROBINSON W.D. (1940) Pellagra in the average population of the northern states. *New Engl. J. Med.*, **223**, 307–315.
FINDLAY G.M. & STERN R.O. (1929) A syndrome in the rat resembling pink disease in man. *Arch. Dis. Childh.*, **4**, 1–11.
FINESTONE A.J. & BOORUJY S.R. (1967) Diabetes mellitus and periodontal disease. *Diabetes*, **16**, 336–340.
FOLLIS R.H., DAY H.G. & MCCOLLUM E.V. (1941) Histological studies of the tissues of rats fed a diet extremely low in zinc. *J. Nutrit.*, **22**, 223–236.
FOLLIS R.H. (1966) The pathology of zinc deficiency. In PRASAD A.S. *Zinc Metabolism*. Chap. 7. Charles C. Thomas, Springfield, Illinois.
FORMICOLA A.J., WEATHERFORD T. & GRUPE H. (1970) The uptake of H^3-estradiol by the oral tissues of rats. *J. periodont. Res.*, **5**, 269–275.
FOROOZAN P. & TRIER J.S. (1967) Mucosa of the small intestine in pernicious anaemia. *New Engl. J. Med.*, **277**, 553–559.
FOSS C.L., GRUPE H.E. & ORBAN B. (1953) Gingivosis. *J. Periodont.*, **24**, 207–219.
FOY H., KONDI A. & MBAYA V. (1966) Serum vitamin B_{12} and folate levels in normal and riboflavin deficient baboons. *Brit. J. Haematol.*, **12**, 239–245.
FRANQUIN J.C., KÖRNER W.F., WEISER H. & BAUME L.J. (1969) L'épithélium de rat blanc soumis à une carence en vitamine A et à une hypervitaminose A. *Rev. mens. Suisse Odonto-stomat.*, **79**, 926–942.
FRANQUIN J.C., BAUME L.J. & KÖRNER W.F. (1970) Influence of vitamin A on the distribution of succinic dehydrogenase in oral epithelium of the white rat. *J. Periodont.*, **41**, 639–643.
FRANQUIN J.C., BAUME L.J. & KÖRNER W.F. (1971) La phosphatase acide dans l'épithélium de la muqueuse alvéolaire du rat soumis à une carence et à un excès de vitamin A. *Schweiz. Monat Zahlheilkinde*, **81**, 363–371.
FRIETAG V., RINDT W. & VOLZ-KINZLER U. (1971) Über die Wirkung von Ovulationshemmern auf rezidivierende Aphthen der Mundschleimhaut. *Dtsch. Zahnärztl., Z.*, **26**, 826–829.
GARDNER F.H. (1956) Observations on the cytology of gastric epithelium in tropical sprue. *J. Lab. clin. Med.*, **47**, 529–539.
GARDNER F.H. (1958) Tropical sprue. *New Engl. J. Med.*, **258**, 791–796, 835–842.
GEIGER E. (1947) Experiments with delayed supplementation of incomplete amino acid mixtures. *J. Nutrit.*, **34**, 91–111.
GERSH I. & CATCHPOLE H.R. (1960) The nature of ground substance of connective tissue. *Perspect. Biol. Med.*, **3**, 282–319.

GILLMAN T. (1970) In CHAMPION R.H., GILLMAN T., ROOK A.J. & SIMS R.T. *An Introduction to the Biology of the Skin*, Chap. 23. F.A. Davis Co., Philadelphia.

GINTER E., ONDREICKA R., BOBEK P. & SIMKO V. (1969) The influence of chronic vitamin C deficiency on fatty acid composition of blood serum, liver triglycerides and cholesterol esters in guinea pigs. *J. Nutrit.*, **99**, 261–266.

GLICKMAN I. & SMULOW J.B. (1964) Chronic desquamative gingivitis—its nature and treatment. *J. Periodont.*, **35**, 31/397–39/405.

GOLDSMITH G.A., GIBBENS J., UNGLAUB W.G. & MILLER O.N. (1956) Studies on niacin requirement in man. III. Comparative effects of diets containing lime-treated and untreated corn in the production of experimental pellagra. *Am. J. Clin. Nutrit.*, **4**, 151–160.

GORLIN R.J. & CHAUDRY A.P. (1960) The oral manifestations of cyclic (periodic) neutropenia. *Archs Derm.*, **82**, 344–348.

GRAHAM R.M. & RHEAULT M.H. (1954) Characteristic cellular changes in epithelial cells in pernicious anaemia. *J. Lab. clin. Med.*, **43**, 235–245.

GREENBERG M.S., BRIGHTMAN V.I., LYNCH M.A. & SHIP I.I. (1969) Idiopathic hypoparathyroidism, chronic candidiasis, and dental hypoplasia. *Oral Surg.*, **28**, 42–53.

GROSS P. (1940) Role of unsaturated fatty acids in acrodynia (vitamin B_6 deficiency) of the rat. *J. invest. Dermat.*, **3**, 505–522.

GUBLER C.J., CARTWRIGHT G.E. & WINTROBE M.M. (1957) Studies on copper metabolism. IX. Enzyme activities and iron metabolism in copper and iron deficiencies. *J. biol. Chem.*, **224**, 533–546.

GÜNTHER S. (1972a) Vitamin A acid in treatment of oral lichen planus. *Archs Derm.*, **106**, 854–857.

GÜNTHER S. (1972b) Topical administration of vitamin A acid in palmar keratoses; callosities, hyperkeratotic eczema, hypertrophic lichen planus, pityriasis rubra pilaris. *Dermatologica*, **145**, 344–347.

GYÖRGY P. (1931) Rachitis und andere Avitaminosen. *Ztschr. f. Ärzt. Fortbild*, **28**, 377, 417.

GYÖRGY P., SULLIVAN M. & KARSNER H.T. (1937) Nutritional dermatoses in rats. *Proc. Soc. exp. Biol. Med.*, **37**, 313–315.

GYÖRGY P. (1941) Dietary treatment of scaly desquamative dermatoses of the seborrheic type. *Arch. Derm. Syph.*, **43**, 230–247.

HAIM G. (1966) Elektronmikroskopische Untersuchungen der Schwangerschaftsveränderungen an der Gingiva. *Les Paradontopathies*, **18**, 197–204.

HALSTED J.A., RONAGHY H.A., ABADI P., HAGHSHENASS M., AMIRHAKEMI G.H., BARAKAT R.M. & REINHOLD J.G. (1972) Zinc deficiency in man. The Shiraz experiment. *Am. J. Med.*, **53**, 277–284.

HANSEN A.E. & WIESE H.F. (1943) Studies with dogs maintained on diets low in fat. *Proc. Soc. exp. Biol. Med.*, **52**, 205–208.

HANSEN A.E. & BURR G.O. (1946) Essential fatty acids and human nutrition. *J. Am. med. Ass.*, **132**, 855–859.

HANSEN A.E., WIESE H.F., BOELSCHE A.N., HAGGARD M.E., ADAM D.J.D. & DAVIS H. (1963) Role of linoleic acid in infant nutrition. *Pediatrics*, **31**, 171–192.

HARRIS I.W. & HORRIGAN D.L. (1964) Pyridoxine responsive anemia—prototype and variations as the theme. *Vitamins Hormones*, **22**, 721–753.

HAUSEMAN J.E. (1970) Toxische Schleimbautveränder ungen bei zytostatischer Therapie. *Dtsch. Zahnärztl. Z.*, **25**, 999–1004.

HAYES K.C., MCCOMBS H.L. & FAHERTY T.P. (1970) The fine structure of vitamin A deficiency. I. Parotid duct metaplasia. *Lab. Invest.*, **22**, 81–89.

HEISS H.B. & GROSS P.B. (1970) Keratosis palmaris et plantaris treatment with topically applied vitamin A acid. *Arch. Derm.*, **101**, 100–103.

HEISS J. & GRASSER H. (1968) Haben Ovulationshemmer Einfluss auf Gingiva und Paradontium? Zytologische, histologische und klinische Untersuchungen. *Dtsch. Zahnärztl. Z.*, **23**, 344–353.

HERMANS P.E., ULRICH J.A. & MARKOWITZ H. (1969) Chronic mucocutaneous candidiasis as a surface expression of deep-seated abnormalities. *Am. J. Med.*, **47**, 503–519.

HERSH E.M., BODEY G.P., NIES B.A. & FREIREICH E.J. (1965) Causes of death in acute leukaemia, a ten year study of 414 patients from 1954–1963. *J. Am. Med. Ass.*, **193**, 105–9.

HICKS R.M. (1969) Nature of the keratohyalin-like granules in hyperplastic and cornified areas of transitional epithelium in vitamin A-deficient rat. *J. Anat.*, **104**, 327–339.

HIGGS J.M. & WELLS R.S. (1972) Chronic muco-cutaneous candidiasis; associated abnormalities of iron metabolism. *Brit. J. Derm.*, **86**, Suppl. 8, 88–102.

HILMING F. (1952) Gingivitis gravidarum. *Oral Surg.*, **5**, 734–751.

HIRSCH E.O. & DAMESHEK W. (1951) Thrombocytopenic purprua due to allergy to quinidine; study of mechanism of thrombocytopenia. *Am. J. Med.*, **9**, 828–833.

HJØRTING-HANSEN E. & BERTRAM U. (1968) Oral aspects of pernicious anaemia. *Brit. dent. J.*, **125**, 266–270.

HODGES R.E., HOOD J., CANHAM J.E., SAUBERLICH H.E. & BAKER E.M. (1970) Clinical manifestations of ascorbic acid deficiency in man. *Am. J. Clin. Nutrit.*, **24**, 432–443.

HOLM-PEDERSEN P. & LÖE H. (1967) Flow of gingival exudate as related to menstruation and pregnancy. *J. periodont. Res.*, **2**, 13–20.

HOOD J., BURNS C.A. & HODGES R.E. (1970) Sjögren's syndrome in scurvy. *New Engl. J. Med.*, **282**, 1120–1124.

HOVE K.A. & STALLARD R.E. (1970) Diabetes and the periodontal patient. *J. Periodont.*, **41**, 53/713–58/718.

HUGOSON A. (1970) Gingival inflammation and female sex hormones. *J. periodont. Res.*, Suppl. **5**, 1–18.

HUGOSON A. (1971) Gingivitis in pregnant women. A longitudinal clinical study. *Odont. Revy.*, **22**, 65–84.

HUGOSON A., WINBERG E. & ÅNGSTRÖM T. (1971) Cytologic findings in vaginal and oral smears from pregnant women. *Odont. Revy.*, **22**, 145–153.

HUNTER W. (1900) Further observations on pernicious anaemia (seven cases): a chronic infective disease. *Lancet*, **1**, 221–224, 296–299, 371–377.

HUNTER W. (1909) In *Severest Anaemias*. Macmillan & Co., London.

HUSAIN S.L. (1969) Oral zinc sulphate in leg ulcers. *Lancet*, **1**, 1069–1071.

IQBAL M. & WYNN C.H. (1970) A comparative study of rat liver, spleen and skin lysosomes. *Enzym. Biol. Clin.*, **11**, 360–368.

IQBAL M. & GERSON S.J. (1971) In SQUIER C.A. & MEYER J. *Current Concepts of the Histology of Oral Mucosa*, Chap. 2, 34. Charles C. Thomas, Springfield, Illinois.
IRVINE V.J., STEWART A.G. & SCARTH L. (1967) A clinical and immunological study of adrenocortical insufficiency (Addison's disease). *Clin. exp. Immunol.*, **2**, 31–69.
IZAK G., RACHMILEWITZ M., ZAN S. & GROSSOWICZ N. (1963) The effect of small doses of folic acid in nutritional megaloblastic anemia. *Am. J. clin. Nutrit.*, **13**, 369–377.
JACOBS A. (1959) Atypical pernicious anaemia. *Postgrad. med. J.*, **35**, 524–525.
JACOBS A. (1960) The buccal mucosa in anaemia. *J. clin. Path.*, **13**, 463–468.
JACOBS A. (1961a) Iron containing enzymes in the buccal epithelium. *Lancet*, **2**, 1331–1333.
JACOBS A. (1961b) Carbohydrates and sulphur-containing compounds in the anaemic buccal epithelium. *J. clin. Path.*, **14**, 610–614.
JACOBS A. (1963) Epithelial changes in anaemic East Africans. *Brit. med. J.*, **1**, 1711–1712.
JACOBS A. (1969a) Tissue changes in iron deficiency. *Brit. J. Haemat.*, **16**, 1–4.
JACOBS A. (1969b) Iron deficiency and the oral mucous membrane. *Brit. J. Derm.*, **81**, 861–862.
JACOBS A. & CAVILL I.A.J. (1968a) The oral lesions of iron deficiency anaemia: pyridoxine and riboflavin status. *Brit. J. Haemat.*, **14**, 291–295.
JACOBS A. & CAVILL I.A.J. (1968b) Pyridoxine and riboflavin status in the Paterson–Kelly syndrome. *Brit. J. Haemat.*, **14**, 153–160.
JACOBSON J.H. (1961) In LYLE D.J. *Clinical Electroretinography*. Charles C. Thomas, Springfield, Illinois.
JAROSHEWSKY A.J., PETROV, V.N., SHCHERBA M.M., KALININ V.I. & MIHAILOVA E.N. (1970) Diagnosis and prophylaxis of iron deficiency in donors. *Haematologia*, **4**, 184–185.
JENSEN H., HJØRTING-HANSEN E. & KJERULF K. (1965) Tongue biopsies in various clinical conditions. *Acta med. Scand.*, **178**, 651–662.
JENSEN H., KJERULF K. & HJØRTING-HANSEN E. (1967) Histochemical examinations in mucosal tongue atrophy. *Acta med. Scand.*, **181**, 281–290.
JOHNSON B.C. (1957) In HEINRICH H.C. *Vitamin B_{12} and Intrinsic Factor*. Ferdinand Enke Verlag, Stuttgart.
JOLLY M. (1967) Vitamin A deficiency; a review. *J. Oral Therapeut. Pharmacol.*, **3**, 364–386.
JONEK J., KONECKI J. & JONEK T. (1970) Effects of estrogens upon the mitotic cycle and DNA synthesis in buccal epithelial cells of castrated mice. *Polish med. J.*, **9**, 1532–1539.
JONES E.H., ARMSTRONG T.G., GREEN H.F. & CHADWICK V. (1944) Stomatitis due to riboflavin deficiency. *Lancet*, **1**, 720–723.
JONSSON G.E. & ÅNGGÅRD E. (1972) Biosynthesis and metabolism of Prostaglandin E_2 in human skin. *Scand. J. Clin. Lab. Invest.*, **29**, 289–296.
JOYNSON D.H.M., JACOBS A., WALKER D.M. & DOLBY A.E. (1972) Defect of cell-mediated immunity in patients with iron-deficiency anaemia. *Lancet*, **2**, 1058–1059.

KALININ V.I. (1970) Tissues of the oral cavity in hypoferric anemia. *Stomatologia (Moscow)*, **49,** 20–22.
KARRING T. & LÖE H. (1973) The effect of age on mitotic activity in rat oral epithelium. *J. periodont. Res.*, **8,** 164–170.
KAUFMAN A.Y. (1969) An oral contraceptive as an etiologic factor in producing hyperplastic gingivitis and a neoplasm of the pregnancy tumor type. *Oral Surg.*, **28,** 666–670.
KELSAY J., BAYSAL A. & LINKSWILER H. (1968) Effect of vitamin B_6 depletion on the pyridoxal, pyridoxamine and pyridoxine content of the blood and urine of men. *J. Nutrit.*, **94,** 490–494.
KELSAY J. (1969) A compendium of Nutritional Status Studies and dietary evaluation studies conducted in the United States, 1958–1967. *J. Nutrit.*, **99,** 119–166.
KENNY F.M. & HOLLIDAY M.A. (1964) Hypoparathyroidism, moniliasis, Addison's and Hashimoto's diseases. *New Engl. J. Med.*, **271,** 708–713.
KEYS A., BROZEK J., HENSCHEL A., MICKELSEN O. & TAYLOR H.L. (1950) In *The Biology of Starvation*. The Univ. of Minnesota Press, Minneapolis.
KIRSCHER C.W. (1973) The epidermal response of developing skin to Prostaglandin-B_1. *Exp. cell. Res.*, **81,** 393–400.
KLEIN A. (1934) Die Veränderung der Mundhöhle der Menstruation. *Zahnärztl. Rdsch.*, **43,** 1531–1539.
KLINGER G. & KLINGER G. (1970) Untersuchungen uber den Einfluss oraler Kontrazeptiva auf die Mund- und Vaginalschleimhaut. *Dtsch. Stomat.*, **20,** 664–669.
KRAMAR J. & LEVINE V.E. (1953) Influence of fats and fatty acids on the capillaries. *J. Nutrit.*, **50,** 149–160.
KRUSE H.D., ORENT E.R. & MCCOLLUM E.V. (1932) Studies on magnesium deficiency in animals. I. Symptomatology resulting from magnesium deprivation. *J. biol. Chem.*, **96,** 519–539.
LAACHE S. (1883) In *Die Anämie*, 144. Malling, Christiania.
LANE M. & ALFREY C.P. (1965) The anemia of human riboflavin deficiency. *Blood*, **25,** 432–442.
LARRABEE A.R., ROSENTHAL S., CATHOU R.E. & BUCHANAN J.M. (1963) Enzymatic synthesis of the methyl group of methionine. IV. Isolation, characterization and role of 5-methyl tetrahydrofolate. *J. biol. Chem.*, **238,** 1025–1031.
LASCHET U. (1961) Die Wirkung von Vitaminen und Hormonen auf das Epithel. *Ztschr. Vitamin. Hormon. Fermentforsch.*, **12,** 1–14.
LAWLER S.D., ROBERTS P.D. & HOFFBRAND A.V. (1971) Chromosome studies in megaloblastic anaemia before and after treatment. *Scand. J. Haemat.*, **8,** 309–320.
LAWRENCE D.J., BERN H.A. & STEADMAN M.G. (1960) Vitamin A and keratinization: Studies on the hamster cheekpouch. *Ann. Otol.*, **69,** 645–660.
LEHRER W.P., WIESE A.C. & MOORE F.R. (1952) Biotin deficiency in suckling pigs. *J. Nutrit.*, **47,** 203–212.
LEWIS G.E. (1930) The smooth tongue: a study in deficiency disease. *Practitioner*, **125,** 749–755.
LINDHE J. & ÅTTSTROM R. (1967) Gingival exudation during the menstrual cycle. *J. periodont. Res.*, **2,** 194–198.

LINDHE J. & BJORN, A-L. (1967) Influence of hormonal contraceptives on the gingiva of women. *J. periodont. Res.*, **2**, 1–6.
LINDHE J. & BRÅNEMARK P-I. (1967a) The effect of sex hormones on vascularization of a granulation tissue. *J. periodont. Res.*, **3**, 6–11.
LINDHE J. & BRÅNEMARK P-I. (1967b) Changes in microcirculation after local application of sex hormones. *J. periodont. Res.*, **2**, 185–193.
LINDHE J. & BRÅNEMARK P-I. (1967c) Changes in vascular permeability after local application of sex hormones. *J. periodont. Res.*, **2**, 259–265.
LINDHE J. & SONESSON B. (1967) The effect of sex hormones on inflammation. *J. periodont. Res.*, **2**, 7–12.
LINDHE J., BIRCH J. & BRÅNEMARK P-I. (1968a) Vascular proliferation in pseudopregnant rabbits. *J. periodont. Res.*, **3**, 12–20.
LINDHE J., BRÅNEMARK P-I. & BIRCH J. (1968b) Microvascular events in cheek-pouch wounds of oöphorectomized hamsters following intramuscular injections of female sex hormones. *J. periodont. Res.*, **3**, 21–23.
LINDHE J., ATTSTRÖM R. & BJÖRN A-L. (1968c) Influence of sex hormones on gingival exudation in gingivitis-free female dogs. *J. periodont. Res.*, **3**, 273–278.
LINDHE J., BRÅNEMARK P-I. & BIRCH J. (1968d) Microvascular changes in cheek-pouch wounds of oöphorectomized hamsters following intramuscular injections of female sex hormones. *J. periodont. Res.*, **3**, 180–186.
LINDHE J., ATTSTRÖM R. & BJÖRN A-L. (1968e) Influence of sex hormones on gingival exudation in dogs with chronic gingivitis. *J. periodont. Res.*, **3**, 279–283.
LINENBERG W.B. (1964) Idiopathic thrombocytopenic purpura. *Oral Surg.*, **17**, 22–29.
LITWACH D., KENNEDY J.E. & ZANDER H.A. (1970) Response of oral epithelia to ovariectomy and estrogen replacement. *J. periodont. Res.*, **5**, 263–268.
LLOYD H.E.D. & GARY J. (1963) Atypical cells in vaginal smears in pernicious anemia. *Am. J. Obst. Gyn.*, **85**, 408–412.
LÖE H. (1965) Periodontal changes in pregnancy. *J. Periodont.*, **36**, 37/209–45/217.
LÖE H. & SILNESS J. (1963) Periodontal disease in pregnancy. *Acta odont. Scand.*, **21**, 533–551.
LOGAN W.S. (1972) Vitamin A and keratinization. *Arch. Derm.*, **105**, 748–753.
LOVE A.A. (1936) Manifestations of leukemia encountered in otolaryngologic and stomatologic practices. *Arch. Otolaryng.*, **23**, 173–222.
LOVESTEDT S.A. & AUSTIN L.T. (1943) Periodontoclasia in diabetes mellitus. *J. Am. dent. Ass.*, **30**, 273–275.
LOW G.C. (1928) Sprue. An analytical study of 150 cases. *Quart. J. Med.*, **21**, 523–534.
LUCIS O.J. & LUCIS R. (1972) Oral contraceptives and endocrine changes. *Bull. Wld. Hlth. Org.*, **46**, 443–450.
LUKACS I., CHRISTOPHERS E. & BRAUN-FALCO O. (1972) Die Wirkung von Vitamin A—Säure auf die Meerschweinchenepidermis und ihre Beeinflussing durch Glucocorticosteroide (Autoradiographische und biochemische Untersuchungen). *Arch. Derm. Forsch.*, **243**, 346–356.

LUNDHOLM I. (1939) Hereditary hypochromic anaemia. A clinical statistical study. *Acta med. Scand.*, Suppl. 102.

LYNCH M.A. & SHIP I.I. (1967a) Oral Manifestations of Leukemia: a postdiagnostic study. *J. Am. dent. Assoc.*, **75,** 1139–1144.

LYNCH M.A. & SHIP I.I. (1967b) Initial oral manifestations of leukemia. *J. Am. dent. Assoc.*, **75,** 932–940.

LYNN B.D. (1967) 'The Pill' as an etiologic agent in hypertrophic gingivitis. *Oral Surg.*, **24,** 333–334.

MACAPINLAC M.P., PEARSON W.N., BARNEY G.H. & DARBY W.J. (1967a) Protein and nucleic acid metabolism in the testes of zinc-deficient rats. *J. Nutrit.*, **95,** 569–577.

MACAPINLAC M.P., BARNEY G.H., PEARSON W.N. & DARBY W.J. (1967b) Production of zinc deficiency in the squirrel monkey. (*Saimini sciureus*). *J. Nutrit.*, **93,** 499–510.

MCCALL K.B., WAISMAN H.A., ELVEHJEM C.A. & JONES E.S. (1946) A study of pyrodoxine and pantothenic acid deficiencies in the monkey (*Maccaca mulatte*). *J. Nutrit.*, **31,** 685–697.

MCCARTHY F.P. & KARCHER P.H. (1946) The oral lesions of monocytic leukemia. *New Engl. J. Med.*, **234,** 787–790.

MACHELLA T.E. (1942) Studies of the B vitamins in the human subject. *Am. J. med. Sci.*, **263,** 114–124.

MACK J.P., LUI N.S.T., ROELS O.A. & ANDERSON O.R. (1972) The occurrence of vitamin A in biological membranes. *Biochim. biophys. Acta*, **288,** 203–219.

MCLAREN D.S. (1966) Present knowledge of the role of vitamin A in health and disease. *Trans. R. Soc. Trop. Med. Hyg.*, **60,** 436–462.

MACMILLAN A.L. & SINCLAIR H.M. (1958) The structural function of essential fatty acids. In SINCLAIR H.M. *Essential Fatty Acids*, Chap. 31. Butterworth Scientific Publications, London.

MAIER A.W. & ORBAN B. (1949) Gingivitis in pregnancy. *Oral Surg.*, **2,** 334–373.

MAIN D.M.G. & RITCHIE G.M. (1967) Cyclic changes in oral smears from young menstruating women. *Brit. J. Derm.*, **79,** 20–30.

MANN A.W., SPIES T.D. & SPRINGER M. (1941) The oral manifestations of vitamin B complex deficiencies. *J. dent. Res.*, **20,** 269–270.

MANSON-BAHR P. & WILLOUGHBY H. (1930) Studies on sprue with special reference to treatment. Based upon an analysis of 200 cases. *Quart. J. Med.*, **23,** 411–442.

MARSH M.E., GREENBERG L.D. & RINEHART J.F. (1955) The relationship between pyridoxine ingestion and transaminase activity. *J. Nutrit.*, **56,** 115–127.

MASROBIAN A.Z. & SHKLAR G. (1968) The effect on gingival wound healing of dietary supplements of zinc sulfate in the Syrian hamster. *Periodontics*, **6,** 224–229.

MASSEY B.W. & KLAGMAN M.I. (1955) Observations on epithelial cells exfoliated from the upper gastrointestinal tract of patients with pernicious anaemia, simple achlorhydria, and carcinoma of the esophagus and stomach. *Am. J. med. Sci*, **230,** 506–514.

MASSLER M. (1951) Oral manifestations during the female climacteric. (The postmenopausal syndrome.) *Oral Surg.*, **4,** 1234–1243.

MASSLER M., SCHOUR I. & CHOPRA B. (1950) Occurrence of gingivitis in suburban Chicago school children. *J. Periodont.*, **21**, 146–164.
MATHUR M., RAMALINGASWAMI V. & DEO M.G. (1972) Influence of protein deficiency on 19S antibody-forming cells in rats and mice. *J. Nutrit.*, **102**, 841–846.
MAYORAL L.G., TRIPATHY K., BOLANOS O., LOTERO H., DUQUE E., GARCIA F.T. & GHITIS J. (1972) Intestinal functional, and morphologic abnormalities in severely protein-malnourished adults. *Am. J. Clin. Nutrit.*, **25**, 1084–1091.
MEAD J.F. & HOWTON D.R. (1958) Interconversions of the unsaturated fatty acids. In SINCLAIR H.M. *Essential Fatty Acids*. Butterworth Scientific Publications, London.
MEDAK H., BURLAKOW P., COHEN L., MCGREW E. & TIECKE R. (1973) Correlation of cytology and clinical findings in pemphigus vulgaris. *J. oral Med.*, **28**, 4–13.
MEULENGRACHT E. (1932) Simple achylic anemia. *Acta med. Scand.*, **78**, 387–426.
MEYER J., MARWAH A. & WEINMANN J.P. (1956) Mitotic rate of gingival epithelium in two age groups. *J. invest. Derm.*, **27**, 237–247.
MILLER D.K. & RHOADS C.P. (1935) The experimental production of loss of hematopoietic elements of the gastric secretion and of the liver in swine with achlorhydrin and anemia. *J. clin. Invest.*, **14**, 153–172.
MILLER J.K. & MILLER W.J. (1962) Experimental zinc deficiency and recovery of calves. *J. Nutrit.*, **76**, 467–473.
MOHAMED A.H. (1972) The microvasculature of the rabbit gingiva as affected by progesterone: an electron microscope and autoradiographic study. Ph.D. Thesis, University of Illinois, Chicago, Illinois.
MÖLLER (no initials) (1851) Klinische Bemerkungen uber revnige weniger Bekannte Krankheiten der Zungen. *Dtsch. Klinik.*, **3**, 273–275.
MONTES L.F., PITTMAN C.S., MOORE W.J., TAYLOR C.D. & COOPER M.D. (1972) Chronic mucocutaneous candidiasis. Influence of thyroid status. *J. Am. Med. Ass.*, **221**, 156–159.
MONTO R.W., RIZEK R.A. & FINE G. (1961) The oral lesions of iron deficiency anaemia. *Oral Surg.*, **14**, 965–974.
MONTO R.W., FINE G. & RIZEK R.A. (1963) Exfoliative cells of the oral mucous membrane in patients receiving chemotherapy for malignant disease. *J. oral Surg.*, **21**, 95–100.
MOORE T. (1957) In *Vitamin A*. Elsevier Publishing Co., London.
MOORE T. (1967) In SEBRELL W.H. & HARRIS R.S. *The Vitamins*, Vol. 1, Chaps. 9A and 11A. Academic Press, New York.
MORLEY A.A. (1966) A neutrophil cycle in healthy individuals. *Lancet*, **2**, 1220–1223.
MORLEY A.A., CAREW J.P. & BAIKIE A.G. (1967) Familial cyclical neutropenia. *Brit. J. Haemat.*, **13**, 719–738.
MUELLER J.F. & VILTER R.W. (1950) Pyridoxine deficiency in human beings induced with desoxypyridoxine. *J. clin. Invest.*, **29**, 193–201.
MÜHLEMANN H.R. (1948) Eine gingivitis intermenstrualis. *Schweiz. Mschr. Zahnheille*, **58**, 865–885.
MÜLLER H. (1877) In *Die progressive perniciöse Anämie*. Caesar Schmidt, Zurich.
NAGARAJU M., ADAMSON D.G. & ROGERS J. (1971) Skin manifestations of folic acid deficiency. *Brit. J. Derm.*, **84**, 32–36.

NAIMAN J.L., OSKI F.A., DIAMOND L.K., VAWTER G.F. & SCHWACHMAN H. (1964) The gastrointestinal effects of iron-deficiency anemia. *Pediatrics*, **33,** 83–99.

NEUMANN A.L., JOHNSON B.C. & THIERSCH J.B. (1950) Crystalline vitamin B_{12} in the nutrition of the baby pig. *J. Nutrit.*, **40,** 403–414.

NIPPERT P.H. & MCGINTY A.P. (1943) Riboflavin deficiency versus perleche. *J. med. Ass. Georgia*, **32,** 295–297.

NOLTE J., BRDICZKA D. & STAUDTE H.W. (1972) Effect of riboflavin deficiency on metabolism of the rat in hyperthyroid and euthyroid state. *Biochim. biophys. Acta*, **268,** 611–619.

NUTLAY A.G., BHASKAR S.N., WEINMANN J.P. & BUDY A.M. (1954) The effect of estrogen on the gingiva and alveolar bone of molars in rats and mice. *J. dent. Res.*, **33,** 115–127.

OATWAY W.H. & MIDDLETON W.S. (1932) Correlation of lingual changes with other clinical data. *Arch. intern. Med.*, **49,** 860–876.

OLIVER W.M., LEAVER A.G. & SCOTT P.G. (1972) The effect of deficiencies of calcium or of calcium and vitamin D on the rate of oral collagen synthesis in the rat. *J. periodont. Res.*, **7,** 29–34.

ORENT E., KRUSE H.D. & MCCOLLUM E.V. (1932) Studies on magnesium deficiency in animals. II. Species variation in symptomatology of magnesium deprivation. *Am. J. Physiol.*, **101,** 454–461.

OSMANSKI C.P. & MEYER J. (1969) Ultrastructural changes in buccal and palatal mucosa of zinc deficient rats. *J. invest. Derm.*, **53,** 14–28.

OTT E.A., SMITH W.H., STOB M. & BEESON W.M. (1964) Zinc deficiency syndrome in the young lamb. *J. Nutrit.*, **82,** 41–49.

PAGE A.R. & GOOD R.A. (1957) Studies on cyclic neutropenia. *Am. J. Dis. Child*, **94,** 623–661.

PAPAZIAN C.E. & KOCH R. (1960) Monilial granuloma with hypothyroidism. *New Engl. J. Med.*, **262,** 16–18.

PARFITT G.J. (1957) A five year longitudinal study of the gingival condition of a group of children in England. *J. Periodont.*, **28,** 26–32.

PEDACE F.J. & STOUGHTON R. (1971) Topical retinoic acid in acne vulgaris. *Brit. J. Derm.*, **84,** 465–469.

PINARD A. & PINARD D. (1877) Treatment of the gingivitis of puerperal women. *Dent. Cosmos.*, **19,** 327.

PLEWIG G., WOLFF H.H. & BRAUN-FALCO O. (1971) Lokalbehandlung normaler und pathologischer memschlicher Haut mit Vitamin A—Säure. Klinische, histologische und elektronenmikroskopische Untersuchungen. *Arch. Klin. exp. Derm.*, **239,** 390–413.

POLLACK H. (1956) Studies on nutrition in the Far East. III. Clinical indicator signs of nutritional insufficiencies before and after enrichment of rice with synthetic vitamins. *Metabolism*, **5,** 231–244.

PORIES W.J., HENZEL J.H., ROB C.G. & STRAIN W.H. (1967a) Acceleration of wound healing in man with zinc sulphate given by mouth. *Lancet*, **1,** 121–124.

PORIES W.J., HENZEL J.H., ROB C.G. & STRAIN W.H. (1967b) Acceleration of healing with zinc sulfate. *Ann. Surg.*, **165,** 432–436.

PORIES W.J. & STRAIN W.H. (1966) Zinc and wound healing. In PRASAD A.S. *Zinc Metabolism*, Chap. 21. Charles C. Thomas, Springfield, Illinois.

PRASAD A.S. (1966) Metabolism of zinc and its deficiency in human subjects. In PRASAD A.S. *Zinc Metabolism*, Chap. 15. Charles C. Thomas, Springfield, Illinois.
PRESS M., KIKUCHI H. & THOMPSON G.R. (1972) Essential fatty acid deficiency secondary to intestinal malabsorption. *Gut*, **13,** 837.
PRUTKIN L. (1967) The effect of vitamin A on hyperkeratinization and the keratoacanthoma. *J. invest. Derm.*, **49,** 165–172.
RAICA N. & SAUBERLICH H.E. (1964) Blood cell transaminase activity in human vitamin B_6 deficiency. *Am. J. Clin. Nutrit.*, **15,** 67–72.
RANDAZZO S.D., CHIARENZA A. & LAZZARO C. (1972) Sui danni della terapia con antifolici nella psoriasi. *Giormale, Ital. Dermatol.*, **47,** 77–81.
RAUCH S. & GORLIN R.J. (1970) In GORLIN R.J. & GOLDMAN H.M. *Oral Pathology*, Chap. 22, 994. C.V. Mosby Co., St Louis.
REID J.T., HUFFMAN C.F. & DUNCAN C.W. (1945) The therapeutic effect of yeast and pyridoxine on poikilocytosis in dairy cattle. *J. Nutrit.*, **30,** 413–423.
REISNER E.H., WOLFF J.A., MCKAY R.J. & DOYLE E.F. (1951) Juvenile pernicious anemia. *Pediatrics*, **8,** 88–106.
REISS F. (1936) A contribution to the cutaneous manifestations of vitamin A deficiency. *Chinese med. J.*, **50,** 945–948.
RESCH C.A. (1940) Oral manifestations of leukemia. *Am. J. Orthodont.*, **26,** 901–907.
RHOADS C.P. & MILLER D.K. (1933) Production in dogs of chronic black tongue with anemia. *J. exp. Med.*, **58,** 585–605.
RICHARDSON D., CATRON D.V., UNDERKOFLEN L.A., MADDOCK H.M. & FRIEDLAND W.C. (1951) Vitamin B_{12} requirement of male weanling pigs. *J. Nutrit.* **44,** 371–379.
RICHMAN M.J. & ABARBANEL A.R. (1943) Effect of estradiol and diethylstilbestrol upon the atrophic human buccal mucosa with a preliminary report on the use of estrogens in the management of sessile gingivitis. *J. Clin. Endocr. Metab.*, **3,** 224–226.
RIETZ P. (1971) On the biological role and metabolism of vitamin A. *Acta Vitamin. Enzymol.*, **25,** 123–134.
RIGGS B.L., RYAN R.J., WAHNER H.W., JIANG N. & MATTOS V.R. (1973) Serum concentrations of estrogen, testosterone and gonadotropins in osteoporotic and nonosteoporotic postmenopausal women. *J. Clin. Endocr. Metab.*, **36,** 1097–1099.
RODRIQUEZ-MOLINA R. (1941) Sprue in Puerto Rico. A clinical study of 100 cases. *Puerto Rico J. Publ. Health Trop. Med.*, **17,** 134–151.
RODRIQUEZ-MOLINA R. (1954) Fundamental concepts in the diagnosis of sprue. *Ann. intern. Med.*, **40,** 33–41.
ROELS O.A. (1966) Vitamin A and lysosomes. *Nutr. Revs.*, **24,** 240–244.
ROSE J.A. (1968) Aetiology of angular cheilosis. Iron metabolism. *Brit. dent. J.*, **125,** 67–72.
ROSE J.A. (1971) Folic acid deficiency as a cause of angular cheilitis. *Lancet*, **2,** 453–454.
ROSEN E.U. & GEEFHUYSIN J. (1971) Immunoglobulin levels in protein calorie malnutrition. *S. Afr. Med. J.*, 980–982.

ROSEN F., HUFF J.W. & PERLZWEIG W.A. (1946) Effect of tryptophane on synthesis of nicotinic acid in rat. *J. Biol. Chem.*, **163**, 343–344.
ROSENBERG M.M., GOLDMAN H.M. & GARBER E. (1961) Effects of experimental thyrotoxicosis and myxedema on periodontium of rabbits. *J. dent. Res.*, **40**, 708–709.
ROTH G.D., LIN H.S. & LIU F.T.Y. (1972) Effect of contraceptive on the periodontal tissue of rats. *J. periodont. Res.*, **7**, 315–322.
ROTHBERG S. (1967) The cultivation of embryonic chicken skin in a chemically defined medium, and the response of the epidermis to excess of vitamin A. *J. invest. Derm.*, **49**, 35–38.
RUBIN C.E. (1959) The diagnosis of gastric malignancy in pernicious anemia. *Gastroenterology*, **29**, 563–587.
RUBRIGHT W.C., HIGA L.H. & YANNONE M.E. (1971) Histological quantification of the biological effects of estradiol benzoate on the gingiva and genital mucosa of castrated rabbits. *J. periodont. Res.*, **6**, 55–64.
RUBRIGHT W.C., TERMAN S.A. & YANNONE M.E. (1973) A comparative study of in vitro ^{3}H-17B-estradiol binding in gingiva, skeletal muscle and uterus of ovariectomized rabbits. *J. periodont. Res.*, **8**, 304–313.
RUSHTON W.A.H. (1962) Visual pigments in man. *Sci. Amer.*, **207**, 120–132, November.
RUSSELL B.G. (1966) Gingival changes in diabetes mellitus. *Acta path. microbiol. Scand.*, **68**, 161–168.
RUSSELL B.G. (1967) The periodontal membrane in diabetes mellitus. *Acta path. microbiol. Scand.*, **70**, 318–319.
RUTLEDGE C.E. (1940) Oral and roentgenographic aspects of teeth and jaws of juvenile diabetics. *J. Am. dent. Ass.*, **27**, 1740–1750.
RYSSEL H.J., BRUNNER K.W. & BOLLAG W. (1971) Die perorale Anwendung von Vitamin A-Säure bei Leukoplakien. Hyperkeratosen und Plattenepithelkarzinom: Ergebnisse und Verträglichkeit. *Schweiz. Med. Wschr.*, **101**, 1027–1030.
SAMUELSSON B. (1972) The synthesis and biological role of prostaglandins. *Biochem. J.*, **128**, 4p.
SAUBERLICH H.E. (1968) In SEBRELL W.H. & HARRIS R.S. *The Vitamins*, Vol. 2, Chap. 9. Academic Press, New York.
SAUBERLICH H.E., CANHAM J.E., BAKER E.M., RAICA N. & HERMAN Y.F. (1972) Biochemical assessment of the nutritional status of vitamin B6 in the human. *Am. J. Clin. Nutrit.*, **25**, 629–642.
SAVILANTI M. (1946) On the pathologic anatomy of the Plummer–Vinson syndrome. *Acta med. Scand.*, **125**, 40–54.
SCHLENK H. (1972) Odd numbered and new essential fatty acids. *Fed. Proc.*, **31**, 1430–1435.
SCHMIDT M.B. (1928) Einfluss eisenreicher und eisenarmer Nahrung auf Blut und Körper. In *Hdb. d. normalen und patholog. Physiologie*, XVI, 2: 1931. Fischer, Jena.
SCHNEIDER H.G. (1965) Die Veräuderungen des Epithels und der dem Attachment dienenden Parodontalgewebe bei Vitamin-A-Mangel (Experimentelle Untersuchungen an Ratten). *Dtsch. Zahnärztl. Z.*, **20**, 989–1000.

SCHNEIDER J.P. & CAREY J.B. (1927) The nature of the glossitis in pernicious anaemia. *Minnesota Med.*, **10**, 214–222.
SCHNEIDER H.G. & POSE G. (1969) Influence of tocopherol on the periodontium of molars in rats fed a diet lacking in vitamin E. *Archs. oral Biol.*, **14**, 431–433.
SCOPP I.W. (1964) Desquamative gingivitis. *J. Periodont.*, **35**, 149–154.
SEBRELL W.H. & BUTLER R.E. (1938) Riboflavin deficiency in man. A preliminary note. *Pub. Health Rep. (U.S.)*, **53**, 2282–2284.
SETHI P., RAMEY E.R. & HOUCK J.C. (1961) Connective Tissue IV. Effect of age upon dermal chemical response to adrenal hormones. *Proc. Soc. exp. Biol. Med.*, **108**, 76–77.
SHEPPARD I.M. (1942) Oral manifestations of diabetes mellitus; study of 100 cases. *J. Am. dent. Ass.*, **29**, 1188–1192.
SHIP I.I., MORRIS A.L., DUROCHER R.T. & BURKET C.W. (1961) Recurrent aphthous ulcerations in a professional school student population. *Oral Surg.*, **14**, 30–39.
SHKLAR G., COHEN M.M. & YERGANIAN G. (1962) Histopathologic study of periodontal disease in the Chinese hamster with hereditary diabetes. *J. Periodont.*, **33**, 14–21.
SILVERMAN S., RENSTRUP G. & PINDBORG J.J. (1963a) Studies in oral leukoplakias. III. Effects of vitamin A, comparing clinical, histopathologic, cytologic and hematologic responses. *Acta odont. Scand.*, **21**, 271–292.
SILVERMAN S., RENSTRUP G. & PINDBORG J.J. (1963b) Studies on oral leukoplakias. VII. Further investigations on the effects of vitamin A on keratinization. *Acta odont. Scand.*, **21**, 553–570.
SILVERMAN S. & SHOUSE C. (1966) Estrogen effects on human oral epithelium. Cytologic, histologic and clinical comparisons. *J. Oral Therapeut. Pharmacol.*, **3**, 87–93.
SINCLAIR H.M. (1952) Essential fatty acids and their relation to pyridoxine. *Biochem. Soc. Symp.*, **9**, 80–99.
SIRCUS W., CHURCH R. & KELLEHER J. (1957) Recurrent aphthous ulceration of the mouth. *Quart. J. Med.*, **26**, 235–250.
SMITH J.F. (1962) Clinical evaluation of massive buccal vitamin A dosage in oral hyperkeratosis. *Oral Surg.*, **15**, 282–292.
SMITH J.H. (1964) Hypervitaminosis A; report of a case. *Oral Surg.*, **17**, 305–307.
SMITH Q.T. & ALLISON D.J. (1966) Changes of collagen content in skin, femur and uterus of 17B-estradiol benzoate treated rats. *Endocrinology*, **79**, 486–492.
SMITH S.E. & ELLIS G.H. (1947) Copper deficiency in rabbits. Achromotrichia, alopecia and dermatosis. *Arch. Biochem.*, **15**, 81–88.
SMITH S.G. & MARTIN D.W. (1940) Cheilosis successfully treated with synthetic vitamin B_6. *Proc. Soc. exp. Biol. Med.*, **43**, 660–663.
SNYDERMAN S.E., HOLT L.E., CARRETERO R. & JACOBS K. (1952) Pyridoxine deficiency in the human infant. *J. Clin. Nutrit.*, **1**, 200–207.
SPERBER G.H. (1969) Oral contraceptive hypertrophic gingivitis. *J. dent. Ass. S. Afr.*, **24**, 37–40.
SPIES T.D., MILANES F., MENÉNDEZ A., KOCH M.B. & MINNICH V. (1946) Observations on the treatment of tropical sprue with folic acid. *J. Lab. clin. Med.*, **31**, 227–241.

SPIES T.D. (guest editor) (1955) Pernicious anemia in relapse (case 9) Edition on—Nutrition and Disease. *Postgrad Med.*, **17**, 20–21, March.

SPRECHER H.W. (1972) Regulation of polyunsaturated fatty acid biosynthesis in the rat. *Fed. Proc.*, **31**, 1451–1457.

SRIVASTAVA S.K., SANWAD G.C. & TEWARI K.K. (1965) Biochemical alterations in rat tissue in iron deficiency anaemia and repletion with iron. *Ind. J. Biochem.*, **2**, 257–266.

STAATS O.J., GOLDSBY J.W. & BUTTERWORTH C.E. (1965) The oral exfoliative cytology of tropical sprue. *Acta Cytol.*, **9**, 228–233.

STAATS O.J., ROBINSON L.H. & BUTTERWORTH C.E. (1969) The effect of systemic therapy on nuclear size of oral epithelial cells in folate related anemias. *Acta Cytol.*, **13**, 84–88.

STAFFORD J.L. (1965) Blood disorders in relation to dentistry. *Ann. R. Coll. Surg. Eng.*, **36**, 280–297.

STARR P. (1928) Results of liver feeding in pernicious anemia. *Am. J. med. Sci.*, **175**, 312–317.

STEFANINI M. (1948) Clinical features and pathogenesis of tropical sprue. *Medicine*, **27**, 379–427.

STEIN G.M. & LEWIS H. (1973) Oral changes in a folic acid deficient patient precipitated by anticonvulsant drug therapy. *J. Periodont.*, **44**, 645–650.

STERN H. (1914) Ein Frühsymptom der perniziösen Anämie. (Wundsein der Zunge und des Gaumens.) *Dtsch. Med. Wochenschr.*, **40**, 1517–1518.

STOKSTAD E.L.R. & KOCH J. (1967) Folic acid metabolism. *Physiol. Rev.*, **47**, 83–116.

STRAUSS K. (1947) Vitamin B_1 therapy in cyclic habitual aphthous stomatitis in women. *Brit. dent. J.*, **83**, 77–80.

SULLIVAN M. & EVANS V.J. (1944) Nutritional dermatoses in the rat. V. Evaluation of the interrelationship of magnesium deficiency and deficiencies of the vitamin B complex. *J. Nutrit.*, **27**, 123–135.

SULLIVAN M., KOLB L. & NICHOLLS J. (1942) Nutritional dermatoses in the rat. *Bull. Johns Hopkins Hosp.*, **70**, 177–192.

SULLIVAN M. & NICHOLLS J. (1942a) Nutritional dermatoses in the rat. VI. The effect of pantothenic acid deficiency. *Arch. Derm. Syph.*, **45**, 917–932.

SULLIVAN M. & NICHOLLS J. (1942b) Nutritional dermatoses in the rat; signs and symptoms resulting from diet containing unheated dried egg white as source of protein. *Arch. Derm. Syph.*, **45**, 295–314.

SUTCLIFFE P. (1972) A longitudinal study of gingivitis and puberty. *J. periodont. Res.*, **7**, 52–58.

SUTTON D.C. & ASHWORTH J. (1940) Interrelationship between the vitamin B complex and the anterior lobe of pituitary gland. *J. Lab. clin. Med.*, **25**, 1188–1192.

SWANSON V.L. & THOMASSEN R.W. (1965) Pathology of the jejunal mucosa in tropical sprue. *Am. J. Path.*, **46**, 511–551.

SWARUP S., GHOSH S.K. & CHATTERJEA J.B. (1967) Aconitase activity in iron deficiency. *Acta Haematol.*, **37**, 53–61.

SYDENSTRICKER V.P., SINGAL S.A., BRIGGS A.P. & DE VAUGHN N.M. (1942) Observations on the 'egg' white injury in man. *J. Am. med. Ass.*, **118**, 1199–1200.

TAFT L.I., HUGHES A. & WOOD I.J. (1958) Tongue biopsy. A technique using a rigid suction tube. *Lancet*, **2**, 69–71.
TAN W.C. & PRIVETT O.S. (1973) Studies on detection and synthesis of prostaglandins in tail skin of the rat. *Lipids*, **8**, 166–169.
TELSEY B. *et al* (1962) Oral manifestations of cyclic neutropenia associated with hypergammaglobulinemia: report of a case. *Oral Surg.*, **15**, 540–543.
TOROK O. & BANOCZY J. (1972) The effect of hydrocortisone on the organ cultures of normal and pathologic mucous membranes of human oral cavity. *Acta Morphol. Acad. Sci. Hung.*, **20**, 119–131.
TROWELL H.C., DAVIES J.N.P. & DEAN R.F.A. (1952) Kwashiorkor. II. Clinical picture, pathology and differential diagnosis. *Brit. med. J.*, **2**, 798–801.
TUCKER H.F. & SALMON W.D. (1955) Parakeratosis or zinc deficiency disease in the pig. *Proc. Soc. exp. Biol. Med.*, **88**, 613–616.
VAN DORP D.A., BEERTHUIS R.K., NUGTEREN D.H. & VAN KEMAN H. (1964) The biosynthesis of prostaglandins. *Biochim. biophys. Acta*, **90**, 204–207.
VAN NIEKERK W.A. (1966) Cervical cytological abnormalities caused by folic acid deficiency. *Acta Cytol.*, **10**, 67–73.
VAN WYCK C.W. (1965) The oral mucosa in kwashiorkor. *J. dent. Ass. S. Afr.*, **20**, 298–302.
VILTER R.W., BIEHL J.P., MUELLER J.F. & FRIEDMAN B.I. (1954) Some abnormalities of vitamin B_6 metabolism in human beings. *Fed. Proc.*, **13**, 776–779.
VILTER R.W., MUELLER J.F., GLAZER H.S., JARROLD T., ABRAHAM J., THOMPSON C. & HAWKINS V.R. (1953) The effect of vitamin B_6 deficiency induced by desoxypyridoxine in human beings. *J. Lab. clin. Med.*, **42**, 335–357.
WADE A.B. & STAFFORD J.L. (1963) Cyclical neutropenia. *Oral Surg.*, **16**, 1443–1448.
WALDENSTROM J. (1938) Iron and epithelium. Some clinical observations. *Acta med. Scand.*, **90** (Suppl.), 380–397.
WAINWRIGHT W.W. & NELSON M.M. (1945) Changes in the oral mucosa accompanying acute pantothenic acid deficiency in young rats. *Am. J. Orthodont.*, **31**, 406–421.
WEISBERGER D. (1941) Lesions of the oral mucosa treated with specific vitamins. *Am. J. Orthodont.*, **27**, 125–127.
WEISSMAN G. & THOMAS L. (1963) Studies on lysosomes. II. The effect of cortisone on the release of acid hydrolases from a large granule fraction of rabbit liver induced by an excess of vitamin A. *J. clin. Invest*, **42**, 661–669.
WENTZ F.M., ANDAY G. & ORBAN B. (1949) Histopathologic changes in leukemia. *J. Periodont.*, **20**, 119–128.
WHITE E.A., FOY J.R. & CERECEDO L.R. (1943) Essential fatty acid deficiency in the mouse. *Proc. Soc. exp. Biol. Med.*, **54**, 301–302.
WILLIAMS R.H. (1943) Clinical biotin deficiency. *New Engl. J. Med.*, **228**, 247–252.
WILLS L. (1948) Treatment of 'pernicious anaemia of pregnancy' and 'tropical anaemia'. *Brit. med. J.*, **1**, 1059–1064.
WILLS L. & EVANS B.D.F. (1938) Tropical macrocytic anaemia: its relation to pernicious anaemia. *Lancet*, **2**, 416–421.
WINTROBE M.M. (1967) *Clinical Hematology*. Lea & Febiger, Philadelphia.

WINTROBE M.M. & BEEBE R.T. (1933) Idiopathic hypochromic anaemia. *Medicine*, **12**, 187–243.
WINTROBE M.M., FOLLIS R.H., ALCAYAGA R., PAULSON M. & HUMPHREYS S. (1943) Pantothenic acid deficiency in swine. *Bull. Johns Hopkins Hosp.*, **73**, 313–333.
WINTROBE M.M., FOLLIS R.H., MILLER M.H., STEIN H.J., ALCAYAGA R., HUMPHREYS S., SUKSTA A. & CARTWRIGHT G.E. (1943) Pyridoxine deficiency in swine. *Bull. Johns Hopkins Hosp.*, **72**, 1–25.
WITTS L.J. (1931) Chronic microcytic anaemia. *Brit. med. J.*, **2**, 883–888.
WOLBACH S.B. & BESSEY O.A. (1942) Tissue changes in vitamin deficiencies. *Physiol. Rev.*, **22**, 233–289.
WOLFF J., SCHWARZ W. & MERKER H.J. (1967) Influence of hormones on the ultrastructure of capillaries. *Bibl. Anat.*, **9**, 334–337.
WOODBURNE A.R. (1941) Herpetic stomatitis (aphthous stomatitis). *Arch. Derm. Syph.*, **43**, 543–547.
WUEPPER K.D. & FUDENBERG H.H. (1967) Moniliasis, 'autoimmune' polyendocrinopathy, and immunologic family study. *Clin. Exp. Immunol.*, **2**, 71–82.
YANG S., OKAMURA H. & BEER A.E. (1973) The effect of estrogen on collagen synthesis at the site of a skin autograph. *Am. J. Obst. Gyn.*, **116**, 694–697.
YOUMANS J.B. (1950) Deficiencies of the water soluble vitamins. *J. Am. med. Ass.*, **144**, 307–314.
ZACHARIAE L. (1966) In ASBOE-HANSEN G. *Hormones and Connective Tissue*, 83, 94. Munksgaard, Copenhagen.
ZALUSKY R. & HERBERT V. (1961) Megaloblastic anemia in scurvy with response to 50 microgm. of folic acid daily. *New Engl. J. Med.*, **265**, 1033–1038.
ZIBOH V.A. & HSIA S.L. (1971) Prostaglandin E_2: Biosynthesis and effects on glucose and lipid metabolism in rat skin. *Arch. biochem. Biophys.*, **146**, 100–109.
ZIBOH V.A. & HSIA S.L. (1972) Effects of prostaglandin E_2 on rat skin: inhibition of sterol ester biosynthesis and clearing of scaly lesions of essential fatty acid deficiency. *J. Lipid Res.*, **13**, 458–467.
ZIL J.S. (1972) Vitamin A acid effects on epidermal mitotic activity, thickness and cellularity in the hairless mouse. *J. invest. Derm.*, **59**, 228–232.
ZISKIN D.E. (1937) The effects of hormonal treatment on the gums and oral mucosa of women. *J. dent. Res.*, **16**, 367–378.
ZISKIN D.E. (1938) Effects of certain hormones on gingival and oral mucous membranes. *J. Am. dent. Ass.*, **25**, 422–426.
ZISKIN D.E. (1946) The effects of large doses of a vitamin D preparation on the oral mucous membranes of human beings. *Am. J. Orthodont.*, **32**, 380–389.
ZISKIN D.E. & BLACKBERG S.N. (1940) The effect of castration and hypophysectomy on the gingival and oral mucous membranes of Rhesus monkeys. *J. dent. Res.*, **19**, 381–390.
ZISKIN D.E., BLACKBERG S.N. & STOUT A.P. (1933) The gingivae during pregnancy. An experimental study and a histopathological interpretation. *Surg. Gynec. Obstet.*, **57**, 719–726.

ZISKIN D.E., BLACKBERG S.N. & SLANETZ C.A. (1936) Effects of subcutaneous injections of estrogenic and gonadotrophic hormones on gums and oral mucous membranes of normal and castrated Rhesus monkeys. *J. dent. Res.*, **15**, 407–428.

ZISKIN D.E. & NESSE G.J. (1946) Pregnancy gingivitis: history, classification etiology. *Am. J. Orthodont.*, **32**, 390.

CHAPTER 6
ORAL CANCER*

W.H. BINNIE

6:0 Introduction

Malignant neoplasms of the oral cavity are relatively rare in most parts of the world. In countries such as the United Kingdom and the United States for example they comprise only 2% to 3% of total malignant tumours. There are exceptions, however, and in various parts of India approximately 40% of all malignant neoplasms are oral. The vast majority are epidermoid (squamous cell) carcinomas, accounting for 90% of all cancers of the oral cavity. The remainder are predominantly malignant tumours of minor salivary tissue and occasionally sarcomata and melanomata. Despite the low incidence of the disease, its importance lies in its high degree of lethality. Even in curable cases there may be severe degrees of dysfunction and mutilation. Unlike carcinoma of the lung, at this time there is no definite link between any single aetiological factor and intraoral carcinoma. Therefore, since one cannot reduce the incidence of the disease one must attempt to reduce the mortality.

It is proposed in this chapter to discuss the clinical features of the disease, examine the extent of the clinical problem in relation to incidence, mortality and factors influencing survival. Much of the epidemiological data is based on a recent survey of oral cancer in England and Wales (Binnie et al 1972) and reference to further sources of information is given in that monograph.

The last section deals with aetiology and examines those factors which from clinical and epidemiological evidence have long been associated with the development of oral cancer.

* The figures in this chapter are adapted from Binnie W. H., Cawson R. A., Hill G. B. & Soaper, Miss A. E., *Oral Cancer in England and Wales* (1972) HMSO, London.

6:1 Clinical Features

Most clinicians are well aware of the clinical appearance of an advanced or late-stage squamous cell carcinoma of the mouth, and have little difficulty in establishing the diagnosis. The lesions may be predominantly exophytic or invasive and destructive. The exophytic lesion is usually a broad-based, elevated mass with rough nodular or warty surfaces. It is indurated at its base and margins and as the tumour becomes more bulky, necrosis may develop so that the central area becomes ulcerated.

The advanced destructive lesion shows a classical crater-like defect with raised, rolled margins. This again is usually highly indurated, due to invasion and preceding inflammation at the periphery.

The clinical appearance of the early epidermoid carcinoma, however, is more important to recognize but, unfortunately, is highly variable. The early lesion may well appear deceptively innocent and simulate many other oral mucosal lesions. It may appear as a white patch, a small polypoid mass with no surface ulceration or associated erythema, a small shallow ulcer or lastly, it may be a flat area of erythematous mucosa. The only way that one can determine the diagnosis with this type of early lesion, which is the important stage to reach a diagnosis, is by first of all being suspicious and secondly biopsying the lesion.

6:1:1 Carcinoma of the lip

Anatomically, the vermilion border of the lip, the muco-cutaneous junction, represents an intermediate zone between skin and mucosa; a transition from one tissue to another. Squamous cell carcinoma of the lip reflects many of the features of its adjacent epithelia but behaviourly tends to lie between the two. As will be seen later, carcinoma of lip has a better prognosis than intraoral carcinoma both with regard to ratio of annual deaths to new cases and to survival. On the other hand it has a poorer prognosis than carcinoma of the facial skin, and Sanderson (1968) claims that vermilion border carcinoma is more aggressive and metastasizes earlier than its equivalent elsewhere on the facial skin.

Early carcinoma of the lip usually appears as a localized thickened area which may have a white or crusted covering. Like skin cancer, lip lesions seldom arise on otherwise healthy-looking tissue. As skin may show elastosis, keratosis, irregular pigmentation and telangiectasia, vermilion border lesions usually arise in leukokeratosis or a lip which shows chronic severe fissuring. Most of these features are due to solar changes and the relationship between lower lip carcinoma and exposure to sunlight and drying are as well known as they are for exposed skin. This association with a definite aetiological agent does not apply to oral mucosal carcinoma.

The early lesion may have been thought by the patient to be a cold sore (herpes labialis) which has persisted rather than healed, and the development of epidermoid carcinoma at the site of previous herpetic infection has been reported (Wyburn-Mason 1957).

Labial carcinoma most often develops on the vermilion border approximately halfway between the midline and commissure and the lower lip is affected in 95% of cases. The lesion is more common in light-skinned people and males are affected much more than females. In the United Kingdom this ratio is approximately 8 to 1. It affects a younger age group than intraoral carcinoma and many patients may be under 40 years of age.

Although the lesion is obvious and usually grows relatively slowly, it may have been ignored, and inevitably a large ulcerating mass develops with extensive invasion of the musculature of the lip. Metastasis, though later to develop, and less frequent than from intraoral sites, does occur and the submental and submandibular lymph nodes are the chief sites of involvement.

Cancer of the upper lip is exceedingly rare and is more likely to arise from minor salivary gland tissue.

6:1:2 Intraoral carcinoma

Carcinoma of the tongue is slightly less common than that of the lip but is by far the most common intraoral site. In contrast to lip cancer it is a highly lethal disease and the prognosis for advanced lesions is exceedingly poor. This is a condition in which the dentist may play a critical role in early detection and provide any possible hope of cure. In the early stages the lesion is usually asymptomatic and careful examination of the tongue is necessary for detection.

Again, this is predominantly a disease of men but not with the same ratio as in the lip. In the United States the ratio is said to be 4 to 1 but other series have shown rates as high as 78% and 87% in males (Frazell & Lucas 1962; Flamant et al 1964). In the United Kingdom, however, the average registrations between 1962 and 1967 showed a ratio of only 3 to 2 male to female. Frazell & Lucas also found that the sex ratio had decreased slightly over a 25-year period and suggested that this was due to the increased use of tobacco and alcohol by women.

Carcinoma of the tongue is a disease of late middle-aged and elderly persons. The most common site is the lateral border towards the ventral surface. Primary lesions of the dorsum are very rare and in the past have been particularly associated with syphilitic glossitis. Lateral border lesions occur in the area of the junction of the anterior two-thirds and posterior third of the tongue, near the site of the foliate papillae and lingual tonsils. The initial appearance may be an area of local thickening or roughness, a white patch, or an area of superficial ulceration or erosion. Advanced carcinomas of the tongue, unlike lip, tend to be deeply invasive and the whole substance of the tongue musculature may become immobilized, resulting in difficulty with speech, dysphagia and severe pain. The lesions metastasize early to the regional lymph nodes possibly involving the contra-lateral side, and in fact the first sign may be a lump in the neck and the consequences may be disastrous.

The floor of the mouth is another important primary site for oral carcinomas, and although less common than carcinoma of the tongue it also carries a poor prognosis. The advanced lesion may be exophytic or ulcerative but the early lesion may well appear simply as an innocuous-looking reddish patch (erythroplakia). However, Pindborg (1971) has reported (and many clinicians have cases they have observed) that many carcinomas of the floor of the mouth in women have an appearance similar to, or have arisen in, that lesion originally described by Cooke (1956) as epithelial naevus. This is an evenly distributed bilateral white patch which may have a thickened, folded appearance but with no erythema or fissuring. These tend to be slowly progressive over a period of years. We have two cases which have been present and frequently biopsied over a period of 10 years which have eventually become highly invasive epidermoid carcinomas.

The advanced lesion of the floor of the mouth may be very difficult to estimate with regard to extent and there may well be early regional lymph node involvement, often bilaterally.

In the United Kingdom the gingival and alveolar mucosae are relatively rare sites for carcinoma compared with tongue or floor of mouth. In the United States, however, where the disease is more common, there is an interesting variation in sex distribution in different parts of the continent. In New York, for instance, a study reported by Martin (1941) showed that 82% of cases occurred in males. In contrast to this, however, in Georgia 45% of alveolar ridge carcinomas affected women and this appeared to be directly proportional to the widespread use of snuff by women in that part of the country (Brown *et al* 1965). The mandible is affected three times more frequently than the maxilla. The lesion is frequently a nodular outgrowth and commonly appears in an area of pre-existing leukoplakia. It is interesting to note that although these lesions tend to be proliferative and spread superficially, it has been shown by Panagopoulos (1959) that there is a high incidence of microscopic bone invasion in spite of negative findings radiographically. It may mimic inflammatory gingival hyperplasia but invades alveolar bone and results in loosening of the teeth (Schreiber & Waldron 1958).

Carcinoma of the buccal mucosa is another less frequent problem in the United Kingdom, but in some parts of the world it is a very common location for primary carcinoma. An unusually high incidence appears to be related to local habits, and this has been well described and illustrated by Mehta et al (1971) in their study of oral cancer in India. Here the site distribution is almost certainly related to the use of betel quids and snuff. Again in these regions where snuff habits are common the disease is as frequent in women as men (Brown et al 1965), but in most parts of the world this is a disease seen with approximately a 4 to 1 frequency in men to women.

Early carcinoma of the buccal mucosa may present as an area of leukoplakia, an irregular patch of erythematous mucosa or a papillomatous overgrowth with roughened surface which is white or pink in colour. Frequently the lesion extends from the buccal mucosa into the labial sulcus. The advanced lesion may be characterized by any of the previously described types. One important special type in this area is verrucous carcinoma, which will be discussed later since it is believed to be a distinct pathological entity.

Like most other sites in the mouth, these lesions tend to be moderate to well-differentiated epidermoid carcinomas and have a slightly better prognosis than other oral sites.

Another distinctive type of lesion must be mentioned in relation to buccal mucosa and this is carcinoma associated with candidal leukoplakia. These lesions are more frequent near the commissural area and the importance of their recognition as a speckled type of leukoplakia and not purely a simple candidal infection has been emphasized by Cawson (1969) and Pindborg (1971).

The hard and soft palate is an exceedingly uncommon area for epidermoid carcinoma in the majority of regions of the world, the one exception being those areas such as India, South America and some of the Pacific islands where the practice of reverse smoking is conducted. In the rest of the world a primary carcinoma of the palate is more likely to be of minor salivary gland origin.

6:1:3 Verrucous carcinoma

This is considered to be a distinctive pathological variety of low-grade squamous cell carcinoma and is not peculiar to the oral cavity, because similar lesions have been described on the dorsum of the hand and mucosa of the penis and vulva (Ackerman & Johnson 1954), larynx and nose (Kraus & Perez-Mesa 1966). The frequency of this condition compared with other forms of oral cancer is difficult to determine but certainly in our experience it is exceedingly rare. Duckworth (1961) has reported that in the United Kingdom verrucous carcinoma represented fewer than 2% of oral carcinomas.

Verrucous carcinoma is found most commonly in the mandibular buccal sulcus and adjacent buccal mucosa and is very much a disease of elderly persons. The average age of patients in a series by Goethals *et al* (1963) was 66 years. It is a widespread proliferating mass of papillary fronds with low degree of invasion and if metastasis does occur it is certainly very late.

It is a condition which is much more common in the United States than in the United Kingdom and has a very strong association with the use of chewing tobacco or snuff (Ackerman 1948). It is frequently preceded by a long-standing area of leukoplakia and develops in a slow indolent fashion. In a way it is similar to many of the carcinomas described by Pindborg in India and South-east Asia in association with betel. In Ackerman's series the disease occurred exclusively in elderly men. However, in the South-eastern United States verrucous carcinoma is seen as often if not more so in elderly women, and again there can be little doubt that this is related to the widespread habit of 'snuff-dipping' in this area, especially in the rural communities, where the lesion was originally referred to as snuff-dipper's cancer (Brown *et al* 1965). Histologically the lesion presents a different appearance from other forms of epidermoid carcinoma in that it is exceedingly well differentiated and in fact shows very little cell atypia. The overall morphological appearance is more important for histological diagnosis but a specific definitive diagnosis may depend on clinical behaviour.

6:2 Incidence and Mortality

The size of the clinical problem of oral cancer is illustrated in Table 6.1, which shows recent annual average numbers of registrations and deaths in England and Wales, with a total population of approximately 48,000,000. Sites are listed using their International Classification of Diseases (ICD)

Table 6.1. Malignant neoplasms of buccal cavity and oral mesopharynx. Average annual registrations and deaths, 1962–1967, England and Wales

ICD No.	Site	Males			Females			Persons		
		Regns.	Deaths	D/R Ratio	Regns.	Deaths	D/R Ratio	Regns.	Deaths	D/R Ratio
140	Lip	548	53	0·1	70	8	0·1	618	61	0·1
141	Tongue	325	258	0·8	206	135	0·7	531	393	0·75
143, 144	Mouth, other	430	201	0·5	225	100	0·4	655	301	0·5
145	Oral mesopharynx	196	130	0·7	72	52	0·7	268	182	0·7
141, 143, 144, 145	Total intraoral	951	589	0·6	503	287	0·6	1454	876	0·6

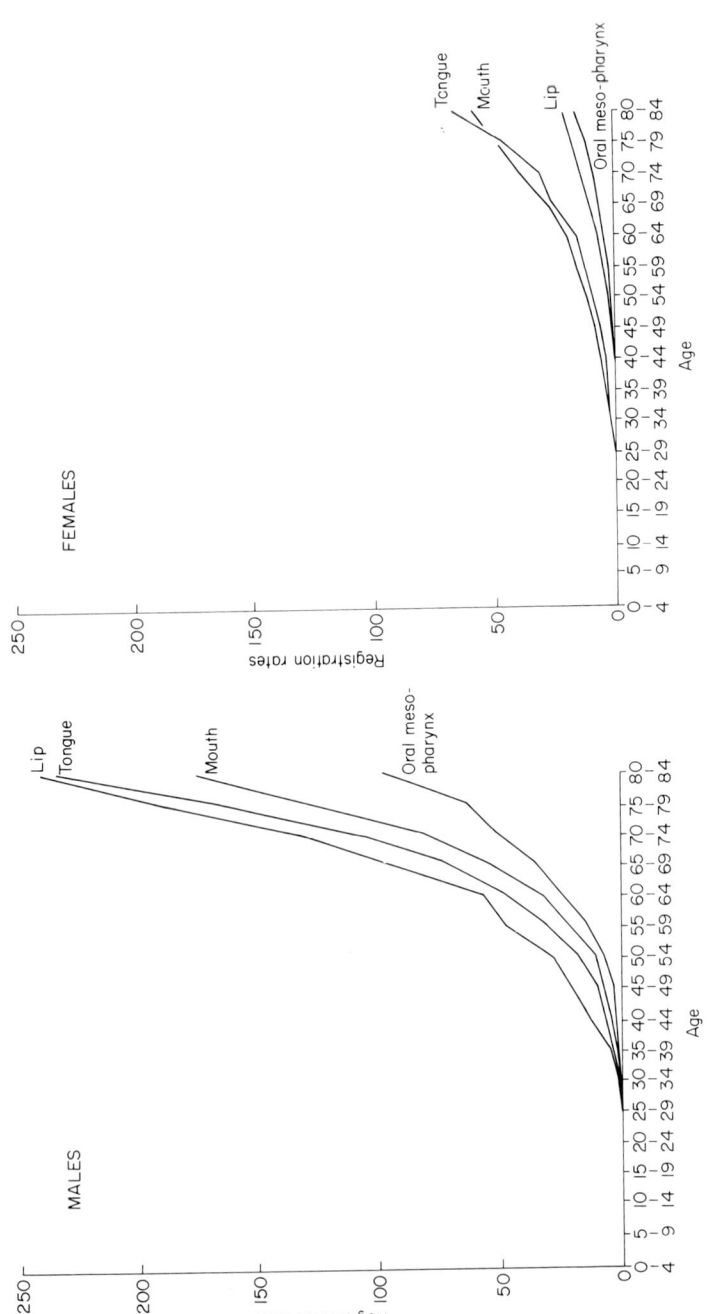

Fig. 6.1. Malignant neoplasms of buccal cavity and oral mesopharynx. Registration rates per million by site, sex and age. 1962–7. England and Wales.

number from the 7th Revision. Because the number of registrations and deaths remains reasonably constant over many years it is interesting to study the ratio (DR) of the two, and these are given in the third columns. This provides a very crude estimate of the lethality of the tumour, or a crude prognostic index. It can be seen from the table that neoplasms

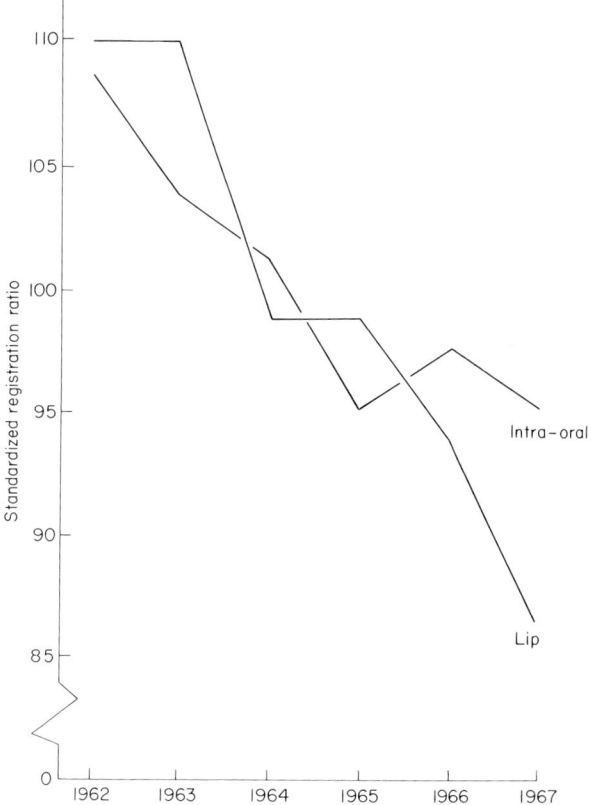

Fig. 6.2. Malignant neoplasms of lip and of tongue, mouth and mesopharynx combined. Standardized registration ratio (average 1962–7 = 100). Males. England and Wales.

arising in the tongue, mouth or oral mesopharynx carry a much worse prognosis than those of the lip. Intraorally the average DR ratio is approximately 0·6 whereas for that of lip it is only 0·1. The prognosis is closely related to the extent of the disease when first recognized, and its accessibility to effective treatment (among other factors). This will be discussed in more detail under Survival.

Study of the sex distribution of lip and intraoral neoplasms in the last few years shows that malignant neoplasms of the lip are eight times more common in men and intraoral cancer is twice as common in men. This is very much an age-related disease and sex/age specific incidence rates based on 1962 to 1967 registrations in England and Wales are shown in Fig. 6.1. For all oral sites it can be seen that rates are low until middle age and then rise steeply with increasing age but more so in males than in females. The overall incidence in the total population is only 1 in 25,000 but, as can be seen, from the graph, in the male population of 80 and over,

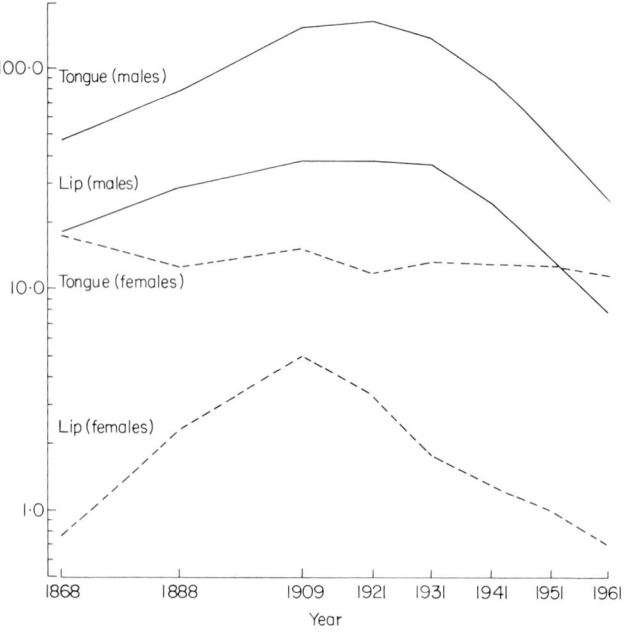

Fig. 6.3. Death rates per million population at ages 35 and over. Cancer of the lip and tongue. England and Wales.

one man in approximately 1,200 will develop an oral neoplasm each year. Ninety-eight per cent of all lip and intraoral carcinomas occur in persons over the age of 40 years.

Trends in incidence of oral neoplasms are difficult to determine, since accurate National Cancer Registry figures are available only from 1962. However, if one studies this as recorded standardized registration ratios, which are shown in Fig. 6.2 for the years from 1962 to 1967, it appears that for both lip and intraoral cancer there is a decrease in incidence of the disease in males.

Mortality from cancer at specific sites was routinely recorded initially by the Registrar General's Office in 1897, but crude death rates at age 35 and upwards were calculated for the years 1868 and 1888 for certain sites (Fig. 6.3). Corresponding figures are also available for 1909. The accuracy of these figures in general may be questioned, but with regard to oral cancer where a diagnosis and death certification are likely to be reasonably accurate, the figures should be of some value. Rates for cancer of the lip in both sexes and for cancer of the tongue in males rose in the latter part of the 19th century and early part of the 20th century and then fell. In contrast to this the rate of cancer of the tongue in females has declined gradually throughout the century. Whether the apparent increase in cancer rates towards the turn of the century was genuine or a reflection of improved diagnosis was a vexed question at the time. King & Newsholme in 1893 thought that the increase was apparent rather than real and due to improvement in diagnosis and more careful certification. Teece (1901), however, concluded that there had been a true increase in cancer mortality and the Registrar General in 1909 pointed out that the rise in mortality from cancer of the tongue could scarcely be explained by improved diagnosis, since it presents little difficulty in recognition and the increase was entirely confined to males. Lacking age-specific data it is not possible to investigate further the apparent increase in mortality rates. The subsequent decrease can, however, be analysed in more detail since comparable age-specific data on cancer of various sites is available after 1911, and this material has been published in a convenient form by McKenzie, Case & Pearson in 1957. In the case of cancer of the lip in males, for example, there is evidence of a fall in mortality beginning about 1930 which affected all ages equally. This is seen from the fact that when age-specific mortality is plotted against date of death the curves turn downwards at more or less the same point in time, but when they are plotted against date of birth they turn downwards at different dates. This is in contrast to the mortality from cancer of the tongue in males, where curves plotted against date of birth turn down at the same point, indicating a downward cohort trend beginning in those men born around 1861. A similar situation emerges from cancer of other parts of the mouth and tonsil. The conclusions for females are very similar except that the gradient of the downward cohort trend for tongue and mouth and tonsil is less than for males. Mortality reflects both incidence and efficacy of treatment and both must be borne in mind when interpreting these trends. Broadly speaking changes in treatment introduced at a given time would tend to affect all ages. The introduction of a new carcinogen into the general environment, e.g. irradiation, would also tend to affect all ages equally. By contrast other kinds of possible aetiological factors, e.g. smoking or alcohol, could affect succeeding generations in turn as they take up the habit or are otherwise exposed. Unfortunately, to assess the role of treatment as it affects trends in mortality can only be clarified if registration data were available over a long period of time, and as stated previously this is not available.

Comparison of incidence and mortality in various countries is shown in Fig. 6.4. There is a wide variation in incidence of malignant neoplasms

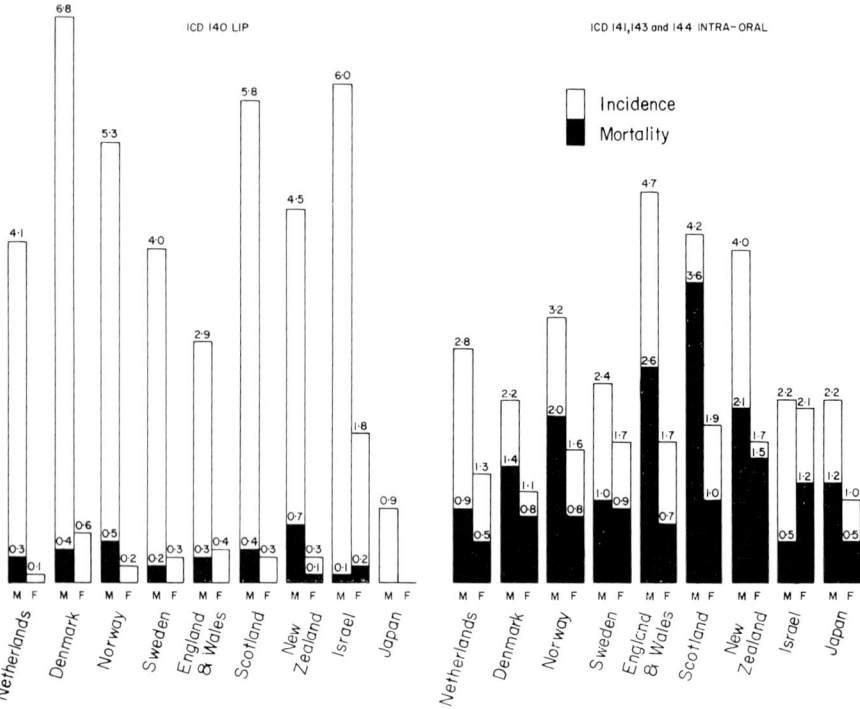

Fig. 6.4. International incidence and mortality rates (per 100,000 population). Malignant neoplasms of buccal cavity and pharynx.

of the lip in men, from 6·8 in Denmark to 0·9 in Japan. The most interesting comparison in this site is that the incidence of the disease in males in Scotland is twice that of England and Wales as a whole, and when one examines regional differences within England and Wales the incidence is highest in the West and East Central areas of England. It is suggested that this is due to occupational differences, as a high proportion of the population in these areas is involved in the agricultural and fisheries industries, and this group shows a significantly higher incidence of the disease when occupational studies are done. In all the countries shown and in others where information is available the incidence in women and mortality in both sexes is very low. Registration data is not available for the Republic of Ireland but in 1962 the mortality rate of cancer of the lip in Ireland was 2·6 per 100,000 in males. This is five or six times that of other countries and indeed approaches the mortality rates for intraoral cancer. By contrast, countries other than Ireland show intraoral cancer mortality rates of at least three times and up to as much as nine times that of lip. The female mortality rate of 0·4 for lip cancer in Ireland is also higher than that of other countries.

Intraoral cancer in all countries studied has a much higher mortality, morbidity ratio than lip cancer. Although England and Wales show the highest incidence of all, Scotland has the highest mortality rate. In the countries listed the incidence in males is at least twice that of females, except in Israel and Sweden. The sex ratio in Israel is equal, while in Sweden the male/female ratio is 3 : 2. This finding could be related to the high incidence in Swedish women of Paterson–Kelly syndrome (sideropenic dysphagia) which has been well documented as a precancerous disease (Ahlbom 1936; Jacobsson 1948; Wynder *et al* 1957). The high incidence of intraoral cancer in Israeli women, however, is less easy to explain, and it has been reported by Botet in 1949 that this syndrome did not affect Jews; but he provides no evidence to this effect. However, if one examines mortality from pharyngeal cancer there is a noticeable difference between Israeli women and Swedish women. Mortality from pharyngeal cancer remains high in Swedish women relative to men, but this is not the case with Jewish women.

It is unfortunate that no incidence figures are available for India and Pakistan as a whole, where it is known that oral cancer is exceptionally common, but varies very widely among the different states (Paymaster 1964; Mehta *et al* 1971). In the Ernakulam district of Kerala, Mehta *et al* found 12 cases of carcinoma in a sample of 10,287 of the population over the age of 15 years. Although not strictly comparable statistically with those in Fig. 6.4, the figures show that the incidence in Ernakulam is at least 20 times higher than in males in England and Wales. Another country on which it would be exceedingly interesting to have data in detail is France. Mortality data shows that the rate of intraoral cancer is 4 per 100,000 and is the highest recorded of all the countries listed. It is also worth noting that in comparison with the United Kingdom where mortality is decreasing it has been rising rapidly in France over the last 10 to 15 years.

The incidence of intraoral cancer is fairly evenly distributed throughout the United Kingdom.

When one examines the incidence and mortality from lip and oral cancer in the 26 occupational orders defined by the Registrar General's Office, one finds that both mortality and morbidity from cancer of the lip are high in farmers, foresters, fishermen, gas, coke and chemical workers and in labourers. The mortality ratio for lip is also high in glass and ceramic workers and crane-drivers, but in this latter group corresponding increases in morbidity index are less noticeable. A high risk in outdoor workers is in keeping with the well-known importance of sunlight in the aetiology of lip cancer and this has been well documented in the United States (Bernier & Clark 1951; Dorn & Cutler 1958). The high figures for gas, coke and chemical workers are interesting in that they may be related to chemical carcinogens in these occupations. The variation in incidence in intraoral cancer in the different occupational categories is less pronounced than that of lip. The one group of workers that did show a high incidence were those in the textile industry. This, although unknown previously in the United Kingdom, has been reported before in the Southern United States by Vogler *et al* in 1962, who noticed a high incidence particularly among women who had worked in the textile mills, where the disease was at least twice as common as cancer in other sites or other non-cancerous oral disease. This did not apply to men from textile mills who had a high incidence of other cancers. However, in each group the numbers were very small and the authors concluded that the finding was not significant. The picture was further complicated by the fact that tobacco chewing was exceedingly common among textile mill workers in this area (Peacock *et al* 1960), since the workers were not allowed to smoke. It is possible of course that in this group in the United Kingdom there is a high incidence of tobacco chewing, but this information is not available at this time and further investigation is necessary to define exactly the job within the occupational category of these textile workers to discover whether it is the group possibly exposed to dyes or other chemicals.

6:3 Survival

Comparison between the numbers of new registrations occurring every year with the number of deaths occurring every year for cancer of the mouth provides a crude indication of the lethality of the disease. In a recent publication the American Cancer Society estimated that in 1973 there would be 7,600 deaths from cancer of the buccal cavity and oropharynx occurring in the United States. They also estimated that the number of new cases would be 15,400; a ratio of 0·5. Since these figures remain reasonably constant each year they provide a prognostic index especially when this is compared with that for other malignant neoplasms. Cancer of the lung for instance causes 72,000 deaths per annum from 79,000 new cases; a ratio of 0·9, and carcinoma of the colon and rectum causes 37,000 deaths from 57,000 new cases; a ratio of 0·6. Both of these tumours therefore are more lethal than that of the mouth and oropharynx. Malignant neoplasms of skin, on the other hand, are much more common than any of the aforementioned sites and the American Cancer Society estimated that in 1973 there would be 120,000 new cases; however, the expected deaths from malignant tumours of the skin, and this includes the sinister malignant melanoma, are only considered to be 5,200. The ratio in this case therefore is only 0.04. Cancer of the skin then presents a very much better prognosis than cancer of the mouth, and if one uses these ratios as a means of comparison, cancer of the mouth and pharynx is twelve times more lethal than cancer of the skin. This grouping of buccal cavity and oropharynx, however, includes many sites among which there may be considerable variation. If one examines data from England and Wales (Fig. 6.1) using the same method of assessment, then individual sites can be studied separately. Lip, for instance, shows a death to registration ratio of only 0·1, whereas tongue is 0·8 and the intraoral sites alone, by which we include tongue, the rest of the mouth and oro-meso-pharynx, show a death to registration ratio of 0·6. It can be seen from this that by means of this prognostic index the lethality of malignant neoplasms of lip lies between that of skin and intraoral cancer.

Interesting as these studies may be, it must be realized that they only provide a very rough estimate of the severity of malignant disease in these various sites, and provide no indication as to the percentage of people surviving and for how many years. A more accurate way to study survival is therefore to start with an initial sample of new registered cases of malignant disease of the oral sites and follow them up every year, and find the number of persons still alive at each follow-up period. This can then be represented in graphic form and provide an accurate record of percentage survival by time. Such a sample is available for cancer registrations in England and Wales. Between 1954 and 1960 all new registrations of cancer of the buccal cavity and pharynx (ICD 140–148, 7th Revision) were accumulated and followed up every year for the first 5 and then after 7 and 10 years. This provided a large initial sample of 17,617 persons (12, 817 males and 4,800 females). Data available allowed analysis of survival by site, sex, age, stage of the lesion and treatment. Some of this data is shown in Figs. 6.5 and 6.6.

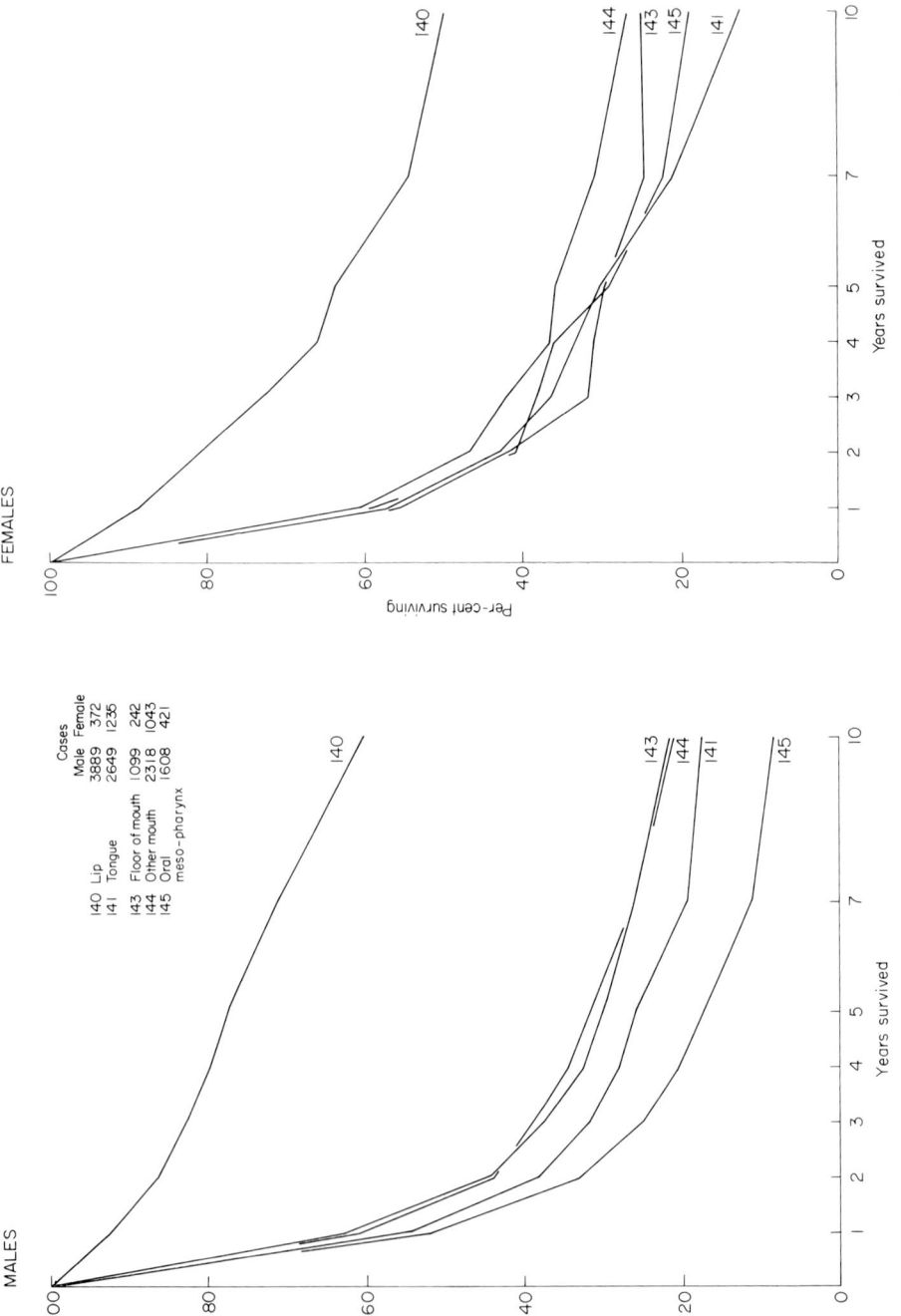

Fig. 6.5. Registrations of 1954–60, ICD 140–145, buccal cavity. Corrected survival rates, all ages, all stages by site.

Where sample sizes are sufficiently large and where a number of these groups can be combined, the survival curves have a smooth and consistent form, and show that there is a relatively rapid deterioration during the first 5 years but thereafter the curve flattens out. Ultimately where it is possible to follow these cases for sufficiently long it would show that at some time after 10 years the survival rate parallels with that of the normal population. This would represent the true cure rate for the different types of oral cancer, as has been shown by Easson & Russell (1968). These

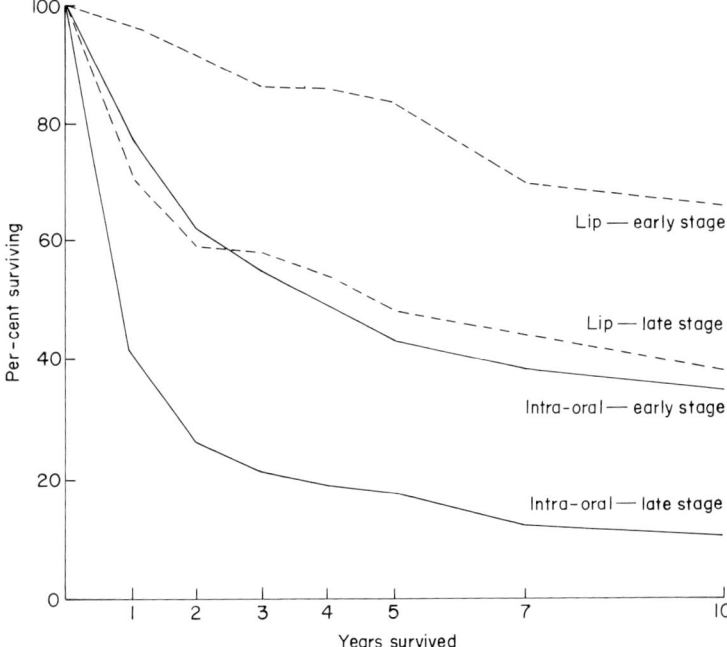

Fig. 6.6. Corrected survival. Intraoral cancer (ICD 141, 143, 144 and 145) compared with lip cancer (ICD 140). Both sexes, all ages by stage.

authors have suggested that survival for 10 years is by and large synonymous with cure.

One of the great advantages of analysing the data in this national survey was that the initial large sample allowed a high degree of statistical validity. Many studies in the past from various institutions suffer from the fact that they cannot accumulate a sufficient initial sample. However, it must be emphasized that the institutional study does have one great advantage, that is accurate and consistent recording of clinical data. Obviously on a national scale there is great variation between the method of recording in different institutions and also variation in registration between the different regional cancer registries. One aspect of this which is probably more important than any of the rest and is exceedingly important when one compares studies from different institutions, is the accurate recording of the stage of the disease at presentation. It is worthwhile to comment on that at this time. Accurate staging has always been the bugbear of accurate comparison between different studies. Many detailed and accurate methods such as those advocated by the U.I.C.C. (1968) known as the TNM method allow for a relatively consistent accurate breakdown of the involvement of the tumour at presentation. On the other hand, it does require effort by the clinician to be accurate and is also somewhat time-consuming. Other institutions may well have their own equally accurate staging methods but this may make comparison between individual institutions very difficult. With regard to the national survey staging was very crude indeed and was defined as Early, where the tumour was localized and less than 4 cm in greatest circumference, or Late, where the lesion was either over 4 cm or showed local involvement of nodes. It will be obvious immediately that this is not a particularly satisfactory method with regard to neoplasms in the mouth, and I think most clinicians would regard a localized neoplasm of the tongue which was approaching 4 cm in diameter to be an advanced lesion. Again, of course, it must be appreciated that the terms Late and Early, although they infer the time span of the neoplasm, do not in fact relate to this but purely mean the extent of involvement of the tumour at presentation. It also means that in those lesions designated as Early stage, there is a wide variation in the degree of involvement of the neoplasm from a small lesion, i.e. 5 mm diameter which may be removed as an excision biopsy, to the lesion involving much deeper tongue muscle which is $3\frac{1}{2}$ cm in diameter and may require gross surgery or extensive radiotherapy. Therefore it must be remembered that these two types of lesions are still included as Early stage. Despite this obvious inaccuracy it can still be seen from the figures shown that there is an obvious wide difference in survival between those lesions designated as Early and those as Late. It should be noted also at this stage that ICD category 142, malignant neoplasms of salivary gland, are not included. This is because there were considered to be wide variations as to which salivary neoplasms were being registered throughout the country and partly because of the inaccuracy of diagnosis.

Examination of the graph shows that for both males and females the prognosis for cancer of the lip is strikingly better than that for any intraoral site. The last three groups, tongue, floor of mouth, and mouth other sites, show a very close correspondence. The reason for the wide difference in prognosis between lip and intraoral tumours is probably related to the extent of the tumour when treatment starts. Further analysis of the survival rates by site, but taking into consideration stage and age, are shown in Fig. 6.6. In view of the close similarity of prognosis for intraoral cancer these figures have been combined where they are compared with Early and Late cancers of the lip. These show that the prognosis of Late cancer of the lip is virtually the same as that for Early intraoral cancer. This sharp difference in survival may possibly be taken to be the result of something other than the difference in stage of the disease at the start of treatment. It may be suggested for instance that intraoral cancer has some special character, e.g. that it spreads more rapidly so that size for size it will respond less well to treatment, than that of the lip. This, however, is pure speculation.

Examination of the effect of age on prognosis shows that there is an obvious deterioration. This is presumably related to the decreasing ability of the older patient to stand up to treatment, whether it be surgery or radiotherapy, to higher incidence of complications such as bronchopneumonia which occur in this group, and loss of immunological competence. Nevertheless, staging as stated earlier is so imprecise in this study that one must accept that among older patients there is the possibility of a higher proportion of more advanced lesions within the nominal category of Early.

The national study also showed that there are differences in survival rates between men and women for the various sites. For the tongue the overall 5-year survival rates are better for women but at 10 years are worse. For floor and rest of mouth the overall 5- and 10-year survival rates are slightly better for women. In the case of cancer of the lip, women show overall a poorer prognosis. It is not possible to explain these irregularities but the findings are surprising in view of those reported by Russell (1954), who found in respect of the tongue, buccal cavity and pharynx 'that a much better response to treatment is manifest in women than in men'. This better prognosis for women continues to be shown at the Christie Hospital (Easson & Russell 1968).

6:4 Aetiological Factors

One of the main objects of epidemiological studies of a disease is to attempt to elicit some causative factor or factors for that disease. Examination of such widespread features as geographical distribution, racial prevalence, occupation, social class, diet, climate, hygiene, use of tobacco and alcohol and many others may produce some evidence—possibly strong or even positive evidence—of linking that feature with the disease. Obvious examples are inhaled tobacco smoke and bronchiogenic carcinoma or actinic radiation in sunny climates and carcinoma of the exposed skin. No such single, clearly recognizable factor has come to light in the case of intraoral cancer.

This is not to say, however, that certain factors have not been implicated. Indeed there is a list which is almost traditional which includes alcohol, smoking, syphilis and oral sepsis. D'Arcy Power in 1918 was in no doubt of their significance. Reviewing cancer of the tongue he concluded:

'Cancer of the tongue has always existed in both men and in animals; the actual cause as yet unknown. Its rapid increase in men within historical times is the result of two causes: The first predisposing, the second exciting. The predisposing cause is the degenerative change taking place as a result of spirochaetal infection, the change being accentuated by lapse of years and indulgence in alcohol. The form in which the alcohol is taken does not seem to be important; beer, spirits and wine are equally harmful. It is the amount consumed, not the quality, which matters. The exciting cause is local irritation. The most effective irritant is tobacco although pyorrhoea and carious teeth often act as minor exciting causes.'

Although he involves the four factors: spirochaetal infection (*T. Pallidum* and not *B. Vincenti*); alcohol—quantity and not type or quality; tobacco—pipe smoking predominantly and not cigarettes or chewing tobacco; and oral sepsis—it was at the time of the 'trench-mouth' epidemic, one of the most interesting facts is the concept of 'co-carcinogenesis'. This has been discussed more recently by Goldhaber (1957) in relation to mouth cancer and involves two distinct phases for development of a malignant neoplasm; initiation and promotion.

In the initiation period, normal cells are converted to tumour cells (i.e. a malignant potential) by a carcinogenic agent in a relatively short time interval. Promotion takes much longer and involves the frequent exposure of the latent tumour cells to an agent which in itself is not a carcinogen, but is referred to as a 'co-carcinogen', and the eventual production of a recognizable neoplasm. Wynder *et al* (1957) apply the terms 'intrinsic' and 'extrinsic' to group factors which act together to produce malignant transformation. Intrinsic factors tend to infer generalized defects from such things as malnutrition from alcoholism and vitamin deficiencies to sideropenia and syphilis. Extrinsic factors are exogenous and have local effects. These include tobacco and sunlight (in the case of lip cancer).

This concept of double or even multiple mechanisms acting to produce neoplasia may well prove to be correct, but at the present time it is purely hypothetical and it is only by implication that any factors are associated at all. It is worthwhile reviewing these factors and assessing how strong their associations are with oral cancer.

6:4:1 Smoking

Over the last 200 years evidence has accumulated to link smoking habits with oral cancer and has been comprehensively reviewed by Clemmeson (1965). There have been attempts to discover the relative effects of different types of smoking on various sites in the mouth with detailed retrospective studies. Incidence figures have been compared with tobacco consumption in large populations. Despite the amount of accumulated evidence by many workers over a long period of time the question is still not satisfactorily answered.

Traditionally, there has been an assumed causal relationship between pipe smoking and cancer of the lip, and from the evidence reviewed by Clemmesen (1965) this would appear to be justified. However, he does explain that early workers considered the development of lip cancer could be due to many factors associated with the pipe-smoking habit, such as tobacco tar, heat from the stem, the drying effect on the mucosa—especially from clay pipes, the ends of which also became jagged with wear. However, more studies (Levin et al 1950; Wynder et al 1957) still support this link. They showed that the incidence of lip cancer in heavy pipe smokers is higher than in non-smokers, and Wynder and his colleagues also suggest an association between pipe smoking and intraoral cancer. It is also important to note that the latter found that pipe and cigar smoking was far more relevant than cigarette smoking. However, it was not possible to isolate the effect of heavy cigarette smoking alone. In another study by Keller (1967) in the United States heavy smoking was linked with the development of cancer of the floor of the mouth and tongue. Again definite evidence of the role of cigarettes could not be isolated. However, this study did relate cigarette smoking to carcinoma of intraoral mucosa, oropharynx and hypopharynx combined.

Care should be taken in analysing studies where cancers of upper respiratory and digestive tracts are combined. Significant relationships between smoking and cancer of these combined sites may not be significant when related to individual sites. The second report of the Royal College of Physicians (1971) on smoking and health claimed that oral cancer was associated with smoking, and used the evidence collected by Doll & Hill (1964a,b). In their prospective studies on British doctors they did find a significant association between mortality from cancer of the mouth, pharynx and nose combined with smoking, but not cigarette smoking. However, when all the cancers of upper respiratory and digestive tracts were combined results showed a significant difference between (a) smokers and non-smokers, (b) heavy smokers and light smokers, but not between continuing smokers and men who have stopped. They stated '. . . unlike lung cancer, the association is less characteristic of cigarette smoking and indeed in several studies the relationship is equally close, or closer with the smoking of pipes and cigars'.

In an earlier prospective study, Dorn (1958) combined deaths from cancers of the mouth, pharynx and oesophagus and found an increased risk for cigarette smokers with a gradient by amount smoked. Kahn (1966) analysed Dorn's data after a longer follow-up period and was able to examine the sites individually. All showed increased risk with strong positive gradients related to number of cigarettes smoked.

Weir & Dunn (1970) reported the mortality experience of 68,153 American men. This prospective study began in 1954 and was primarily concerned with cigarette smoking, occupation and lung cancer, but other causes of death were also studied. The total number observed deaths from cancer of the mouth (ICD 141, 143, 144) was 19. The relative risk for all cigarette smokers was 2·76 compared with non-smokers. For men smoking 30 or more cigarettes per day the risk was 5·32 times greater. Despite the fact that the absolute numbers are small, the analyses appear significant, especially when one realizes that, because the study was concerned primarily with cigarettes and lung cancer, the 'non-smokers' group included 'pipe only and/or cigar smokers'.

In studies which follow up treated or 'cured' cancer cases the findings are contradictory. Moore (1964) observed two matched groups of patients with treated oral or laryngeal cancer depending on whether they continued to smoke after treatment or not. Only one of the 29 who had stopped smoking developed a second cancer, but 17 of the 49 who continued to smoke developed a second cancer. The observation time was at least three years. However, in a similar follow-up study by Castigliano (1968) no such reduction in second cancers was found.

Very few studies have isolated cigars specifically as an aetiological agent. Recently, however, Pindborg *et al* (1972) reported that leukoplakias of the floor of the mouth in Danish women were more frequently associated with cheroot smoking than leukoplakias of other intraoral sites. Follow-up of these leukoplakias is needed in order to assess their malignant potential.

One of the most significant factors in relation to type of smoking habit and oral cancer has been the change in pattern of tobacco consumption. Although there has been a steady decline in registrations of oral cancer in England and Wales and in the United States (McComb & Fletcher 1967; Pelton 1969) there has been an increase in tobacco consumption. This is due to a great increase in cigarette smoking and there has been a steady decline in consumption of other tobacco products. The change in relative incidence of oral cancer in men and women must also be considered. The decline in oral cancer rates in men has been associated with a decline in other forms of tobacco especially of pipe smoking. This particular change in smoking habit does not, of course, apply to women whose incidence of oral cancer has declined less rapidly than it has in men. However, this decline has been associated with a similar increase in cigarette smoking.

It would seem therefore from the evidence available that there is an association between pipe, and possibly cigar, smoking and oral cancer. There is, however, conflicting opinion with regard to cigarette smoking.

Finally, there is evidence to show that in some parts of the world where the habit of smoking cigarettes and tobacco in various forms with the burning end inside the mouth there is a high incidence of oral cancer. However, this relationship is by no means universal. In the state of Andhra Pradesh in India reverse smoking is related to cancer of the palate, normally one of the rarest sites for squamous cell carcinoma to develop (Kini & Rao 1937; Khanolkar & Suryabai 1945; Reddy & Rao 1957; Pindborg et al 1971; Mehta et al 1971). In Colombia, the evidence is less definite. The habit is practised predominantly by women, and in Colombia the incidence of intraoral cancer in females approached that of males (Doll et al 1970) and was reported by Smith (1973) to be possibly higher. In the Caribbean, however, extensive studies by Quigley et al (1964, 1966) have shown no such association between reverse smoking and oral cancer. The reason for the differences are unknown.

6:4:2 Tobacco chewing habits

The use of tobacco to chew or hold in the mouth, although rare in the United Kingdom, is common in many parts of the world and has strong associations with leukoplakia and carcinoma.

This has been recognized in the United States for some time and is often referred to as 'snuff-dippers' cancer', particularly in the South-eastern States. The type of lesion associated with chewing tobacco or snuff is invariably a verrucous type of carcinoma (Ackerman 1948) following long-standing leukoplakia at the site where the tobacco was most commonly placed. This is normally the mandibular buccal sulcus. A comprehensive review of verrucous carcinoma and its relationship with tobacco is provided by Waldron (1970), who points out that in many areas the disease and habit are more common in women than men.

The habit, in various forms, also accounts for many oral cancers in South-east Asia and India (Clemmesen 1965). The tobacco is blended in various forms; often with lime and rolled in a betel leaf to form a quid (the variations in tobacco preparation are illustrated by Mehta *et al* 1971), and habitual users may well have a quid in the mouth for 24 hours per day. The lesions produced are similar to those in the United States. A papilliferous, ulcerated growth at the site where the quid is held develops after many years of leukoplakia. It is interesting to note that although the strong link is with tobacco (Muir & Kirk 1960; Wahi 1968) it has been suggested by Atkinson *et al* (1964) that the aetiological agent may be the lime. This is supported by the fact that the oral cancer incidence is high in Papua, New Guinea, where lime is used with betel nut but without tobacco, but low in Afghanistan and Nigeria, where tobacco is chewed without lime (Hirayama 1966). However, as has been noted by Pindborg *et al* (1968) and Cooke (1969), although the Papuans may not chew tobacco with their betel and lime, they smoke considerable amounts. It should also be borne in mind that tobacco held in the mouth may vary considerably in different areas. In the United States for instance chewing tobacco or snuff is produced commercially for that purpose with various additives and flavouring agents, and the final product will bear little resemblance to that used in Papua or Nigeria.

In the United Kingdom, tobacco is chewed on a very small scale. No figures are available since no tobacco is produced specifically for that purpose. The few habitués use pipe tobaccos and usually are employed in occupations where smoking is prohibited. This probably accounts for the low incidence of verrucous carcinoma (2% of oral carcinomas) reported by Duckworth (1961), although it must be noted that chewing tobacco is by no means a prerequisite for verrucous carcinoma (Geothals *et al* 1963).

6:4:3 Alcohol

The role of alcohol consumption in the development of oral cancer is difficult to assess. This is partly due to the fact that it has been difficult to assess in isolation because many consumers are also smokers. In contrast to this it has been noted that there is a much lower mortality rate in Seventh Day Adventists who abstain from both alcohol and tobacco. Two important studies implicating alcohol with oral cancer (Wynder et al 1957; Schwartz et al 1962) drew attention to this difficulty. Wynder et al (1957) reported that frequent, heavy drinkers, especially of whisky (American), are at risk and this is increased further when combined with smoking. Schwartz et al (1962) interviewed 3,937 French males with cancer of various sites and compared them with matched controls. Analyses showed an association between alcohol consumption and cancer of the tongue, hypopharynx, larynx and oesophagus and probably with buccal cavity and oropharynx. This excluded the possible overlapping influence of smoking.

France has a very high mortality rate for both oral and oesophageal cancer and, unlike the situation in the United Kingdom, both are increasing. Massé (1972) has demonstrated that by far the highest incidence of oesophageal cancer in France is found in the apple-growing areas of Brittany and Normandy and, having examined many factors, is convinced this is due to consumption of crude, home-distilled spirits from pressed apples—a crude 'calvados'. It would be interesting to know if the same geographical pattern also applies to oral cancer.

The exceptionally high mortality from oral cancer in France is also associated with a high incidence of cirrhosis of the liver. This link between a high alcohol consumption or liver cirrhosis and oral cancer has been noted by several authors (Trieger et al 1958; Trieger et al 1959; Vincent & Marchetta 1963; Keller 1967; Vincent et al 1964; Martinez 1969). The association between the two diseases in England and Wales is not as close as in France or, as would appear, in the United States. Although spirit consumption in the U.K. dropped dramatically from 1900 to 1940 it then began to rise steadily. This has been associated in the last 15 years not with an increase but with a mild decrease in oral cancer incidence.

It is difficult to explain the apparent contrast in findings in France and the United States on one hand with those in England and Wales on the other. Although many factors at present unknown could be involved it is possible that prohibition in the U.K. of unmatured, pot-still spirits containing toxic by-products has been a preventive measure in oral carcinogenesis. Certainly within the U.K. quantitative differences in alcohol consumption do not reflect proportionate differences in incidence. Although no figures are available for the amount consumed there can be little doubt that there is more alcohol drunk *per capita* in Scotland than in England and Wales. Recent official reports (Erroll 1972; Clayson 1973) show that hospital admissions for alcoholism are seven times as high for men and five times as high for women in Scotland than in England and Wales. Death rates from alcoholism are six times and twice as high respectively. Convictions for drunkenness and deaths from hepatic cirrhosis also point towards higher average consumption. However, although mortality rates for intraoral cancer are higher in Scotland (3·6 compared with 2·6 per 100,000), incidence is slightly less (4·2 to 4·7 per 100,000).

If alcohol is a contributing factor in the development of oral cancer, and it would appear that it is, it would seem that type and quality may be more important than simply quantity. It would also seem important to establish whether its role is systemic or local. Studies by Protzel et al (1964) suggest that its effect is systemic.

6:4:4 Syphilis

There are frequent reports since the last century of an association between syphilis and oral cancer, particularly cancer of the tongue, and once again we are indebted to Clemmesen (1965) for a comprehensive review of the literature. This association has been reported at various time periods, in widely differing situations and by many methods. In a well-documented, controlled study by Fry in 1929, the incidence of a positive Wassermann reaction (WR) in cancer patients was compared with that in patients without malignant disease. The relative risk of cancer of the tongue for patients with a positive WR was found to be 3·1. A very similar figure of 2·6 was reported by Wynder et al (1957), who also managed to eliminate the possibility of other factors such as alcohol and smoking confusing the association. Levin et al (1942) compared registrations of syphilis with registrations of cancer of many sites in white males in New York State. Despite a low overall incidence of syphilitic infection, there was serological and clinical evidence five times greater in patients with lingual cancer than in those with other forms of malignant neoplasms. Moreover the expected number of cases of lingual cancer was exceeded fourfold by the actual number found among the registered syphilitics.

In England and Wales, although there has been an increase in venereal disease in recent years, the mortality from syphilis and incidence of late syphilitic disease has been falling steadily as has oral cancer, if at a much slower rate. The site commonly associated with syphilitic-linked leukoplakia or carcinoma is the dorsum of the anterior two-thirds of the tongue, which is nowadays an unusual cancer site, relative to the lateral border, ventral surface or posterior third.

Despite the fact that the evidence favours a strong association between the two diseases it by no means infers proof of syphilis being a causative factor in lingual cancer. It may well be for instance that substances used in the treatment of syphilis before penicillin, such as various preparations of arsenicals and heavy metals, were more influential as carcinogenic agents than the infection itself. However, there is no positive evidence that the widespread introduction of penicillin has been responsible for the decrease in oral cancer in those countries where this has been the case. There certainly has been no period in the last 25 years which has shown a sharp drop in incidence or mortality from oral cancer. There have been no recent figures available for the association between the two diseases and it is unlikely now that more conclusive epidemiological evidence will emerge.

6:4:5 Iron deficiency

In 1919, at the Summer Congress of the Laryngological Section of the Royal Society of Medicine, papers were read quite independently by D.R. Paterson and A. Brown Kelly describing a type of chronic dysphagia most commonly found in middle-aged women. They also described the atrophic appearance of the mucosa of the upper gastrointestinal tract and such lesions as commissural fissures, atrophic glossitis, a pale smooth pharyngeal mucosa and web-like deformities at the pharyngeal oesophageal junction. Brown Kelly also noted that some of his patients had a history of anaemia, and Vinson (1922), despite the fact that he considered the dysphagia to be 'hysterical', reported that 37 of his 63 patients had haemoglobin values of less than 60%. It was not until 1939, however, that Waldenstrom & Kjellberg pointed out the significance of diminished body iron stores associated with low serum iron levels and the absence of stainable bone-marrow iron, and introduced the term 'sideropenic dysphagia' to describe the disease complex.

It is interesting to note that in his original paper Paterson (1919) was aware of '. . . the not infrequent super-vention in such cases of malignant disease of the mouth and gullet'. But, in fact, Watts (1961) points out that it was probably Logan Turner in 1913 who was the first to observe the neoplastic potential of the mucosal lesion seen in this syndrome, noting the very high preponderance in women. Most of the definitive data, however, has come from Scandinavia, and Ahlbom (1936, 1937), apart from confirming the importance of sideropenic dysphagia in the development of carcinoma of the meso- and hypo-pharynx, showed that this also applied to the buccal mucosa, tongue and all levels of the oesophagus. The condition appears to affect Swedish women in particular and probably accounts for the low male : female ratio of oral and pharyngeal cancer mortality in that country. Wynder & Fryer (1958) in an extensive investigation of aetiological considerations of sideropenic dysphagia in Swedish women suggest that the condition is decreasing.

It would be interesting to know the prevalence of iron deficiency in the U.K. and its association with oral mucosal changes. Lack of information in the past is partly due to the fact that iron was only assessed by haemoglobin estimation and not by serum and marrow estimations. Richards (1969) drew attention to the high prevalence of post-cricoid carcinoma in Wales—double the mortality rate of the highest areas in England. Of 266 cases in women 35% had a complaint of dysphagia for at least five years before the diagnosis of the carcinoma was made. How many patients with oral cancer in the U.K. have chronically low serum iron levels?

Cawson (1969) and Pindborg (1971) have drawn attention to the possible relationship between chronic hyperplastic candidiasis, the so-called 'speckled' form of leukoplakia and the development of oral cancer. It is of interest that many cases of chronic oral muco-cutaneous candidosis occur in patients who are sideropenic (Higgs & Wells 1972).

6:4:6 Dental factors

Long-standing neglect of the teeth and periodontal tissues has often been considered as an important predisposing or exciting factor in the development of oral cancer (Raven 1969). Mechanical irritation from sharp broken teeth, jagged restorations and poorly fitting dentures may be found to be immediately related to a carcinoma of tongue, lip or buccal sulcus, but this may be purely coincidental since the frequency of these irritant factors in the general population is high. The relationship is very difficult to assess on a scientific basis. Patients examined who have well-established cancer, and this unfortunately, as we have seen, is the majority, may be expected to have poor oral hygiene, and this does not indicate what their past standards were. It is also difficult to estimate with any degree of accuracy retrospectively. The unreliability of dental histories both from patients and their records makes a valid scientific study almost impossible.

Similar difficulties appear when one tries to study the possible influences of dentures. Information must be obtained concerning duration, standard of fit, extension of flanges and relationship to the neoplasm. Apart from the fact that it appears difficult to define what constitutes a satisfactory denture it may be impossible to examine the denture *in situ* when the patient presents with cancer. Vogler *et al* (1962) could find no correlation between oral cancer and presence or fit of dentures in their study. Wynder *et al* (1957) found that twice as many oral cancer sufferers were edentulous than age-matched controls, but this could well be explained by the cancer patients having had their mouths prepared for surgery or radiotherapy.

Dentures are certainly responsible for the production of large amounts of hyperplastic tissue. Chronic irritation due to mechanical trauma from denture bases causes chronic inflammatory fibrous hyperplasia, and Lucas (1972) has remarked that if this type of trauma was associated with the development of oral cancer one would expect to see it more often in this redundant tissue. In fact it must be very rare indeed to find squamous cell carcinoma in specimens submitted for histological examination which were considered clinically to be denture hyperplasia.

Wood (1961), discussing the treatment of oral cancer by irradiation, implied that improved dental health was associated with the decrease in oral cancer incidence. Personal inquiry shows this to be a widely held belief among cancer therapists. Most are quick to point out that they have no evidence for this but still believe it to be the single most important factor. They may be right, but at present there is very little evidence to link the two. On the other hand, there is no evidence which disproves the association either.

Concluding Remarks

This chapter has been an attempt to present certain aspects of squamous cell carcinoma as it affects the lip and oral mucosa. It is hoped that the clinical, epidemiological and aetiological information may provide a perspective of the problem for those clinicians who are less intensely involved with the oral cavity than the dental profession.

In the Western hemisphere, although oral cancer is a minor problem compared with cancer of lung, colon, breast or uterus, it nevertheless is a highly lethal disease. Only lung cancer shows a consistently higher mortality/morbidity ratio. For those survivors, treatment may produce distressing sequelae.

In reviewing the aetiological factors which have claimed most interest in the past, it is obvious that further investigation is necessary to clarify the situation. Unlike lip and skin cancer with their definite relationship to actinic radiation, no causative agent is identifiable for malignant transformation of the human oral mucosa. It is to be hoped that the causes will be found (and myths dispelled) and their influence eliminated; the proof would be a reduction in incidence of the disease. However, as Smith (1973) concluded, the persuasion of those at risk to protect themselves may be the most difficult aspect of the exercise.

At the present time, since we cannot hope greatly to reduce the incidence, and since all evidence shows that prognosis is most closely related to the stage of the disease at time of diagnosis regardless of type of treatment, we must concentrate on reducing mortality. This can best be achieved by earlier diagnosis and institution of treatment.

6:5 References

ACKERMAN L.V. (1948) Verrucous carcinoma of the oral cavity. *Surgery*, **23**, 670.
ACKERMAN L.V. & JOHNSON R. (1954) Present day concepts of intra-oral histopathology. In *Proceedings of the Second National Cancer Conference*. American Cancer Society, Inc., New York.
AHLBOM H.E. (1936) Simple achlorhydric anaemia, Plummer–Vinson syndrome, and carcinoma of the mouth, pharynx and oesophagus in women. *Brit. med. J.*, **2**, 331.
AHLBOM H.E. (1937) Pradisponierende faktoren fur plattenepithelkarzinom in mund hals und speiserohre. *Acta radiol. (Stockh.)*, **18**, 163.
AMERICAN CANCER SOCIETY (1973) *Cancer Facts and Figures*. American Cancer Society, Inc., New York.
ATKINSON L., CHESTER I.C., SMYTH F.G. & TEN SELDAM R.E.J. (1964) Oral cancer in New Guinea: A study in demography and aetiology. *Cancer*, **17**, 1289.
BERNIER J.L. & CLARK M.L. (1951) Squamous cell carcinomas of the lip. *Milit. Surg.*, **109**, 379.
BINNIE W.H., CAWSON R.A., HILL G.B. & SOAPER (MISS) A.E. (1972) *Oral Cancer in England and Wales: A national study of morbidity, mortality, curability and related factors*. Office of Population Censuses and Surveys: Studies on Medical and Population Subjects No. 23. H.M.S.O., London.
BOTET J.M.F. (1949) Considerations sur le syndrome de Plummer–Vinson. *Ann. Oto-laryng. (Paris)*, **66**, 23.
BROWN R.L., SUK J.M., SCARBOROUGH R.R., WILKINS S.A. & SMITH R.R. (1965) Snuff dippers' intra-oral cancer; clinical characteristics and response to therapy. *Cancer*, **18**, 2.
BROWN KELLY A. (1919) Spasm of the entrance to the oesophagus. *J. Laryng.*, **34**, 285.
CASTIGLIANO S.G. (1968) Influence of continued smoking on the incidence of second primary cancers involving the mouth, pharynx and larynx. *J. Am. dent. Ass.*, **77**, 580.
CAWSON R.A. (1969) Leukoplakia and oral cancer. *Proc. R. Soc. Med.*, **62**, 610.

CLAYSON C.W. (1973) *Report of the Departmental Committee on Scottish Licensing Law.* H.M.S.O., Edinburgh.
CLEMMESEN J.C. (1965) *Statistical Studies in the Aetiology of Malignant Neoplasms*, Vol. 1, 59. Munksgaard, Copenhagen.
COOKE B.E.D. (1956) Leukoplakia buccalis and oral epithelial naevi; a clinical and histological study. *Brit. J. Derm.*, **68,** 151.
COOKE R.A. (1969) Verrucous carcinoma of the oral mucosa in Papua, New Guinea. *Cancer*, **24,** 397.
DOLL R. & HILL A.B. (1964) Mortality in relation to smoking: ten years' observations of British doctors. *Brit. med. J.*, **1,** 1399-1410, 1460-1467.
DOLL R., MUIR C.S. & WATERHOUSE J.A.H. (1970) *Cancer Incidence in Five Continents*, Vol. II. U.I.C.C., Geneva.
DORN H.F. & CUTLER S.J. (1958) *Morbidity from Cancer in the United States.* Public Health Monograph No. 56, U.S. Department of Health, Education and Welfare, Washington D.C.
DUCKWORTH R. (1961) Verrucous carcinoma presenting as mandibular osteomyelitis *Brit. J. Surg.*, **49,** 332.
EASSON E.C. & RUSSELL M.H. (1968) *The Curability of Cancer in Various Sites.* Pitman Medical Press, London.
ERROLL, LORD (1972) *Report of the Departmental Committee on Liquor Licensing.* H.M.S.O., London.
FLAMANT R., HAYEM M., LAZAR P. & DENOIX P. (1964) Cancer of the tongue; study of 904 cases. *Cancer*, **17,** 377.
FRAZELL E.L. & LUCAS J.C. JR (1962) Cancer of the tongue. *Cancer*, **15,** 1085.
FRY H.J.B. (1929) Syphilis and malignant disease: a serological study. *Brit. J. Hygiene*, **29,** 313.
GEOTHALS P.L., HARRISON E.G. & DEVINE K.D. (1963) Verrucous squamous carcinoma of the oral cavity. *Am. J. Surg.*, **106,** 845.
GOLDHABER P. (1957) The role of saliva and other environmental factors in oral carcinogenesis. *J. Am. dent. Ass.*, **54,** 517.
HIGGS J. & WELLS R.S. (1972) Chronic muco-cutaneous candidiasis: associated abnormalities of iron metabolism. *Brit. J. Derm.*, **86,** Suppl. 8, 88.
HIRAYAMA T. (1966) An epidemiological study of oral and pharyngeal cancer in Central and South-East Asia. *Bull. Wld. Hlth. Org.*, **34,** 41.
JACOBSSON F. (1948) Cancer of the tongue: clinical study of 227 cases treated at Radiumhemmet 1931-1942. *Acta Radiologica*, Suppl. **68,** 107.
KAHN H.A. (1966) *National Cancer Institute Monograph*, **19,** 1.
KELLER A.Z. (1967) Cirrhosis of the liver, alcoholism and heavy smoking associated with cancer of the mouth and pharynx. *Cancer*, **20,** 1015.
KHANOLKAR V.R. & SURYABAI B. (1945) Cancer in relation to usages. Three new types in India. *Arch. Path.*, **40,** 351.
KING G. & NEWSHOLME A. (1893) On the alleged increase of cancer. *Roy. Soc. London*, **53,** 405.
KINI M.G. & RAO K.V.S. (1957) The problem of cancer. *Indian Med. Gaz.*, **72,** 677.
KRAUS F.T. & PEREZ-MESA C. (1966) Verrucous carcinoma. *Cancer*, **19,** 26.
LEVIN M.L., KRESS L.C. & GOLDSTEIN H. (1942) Syphilis and Cancer. *New York State J. Med.*, **42,** ii, 1737.

LEVIN M.L., GOLDSTEIN H. & GERHARDT P.R. (1950) Cancer and tobacco smoking. *J. Am. med. Ass.*, **143**, 336.
LOGAN TURNER A. (1913) Malignant disease of the oesophagus with special reference to carcinoma of the upper end: a clinical study based upon analysis of 68 cases of tumour. *J. Laryng.*, **28**, 281.
LUCAS R.B. (1972) *Pathology of Tumours of the Oral Tissues*, 2nd edition, 124. Churchill Livingstone, Edinburgh and London.
McCOMB W.S. & FLETCHER G.H. (1967) *Cancer of the Head and Neck*. Williams & Wilkins Co., Baltimore.
MACKENZIE A., CASE R.A.M. & PEARSON J.T. (1957) *Cancer Statistics for England and Wales. 1951–1955* General Register Office Studies on Medical and Population Subjects No. 13. H.M.S.O., London.
MARTIN H.E. (1941) Cancer of the gums. *Am. J. Surg.*, **54**, 765.
MARTINEZ I. (1969) Factors associated with cancer of the oesophagus, mouth and pharynx in Puerto Rico. *J. nat. Cancer Inst.*, **47**, 1069.
MASSÉ L. (1972) Epidemiology of cancer of the oesophagus in Brittany. Typescript of special lecture in the University of London.
MEHTA F.S., PINDBORG J.H. & HAMNER J.E. (1971) *Oral Cancer and Precancerous Conditions in India*. Munksgaard, Copenhagen.
MOORE C. (1964) Smoking and mouth–throat cancer. *Am. J. Surg.*, **108**, 565.
MUIR C.S. & KIRK R. (1960) Betel, tobacco and cancer of the mouth. *Brit. J. Cancer*, **14**, 597.
PANAGOPOULOS A.P. (1959) Bone involvement in maxillofacial cancer. *Am. J. Surg.*, **98**, 898.
PATERSON D.R. (1919) A clinical type of dysphagia. *J. Laryng.*, **34**, 289.
PAYMASTER J.C. (1964) Cancer and its distribution in India. *Cancer*, **17**, 1026.
PEACOCK E.E., GREENBERG B.G. & BRAWLEY B.W. (1960) The effect of snuff and tobacco on the production of oral carcinoma. *Annals of Surgery*, **151**, 542.
PELTON W.J. (1969) *Epidemiology of Oral Health*. Harvard University Press.
PINDBORG J.J., BARMES D.E. & ROED-PETERSEN B. (1968) Epidemiology and histology of oral leukoplakia and leukodema among Papuans and New Guineans. *Cancer*, **22**, 379.
PINDBORG J.J. (1971) Oral leukoplakia. *Austr. dent. J.*, **16**, 83.
PINDBORG J.J., MEHTA F.S., GUPTA P.C., DAFTARY D.K. & SMITH C.J. (1971) Reverse smoking in Andhra Pradesh, India. A study of palatal lesions among 10,169 villagers. *Brit. J. Cancer*, **25**, 10.
PINDBORG J.J., ROED-PETERSEN B. & RENSTRUP G. (1972) Role of smoking in floor of mouth leukoplakias. *J. oral Path.*, **1**, 22.
POWER D'ARCY (1918) On cancer of the tongue. *Brit. J. Surg.*, **6**, 336.
PROTZEL M., GIARDINA A.C. & ALBANO E.H. (1964) The effect of liver imbalance on the development of oral tumours in mice following the application of benzpyrene or tobacco tar. *Oral Surg.*, **18**, 622.
QUIGLEY L.F., COBB C.M., SCHOENFELD S., HUNT E. & WILLIAMS P. (1964) Reverse smoking and its oral consequences in Caribbean and South American peoples. *J. Am. dent. Ass.*, **69**, 427.
QUIGLEY L.F., SHKLAR G. & COBB C.M. (1966) Reverse cigarette smoking in Caribbeans: clinical, histologic and cytologic observations. *J. Am. dent. Ass.*, **72**, 867.

RAVEN W. (1969) Carcinoma of the mouth and pharynx. *Brit. med. J.*, **2**, 1408.
REDDY D.K. & RAO V.K. (1957) Cancer of the mouth in coastal Andhra due to smoking cigars with the burning end inside the mouth. *Indian J. Med.*, **11**, 791.
RICHARDS S. (1969) Premalignant lesions affecting the mouth, pharynx and larynx. Report of the Summer meeting of the Association of Head and Neck Oncologists of Great Britain. *Brit. med. J.*, **1**, 570.
ROYAL COLLEGE OF PHYSICIANS (1971) *Smoking and Health Now*. Pitman Medical and Scientific Publishing, London.
RUSSELL M.H. (1954) Cancer of the mouth, tongue and pharynx: sex differences in prognosis following radiotherapy. *Brit. med. J.*, **1**, 430.
SANDERSON K.V. (1968) Tumours of the skin. In ROOK A., WILKINSON D.S. & EBLING F.J.G. *Textbook of Dermatology*, Vol. 2, Chap. 57, 1713. Blackwell Scientific Publications, Oxford and Edinburgh.
SCHRIEBER H.R. & WALDRON C.A. (1958) Carcinoma of the gingiva simulating gingival hyperplasia. *J. Periodont.*, **29**, 196.
SCHWARTZ D., LELLOUCH J., FLAMANT R. & DENOIX P.F. (1962) Alcoolet cancer. Resultats d'une enquête retrospective. *Revue Français des Etudes Clinique et Biologique*, **7**, 590.
SMITH C.J. (1973) Global epidemiology and aetiology of oral cancer. *Int. dent. J.*, **23**, 82.
TEECE R. (1901) The increase of cancer. *J. Inst. Actuaries*, **36**, 89.
TRIEGER N., SHIP I.I., TAYLOR G.W. & WEISBERGER D. (1958) Cirrhosis and other predisposing factors in carcinoma of the tongue. *Cancer*, **11**, 357.
TRIEGER N., TAYLOR G.W. & WEISBERGER D. (1959) The significance of liver dysfunction in mouth cancer. *Surg. Gynac. Obst.*, **108**, 230.
UNION INTERNATIONALE CONTRE LE CANCER (1968) *TNM Classification of Malignant Tumours*. U.I.C.C., Geneva.
VINCENT R.G. & MARCHETTA F.A. (1963) The relationship of the use of tobacco and alcohol to oral cancer. *Am. J. Surg.*, **106**, 501.
VINCENT R.G., MARCHETTA F.A. & NIGOGOSYAN G. (1964) Incidence of cirrhosis in oral cancer. *New York State J. Med.*, **64**, 2174.
VINSON P.P. (1922) Hysterical dysphagia. *Minn. Med.*, **5**, 107.
VOGLER W.R., LLOYD J.W. & MILMORE B.K. (1962) a retrospective study of etiological factors in cancer of the mouth, pharynx and larynx. *Cancer*, **15**, 246.
WAHI P.N. (1968) The epidemiology of oral and oropharyngeal cancer. A report of the study in Mainpuri district, Uttar Pradesh, India. *Bull. Wld. Hlth. Org.*, **38**, 495.
WALDENSTROM J. & KJELLBERG S.R. (1939) The roentgenological diagnosis of sideropenic dysphagia. *Acta Radiol.*, **20**, 618.
WALDRON C.A. (1970) Oral epithelial tumours. In GORLIN R.J. & GOLDMAN H.M. *Thoma's Oral Pathology*, 6th edition, Chap. 19. C.V. Mosby Co., St Louis.
WATTS J.McK. (1961) The importance of the Plummer–Vinson syndrome in the aetiology of carcinoma of the upper gastro-intestinal tract. *Postgrad. med. J.*, **37**, 523.
WEIR J.M. & DUNN J.E. (1970) Smoking and mortality: a prospective study. *Cancer*, **25**, 105.

WOOD C.A.P. (1961) The treatment of malignant disease of the jaws by radiation. *Brit. dent. J.*, **110,** 234.
WYBURN-MASON R. (1957) Malignant change following herpes simplex. *Brit. med. J.*, **2,** 615.
WYNDER E.L., BROSS I.J. & FELDMAN R.M. (1957) A study of the etiological factors in cancer of the mouth. *Cancer*, **10,** 1300.
WYNDER E.L. & FRYER J.H. (1958) Etiologic considerations of Plummer–Vinson (Paterson–Kelly) syndrome. *Ann. intern. Med.*, **49,** 1106.

CHAPTER 7
PREMALIGNANT LESIONS OF ORAL EPITHELIUM

D. GORDON MACDONALD

7:0 Introduction—The Concept of Premalignancy

Binnie, in Chapter 6, has indicated the problems of the not inconsiderable morbidity and mortality caused by oral cancer. The best solution to these problems would undoubtedly be the prevention of the disease. As was also indicated in the preceding chapter, our present knowledge of the causation of oral cancer is very incomplete and it is unlikely that satisfactory procedures for prevention will be formulated in the absence of a much better understanding of the aetiology of the disease. In the short term, adequate therapy of oral cancer probably offers the best chance of success and, as Binnie *et al* (1972) stressed, the chances of successful treatment are greatly improved by early diagnosis. These chances would be further improved if it were possible to make the diagnosis before the development of overt malignancy. In other words if the diagnosis could be established while the lesion was at a premalignant stage.

In most textbooks dealing with oral cancer a section on premalignant lesions precedes the discussion of oral cancer. This frequently creates an impression that all oral epithelial cancer is preceded by some recognizable premalignant condition. Furthermore, detailed descriptions of the histological changes of premalignancy and malignancy may be closely linked, implying often that they differ only in degree. This present account of premalignant lesions follows the discussion of oral cancer to highlight the need to examine alleged premalignant lesions, at least initially, as a separate entity and avoid creating the impression that these represent merely a transitional stage of epithelium *en route* to malignant neoplasia.

This present chapter is an attempt to examine premalignant lesions of oral epithelium from two viewpoints. Firstly, the concept of premalignancy and oral lesions which appear to be premalignant will be discussed and the possible significance of these lesions in relation to oral cancer will be reviewed. Secondly, the diagnosis of these premalignant lesions will be investigated with particular reference to the problem of the recognition of factors which would help in indicating malignant potential.

The Concept of Premalignancy

Prior to the discussion of possibly premalignant lesions it is important to ask the general question 'What is meant by a premalignant lesion?' Clinical observation indicates that in a proportion of cases of squamous cell carcinoma in the mouth the tumours are preceded by or co-exist with other distinctive oral epithelial lesions. It is suggested that these associations of lesions occur more frequently than would be expected to arise by chance alone and the implication is that the other lesions may be precursors of malignant tumours. These precursor lesions are the ones which have been designated as premalignant.

Epidemiological evidence of human cancer related to environmental factors such as occupation has demonstrated that a long latent period, usually 5 to 20 years, occurs between the commencement of exposure and the appearance of the tumour. Furthermore, occupational tumours may arise many years after cessation of the hazardous occupation. Experimental work in animal skin and oral mucosa has produced similar findings and prompted the development of a 'two-stage mechanism' hypothesis of carcinogenesis (see Berenblum 1970a). This hypothesis suggests that cells are firstly changed from normal to 'dormant' tumour cells, by some carcinogenic influence. This is the phase of initiation and at this stage the tissue may be clinically and histologically normal. Subsequently, exposure of the initiated tissue to other agents may result in the promotion of the dormant tumour cells so that a visible tumour is produced. While a few substances such as urethane are known to have only initiating effects upon skin, most skin and oral mucosal carcinogens tested experimentally have been found to have both initiating and promoting effects.

The effect of promoting agents is usually to cause hyperplasia. Thus a complex situation exists in which the initiating action of a carcinogen may not cause morphological change but the promoting action of that same carcinogen may cause hyperplasia. Berenblum (1970b) summarizes this problem by stating that 'pathological changes in the tissue during the latent period have always been considered to represent a precancerous state, yet according to recent experimental evidence they may after all constitute a side reaction unconnected with the neoplastic process. Most carcinogens are toxic apart from being carcinogenic.'

On *a priori* grounds it would seem reasonable to suppose that more than one type of premalignant lesion might exist. One type of lesion might render the oral epithelium more susceptible to the action of carcinogens. The available evidence about the aetiology of oral cancer indicates that environmental carcinogenic factors are important; therefore oral lesions which make the tissues more susceptible than usual to these carcinogens would appear clinically to be premalignant. Such lesions may be more accurately described as predisposing conditions which are of themselves not truly preneoplastic. Alternatively lesions could exist which are actually a stage in the development of oral malignancy, in other words lesions undergoing promotion. It seems unlikely that a single sudden event is responsible for the development of malignant neoplasia. A progressive loss of, or diminished effectiveness of normal control mechanisms seems a more likely cause. However, even if a single somatic mutation were the cause of neoplasia it would take time for the development of a clone of malignant cells large enough to be evident clinically as a neoplasm. In either event it is reasonable to suppose that a stage would exist in which the epithelium was demonstrably abnormal, but had not invaded the underlying tissues. This stage could also be called a premalignant lesion or might even be better called precancer. Such a lesion could arise from a previously normal epithelium or from a predisposing lesion.

7:1 Lesions of Oral Epithelium which may be Premalignant

The decision that a particular type of lesion is premalignant can be arrived at in two main ways. Patients with supposed premalignant lesions can be followed up directly to observe the incidence of malignant transformation. Alternatively patients with carcinomas can be studied to discover the proportion of cases in whom co-existing alleged premalignant lesions are present. This latter approach should also provide data about the importance of premalignant lesions in relation to the overall clinical problem of oral cancer.

7:1:1 Leukoplakia

The most frequent of the allegedly premalignant lesions of oral epithelium is leukoplakia. The term leukoplakia is now being generally accepted as a clinical descriptive one carrying no histological connotation. Leukoplakia is defined as a raised white patch on the oral mucosa, measuring 5 mm or more, which cannot be scraped off and which cannot be attributed to any other diagnosable disease (Mehta *et al* 1971). Some authors omit the concept of a minimal size in the definition of leukoplakia (Waldron 1970a).

On clinical grounds leukoplakia may be further subdivided into several variants. The most frequent of these is homogeneous leukoplakia, in which the lesions appear as fairly uniform plaques. Ulceration may occur in these plaques, in which case the term ulcerated leukoplakia may be used. In 1963, Pindborg *et al* identified a type of leukoplakia which presented as white nodular patches intermingled with erythematous areas, and this variant was designated as speckled leukoplakia. Other authors distinguish slightly different variants of leukoplakia; for example Bánóczy & Sugár (1972) described three types. These were leukoplakia simplex, showing simple keratinization or hyperkeratinization; leukoplakia verrucosa, in which there is verrucous proliferation, and thirdly, leukoplakia erosiva which appears to correspond approximately to the speckled leukoplakia of Pindborg.

Malignant change in leukoplakia has been extensively studied. Older investigations of the incidence of oral cancer in leukoplakia gave a wide range of values with an average of about 30% malignant transformation (Shafer & Waldron 1961). These values were often derived from small highly selected groups. More recently, larger series of patients with leukoplakia have been followed up carefully in several countries. Pindborg *et al* (1968) reported upon a series of Danish patients followed for 3 months to 9 years and noted a 4·4% incidence of malignant transformation. Silverman & Rozen (1968), reporting upon a study on patients in the United States, used a slightly different clinical definition of leukoplakia which included only those lesions remaining after the removal of irritants. Of these persistent leukoplakias approximately 6% became squamous cell carcinomas between 1 and 11 years. Einhorn & Wersäll (1967) studied 782 patients with leukoplakia in Sweden over a prolonged period and noted that oral carcinoma developed in 2·4% after 10 years and 4% within 20 years. In Hungary, Bánóczy & Sugár (1972) demonstrated a 5·9% incidence of malignant transformation in 520 patients. These figures from several parts of the world are fairly comparable, and would certainly support the conclusions reached by Cawson (1969) that 90–95% of cases of leukoplakia will not develop cancer in a 5-year period. None the less Einhorn & Wersäll (1967) emphasized that the incidence of cancer in leukoplakia is probably 50 to 100 times greater than that arising in normal mucosa. In India, Gangadharan & Paymaster (1971) indicated that the increased risk in leukoplakia was somewhat lower, being only about 6 or 7 times greater than in the general population.

Since several clinical types of leukoplakia are described it is pertinent to ask if these are all equally likely to undergo malignant change. Pindborg et al (1963) indicated that speckled leukoplakias had a more sinister prognosis than homogeneous leukoplakia. In a later study Pindborg et al (1968) confirmed that malignant change occurred more frequently in speckled leukoplakias. Bánóczy & Sugár (1972), in their carefully documented study of 520 patients, showed that of 265 patients with leukoplakia simplex none developed carcinomas. Of 173 patients with leukoplakia verrucosa 8 developed carcinomas. However, 23 out of 82 patients with leukoplakia erosiva (speckled leukoplakia) developed carcinomas. In other words 74% of cases of leukoplakia subsequently undergoing malignant transformation presented initially as speckled leukoplakias. The demonstration that leukoplakia verrucosa is of more serious portent than leukoplakia simplex would seem ample justification for dividing the homogeneous leukoplakia of Scandinavian workers into two categories.

Few authors have attempted epidemiologic studies of the prevalence of leukoplakia in population groups. Data are available, however, for Hungary and for India. In Hungary the incidence of leukoplakia has been reported as varying between 0·6% and 3·6% in eight different parts of the country (Bánóczy et al 1969; Bruszt 1962). In India Mehta et al (1971), examining individuals aged 15 and over in five separate districts, found the incidence of leukoplakia varied from 0·2% to 4·9%. Mehta et al (1961), in a study of 4,734 Bombay policemen, reported a 3·5% incidence of leukoplakia, and in a later follow-up study of the same group a further incidence of 2·8% in a 10-year period was observed (Mehta et al 1972). These figures indicate that leukoplakia is much more frequent than oral cancer and support the conclusion that only a small proportion of leukoplakias undergo malignant transformation.

Having decided that leukoplakia can proceed to cancer in a proportion of cases, it is important to ask what proportion of carcinomas do appear to arise from leukoplakia. The answer to this question is complicated by several variables. Authors sometimes fail to define their terms and it may be impossible to interpret data, because for example the way in which a term such as leukoplakia is used is not stated. Interpretation of available data is further complicated by the fact that squamous cell carcinomas may present identical clinical appearances to premalignant lesions. Despite these difficulties, however, it is possible to give some information on the incidence of carcinomas which appear at the time of examination to co-exist with leukoplakia.

Reports of the frequency of oral cancer co-existing with leukoplakia show a wide variation. Shafer & Waldron (1961) quote values from 2 to 75%. Weisberger (1957) studied 275 patients with oral cancer and reported that '60% had carcinoma at the site of leukoplakia'. This value is often quoted, but in so far as the author fails to define leukoplakia or indicate that he discriminates between leukoplakia and actual carcinoma presenting as a white patch it is not possible to interpret the statement about incidence. Silverman *et al* (1963), reporting on a large series of patients in the U.S.A., noted 19% had leukoplakia associated with carcinoma. In Norway, Hobaek (1946) found 16% of carcinomas arising in leukoplakia, while in India, Paymaster (1962) found a 32% incidence. These last two studies were of 1,272 and 10,580 cases respectively, and probably give a better overall impression of the frequency of co-existing leukoplakia and cancer than do small series of patients with restricted distribution of lesions with regard to site. As will be discussed shortly there is a variation at different oral sites in the proportion of carcinomas co-existing with leukoplakia. In summary it can be stated that the majority of oral carcinomas arise in epithelium which does not show leukoplakia.

7:1:2 Candidal leukoplakia

The association of chronic candidal infection and leukoplakia was discussed by Cawson (1966), who noted 15 cases of chronic candidosis in 138 biopsy specimens of leukoplakia. Cawson & Lehner (1968) found that it was not possible to point to any clinical features which reliably differentiated those lesions in which candida was present. However, candidal infection is proportionately more frequent in speckled than in homogeneous leukoplakias. Roed-Petersen *et al* (1970) subdivided speckled leukoplakias by distinguishing a nodular variant which they called candida-suspect. This type of leukoplakia presents as a greyish-white, diffusely demarcated patch in which the central part shows white raised nodules on an erythematous background.

Renstrup (1970), studying a group of 235 patients with leukoplakia, found overall a 23% incidence of candidal infection. Sixty-one per cent of speckled leukoplakias showed candidal infection, whereas only 3% of homogeneous leukoplakias contained fungi. Bánóczy & Sugár (1972) also found a 61% incidence of candida in their cases of speckled leukoplakia.

Daftary *et al* (1972), reporting on the presence of candida in oral leukoplakias in India, found only a 6·3% incidence overall. Of these, proportionately more were found in speckled leukoplakias and ulcerated leukoplakias than in homogeneous leukoplakias. These authors noted that candida was not observed in the palatal leukoplakia associated with reversed smoking or the labial leukoplakia associated with clay-pipe smoking. In both these instances the excessive heat caused by the smoking habits might have been related to the lack of fungal invasion.

The question of the aetiologic significance of candidosis is not yet settled. Cawson (1969) argues convincingly that candidosis is a cause of leukoplakia and chronic candidosis is known to produce epithelial proliferation. He also noted that of 10 patients with chronic hyperplastic candidosis 6 developed carcinomas. Whether or not the candida is related to the critical step of malignant transformation is yet to be decided, but the high incidence of candidosis in those leukoplakias with the poorest prognosis would suggest that it should be regarded with grave suspicion. There do not appear to be any reports of the frequency of candidal invasion in squamous cell carcinomas although Bánóczy & Sugár (1972) do record that candida was present in 65% of their cases of leukoplakia undergoing malignant transformation. It is not possible to estimate the overall significance of candidal leukoplakia as a premalignant lesion.

7:1:3 Nicotine stomatitis

Nicotine stomatitis (stomatitis nicotina) is a lesion of the palate which was described by Thoma (1941). Some authors consider it merely as a type of leukoplakia, but Pindborg *et al* (1971) distinguished between leukoplakia of the palate and what they call leukokeratosis nicotina palati, which presented as white patches with red umbilicated centres which are the orifices of minor salivary glands. The lesion may involve the whole palate or may be restricted to the posterior part of the hard palate. Several authors have shown that nicotine stomatitis is directly related to smoking, especially to pipe smoking or to reverse smoking, in which the lighted end of a cigar or cigarette is held within the mouth. In individuals practising reverse smoking the effects of heat will be added to the effects of the tobacco smoke.

It is generally felt that nicotine stomatitis is not a significant premalignant condition (Waldron 1970b). Epidemiological evidence of the frequency of nicotine stomatitis in European countries or in the United States is not available and follow-up studies to determine the rate of malignant transformation are similarly lacking. It is known, however, that carcinoma of palate is rare in these countries.

In India, Mehta et al (1971) found a prevalence of leukokeratosis nicotina palati of between 0 and 0.3% except in the state of Andhra Pradesh in South India, in which reverse smoking is practised extensively. Pindborg et al (1971), describing this study, reported a prevalence of leukokeratosis nicotina palati of 9.5% in a study of 10,169 villagers of whom 43.8% were reverse smokers. Among these reverse smokers 17.9% had leukokeratosis nicotina palati. The great majority of oral carcinomas in this population occurred in the palate. Ramula et al (1973) also studied a population with a high incidence of reverse smoking. They noted that of 250 cases of intraoral cancer, 154 were located on the hard palate and the majority were related to reverse smoking of chuttas, a form of small homemade cigars. Ramula et al (1973) concluded that there was a close relationship between reverse smoking, nicotine stomatitis and carcinoma of the hard palate, and that nicotine stomatitis could be considered precancerous.

7:1:4 Erythroplakia

Erythroplakia has been defined as a well-demarcated red, often fiery-red, patch which cannot be attributed to other causes (Mehta et al 1971). Shear (1972) pointed out that the term erythroplakia is of fairly recent origin. The term erythroplasia has been used for a longer period and is an attempt at translation of the word *erythroplasie* used by Queyrat (1911) to describe sharply defined, red lesions on the glans penis. Shear (1972) indicated that erythroplakia is a more appropriate translation especially as it is used in contradistinction to the term leukoplakia.

Three clinical variants of erythroplakia have been described (Shear 1972). These are homogeneous erythroplakia, erythroplakia interspersed with patches of leukoplakia and granular or speckled erythroplakia. Speckled erythroplakia is identical with the previously defined speckled leukoplakia (Shear 1972). Kramer (1969) suggested that speckled leukoplakia would be better called speckled erythroplakia. However, the nomenclature of oral mucosal lesions is sufficiently confusing already without trying to change a well-understood term such as speckled leukoplakia which has been in use for over a decade.

Erythroplakia is much rarer than leukoplakia, and in the entire survey of 50,915 Indian villagers reported by Mehta et al (1971) only 9 cases of erythroplakia were found. These authors regarded erythroplakia as undoubtedly the most severe of the oral precancerous lesions. Kramer (1969) was similarly impressed by the seriousness of this lesion and noted that a persistent velvety-red patch on oral mucosa was often at an advanced stage of development towards invasive malignancy in that it warranted the diagnosis of carcinoma *in situ*.

The rate of malignant transformation of cases of erythroplakia has not been reported. Also, the proportion of oral carcinomas co-existing with or appearing to arise from areas of erythroplakia does not appear to have been documented.

7:1:5 Lichen planus

Lichen planus is a chronic disease of oral mucosa and skin and is of unknown aetiology. It gives a variety of clinical appearances associated with keratosis or hyperkeratosis of oral mucosa (Andraesen 1968). Kovesi & Bánóczy (1973) state that about 110 cases are recorded of oral carcinoma developing in lichen planus. In the series of 326 patients with lichen planus reported by these authors only one developed a carcinoma. Shklar (1972) in a larger series of cases found only three instances of carcinoma developing in over 600 patients with lichen planus.

Shklar (1972) considered that oral carcinoma was a relatively common disease and suggested that it was seen four times as often as lichen planus. He further suggested that any co-existence of lichen planus and oral carcinoma would tend to be coincidental. This is a purely subjective view and does not take account of the published data on the incidences of these two conditions. Few studies of the incidence of lichen planus in a large population have been made. Mehta *et al* (1971) found the frequency of lichen planus to be between 100 and 1000 per 100,000 population in Indian villagers over the age of 15. Kovesi & Bánóczy (1973) reported the incidence as 600 per 100,000 population in Hungary. Mehta *et al* (1971) reported the incidence of oral cancer at 53 per 100,000 in the Indian villagers. The incidence of oral cancer in adults in Europe is likely to be less than half this figure. Thus lichen planus probably occurs some two to ten times more frequently than oral cancer. Cancer occurs in approximately 0·4–0·5% of cases of oral lichen planus (Shklar 1972; Kovesi & Bánóczy 1973). Put another way this means that the likelihood of oral cancer developing in lichen planus is 10 to 20 times as great as that occurring in the population generally. This difference is statistically highly significant, although this does not of course prove a cause and effect relationship between these two diseases.

Although the aetiology of lichen planus is unknown, it is felt by many authors that stress is a contributory factor. If this is so, it might be expected that patients with oral malignancy and suffering from related stress might develop lichen planus. The frequency with which lichen planus is found in patients with oral cancer does not appear to have been studied. At least two patients in Glasgow being followed up after successful treatment of oral squamous cell carcinomas have developed typical clinical and histological lesions of lichen planus.

As noted previously, lichen planus can present in a number of clinical variants. Andraesen & Pindborg (1963) recorded 16 cases of malignant change in erosive lichen planus and 11 in plaque lesions. Other authors subsequently have stressed that malignancy may supervene in erosive and atrophic lichen planus (Kovesi & Bánóczy 1973).

7:1:6 Squamous cell papilloma

The squamous cell papilloma is a benign neoplasm which is said to be a common tumour of oral mucosa (Lucas 1972a). Opinion varies as to whether or not it should be considered premalignant. For example McCarthy & Shklar (1964) and Shklar (1965) grouped this lesion with others which they considered premalignant because of the frequency with which histological features suggestive of premalignancy may be observed in papillomas. No epidemiological data are available to indicate either the frequency of occurrence of squamous cell papillomas or the incidence of malignant transformation of these lesions. Similarly no data are available to suggest what proportion of squamous cell carcinomas might have arisen from papillomas.

In animal experimental studies oral squamous cell carcinomas frequently appear to arise by invasion in the base of papillomas. In studies on hamster cheek pouch painted with chemical carcinogen Salley (1954) noted that the sequential response to the carcinogen was hyperplasia followed by papilloma formation prior to the development of carcinomas. The type of papilloma seen in the hamster cheek pouch and at other intraoral sites in the hamster differs from that seen in man in that it shows more acanthosis and presents as a bulbous overgrowth rather than the multiple fronds of the usual human lesion.

The situation regarding the malignant potential of human oral squamous cell papillomas is as yet unresolved but the consensus of opinion would appear to be that papillomas are not premalignant lesions.

7:1:7 Chronic ulceration and mechanical irritation

Chronic ulcers and fissures of oral epithelium are often cited as potentially malignant lesions (Lucas 1972b). A distinction has to be made between ulcers arising in otherwise normal epithelium and ulcers superimposed upon other lesions such as leukoplakia. Persistent ulceration of leukoplakia has long been regarded as a serious prognostic indicator often suggesting that malignant transformation has already occurred.

In experimental animals, Renstrup *et al* (1962) showed that chronic mechanical irritation producing ulceration in the hamster cheek pouch did not of itself produce tumours but did hasten the development of carcinomas induced by topically applied carcinogen. Fujita *et al* (1973), working with hamster tongue, showed that application of chemical carcinogen alone produced few tumours whereas scratching with a barbed broach in conjunction with carcinogen produced a high tumour yield.

No detailed study in man has been made of the relationship of chronic ulceration to the development of oral carcinomas. Oral cancers frequently present as ulcerated lesions but by that stage it is impossible to state whether the ulceration contributed to the development of the neoplasm or occurred secondarily. While the importance of chronic ulceration as a premalignant condition must remain in doubt, it should be emphasized that chronic ulcers, especially if present in relation to other possibly premalignant lesions, should be regarded with grave suspicion as they may represent already malignant lesions.

7:1:8 Oral epithelial atrophy

Atrophy of oral epithelium is a feature of several diseases. In some of these there is a tendency for leukoplakia to develop in the atrophic epithelium and these cases of leukoplakia often have a poor prognosis. The conditions causing epithelial atrophy which seem to be important in this regard are syphilis, oral submucous fibrosis, Kelly–Paterson syndrome and possibly some vitamin deficiencies.

7:1:8a SYPHILIS AND LEUKOPLAKIA

Although many authors comment rather vaguely upon the possible importance of syphilis and oral cancer generally, it is probably only of importance in tongue lesions. In tertiary syphilis a chronic interstitial glossitis can occur, and associated with this there is loss of papillae and atrophy of the dorsum of the tongue. Leukoplakia may then occur and involve much of the dorsum of the tongue. This leukoplakia is often verrucous in type and ulceration is frequent. Cawson (1969) felt that this type of leukoplakia was particularly prone to undergo malignant transformation. Weisberger (1957) noted that of 14 patients with leukoplakia and syphilis all developed oral malignancy. No large follow-up study of syphilitic leukoplakias has been made from which accurate data about the incidence of malignant transformation can be derived.

In older literature (see Hobaek 1946 for review) syphilis was considered to be a very important cause of leukoplakia, and in several studies of leukoplakia incidences of syphilis as high as 100% were recorded. Kramer (1969) felt that it was probable that syphilitic leukoplakia was now less frequent because of the decline in the incidence of syphilis. Renstrup (1958) found only 3 of 90 patients with leukoplakia had a positive Wassermann reaction. Bánóczy & Sugár (1972) found a 2·5% incidence of syphilis in leukoplakia but a 10% incidence in cases of carcinomas arising in leukoplakias, thus confirming the view that leukoplakia occurring in a patient with syphilis should be regarded with particular suspicion.

Smith (1973), discussing syphilis in relation to the aetiology of oral cancer, raised the important point that the possible influence of medicaments had not been considered. Older treatments for syphilis included the use of arsenicals and heavy metals. Newbold (1972) included arsenic as one of the major factors related to precancer and the skin, but its effect on oral epithelium is not documented.

7:1:8b ORAL SUBMUCOUS FIBROSIS

Submucous fibrosis is a disease which occurs almost exclusively in Indians. It is an insidious chronic affliction which may involve any part of the oral mucosa and is characterized by inflammatory and fibro-elastic changes in the connective tissue followed by epithelial atrophy. Leukoplakia may arise in this atrophic epithelium. Paymaster (1956) was the first to mention this as a possibly premalignant lesion.

Pindborg (1965) and Pindborg et al (1970) reported that of a series of 101 patients with submucous fibrosis in North India 26·9% showed oral leukoplakia. This contrasted with an incidence of leukoplakia of 3% in 19,899 patients without submucous fibrosis. Pindborg et al (1970) conceded that most studies of submucous fibrosis had been made on selected population groups. However, in the epidemiological study of 50,915 Indians Mehta et al (1971) found that 12·7% of individuals with submucous fibrosis had oral leukoplakia in contrast to 2·0% in the overall population studied.

Paymaster (1962) stated that carcinoma developed in 30% of cases of submucous fibrosis seen in the state of Bombay. This is probably an overestimate based on selected cases of submucous fibrosis, although it does add considerable support to the concept of submucous fibrosis as a premalignant lesion. Pindborg (1965) found that 6% of 101 cases of submucous fibrosis in North India had histologic evidence of oral cancer. It is not yet possible to give an accurate figure for the rate of malignant transformation based on follow-up studies of submucous fibrosis.

Further evidence of the premalignant nature of submucous fibrosis came from Pindborg & Zachariah (1965), who demonstrated co-existing submucous fibrosis in 40 of 100 patients with oral cancer in South India.

Pindborg (1972) summarized a large volume of previous work and concluded that comparison of individuals with submucous fibrosis and the Indian population generally showed a higher incidence of leukoplakia and oral carcinoma in those with submucous fibrosis. Furthermore, submucous fibrosis was frequent in cases of oral cancer. He concluded that submucous fibrosis was a premalignant condition.

7:1:8c KELLY–PATERSON SYNDROME

This syndrome, also known as Plummer–Vinson syndrome or sideropaenic dysphagia, consists of anaemia, glossitis and post-cricoid dysphagia. Atrophy of oral mucosa occurs in this condition and this may be followed by leukoplakia with a particular predisposition to malignant transformation.

Kelly–Paterson syndrome is almost always found in females of middle age and is a major disorder involving haemopoiesis and epithelia of the upper gastrointestinal tract. The haematologic findings in Kelly–Paterson syndrome are variable. Elwood et al (1964) reported hypochromic anaemia in roughly 50% of cases, but some patients although iron-deficient do not exhibit anaemia. Classically this syndrome is associated with post-cricoid carcinoma, but Wynder & Fryer (1958) found 18% of cancer in Kelly–Paterson syndrome was oral cancer.

The incidence of Kelly–Paterson syndrome is said to be highest in Sweden and this is said to correlate with the higher female oral cancer rates in Sweden (Watts 1961). In other countries this syndrome is uncommon. The incidence of malignant transformation in Kelly–Paterson syndrome is not known nor is the frequency of the syndrome in patients with oral cancer known in detail.

7:1:8d ATROPHY IN IRON DEFICIENCY AND
VITAMIN B DEFICIENCY

Atrophy of oral epithelium can occur in iron deficiency other than in Kelly–Paterson syndrome and in B group vitamin deficiencies. It is often said that the atrophy is seen in iron-deficiency anaemia and in megaloblastic anaemia. The interrelationship of the anaemia and the mucosal changes has not yet been clarified, but it seems more likely that the mucosal changes are the result of the deficiencies manifested in a tissue of high turnover rather than secondary effects of the anaemia.

The relevance of mucosal atrophy in iron and vitamin deficiencies to the development of oral premalignant lesions and oral cancer has not yet been elucidated. One of the problems is that in humans single deficiencies seldom occur and, as Foy *et al* (1972) pointed out, the integrity of stratified squamous epithelia depends upon a variety of dietary constituents. These authors studied riboflavin deficiency in baboons and indicated that deficiency of this vitamin resulted in a high incidence of oral and skin lesions with the histological features of premalignancy. Much more work is obviously required in this area of oral mucosal integrity related to dietary factors.

7:2 Further Factors of Relevance to Premalignant Lesions and Malignant Transformation

In the preceding section a broad superficial view of premalignant lesions and their relationship to oral malignancy was presented. Several other factors require to be discussed as modifying influences in premalignancy. Leukoplakia, as was noted previously, is much the most frequent of the premalignant lesions and has been the most investigated. It is in relation to leukoplakia that the effects of site, age and sex require to be considered.

7:2:1 Site

Squamous cell carcinomas at different sites in oral epithelium are known to have widely differing biological behaviour in terms of invasiveness and the tendency to metastasize. Lip lesions for example are much less aggressive than tongue lesions. It would be reasonable therefore to expect variations in the leukoplakias seen at different sites.

The site distribution of leukoplakias varies considerably in different populations and often this can be related to particular local factors such as tobacco habits. It is difficult to correlate the results of different workers because of variations in the sites quoted and the fact that many authors do not give their criteria for the delineation of particular sites. Furthermore, most of the available studies are of patients attending institutions for treatment, and this clearly influences the types of cases presenting and the proportions of lesions at different sites seen. Hobaek (1946), reporting from the Norwegian Radium Hospital, showed a 50·7% incidence of leukoplakias of lip, whereas Shafer & Waldron (1962), reporting on Dental School cases in the United States, saw only 7·8% of their cases with lip involvement.

In India the buccal mucosa is generally reported as much the most frequent site of leukoplakia. Paymaster (1962) reported a 46% incidence in cheek. In a more recent survey in Bombay, Roed-Petersen et al (1972) found 42·8% of leukoplakia in the labial commissure and 41·9% on buccal mucosa. These authors also demonstrated that the topographical distribution of leukoplakia was mainly attributable to tobacco habits.

In European studies also the commissures have usually been reported as the most frequent sites of leukoplakia (Renstrup 1958; Pindborg et al 1962; Bánóczy & Sugár 1972).

A few authors have compared the incidence of leukoplakia at particular sites with the incidence of malignant change. Bánóczy & Sugár (1972) in Hungary found that despite the high frequency of leukoplakia involving the commissures and buccal mucosa (62·8% of cases) only 19·4% of carcinomas occurred at these sites. In contrast, the tongue, in which 38·8% of cancers occurred, accounted for only 8·5% of leukoplakias. As the carcinomas described in this study were those arising from leukoplakia, it indicated a much higher rate of malignant transformation in tongue lesions. Roed-Petersen (1971), in Denmark, found an even greater difference, in that 44·4% of cancers occurred at the margin of the tongue whereas only 1·7% of leukoplakias were present at this site.

In India, Gangadharan & Paymaster (1971) found a much smaller discrepancy between the proportions of leukoplakias and carcinomas occurring at different sites when comparison was made with all oral cancer cases. This finding is probably related to the different aetiological factors found in India.

The frequency with which carcinomas at different sites are associated with leukoplakia has been less well documented. Hobaek (1946) showed that 25·8% of carcinomas of buccal mucosa developed in leukoplakia whereas only 13·1% of tumours of tongue and sublingual region were related to leukoplakia.

This brief discussion indicates that the site of leukoplakic lesions is important. It also highlights the fact that the importance of leukoplakia as a premalignant lesion varies at different sites both in terms of the frequency of malignant transformation and the proportion of carcinomas associated with leukoplakia.

7:2:2 Age

Leukoplakia is a chronic affliction, and as might be expected the incidence in the great majority of studies rises with age to become maximal in an over-50 age group. The immediate implication of this is that the duration of exposure to aetiologic factors such as tobacco is probably important. However, many other factors may be relevant. Habits may change with age (Roed-Petersen 1972). Age-related changes occur in the tissues, and the oral environment generally changes with alterations in the natural dentition and the periodontal status. The importance of dentures is also likely to increase with age. Hormonal status will change, especially in females, and diet may also change. The incidence of systemic disease, such as cardiovascular disease, will rise with age and this may affect the nutrition and respiration of oral mucosa. It is not clear which, if any, of these factors is important in oral leukoplakia but it is probable that the increasing incidence with age is a function of many interacting variables about which there is little detailed information.

7:2:3 Sex

It is well known that leukoplakia and oral cancer are more common in males than in females. Renstrup (1958), studying leukoplakia, found a 2 : 1 ratio in favour of males in Denmark, and Shafer & Waldron (1961) found a similar ratio in the United States. In Hungary, Bánóczy & Sugár (1972) found a 3 : 1 ratio, and in India, Gangadharan & Paymaster (1971) found the ratio even more biased in favour of males with a 4·3 : 1 ratio.

The sex ratio of leukoplakias at different sites also varies in many studies, but interpretation of these differences is rendered difficult because of the factors mentioned previously in relation to site variations generally. In India, Roed-Petersen et al (1972) found that the major part of the sex variation with regard to site of occurrence of leukoplakia was explicable on the basis of different tobacco habits. Similarly Pindborg et al (1972) were able to account for the higher incidence of floor-of-mouth lesions in Danish women as related to cheroot smoking. Lip lesions are more common in Caucasian males and this has been related to actinic radiation in outdoor workers, of whom a greater proportion are males.

Studies of the sex ratio of oral cancer, however, have shown a smaller discrepancy between the sexes. Gangadharan & Paymaster (1971) found the male to female ratio for oral cancer to be 2·3 : 1, in contrast to the 4·3 : 1 ratio for leukoplakia. A higher rate of malignant transformation in leukoplakias has been found in women than in men. Roed-Petersen (1971) found the malignant transformation rate to be 5·8% for females, but only 2·1% for males. Bánóczy & Sugár (1972) found rates of 7·2% for females and 5·5% for males. These authors also found that malignant transformation in males was found at all the intraoral sites recorded, but was most common in lip, accounting for nearly 23% of instances. In contrast 8 of 9 cases of malignant transformation in females occurred in the tongue.

7:2:4 Size of lesion and lack of predisposing factors

Roed-Petersen (1971) mentioned two further factors of importance in relation to malignant transformation of leukoplakias. Leukoplakias which were larger than 5·5 cm² in size more often became malignant. Also, leukoplakias in patients without tobacco habits or who only smoked occasionally became malignant five times more frequently than in those with daily smoking habits.

7:2:5 Natural history of allegedly premalignant lesions

As was indicated in the foregoing discussion, several authors have followed up series of patients with leukoplakia over many years. So far only those lesions which have progressed to malignancy have been discussed. The other possible outcomes are that the lesion could remain static, could increase in size or could decrease in size. The outcome may also be influenced by treatment, which has in most cases been either surgical removal, elimination of irritants or a combination of both.

Regression of leukoplakia is not infrequent. Pindborg et al (1968) reported that of 214 patients with leukoplakia 20·1% showed complete regression of lesions while in 17·8% the lesions decreased in size. Mehta et al (1972), in a follow-up study of Bombay policemen, found that 42·4% of lesions seen at the beginning of the study had regressed to normal in a period of 10 years. These figures indicate that the incidences of regression and of disappearance of leukoplakia are much higher than the incidence of malignant transformation.

Mehta et al (1972) found 41·5% of lesions persisted over a 10-year period, but did not state whether or not these lesions changed in size. Pindborg et al (1968) found 45·3% of lesions unchanged in their follow-up study and only 3·3% of lesions increased in size. Bánóczy & Csiba (1972) also found only a minority of about 9% of leukoplakias increased in size, and these were almost all cases in which the aetiologic factors thought to be involved remained unchanged.

In relation to treatment Bánóczy & Csiba (1972) showed that the most important factor was probably removal of aetiologic factors, and also that surgical treatment produced a better outcome when combined with elimination of aetiologic factors. The data of Pindborg et al (1968) suggest that surgical removal is only rarely followed by recurrence. Despite these encouraging results the studies of Einhorn & Wersäll (1967) indicated that there was no evidence that the incidence of carcinoma in leukoplakia was diminished by surgical intervention. However, these authors did not feel that surgical treatment should be abandoned. Probably their findings were influenced by selection in that only clinically more suspicious cases were submitted to surgery.

7:3 Aetiology of Premalignant Lesions

Many of the aetiologic factors thought to be of importance in premalignant lesions have already been discussed. It is important to try to take an overall view of these factors and to consider them in relation to the ideas about the concept of premalignancy expressed previously. It is also important to realize that malignant transformation occurs in only a small proportion of premalignant lesions and this would suggest that the aetiologic factors responsible for malignant transformation may differ from those responsible for the original lesions. The aetiology of erythroplakia and of lichen planus is unknown. However, some information is available about leukoplakia.

Leukoplakia

Leukoplakia, the most frequent of the premalignant lesions, can arise from apparently normal or previously abnormal epithelium. It is probable that the effects of syphilis, submucous fibrosis and Kelly–Paterson syndrome are to render the epithelium less resistant to the causative agents of leukoplakia.

Tobacco habits in a variety of forms have been quoted as the most frequent cause of oral leukoplakia. Roed-Petersen *et al* (1972) found the most important aetiological factors in leukoplakia seen in Bombay Dental College were both smoking and age. They concluded, however, that other factors, so far unrecognized, may also play a role. Bánóczy & Sugár (1972) found smoking to be a less frequent aetiological agent in leukoplakias undergoing malignant transformation than in leukoplakias generally.

A major problem related to tobacco carcinogenesis is the large number of active constituents which can be derived from tobacco (Wynder & Hoffmann 1972; Bock 1972). Some of these are initiators and some are promotors. Some substances, in addition to a promoting effect, can enhance carcinogenesis by a number of actions such as facilitating absorption. It is not yet known which elements of tobacco or tobacco smoke are of importance in the aetiology of leukoplakia or of malignant transformation.

Bánóczy & Sugár (1972) gave a detailed analysis of the aetiologic agents in leukoplakia and contrasted all leukoplakias with those undergoing malignant transformation. In addition to smoking, these authors listed as aetiologic factors mechanical factors, alcohol, syphilis, electrical potential difference, and candida. In over half the cases of malignant transformation several factors appeared operative. However, all these additional factors were more frequent in the malignant transformation group. It is noteworthy that none of these factors individually was found in all cases of leukoplakia or of malignant transformation. In 4·2% of leukoplakias and 3·2% of cases of malignant transformation, no aetiological factor was found.

Lehner and his colleagues have recently published observations on immunological changes in leukoplakias and a possible aetiologic factor related to herpes virus infection, and it is pertinent to examine these in some detail at this point.

Lehner (1970) observed that a mononuclear cell infiltration had been noted in leukoplakia by most workers, but that they had associated little importance to it. On the assumption that the presence of these cells might suggest that immunological changes were occurring, Lehner (1970) conducted a study on cell-mediated immunity in patients with clinical leukoplakia including some who were later shown to have carcinoma or carcinoma *in situ* on histological examination. Quantitation of the mononuclear cell infiltrate in the lamina propria related to leukoplakia was also undertaken. Lymphocyte transformation by antigens derived from autologous leukoplakia was depressed in cases of carcinoma and carcinoma *in situ* and to a lesser extent in cases with acanthosis and epithelial atypia. Pyroninophilic cells, that is cells with the cytoplasmic staining suggestive of plasma cells, were increased in these same groups. Lehner (1970) thus suggests two new criteria to be used in the evaluation of premalignancy; namely selective depression of lymphocyte transformation, and increased pyroninophilic cell count in the area of the lesion. The selective depression of lymphocyte transformation by autologous leukoplakia could be evaluated sequentially on tissue stored from the original biopsy. The great problem with a study of this nature is the complexity of antigens which may be present in the biopsy tissue. Despite all attempts at cleaning the tissue it is likely to contain many microbial antigens.

In later studies Lehner *et al* (1973a,b) investigated cell-mediated immunological reactions to *Herpesvirus hominis* type 1 (HVH1) in groups of patients with epithelial atypia and carcinoma. Cases with oral carcinoma were found to have non-specific depression of cell-mediated immune responses. A specific increase in cell-mediated immunity to HVH1 was demonstrated in leukoplakia with epithelial atypia and sequential studies revealed fluctuations in the lymphocyte stimulation index to HVH1 with a fall associated with malignant transformation. Lehner *et al* (1973b) felt that these results might indicate the involvement of HVH1 in the pathogenesis of some leukoplakias and suggested that the development of the histological features of premalignancy and subsequent carcinoma might be related to cell-mediated immune responses to this virus.

The possible role of HVH1 in carcinogenesis is not clear. This virus has not been proven to have oncogenic properties. However, Lehner *et al* (1973a) cite experimental work to suggest that the virus may enhance papilloma or carcinoma formation in mouse skin when administered with a chemical carcinogen (Tanaka & Southam 1965; Southam *et al* 1969). This effect is not due to either initiation or promotion by the virus. It appears that the virus causes epithelial hyperplasia which potentiates the effect of the chemical carcinogen. An alternative explanation of the mode of action of HVH1 is that the virus might cause derepression of latent endogenous RNA oncogenic viruses (Heubner & Todaro 1969). Lehner *et al* (1973a) also suggested that malignant transformation which results in invasion may be associated with non-specific impairment of cell-mediated immunity, possibly as a result of prolonged viral stimulation.

These developments relating to immunology and virology have extended knowledge of possible aetiologic agents in leukoplakia and oral malignancy. They also suggest the possibility of useful diagnostic tests in the evaluation of premalignancy.

Premalignant lesions—some unifying thoughts

In the absence of detailed knowledge of particular aetiologic agents it is not possible to analyse premalignant lesions accurately in terms of theoretical considerations such as initiation and promotion. Some general observations are possible. Examination of the various allegedly premalignant conditions indicates that in all of these at least one, if not both of two changes, are likely to have occurred. These changes are an increase in new cell production with an enlarged progenitor cell compartment, and an increased permeability of epithelium because of ulceration, erosion or atrophy. Oehlert (1973), reviewing cellular proliferation in carcinogenesis, stressed that a high proliferative activity at the time of carcinogen application intensified the effect of carcinogens. Only cells with the ability to proliferate can form the stem cells of tumours. Thus a lesion with more proliferating cells may be more likely to undergo malignant change. Oehlert (1973) observed that a large volume of evidence supported the concept that the only change which was characteristic for the effect of carcinogens was the disturbance of the mitotic process.

In normal oral epithelium the progenitor cell compartment is confined to the deeper cell layers of the epithelium. It seems likely that these cells are much better protected from environmental influences, whether or not these are carcinogenic, than are the progenitor cells in ulcerated or atrophic epithelia. The importance of lesions such as syphilis or submucous fibrosis is that they probably render the epithelium more permeable to hyperplasiogenic substances which produce an increased proliferative pool.

The foregoing remarks would suggest that the great majority of allegedly premalignant lesions, including the small proportion in which malignant transformation occurs, are probably predisposing conditions rather than precancerous in terms of the ideas discussed previously in the section on the concept of premalignancy. Since the great majority of oral carcinomas arise in the absence of preceding lesions it is likely that the aetiologic factors responsible for them differ from those causing the premalignant lesions. There appear to be two areas which have to date been largely ignored and which may well prove important sources of carcinogens. These are food and the metabolic products of oral bacteria. Of these, the bacterial metabolites may prove the more significant and this may be a factor in the alleged higher incidence of oral malignancy related to poor oral hygiene.

7:4 Diagnosis of Premalignant Lesions

It is not possible on clinical grounds alone to decide if a lesion presenting with the features of premalignancy already described is a squamous cell carcinoma, a premalignant lesion or an entirely benign lesion. This is a decision which has to be made at present largely on histological grounds and as such is in the domain of the diagnostic pathologist. Nevertheless the clinician should know the basis upon which the decision is made and the limitations of the histopathologist.

The foregoing part of this chapter was written with a broad readership of both clinicians and pathologists in mind. This present section is written mainly for the benefit of clinicians, and the diagnostic pathologist will not find in it the detailed knowledge required for histological diagnosis.

The single most important histological criterion in the diagnosis of squamous cell carcinoma of the mouth is invasion of the underlying tissues by the tumour. The tumours can also exhibit a wide range of other histological changes in cell appearances. Similar changes can be seen in lesions which lack the critical feature of invasion, and it is these lesions which are recognized as premalignant on histological grounds.

The histological abnormalities thought to characterize epithelial premalignancy have been grouped together under a number of headings. In older literature the term dyskeratosis is used. Strictly speaking, this term refers to an abnormality in keratinization but by common usage it has been extended to include all the features suggestive of premalignancy. In the gynaecologic literature and occasionally in oral pathology the term dysplasia is used. In so far as this term implies abnormal formation it is probably more appropriate than dyskeratosis. In the Scandinavian literature the terms epithelial atypia or cellular atypia have been used for many years to describe the same changes as other authors describe for dyskeratosis or dysplasia. Atypia is the term which has been adopted by the World Health Organization Study Group on Oral Premalignant Lesions.

7:4:1 Epithelial atypia

The precise designation of the histological changes which constitute epithelial atypia shows minor variations in different authors' writings. However, the 13 changes suggested by Smith & Pindborg (1969) would probably satisfy most investigators. These authors described five abnormalities relating to the proportions of different cell compartments in the epithelium and the arrangement of cells. These features were basal cell hyperplasia, drop-shaped rete ridges, irregular epithelial stratification, loss of polarity and loss of intercellular adherence. Of these features, basal cell hyperplasia describes an increase in the size of the progenitor cell compartment, and drop-shaped rete ridges are also a function of an increased progenitor cell compartment which forms downgrowths into the lamina propria. Irregular stratification of cells probably relates to altered migration kinetics, and loss of polarity, a term used to describe irregular orientation of cells especially in the progenitor cell compartment, is probably a manifestation of altered cell production kinetics and migration kinetics. It might also be due to a disturbance of the bivalent cell division mechanism which is probably present in complex epithelia such as human oral epithelium (Oehlert 1973). Loss of intercellular adherence may be related to inflammatory changes but probably is also affected by altered cell production and migration kinetics.

The keratinization pattern may alter in epithelial atypia in that keratinization can occur below the normal keratinized layer. This is probably due to a disturbance in cell maturation. The surface characteristics of the epithelium are not usually included as a feature of atypia but lesions showing obvious atypia are usually para-keratinized or non-keratinized rather than ortho-keratinized.

Three features of atypia describe cytological abnormalities. These are hyperchromatic nuclei, anisocytosis and anisonucleosis and pleomorphism of cells and nuclei. The hyperchromatic nuclei may represent an increase in nuclear material either in normal cells in the G2 phase of the cell cycle (the premitotic–postsynthetic gap—see Chapter 1) or they may be abnormal nuclei. The abnormal variation in sizes and shapes of cells and nuclei probably relates to disturbances in both cell production and cell maturation.

Three histological changes described under epithelial atypia refer to cell division. These are increased mitotic activity, mitoses at an abnormally superficial level in the epithelium and the presence of bizarre mitoses. Mitoses at an abnormally superficial site reflect a reduced chalone level in the epithelium (Bullough 1972) and an increase in the size of the progenitor cell compartment.

Pindborg and his co-workers have used as their criterion for atypia, the presence of two or more of these 13 histological changes.

7:4:2 Epithelial atypia as an indicator of premalignancy

The importance of epithelial atypia as an indicator of premalignancy has been debated. As noted previously, Berenblum (1970b) observed that many of the histological changes in supposed premalignant lesions are unconnected with the neoplastic process. Cawson (1969) indicated that atypia should not be assumed as a usual or inevitable preliminary of invasive carcinoma. This is clearly relevant in relation to verrucous carcinomas which classically do not exhibit atypia.

Speckled leukoplakias are known to have a poorer prognosis than homogeneous leukoplakias. Pindborg et al (1963) found that 51% of their cases of speckled leukoplakia showed atypia. In a larger series of 723 cases, Mehta et al (1969) found atypia in 8·4% of homogeneous leukoplakias and 59·1% of speckled leukoplakias. Thus the incidence of atypia is substantially greater in the type of leukoplakia known to have a poorer prognosis. This fact alone, however, does not necessarily prove that these two observations are related.

Pindborg et al (1970), in a study of atypia in 51 cases of submucous fibrosis, observed that 22·6% exhibited atypia. In cases developing carcinomas, atypia was noted in 71·4% of histological sections from areas adjacent to the carcinomas, whereas it was recorded in only 11·5% of areas of submucous fibrosis remote from the carcinomas (Pindborg et al 1967).

A follow-up study on patients with atypia was presented by Mincer et al (1972). The results showed that atypia did not invariably proceed to malignancy but that indeed just over 10% of lesions reduced in size or disappeared without surgery. However, 35% of cases recurred after surgery, 11·1% showed increased severity of atypia and 11·1% underwent malignant transformation. These authors concluded that the presence of epithelial atypia in a biopsy indicated a significant likelihood that frank malignancy would develop.

Although this is an area which is still being debated, the consensus of opinion is probably that, while carcinomas may develop without preceding lesions which show epithelial atypia on biopsy, there is an increased chance of malignant transformation in lesions which do show atypia. The individual histological changes which together give rise to the diagnosis of epithelial atypia are not exclusively found in the types of lesions considered to be premalignant. MacDonald & Rennie (1975) for example indicated the frequent occurrence of these histological changes in denture induced hyperplasia. As Mincer et al (1972) pointed out, the difficulty in diagnosis lies in the failure of the present techniques to distinguish reversible atypia from that which will proceed to neoplasia.

7:4:3 The evaluation of epithelial atypia

Most diagnostic pathologists assess epithelial atypia subjectively and there is considerable individual variation in the importance different pathologists attach to particular features of atypia. The general assumption is made that the risk of malignant transformation increases with increasing severity of atypia, although this is an assumption which has probably not been adequately tested.

Kramer (1969) and Kramer et al (1970a,b) discussed the problems of subjective histological interpretation and presented details of an objective computer-assisted system for evaluating some oral lesions. Leukoplakic lesions which subsequently underwent malignant transformation were compared with leukoplakias not progressing to malignancy. Kramer (1969) listed eight features which were given the highest values in the discriminant analysis of these two groups of leukoplakic lesions. Six of these are features of epithelial atypia mentioned previously. In addition the presence of enlarged nucleoli in epithelial cells appeared important, but of particular interest was the finding that the presence of Russell bodies in the connective tissue was important. These are derived from plasma cells and consist of distended cysternae of rough endoplasmic reticulum containing immunoglobulin. This lends support to the idea that immunological changes are important features of malignant transformation.

The discriminant analysis also confirmed the importance of abnormal mitoses (Kramer 1969) but unfortunately details of what constitutes an abnormal mitosis are lacking. The decision that an individual mitotic figure is abnormal is a subjective one and this is an area which requires more study.

The use of computer-assisted diagnosis must at present be limited to a few centres and be used mainly as a research tool. The more immediate requirement is for a simple objective grading system of epithelial atypia.

In 1969 Smith & Pindborg produced a monograph describing an objective system for the histological grading of epithelial atypia based on comparison of the specimen being studied with a standard series of photographs to produce a numerical score or index of atypia. This system has not been fully evaluated on human material but MacDonald (1973) tested it on experimental hamster cheek pouch lesions. He showed that

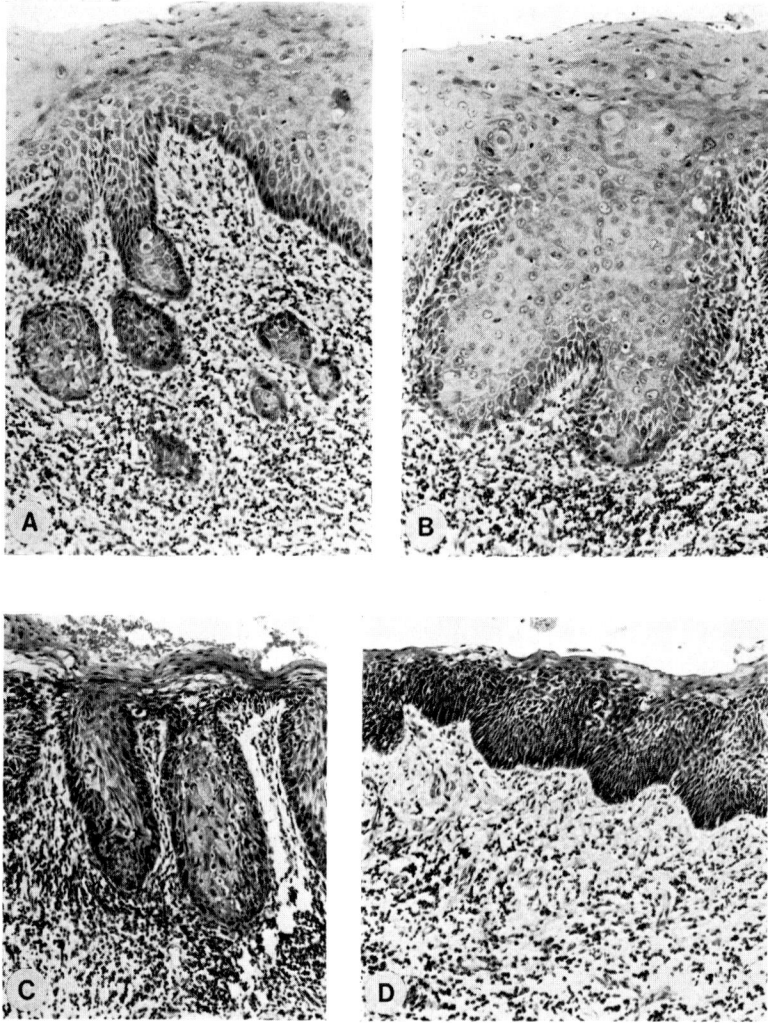

Fig. 7.1. Four areas from a lesion of buccal and lower labial mucosa. These examples are all from the same patient and are photographed at the same magnification of ×96.

   A. Early invasive squamous cell carcinoma.

   B. Acanthosis with atypia showing loss of polarity, irregular stratification of stratum spinosium cells and premature keratinization.

   C. Irregular atrophy and acanthosis with drop-shaped rete ridges showing atypia.

   D. Atypia with marked basal cell hyperplasia and irregular stratification. Note the small cell size compared to the other illustrations. This type of atypia is classified as carcinoma *in situ* by some authors.

premalignant lesions proceeding to malignancy had significantly higher atypia scores than lesions which did not undergo malignant transformation.

Problems of histological evaluation of epithelial atypia

The evaluation and interpretation of epithelial atypia is made difficult because of the facts that histological changes may be restricted to small foci and individual areas even in a single specimen may show very varied appearances.

The focal nature of epithelial atypia is illustrated in Fig. 7.1, which shows four separate areas all from the labial and buccal mucosa of one patient. This presents a considerable sampling problem to the clinician, who must decide which areas of a lesion to biopsy. In general speckled, ulcerated or eroded areas of lesions are likely to show the most severe changes and should be selected for biopsy. The pathologist must then sample the biopsy tissue adequately and it is usually necessary for him to examine many sections, as the histological picture can change dramatically in sections even as little as a millimetre apart. Even with careful sampling it is possible to miss foci of atypia and this may account for some cases in which malignant change has occurred in lesions, thought not to exhibit atypia.

The widely varying appearances of different foci of atypia presents a more difficult problem which is as yet unresolved. It is not known for example whether the atypia seen in Fig. 7.1B has a better prognosis than that seen in Fig. 7.1C. Four foci of early invasive squamous cell carcinoma were found in this same patient and one of these is shown in Fig. 7.1A. This lesion exhibits quite a different pattern from that seen in the other illustrations and shows little atypia. This may indicate the presence of some different factor related to the malignant transformation.

7:4:4 Carcinoma in situ

Carcinoma *in situ* is a term which is used variously by different authors. Kramer (1973) indicated that if epithelial atypia were severe a histological diagnosis that the lesion is malignant may be reached even if no invasion is present. Some oral pathologists use the term carcinoma *in situ* for any case of severe epithelial atypia, whereas others have adopted the criteria used for lesions of the uterine cervix as proposed by the International Committee for Histological Definitions in 1961 (see Langley & Crompton 1973, for review). This laid stress on the changes involving the whole thickness of the epithelium with no differentiation of cells from progenitor to more superficial cells. Kramer (1973) pointed out that some superficial maturation may be allowed in oral lesions without negating the diagnosis. This type of lesion is illustrated in Fig. 7.1D, but there is as yet no evidence that this type of atypia has a worse prognosis than other combinations of the features of atypia.

If carcinoma *in situ* is the term to be used for lesions which are believed to have undergone a malignant change but not yet become invasive, then this in theory is a worthwhile group of lesions to distinguish by a separate name. In our present state of knowledge it is not possible to state on either histological or clinical grounds which lesions fall into this category, and therefore the use of the term carcinoma *in situ* is confusing and is probably best avoided until the prognosis of lesions exhibiting different types of atypia is better understood.

7:4:5 Other possible aids to diagnosis of premalignant lesions

It is clear from the discussion of the problems of diagnosing premalignant lesions that histopathological studies alone are not entirely satisfactory. Much effort has been expended on the search for other aids to diagnosis. Although these have in some instances extended knowledge about carcinogenesis, they have not yet produced more accurate diagnostic tests. Only a brief review of these other studies will be given; because, with the exception of cytology, no properly executed evaluation of the diagnostic potential of these additional techniques has been carried out.

Cytology

Study of cells either exfoliated into the oral cavity or scraped from suspicious lesions has been much publicized as a simple diagnostic test for premalignant lesions. It has the disadvantage that only the superficial cell layers can be examined and the best that it can do is to indicate that a biopsy of a particular area should be taken. An important disadvantage of cytology is the incidence of false negative results in malignant lesions (Shklar *et al* 1968). Cytology may be used as an adjunct to clinical examination to select the site for biopsy but it is certainly not a substitute for proper histopathological examination.

Quantitation in histopathology

Increased mitotic activity appears to be important in premalignant lesions. El-Labban *et al* (1971) reported on the frequency of mitoses in the same material as was reported by Kramer *et al* (1970a,b) and the mitotic values in premalignant leukoplakias were found to differ from those in simple keratosis or lichen planus. Alvares *et al* (1972) used an *in vitro* labelling technique with tritiated thymidine to demonstrate that homogeneous leukoplakias showed faster cell renewal and mitotic cycles than normal epithelia. The practical application of this work to the diagnostic situation raises several problems which have yet to be solved.

Histochemistry and biochemistry

Many studies have been reported on the histochemistry of human and experimental premalignant and malignant oral lesions. These have confirmed the general finding in neoplastic lesions of a tendency for a change from aerobic to anaerobic glycolysis with a change in enzyme patterns. No practical diagnostic test has emerged from this work, but quantitative histochemical studies such as those of Cabrini (1973) indicate that this may develop in the future.

The total lactic dehydrogenase level in carcinomas is increased and there is a change in the isoenzyme patterns. Langvad & Roed-Petersen (1969, 1970) and Langvad *et al* (1970) have demonstrated the altered isoenzyme patterns of lactic dehydrogenase in leukoplakias in Denmark and in India. This has not yet been evaluated as a diagnostic tool.

Electron microscopy

Several authors have reported ultrastructural alterations in leukoplakic epithelium. The most significant changes appear to occur at the epithelial connective tissue interface. Frithiof (1972) summarized his previous work, indicating that most of these changes were not specifically preneoplastic, but suggested that a type of long thin cytoplasmic process of basal cells extending into the connective tissues might be a specific indicator of malignancy. Smith (1972) and Tarin (1972) emphasized that the critical changes in malignancy occur in the junctional zone of epithelium and connective tissue but a full evaluation of the diagnostic potential of these tissue changes has yet to be made.

Immunology

The work of Lehner and his colleagues on immunologic changes in leukoplakia has already been discussed. One further possible diagnostic tool involving immunology concerns the alteration of epithelial cell surface antigens. Dabelsteen & Fulling (1971) demonstrated that in normal oral epithelia blood group substances A and B were found on all cells above the basal layer. In atypia these substances were absent or had a patchy distribution and this was correlated with the degree of atypia.

Conclusions

Squamous cell carcinomas of oral epithelium can be preceded by other clinically and histologically distinctive lesions. However, only a minority of carcinomas appear to be associated with these lesions and the role of premalignant conditions has probably been overemphasized to the detriment of the study of other factors in oral carcinogenesis. Nevertheless, patients do present with premalignant lesions and the work reviewed in this chapter has indicated the likelihood of malignant transformation of these lesions and the particular features which seem to be associated with a poor prognosis. The histopathological diagnosis of premalignant lesions remains a major problem, but advances are occurring in this field and there are possibilities for the development of several other diagnostic aids.

7:5 References

ALVARES O., SKOUGARD M.R., PINDBORG J.J. & ROED-PETERSEN B. (1972) In vitro incorporation of tritiated thymidine in oral homogeneous leukoplakias. *Scand. J. dent. Res.*, **80,** 510–514.

ANDRAESEN J.O. (1968) Oral lichen planus 1. A clinical evaluation of 115 cases. *Oral Surg.*, **23,** 31–42.

ANDRAESEN J.O. & PINDBORG J.J. (1963) Cancerudvikling i oral lichen planus. *Nord. Med.*, **70,** 861–866.

BÁNÓCZY J. & CSIBA A. (1972) Comparative study of the clinical picture and histopathologic structure of oral leukoplakia. *Cancer*, **29,** 1230–1234.

BÁNÓCZY J., RADNAI I. & REMÉNYI I. (1969) Módszertani tapasztalataink Dunakeszi és Felsögöd lakosságán végzeti stomatoonkolagiai szürövizsglalátok alapján. *Fogorvosi Szemle*, **62,** 118–122, cited by Bánóczy & Sugár 1972.

BÁNÓCZY J. & SUGÁR L. (1972) Longitudinal studies in oral leukoplakias. *J. oral Path.*, **1,** 265–272.

BERENBLUM I. (1970a) The study of tumours in animals. In FLOREY H.W. *General Pathology*, 770. Lloyd-Luke Ltd, London.

BERENBLUM I. (1970b) The epidemiology of cancer. In FLOREY H.W. *General Pathology*, 732. Lloyd-Luke Ltd, London.

BINNIE W.H., CAWSON R.A., HILL G.B & SOAPER A.E. (1972) *Oral Cancer in England and Wales.* H.M.S.O., London.

BOCK F.G. (1972) The nature of tumour-promoting agents in tobacco products. In *Carcinogenesis: Recent Investigations*, 92–106. M.S.S. Information Corporation, New York.
BRUSZT P. (1962) Stomato-onkologische Reihenumtersuchungen in sieben Gemeinden Sudungerns. *Schwiez Monatsschrift für Zahnheilkunde*, **72**, 758–766, cited by Bánóczy & Sugár 1972.
BULLOUGH W.S. (1972) The control of epidermal thickness. *Brit. J. Derm.*, **87**, 187–199, 347–354.
CABRINI R.L. (1973) Histochemistry of early oral cancer. *Int. dent. J.*, **23**, 100–107.
CAWSON R.A. (1966) Chronic oral candidosis and leukoplakia. *Oral Surg.*, **22**, 582–591.
CAWSON R.A. (1969) Leukoplakia and oral cancer. *Proc. R. Soc. Med.*, **62**, 610–615.
CAWSON R.A. & LEHNER T. (1968) Chronic hyperplastic candidiasis—candidal leukoplakia. *Brit. J. Derm.*, **80**, 9–16.
DABELSTEEN E. & FULLING H.J. (1971) A preliminary study of blood group substances A and B in oral epithelium exhibiting atypia. *Scand. J. dent. Res.*, **79**, 387–393.
DAFTARY D.K., MEHTA F.S., GUPTA P.C. & PINDBORG J.J. (1972) The presence of Candida in 723 oral leukoplakias among Indian villagers. *Scand. J. Dent. Res.*, **80**, 75–79.
EINHORN J. & WERSÄLL J. (1967) Incidence of oral carcinoma in patients with leukoplakia of the oral mucosa. *Cancer*, **20**, 2189–2193.
EL-LABBAN N., LUCAS R.B. & KRAMER I.R.H. (1971) The mitotic values for the epithelium in oral keratosis and lichen planus. *Brit. J. Cancer*, **25**, 411–416.
ELWOOD P.C., JACOBS A., PITMAN R.G. & ENTWISTLE C.C. (1964) Epidemiology of the Paterson–Kelly syndrome. *Lancet*, **2**, 716–720.
FOY H., GILLMAN T. & KONDI A. (1972) Histological changes in the skin of baboons deprived of riboflavin. In *Medical Primatology 1972*. Proceedings of 3rd Conference on Experimental Medicine & Surgery in Primates, Part 11, 159–168. Karger, Basel.
FRITHIOF L. (1972) Ultrastructural changes at the epithelial–stromal junction in human preinvasive and invasive carcinoma. In TARIN D. *Tissue Interactions in Carcinogenesis*, 161–189. Academic Press, London.
FUJITA K., KAKU T., SASAKI M. & ONOE T. (1973) Experimental production of lingual carcinomas in hamsters by local application of 9,10-dimethyl-1,2-benzanthracene. *J. dent. Res.*, **52**, 327–332.
GANGADHARAN P. & PAYMASTER J.C. (1971) Leukoplakia—an epidemiologic study of 1504 cases observed at the Tata Memorial Hospital, Bombay, India. *Brit. J. Cancer*, **25**, 657–668.
HEUBNER R.J. & TODARO G.J. (1969) Oncogenes of RNA tumor viruses as determinants of cancer. *Proc. nat. Acad. Sci. (Wash.)*, **64**, 1087–1094.
HOBAEK A. (1946) Leukoplakia oris. *Acta odont. Scand.*, **2**, 61–91.
KÖVESI G. & BÁNÓCZY J. (1973) Follow-up studies in oral lichen planus. *Int. J. oral Surg.*, **2**, 13–19.
KRAMER I.R.H. (1969) Precancerous conditions of the oral mucosa. *Ann. R. Coll. Surg. Engl.*, **45**, 340–356.
KRAMER I.R.H. (1973) Carcinoma-in-situ of the oral mucosa. *Int. dent. J.*, **23**, 94–99.

KRAMER I.R.H., LUCAS R.B., EL-LABBAN N. & LISTER L. (1970a) The use of discriminant analysis for examining the histological features of oral keratosis and lichen planus. *Brit. J. Cancer*, **24**, 673–683.

KRAMER I.R.H., LUCAS R.B., EL-LABBAN N. & LISTER L. (1970b) A computer-aided study on the tissue changes in oral keratosis and lichen planus and an analysis of case groupings by subjective and objective criteria. *Brit. J. Cancer*, **24**, 407–426.

LANGLEY F.A. & CROMPTON A.C. (1973) Epithelial abnormalities of the cervix uteri. In *Recent Results in Cancer Research*, **40**, 58–61. William Heinemann Medical Books Ltd, London.

LANGVAD E. & ROED-PETERSEN B. (1969) Studies in oral leukoplakias XVII. Lactate dehydrogenase isoenzyme patterns in oral leukoplakia. *Acta path. microbiol. scand.*, **75**, 193–200.

LANGVAD E. & ROED-PETERSEN B. (1970) Lactate dehydrogenase isoenzyme patterns in oral leukoplakias and in clinically uninvolved oral mucosa of the same persons. *Acta path. microbiol. scand.*, **78**, 505–508.

LANGVAD E., ZACHARIAH J. & PINDBORG J.J. (1970) Lactate dehydrogenase iso-enzyme patterns in leukoplakia, submucous fibrosis and carcinoma of the oral mucosa in South Indians. *Acta path. microbiol. scand.*, **78**, 509–515.

LEHNER T. (1970) Immunopathology of oral leukoplakia. *Brit. J. Cancer*, **24**, 442–446.

LEHNER T., WILTON J.M.A., SHILLITOE E.J. & IVANYI L. (1973a) Cell-mediated immunity and antibodies to Herpesvirus hominis type 1 in oral leukoplakia and carcinoma. *Brit. J. Cancer*, **27**, 351–361.

LEHNER T., SHILLITOE E.J., WILTON J.M.A. & IVANYI L. (1973b) Cell-mediated immunity to Herpesvirus type 1 in carcinoma and pre-cancerous lesions. *Brit. J. Cancer*, **28**, Suppl. I. 128–134.

LUCAS R.B. (1972a) in *Pathology of Tumours of the Oral Tissues* 2nd edition. Edinburgh, Churchill-Livingstone, p. 121.

LUCAS R.B. (1972b) in *Pathology of Tumours of the Oral Tissues* 2nd edition, Edinburgh, Churchill-Livingstone, p. 125.

MACDONALD D.G. (1973) Experimental oral carcinogenesis. Ph.D. Thesis, University of Glasgow.

MACDONALD D.G. & RENNIE J.S. (1975) Oral epithelial atypia in denture induced hyperplasia, lichen planus and squamous cell papilloma. *Int. J. oral Surg.*, **4**, 40–45.

MCCARTHY P.L. & SHKLAR G. (1964) in *Diseases of the Oral Mucosa* 2nd edition, New York, McGraw-Hill Book Company, pp. 298–300.

MEHTA F.S., PINDBORG J.J., GUPTA P.C. & DAFTARY D.K. (1969) Epidemiologic and histologic study of oral cancer and leukoplakia among 50,915 villagers in India. *Cancer*, **24**, 832–849.

MEHTA F.S., PINDBORG J.J. & HAMNER J.E. (1971) *Oral Cancer and Precancerous Conditions in India*. Munksgaard, Copenhagen.

MEHTA F.S., SANJANA M.K., SHROFF B.C. & DOCTOR R.C. (1961) Incidence of leukoplakia among 'pan' (betel leaf) chewers and 'bidi' smokers. A study of a sample survey. *Ind. J. med. Res.*, **49**, 393–399.

MEHTA F.S., SHROFF B.C., GUPTA P.C. & DAFTARY D.K. (1972) Oral leukoplakia in relation to tobacco habits. *Oral Surg.*, **34**, 426–433.

MINCER H.H., COLEMAN S.A. & HOPKINS K.P. (1972) Observations on the clinical characteristics of oral lesions showing histologic epithelial dysplasia. *Oral Surg.*, **33**, 389–399.
NEWBOLD P.C.H. (1972) Pre-cancer and the skin. *Brit. J. Derm.*, **86**, 417–434.
OEHLERT W. (1973) Cellular proliferation in carcinogenesis. *Cell Tissue Kinet.*, **6**, 325–335.
PAYMASTER J.C. (1956) Cancer of the buccal mucosa. A clinical study of 650 cases in Indian patients. *Cancer*, **9**, 431–435.
PAYMASTER J.C. (1962) Some observations on oral and pharyngeal carcinomas in the state of Bombay. *Cancer*, **15**, 578–583.
PINDBORG J.J. (1965) Frequency of oral submucous fibrosis in North India. *Bull. Wld. Hlth. Org.*, **32**, 748–750.
PINDBORG J.J. (1972) Is submucous fibrosis a precancerous condition in the oral cavity? *Int. dent. J.*, **22**, 475–480.
PINDBORG J.J., JØLST O., RENSTRUP G. & ROED-PETERSEN B. (1968) Studies in oral leukoplakia: A preliminary report on the period prevalence of malignant transformation in leukoplakia based on a follow-up study of 248 patients. *J. Am. dent. Ass.*, **76**, 767–771.
PINDBORG J.J., MEHTA F.S. & DAFTARY D.K. (1970) Occurrence of epithelial atypia in 51 Indian villagers with oral submucous fibrosis. *Brit. J. Cancer*, **24**, 253–257.
PINDBORG J.J., MEHTA F.S., GUPTA P.C., DAFTARY D.K. & SMITH C.J. (1971) Reverse smoking in Andhra Pradesh, India: a study of palatal lesions among 10,169 villagers. *Brit. J. Cancer*, **25**, 10–20.
PINDBORG J.J., POULSEN H.E. & ZACHARIAH, J. (1967) Oral epithelial changes in thirty Indians with oral cancer and submucous fibrosis. *Cancer*, **20**, 1141–1146.
PINDBORG J.J., RENSTRUP G., POULSEN H.E. & SILVERMAN S. (1963) Studies in oral leukoplakias V. Clinical and histologic signs of malignancy. *Acta odont. Scand.*, **21**, 407–414.
PINDBORG J.J., ROED-PETERSEN B. & RENSTRUP G. (1972) Role of smoking in floor of the mouth leukoplakias. *J. oral Path.*, **1**, 22–29.
PINDBORG J.J. & ZACHARIAH J. (1965) Frequency of oral submucous fibrosis among 100 South Indians with oral cancer. *Bull. Wld. Hlth. Org.*, **32**, 750–753.
QUEYRAT L. (1911) Erythroplasie du Gland. *Bull. Soc. franc. de dermat et syph.*, **22**, 378–382.
RAMULA C., RAJU M.V.S., VENKATARATHNAM G. & REDDY C.R.R.M. (1973) Nicotine stomatitis and its relation to carcinoma of the hard palate in reverse smokers of chuttas. *J. dent. Res.*, **52**, 711–718.
RENSTRUP G. (1958) Leukoplakia of the oral cavity. *Acta odont. Scand.*, **16**, 99–111.
RENSTRUP G. (1970) Occurrence of Candida in oral leukoplakias. *Acta path. microbiol. Scand.*, **78**, 421–424.
RENSTRUP G., SMULOW J.B. & GLICKMAN I. (1962) Effect of chronic mechanical irritation of chemically induced carcinogenesis in the hamster cheek pouch. *J. Am. dent. Ass.*, **64**, 770–777.
ROED-PETERSEN B. (1971) Cancer development in oral leukoplakia: follow-up of 331 patients. *J. dent. Res.*, **50**, 711 (abstract).

ROED-PETERSEN B., GUPTA P.C., PINDBORG J.J. & SINGH B. (1972) Association between oral leukoplakia and sex, age and tobacco habits. *Bull. Wld. Hlth. Org.*, **47,** 13–19.

ROED-PETERSEN B., RENSTRUP G. & PINDBORG J.J. (1970) Candida in oral leukoplakias. *Scand. J. dent. Res.*, **78,** 323–328.

SALLEY J.J. (1954) Experimental carcinogenesis in the cheek pouch of the Syrian hamster. *J. dent. Res.*, **33,** 253–262.

SHAFER W.G. & WALDRON C.A. (1961) A clinical and histopathologic study of oral leukoplakia. *Surg. Gynec. Obstet.*, **112,** 411–420.

SHEAR M. (1972) Erythroplakia of the mouth. *Int. dent. J.*, **22,** 460–473.

SHKLAR G. (1965) The precancerous oral lesion. *Oral Surg.*, **20,** 58–70.

SHKLAR G. (1972) Lichen planus as an oral ulcerative disease. *Oral Surg.*, **33,** 376–387.

SHKLAR G., MEYER I., CATALDO E. & TAYLOR R. (1968) Correlated study of oral cytology and histopathology. *Oral Surg.*, **25,** 61–70.

SILVERMAN S., RENSTRUP G. & PINDBORG J.J. (1963) Studies in oral leukoplakias III. Effects of vitamin A comparing clinical, histopathologic, cytologic and hematologic responses. *Acta odont. scand.*, **21,** 271–292.

SILVERMAN S. & ROZEN R.D. (1968) Observations on the clinical characteristics and natural history of oral leukoplakia. *J. Am. dent. Ass.*, **76,** 772–777.

SMITH C.J. (1972) The epithelial–connective tissue junction in the pathogenesis of human and experimental oral cancer. In TARIN D. *Tissue Interactions in Carcinogenesis*, 191–225. Academic Press, London.

SMITH C.J. (1973) Global epidemiology and aetiology of oral cancer. *Int. dent. J.*, **23,** 83–93.

SMITH C.J. & PINDBORG J.J. (1969) *Histological Grading of Oral Epithelial Atypia by the Use of Photographic Standards.* C. Hamburgers Bogtrykkieri, Copenhagen.

SOUTHAM C.M., TANAKA S., ARATA T. & SIMKOVIC D. (1969) Enhancement of responses to chemical carcinogens by nononcogenic viruses and antimetabolites. *Progress in Experimental Tumour Research II*, 194. Karger, Basel/New York.

TANAKA S. & SOUTHAM C.M. (1965) Joint action of Herpes Simplex virus and 3-methylcholanthrene in production of papillomas in mice. *J. nat. Cancer Inst.*, **33,** 441–451.

TARIN D. (1972) Morphological studies on the mechanism of carcinogenesis. In TARIN D. *Tissue Interactions in Carcinogenesis*, 227–289. Academic Press, London.

THOMA K.N. (1941) Stomatitis nicotina and its effect on the palate. *Am. J. Orthodont.*, **27,** 38–47.

WALDRON C. (1970a) In GORLIN R.J. & GOLDMAN H.M. *Thoma's Oral Pathology*, 6th edition, 810. C.V. Mosby Co., St Louis.

WALDRON C. (1970b) In GORLIN R.J. & GOLDMAN H.M. *Thoma's Oral Pathology*, 6th edition, 818. C.V. Mosby Co., St Louis.

WATTS J.McK. (1961) The importance of the Plummer–Vinson syndrome in the aetiology of carcinoma of the upper gastro-intestinal tract. *Postgrad. Med. J.*, **37,** 523–533.

WEISBERGER D. (1957) Precancerous lesions. *J. Am. dent. Ass.*, **54,** 507–508.
WYNDER E.L. & FRYER J.H. (1958) Etiologic considerations of Plummer–Vinson (Paterson–Kelly) Syndrome. *Ann. int. Med.*, **49,** 1106–1128.
WYNDER E.L. & HOFFMANN D. (1972) A study of tobacco carcinogenesis X. Tumour promoting activity. In *Carcinogenesis: Recent Investigations*, 107–119. M.S.S. Information Corp., New York.

CHAPTER 8
BACTERIAL AND VIRAL DISEASES AND THE ORAL MUCOSA

J.C. SOUTHAM

8:1 Bacteria

8:1:1 Introduction—Bacterial ecology of the oral mucosa

The ecological balance between the commensal bacteria of the mouth and host may fluctuate naturally over short periods of time, but its overall stability is in many ways remarkable. Various factors may upset the balance, and diseases of the oral mucosa caused by normal commensal bacteria may follow either an alteration in the bacterial flora (i.e. antibiotic stomatitis) or an alteration in the host (i.e. acute ulcerative gingivitis, actinomycosis). Commensal oral bacteria may also be important in the pathogenesis of disease elsewhere in the body (i.e. infective endocarditis). Local environmental factors are generally able to prevent the potentially pathogenic bacteria normally present in the mouth from causing diseases of the oral mucosa (Ross 1972; MacFarlane & Mason 1972a) but pathogenic bacteria not normally present in the mouth may cause diseases of the mucosa (i.e. tuberculosis, leprosy, syphilis).

Since effective chemotherapeutic agents were introduced into clinical medicine over 30 years ago, the development of bacterial resistance to their activity has been a constant problem. An understanding of the mechanisms of bacterial antibiotic resistance is essential if chemotherapy is to be successful. Bacteria may be naturally resistant to a chemotherapeutic agent or resistance may arise in initially sensitive strains or species in two main ways.

8:1:2 Mutation and infective transfer

8:1:2a MUTATION

Bacterial mutations occur spontaneously and antibiotic-resistant mutants originate as readily in the absence of an antibiotic as in its presence.

Mutants have a lower survival time than the parent strain, but if an antibiotic is present the mutant-resistant strain may flourish at the expense of the parent-sensitive strain (therapeutic selection). The rate at which resistance develops by this method partly depends on the dosage of the antibiotic but also varies with different antibiotics, being slow with penicillin, tetracyclines and sulphonamides, faster with erythromycin and rapid with streptomycin. On prolonged growth in the absence of the drug regression to sensitivity usually occurs but is often incomplete.

8:1:2b INFECTIVE TRANSFER

This involves the transfer of genetic material from a resistant to a sensitive bacteria either by conjugation or translocation. Conjugation involves the transmission of a resistance or R factor between resistant and sensitive strains when they grow together and requires cell-to-cell contact, as the factor cannot be demonstrated in the cell-free state. Multiple resistance can be transferred by this method, and in many cases it appears to involve a decrease in the permeability of the bacteria to the drug. A bacteria may lose its capacity to transfer R factor even though it remains resistant, or it may lose both R factor and its resistance. Resistance due to conjugation is encountered almost entirely in commensal coliform bacteria but it is capable of being transferred to highly pathogenic bacteria such as salmonellae and shigellae. Transduction involves the transference of antibiotic resistance by bacteriophage. Originally the transference of a capacity to produce penicillinase to penicillin-sensitive staphylococci was demonstrated, but it has now been shown that staphylococcal resistance to a number of antibiotics can be transferred by this method. It is not known whether or to what extent transduction is responsible for antibiotic resistance in clinical practice but there is a high possibility that it is very important. Drug resistance can also be transferred between coliform organisms by this method, but owing to the limited host range of phages transfer can occur only within a bacterial species.

Only those bacterial diseases specifically mentioned in the introduction will be discussed in this chapter; non-specific bacterial diseases of the oral mucosa due to alterations in host resistance (e.g. blood dyscrasias, immunological deficiencies) are more appropriately discussed in Chapters 5 and 9.

8:1:3 Antibiotic stomatitis

Stomatitis is an occasional complication of systemic antibiotic therapy, the usual explanation given for this being that antibiotics administered either orally or parenterally are excreted in saliva with consequent suppression of the normal oral flora and its replacement by resistant species such as coliform organisms and *Candida albicans* (Garrod & O'Grady 1971). However, Stephen & Speirs (1972) have failed to find evidence of antibiotic activity in either parotid or mixed human saliva after single dose administration of various antibiotics in normal volunteers. They suggest that the most likely source of antibiotic activity in the mouth is the gingival sulcus. In a patient receiving systemic antibiotic therapy the gingival fluid will contain the antibiotic in near-serum concentrations and will constantly bathe the bacteria in the sulci with subsequent changes in the flora both of the sulci and of the mouth generally.

The oral flora may change within 24 hours of antibiotic therapy being given. Garrod & Waterworth (1962) showed that one day after penicillin is given almost all streptococci have disappeared from the mouth but after two days large numbers of resistant streptococci are present. Increased numbers of Gram −ve bacilli are found after three or four days of treatment (Long 1947). With long-term antibiotic therapy Handelman & Hawes (1965) found that although there was no difference in the total cultivable count of bacteria on aerobic or anaerobic incubation, the facultative streptococcal population was reduced by 24%, this reduction particularly affecting *Strep. salivarius*. Antibiotic-resistant strains of other bacterial species may be found (Spencer *et al* 1970), although the type and dosage of the antibiotic will affect the numbers of resistant organisms present (*Brit. med. J.* 1971a). The change in oral flora with antibiotic therapy is important in the prevention of infective endocarditis (*vide infra*) and is a possible preventive measure in dental caries (Scherp 1971) and chronic periodontal disease (Löe 1970). In view of the potential dangers of prolonged antibiotic therapy, the effects of other antibiotic agents on the oral flora have been investigated. Twice-daily chlorhexidine mouth rinses have been shown to reduce the number of bacteria in saliva by 95% after 5 days (Schiott *et al* 1970), and although the bacteria were not studied in detail all the main groups of bacteria were still present. Significantly stomatitis was not described in volunteers after 40 days' medication, suggesting that the bacterial suppression affected all species.

8:1:4 Acute ulcerative gingivitis (AUG)

The typical clinical features seen in AUG are necrosis and ulceration of the interdental papillae with crater-like, punched-out ulcers which may also involve the gingival margins. The ulcers are covered with a greyish-green pseudomembrane demarcated from the surrounding mucosa by a linear erythema. There is usually a short history of bleeding and soreness of the gums following minor trauma. It is often said that malaise, cervical lymphadenopathy and fever are also present but they are not specific to the disease and probably occur only in some advanced cases. The recurrence rate of AUG is high, one survey showing a 25% recurrence rate when patients were re-examined up to six months after the initial attack (Smitt 1965).

Histological examination of the lesions shows that the surface epithelium of the papillary and marginal gingiva is destroyed and replaced by a meshwork variably composed of fibrin, necrotic epithelial cells, red and white blood cells, bacteria and cellular debris. The underlying connective tissue shows marked acute inflammatory changes. Evidence suggests that the initial breach in the epithelium occurs about midway between the crest and the bottom of the gingival pocket (Stammers 1946) and interproximally rather than the tip of the papilla (Blake 1968). Smears of the pseudomembrane stained with Gram after heat fixing show a multiplicity of organisms with a great preponderance of spirochaetes and fusiform organisms. In smears examined by phase contrast microscopy motile amoebae and trichomonas organisms are also frequently seen (Blake 1968). Light microscopy shows bacteria present in both the pseudomembrane and superficial layers of living tissue (Stammers 1946; Schaffer 1953), but accurate interpretation of the appearances is difficult. Electron microscopy shows spirochaetes in the connective tissue up to 250 μ beneath the surface of the ulcer and also in the intercellular spaces of the epithelium adjacent to the ulcer (Listgarten 1965). Fusiform bacilli are also present but are sparse in the deeper areas of spirochaete penetration (Heylings 1967).

After more than 70 years of investigations the precise role of the various types of bacteria present in AUG remains unclear. The disease is associated with a mixed bacterial population (the fusospirochaetal complex) which at different times has been said to include vibrios, diphtheroids, motile Gram −ve rods, cocco-bacilli and cocci as well as spirochaetes and fusiform bacilli (Heylings 1967). Overgrowth of a particular bacterial species indigenous to an area, however, does not necessarily indicate responsibility for that disease, and further information is required to show the aetiological role, if any, of the different types of bacteria. Apart from isolated case reports there is no evidence that AUG is a communicable disease and so in the past doubt has been expressed as to whether bacteria are necessary for AUG to develop. In view of the clinical response to chemotherapy there can now be little doubt that bacteria are involved in the production of the clinical symptoms, but whether as a primary cause or only as secondary invaders is uncertain.

Experimental abscesses have been produced by the intracutaneous injection of live or dead spirochaetes (Hampp & Mergenhagen 1961) and fusobacteria (Hampp & Mergenhagen 1963), but MacDonald et al (1963) point out that the abscesses produced were foreign body reactions rather than true infections because a very high dose of bacteria was required and the bacteria died soon after injection. Individual cultures of other organisms of the fusospirochaetal complex are generally non-infective when injected subcutaneously in experimental animals but combinations of some of these organisms are infective. MacDonald et al (1956) found that while a number of combinations of organisms were infective a minimum of four different organisms was required, namely two bacteroides species (one of which was *Bacteroides melaninogenicus*), a motile Gram −ve anaerobe and a facultative diphtheroid. Later work suggested that *Bacteroides melaninogenicus* is the primary pathogen in these experimental mixed infections (MacDonald et al 1963). This organism produces a collagenolytic enzyme and cell-free extracts of the organism potentiate the pathogenicity of experimental fusobacterial infections (Kaufman et al 1972). Similar experimental infections have not been produced in the gingiva and so their significance in relation to the aetiology of AUG is dubious. The spirochaetes and fusiform organisms seen in the lesions of AUG with the electron microscope are morphologically different from the cultivated strains and there is a possibility that the primary pathogens have not been investigated in the experimental infections with organisms of the fusospirochaetal complex.

The immunological changes in acute ulcerative gingivitis have been investigated by Lehner and colleagues (Lehner & Clarry 1966; Lehner 1969; and Wilton et al 1971). A significantly depressed serum IgG level and raised serum IgM level have been found in the first few days after the onset of clinical symptoms in both primary and recurrent attacks of AUG, the IgG then showing a rise to a normal level during the first month while the raised IgM level was maintained. No significant elevation in serum immunoglobulin levels against *Odontomyces viscosus, Fusobacterium fusiforme, Veillonella alcalescens* and *Bacteroides melaninogenicus* occurred between the first day of attendance of the patients and up to one month after the onset of symptoms. Both serum and salivary IgA levels failed to show a significant difference between patients and controls. Cell-mediated immunity as measured by the lymphocyte transformation test (see Chapter 10) was significantly raised against the same four organisms, but the response against *Fusobacterium fusiforme* was the only one which was significant compared with the findings in chronic marginal gingivitis (CMG). Lehner interprets these findings as indicating that none of the Gram −ve anaerobes investigated has a primary role in AUG. The similarity of the cell-mediated immune response in AUG and CMG suggests that AUG is superimposed on CMG, the significantly greater response to *Fusobacterium fusiforme* suggesting that this organism might be involved in the change from the chronic to the acute disease. The immunological response to purified endotoxins and other bacteria, notably spirochaetes, still requires investigation.

The concept is now developing that reduced host resistance, at a local or general level, associated with tissue damage, facilitates the growth of endogenous organisms, particularly those of the fusospirochaetal complex. In AUG, fusiform and possibly spirochaetal organisms may be particularly significant in conferring special features on the character of the infection. The migration of spirochaetes and fusiform organisms into vital tissue as seen with the electron microscope may follow depolymerization of the ground substance by hyaluronidase and chondroitinase of bacterial origin, but these organisms themselves may so alter the tissue that growth or invasion of other organisms of the fusospirochaetal complex are encouraged with subsequent pathological results. It is not known whether the immunological changes have a predominantly protective or pathogenic function. Known predisposing factors to AUG such as poor oral hygiene, pre-existing gingivitis, local trauma and general factors such as intercurrent illness, fatigue and emotional stress are consistent with this concept of reduced host resistance and tissue damage.

In Europe and North America AUG is almost entirely a disease of young adults and is virtually never seen in children. AUG is however commonly seen in children in underdeveloped and remote areas of Africa, Asia and South America, a prevalence of up to 26% in the age group 2–6 years recorded in parts of Nigeria (Sheiham 1966). Predominantly confined to these areas is noma or cancrum oris, a disease most frequently seen in children with an acute onset and the rapid development of an area of demarcated gangrene. The histological and bacteriological features are similar to those of AUG, and Emslie (1963) considered that all the cases which he saw in Nigeria were an extension of AUG. Other investigations have found no direct relationship between the two conditions (Pindborg et al 1967) but do not exclude the possibility of a similar pathogenesis. Almost all cases of cancrum oris appear to develop in malnourished children whose nutritional status has been still further lowered by an infection such as measles, herpetic stomatitis or malaria (Tempest 1966; Enwonwu 1972).

8:1:5 Actinomycosis

Actinomyces are bacteria (Rippon 1972) which are normal inhabitants of the oral cavity. Two pathogenic species are described: israeliae, the human strain, and bovis, the bovine strain, but they are not host specific and can only be differentiated serologically. About 60% of all infections associated with actinomyces occur in the cervico-facial region and other bacteria (mainly staphylococci and streptococci) can usually be isolated from these infections also (Holm 1950). It is impossible to assess accurately the individual roles of the various organisms in such mixed infections, but it is likely that the combination of other organisms found in the lesions provide improved conditions for anaerobic growth of actinomyces by reducing the oxygen tension of the involved tissues and by lowering host resistance. Attempts to produce experimental infections with actinomyces in man have failed, thus supporting the idea that the associated bacteria are important, but experimental intraperitoneal infections in mice have been successfully produced (Brown & Lichtenberg 1970).

In cervico-facial actinomycosis, the soft tissues of the submaxillary area and neck are involved. Clinically the lesions are characterized by the development of firm swellings which often recur and which after months or years soften and are accompanied by the formation of multiple sinuses and fibrosis of the surrounding tissue. The regional lymph nodes are only involved by direct spread. In about half the cases there is a history of previous trauma, most commonly the extraction of a mandibular third molar (Mitchell 1966). Infection is endogenous and it is usually claimed that either a tooth socket or an infected root canal are the portals of entry for the organisms. However, the infections are almost always confined to soft tissue and clinical involvement of bone is rare, presenting as either periostitis (Norman 1970) or osteomyelitis (Nathan et al 1962). Actinomyces have been described as a chance finding in apical granulomas

(Browne & O'Riordan 1966) but there is no direct evidence that such infections spread more widely. Infections of the tongue and salivary glands are occasionally described.

Actinomyces can also be isolated from some acute or subacute cervical abscesses, clinically indistinguishable from the common dental abscess. Clinical experience suggests that these lesions are acute dental abscesses with the actinomyces behaving as colonizing opportunists and the lesions can be treated as dental abscesses and not as cases of cervico-facial actinomycosis (Mitchell 1966).

Histologically actinomycotic lesions are thought to develop as areas of diffuse oedema and leucocytic infiltration that is mainly mononuclear with surrounding fibrovascular proliferation. Phagocytic cells may transport some of the organisms to adjacent parts, causing fresh foci of infection near the primary one. A central area of suppurative necrosis may develop in each focus, in which a tangled mesh of Gram +ve filaments of actinomyces is present with radiating, sometimes terminally clubbed and often Gram −ve filaments projecting on the surface.

Suspicion is possibly the most important factor in the diagnosis of actinomycosis. If pus from a lesion is allowed to drip down the side of a glass tube, 'sulphur granules' consisting of a tangled mesh of filaments may be seen and should be crushed between two glass slides and stained by Gram's method. The laboratory isolation of actinomyces is described by Cruickshank (1965). Surgical drainage of abscesses and prolonged chemotherapy are the essentials of treatment (Norman 1970).

8:1:6 Tuberculosis

Although there has been a dramatic decrease in the prevalence of tuberculosis in Britain since effective chemotherapy was introduced, tuberculosis is not a rare disease, over 11,000 cases being notified in England and Wales in 1970 (Springett 1972). It occurs most often in the elderly British male but Asian immigrants have a notification rate up to 26 times higher than the native-born British population (British Tuberculosis Association 1966). Two basic patterns of tuberculous disease can be recognized. Primary or 'childhood' type tuberculosis is seen in patients infected for the first time (whether children or adults) and is usually a subclinical infection. It is characterized by a small focus at the site of infection (usually the lung) and prominent involvement of the regional lymph nodes, as there is free lymphatic drainage of tubercle bacilli for 10 to 14 days. At about this time an immune reaction develops which includes delayed type hypersensitivity and cellular immunity to tuberculoprotein. The primary infection usually heals by fibrosis and in some cases viable bacilli may persist in the lesions for months or years. Reinfection, 'adult' or secondary tuberculosis follows a reactivation of the primary infection or is a reinfection of a previously exposed individual. It is characterized by a prominent local focus and there is no spread to the regional lymph nodes, as the delayed type hypersensitivity and cellular immunity to tuberculoprotein developed during the primary infection prevent the spread of the infection to the lymph nodes. Various kinds of antibodies against the protein and carbohydrate constituents of the tubercle bacilli are formed, but the cell wall appears to be resistant to their activity and there is no evidence that humoral factors play any part in immunity to tuberculosis.

The injection of attenuated living tubercle bacilli (BCG) into a non-immune patient produces a relative immunity to subsequent tuberculous infection. The relative immunity to tuberculosis which follows either natural infection or BCG injection can be demonstrated by the Mantoux reaction, which consists of the intradermal injection of tuberculo-protein. The reaction usually becomes positive about 2 weeks after the primary infection or BCG injection but may remain negative for up to 6 weeks, especially in the presence of an overwhelming infection. In later life it may become negative when tuberculin hypersensitivity falls.

Most forms of non-respiratory tuberculosis are now rare in Britain but they occur particularly in Asian immigrants. Tuberculosis of the mouth and throat may present in one of several ways (Cawson 1960).

1 Primary tuberculosis of the oral mucosa. This is uncommon and usually occurs in children and adolescents as an indolent painless ulcer associated with enlarged regional lymph nodes. Cases in adults have been reported (O'Neil 1963).

2 Primary tuberculosis of the tonsils. The tonsillar lesion is usually minimal and found only on histological examination, the infection presenting clinically with cervical lymphadenitis.

3 Secondary tuberculosis of the oral mucosa associated with pulmonary tuberculosis. The tongue is the commonest site. Ulceration is the usual presenting feature but there is great variation in the types of ulcer described in reported cases. Characteristically the ulcers are described as painful but this is by no means invariable. Spread from the lungs is probably via the sputum but haematogenous spread cannot be excluded.

4 Secondary tuberculosis of the mandible or maxilla associated with pulmonary tuberculosis. Clinically these lesions may be indistinguishable

from non-specific infections such as periapical granulomas and abscesses and may present as facial sinuses (Sowray 1967).
5 Very rarely lupus vulgaris of the face extends to the oral mucosa.

Diagnosis of these lesions is made on histological examination of a biopsy. Caseation is usually either absent or minimal in tuberculous lesions of the oral mucosa, and suspicion is raised by the presence of epithelioid cells and Langhan's type multinucleate giant cells in the inflamed base of an ulcer. The diagnosis is confirmed by finding acid- and alcohol-fast bacilli on Ziehl–Neelsen staining, and further bacteriological methods of diagnosis are rarely indicated. When the diagnosis has been made, the patient must always be referred to a physician for treatment.

8:1:7 Leprosy

At the present time leprosy is largely confined to tropical countries, as only in these areas do living habits and hygiene allow persistent and repeated contact with affected patients for the transmission of infection to occur. Occasional cases of leprosy are seen in Western countries in immigrants or in people who have lived in the tropics for a number of years. For a review of the pathology of leprosy with special reference to the oral manifestations, see Southam & Venkataraman (1973).

Leprosy is usually transmitted by droplet infection, the source of the infection being an individual who is harbouring living organisms in the mucosa of the upper respiratory tract. Clinical disease develops after an incubation period varying between 2 and 7 years and can be separated into a number of types depending on the immune status of the individual. At one extreme is the tuberculoid type which is associated with a cell-mediated immune reaction to leprosy bacilli as shown by the lepromin test. This test is similar to the Mantoux test and consists of the intradermal injection of a suspension of heat-killed leprosy bacilli. Bacilli are found only with great difficulty after prolonged searching in lesions of tuberculoid leprosy. At the other extreme lepromatous leprosy is associated with no cell-mediated immune reaction to leprosy bacilli as shown by the lepromin test, and masses of bacilli are present in the lesions of lepromatous leprosy. The other types of leprosy are associated with different degrees of cell-mediated immunity and show different combinations of the features seen in the two polar types (Ridley & Jopling 1966).

The clinical features of tuberculoid leprosy are neural and dermal. Hyperaesthesia or paraesthesia may follow the local proliferation of Schwann cells in a nerve infected with bacilli after haematogenous spread, and the dermal lesions consist of isolated, well-defined plaques with raised borders. Involvement of the oral mucosa by tuberculoid leprosy has never been described, but the neurological features may involve the mouth and face. It is usually impossible to demonstrate leprosy bacilli in affected tissues, and histological examination shows an appearance indistinguishable from tuberculosis except that caseation never occurs.

Dermal lesions may also occur in lepromatous leprosy and appear as multiple, symmetrical, bilateral, macules, papules and nodules. Nerve degeneration occurs late in the disease with resultant anaesthesia or muscle wasting, and may be followed by atrophy of phalanges and metatarsal bones with associated deformity. Similar atrophy of the anterior nasal spine and adjacent maxillary alveolus may result in a saddle nose and loss or loosening of the maxillary incisors. Lepromatous nodules may occur in the oral mucosa, and they often ulcerate and become atrophic and scarred with shrinkage deformities of the tissues. On histological examination the mucosal lesions show in the submucosa masses of histiocytes with only scanty lymphocytes. Numerous Gram +ve and acid- and alcohol-fast leprosy bacilli are also present, and as they are engulfed the macrophages may accumulate fat in their cytoplasm (lepra cells). The lesions of lepromatous leprosy are relatively highly infectious when compared with the lesions of tuberculoid leprosy.

8:1:8 Syphilis

Treponema pallidum is a slender, spiral, motile organism up to 20 μ in length and 0·2 μ in thickness. Acquired syphilis is almost invariably transmitted by sexual contact and primary lesions (chancres) occasionally occur on the lips or oral mucosa. Typically a chancre is described as a clean-based, painless, shallow ulcer on a slightly elevated papule with marked induration of the subjacent connective tissue. Superimposed secondary infection may alter this typical picture and make recognition difficult. Histologically the lesion consists of ulcerated granulation tissue with a dense mononuclear cell infiltrate chiefly composed of plasma cells. In the deeper tissues the inflammatory infiltrate is less dense and perivascular in distribution, and the walls of many vessels show concentric fibroblastic and endothelial proliferation (endarteritis obliterans). Silver staining may show numerous spirochaetes in the areas of active inflammation. The intense inflammatory reaction of oral ulceration usually obscures the perivascular pattern and makes the histological appearance non-specific. The chancre heals spontaneously within two months with reepithelialization of the surface wound. Early in the primary infection spirochaetes can be found in the blood and without treatment the spirochaetaemia may persist for weeks, months and even years. There is a powerful humoral antibody response by the end of the primary infection which appears to have little effect on the spirochaetaemia.

Two or three months after the primary infection, the development of secondary syphilis is shown by a generalized skin rash which occasionally may be accompanied by involvement of mucous membranes. In the mouth there may be a diffuse erythema or the characteristic mucous patch, which is a necrotic slough covering an area of chronic inflammation. The mucous patch heals very slowly and teems with spirochaetes but otherwise histological examination shows no distinguishing features. Secondary syphilis has many of the features of an immune complex disease (Turk 1972).

Over 80% of the lesions of tertiary syphilis involve the central nervous or cardiovascular systems, the lesions presenting clinically many years after the secondary infection. The other lesion seen in the tertiary stage is the gumma, which most commonly develops in muco-cutaneous tissues, bone, liver and testes. A gumma varies in size from a microscopic focus to a large tumorous mass. Histologically it consists of a central mass of avascular, coagulated necrotic material surrounded by tissue containing prominent fibroblasts, lymphocytes and plasma cells. Spirochaetes are very scanty or absent. Intraoral gummas usually occur in the midline of the tongue or palate, and initially are indurated swellings which subsequently often become ulcerated and necrotic to form deep painless ulcers with an ischaemic slough at the base, which in the palate leads to perforation. Endarteritis obliterans is thought to cause the atrophic glossitis which may also be seen in tertiary syphilis, the smooth surface of the tongue being broken up by fissures resulting from atrophy of the tongue musculature. Leukoplakia frequently follows and carcinoma of the tongue develops with far greater frequency than coincidence would permit (Meyer & Shklar 1967). In the latent phase between the secondary and tertiary manifestations of syphilis a delayed hypersensitivity skin reaction to treponemal antigens develops and a balance appears to be struck with the infecting organism. Tertiary manifestations of infection possibly follow a decrease in cellular immunity and immune complex deposition (Turk 1972).

Congenital syphilis may occur if there is a maternal spirochaetaemia during foetal life. The treponemes are said not to invade the placenta or foetus until the fifth month of intrauterine life, and the severity of the disease in the foetus presumably depends on the degree of spirochaetaemia in the mother. Severe infections lead to abortions and stillbirths. Less severe infections result in muco-cutaneous lesions during infancy, an extensive desquamative rash with sloughing being characteristic. Syphilitic osteochondritis and perichondritis result in destruction of the vomer with collapse of the bridge of the nose and the characteristic saddle deformity. Involvement of the developing tooth germs of the permanent incisors and first molars produces the well-known Hutchinsonian incisors and Moon's molars (Bradlaw 1953).

Diagnosis of primary and secondary lesions of syphilis may be made by finding the causative organism in smears of the lesions examined by dark ground microscopy. Intraoral lesions are more likely to be biopsied and diagnosis made by silver staining. Otherwise serological methods of diagnosis are used. Three distinct antibodies appear in the serum after a syphilitic infection. The first, a reagin, reacts with an antigen composed of an alcoholic extract of heart muscle and can be demonstrated either by complement fixation (Wassermann reaction) or by flocculation (Kahn or VDRL tests). These tests usually become positive towards the end of the primary infection. In general the flocculation tests are more sensitive but less specific than the complement fixation tests. False positive reactions occur most frequently in malaria, leprosy, collagen diseases such as lupus erythematosis, infectious mononucleosis, measles and rubella, and the reactions are always positive in other tropical spirochaetal diseases such as yaws.

A second antibody reacts with a protein component of a non-pathogenic strain of *Tr. pallidum* and can be demonstrated in the Reiter Protein Complement Fixation Test (RPCF). This test is more specific and more sensitive than the previous tests. The third antibody reacts directly with a pathogenic strain of *Tr. pallidum* in the Treponema Immobilization (TPI) and Fluorescent Treponemal Antibody (FTA) tests. These tests are the most specific for syphilis and the FTA test has technical and economic advantages over the TPI test. At the present time the WR and VDRL or Kahn tests are used in routine diagnosis with the RPCF and FTA tests mainly used as confirmatory tests.

Tr. pallidum is very susceptible to antibiotics. In Western countries most people receive some treatment for the primary infection and secondary syphilis is seldom seen, although it may be common in other parts of the world. The treatment, however, may not be adequate for a permanent cure and tertiary features may subsequently be seen. The serological reactions may occasionally remain positive even after apparently adequate antibiotic treatment, and conversely may become negative when antibiotic treatment is insufficient to effect a permanent cure although the FTA and TPI tests are likely to remain positive in such cases.

8:1:9 Infective endocarditis—the role of oral bacteria

There is a growing tendency for the classification of endocarditis into acute and subacute forms to be replaced by naming the responsible organism, and the general term infective endocarditis is being increasingly adopted. In pre-penicillin days 95% of cases of infective endocarditis were caused by *Streptococcus viridans*, while during the period 1959–68 only 50% of cases were caused by this organism (Ridley 1970). Ever since the suggestion early this century that bacteria from infected teeth might be a source of the infection in infective endocarditis (Horder 1909), most people have accepted that there is a causal relationship between dental disease and *Streptococcus viridans* (SV) endocarditis, but it must be realized that such a relationship has not been proved. Okell & Elliot (1935) were the first to demonstrate bacteraemia associated with the extraction of teeth, and since then bacteraemia has been demonstrated with gingivectomy (Bender *et al* 1963), subgingival curettage (Rogosa *et al* 1960), intraoral suture removal (King & Crawford 1973), endodontic treatment when the reamer reached the periapical area (Bender *et al* 1963), tooth brushing (Sconyers *et al* 1973), and chewing hard food (Cobe 1954) or paraffin wax (Murray & Moosnick 1941). Bacteraemia due to dental procedures must therefore be a common occurrence but infective endocarditis is uncommon, Hilson (1970) estimating that the risk of bacterial endocarditis developing is about 1:3,000 per extraction in susceptible patients. Other factors must influence whether endocarditis follows bacteraemia, and Hook & Kaye (1962) consider these to be the number and type of bacteria in the blood, and the duration, status and type of the heart disease. At least 1,000 to 10,000 bacteria are needed to enter the blood to give even intermittently positive blood cultures (Hilson 1970), but the number of bacteria in the blood following different dental procedures has never been investigated. The finding of Sconyers *et al* (1973) that bacteraemia occurred in only 16% of patients with periodontitis after tooth brushing, but in all patients after the extraction of teeth could well be due to the relative number of bacteria in the blood following the two procedures, and bacteria may in fact be present more frequently after tooth brushing than these figures suggest. Rogosa *et al* (1960) showed that in patients undergoing dental extraction, curettage and gingivectomy, one-third of the isolations from the blood were streptococci, one-third diphtheroids, and one-third other organisms. Some other factors must then be responsible for the streptococci being far more frequently isolated from the lesions of infective endocarditis than diphtheroids or the other organisms, and for some species of streptococci present in the mouth only rarely causing infective endocarditis (Philips 1972). Anaerobic bacteria outnumber aerobes in dental plaque but only a few reports mention anaerobes in bacteraemia after dental procedures, probably because satisfactory anaerobic cultures were not used. The incidence of anaerobes in bacterial endocarditis is however less than 1% (Werner et al 1967). When living bacteria are injected into the veins of an experimental animal, except for some virulent encapsulated strains the bacteria are largely cleared within 10 minutes, most of the bacteria being found in the macrophages of the liver and spleen. A few bacteria may persist for some time, but all disappear completely within an hour or two. Virulent encapsulated strains are also rapidly removed from the blood if specific antibody is present in the serum. Most patients have high levels of circulating antibody to *Streptococcus viridans* and if SV endocarditis is to develop, the bacteria must rapidly enter the mesh of fibrin and platelets constituting the vegetation, where they are presumably isolated from phagocytic activity and able to proliferate. It is probable that a variable immunological response to the infection, rather than the bacteraemia itself, is the more important factor determining whether or not endocarditis is to develop (Hayward 1973). The antibiotic cover given for the prophylaxis of infective endocarditis does not prevent bacteraemia but assists in the more rapid and effective removal of bacteria from the blood and vegetation.

Congenital, rheumatic or atherosclerotic cardiac abnormalities are liable to develop endocarditis (Hayward 1970), and there is an increasing incidence of endocarditis following cardiac surgery, particularly the insertion of valve prostheses. Endocarditis occurs more frequently with some lesions than others, and Rodbard (1963) explains this in terms of haemodynamics, vegetations occurring most frequently where a high-pressure source (e.g. aorta, left ventricle) forces blood at a high velocity through a narrow orifice (e.g. stenosed valve) into a low-pressure sink (e.g. pulmonary artery, atrium) and so are often associated with regurgitation.

It is widely accepted that the mouth is the main source of the organisms found in SV endocarditis, and the decline in the incidence of this disease since the pre-antibiotic days is presumably related to improved oral hygiene and the use of an antibiotic cover for dental procedures in susceptible patients. It is unlikely that SV endocarditis can ever be eliminated as a disease because bacteraemia may follow such frequent procedures as tooth brushing, and the disease may occur without previous knowledge or evidence of cardiac abnormality (Steiner *et al* 1973). Dental procedures have been implicated in about 16% of cases of infective endocarditis reported since 1947 (Leinbach 1965), and so procedures such as mastication and tooth brushing probably accounted for most of the other cases of SV endocarditis. It has been suggested that the low incidence of SV endocarditis in Uganda reflects the healthy state of the teeth and the rarity of dental manipulations in the Ugandan population (Somers *et al* 1972). SV endocarditis has been described in edentulous patients (Simon & Goodwin 1971), oral ulceration related to dentures being the likely source of infection.

The protective measures against infective endocarditis in susceptible patients should include antibiotic cover for the extraction of teeth, sub-gingival currettage, gingivectomy and other surgical procedures. Although theoretically indicated for other dental procedures, an antibiotic cover is rarely given in practice. Details of suitable methods for antibiotic prophylaxis are given by Kay (1972) and Fleming (1970) and their effectiveness investigated in experimental streptococcal endocarditis by Duracks & Petersdorf (1973). The importance of using another antibiotic if a course of penicillin has been given any time during the previous 4 weeks must be stressed (*Brit. med. J.* 1971a) as a penicillin-resistant flora in the mouth may rapidly follow penicillin therapy and persist for some time after the cessation of treatment (Garrod & Waterworth 1962). Cooke (1970) advises that only one tooth should be extracted at a time in susceptible patients, but Kraus (1958) states that the risk of bacteraemia is increased little with multiple as compared with single extractions. There is no evidence to say whether infected teeth in an already established case of endocarditis should be extracted before, during or after a course of treatment for the endocarditis.

Regular dental treatment should be maintained for all susceptible patients so that all treatment can be elective. It is important that the fit of dentures be checked at regular intervals and the patient advised to report immediately if an ulcer develops. In view of the rarity of SV endocarditis in edentulous patients Beeley (1969) recommends the extraction of all remaining teeth in patients with bacterial endocarditis to prevent a recurrence, but Croxson *et al* (1971) only recommend such a course of action in the small group of patients who have had more than one recurrence.

It might be thought that the necessity for an antibiotic cover for surgical procedures in susceptible patients would be well known by the dental and medical professions and by the patients themselves. Surprisingly, investigations by McGowan & Tuohy (1968) and Caldwell *et al* (1971) show that this is not so.

8:2 Viruses

8:2:1 Mechanisms of viral disease

Viruses are the smallest of all micro-organisms, varying in size from 20 to 200 μ in diameter. They have a distinctive chemical structure, with a basic ingredient of a nucleic acid (either DNA or RNA but never both) surrounded by a protein shell (capsid). Some viruses are ensheathed in one or more outer membranes or envelopes which are predominantly composed of lipid, and the larger viruses may also contain carbohydrates and even some enzymes such as phosphatase and lipase. Electron microscopy and x-ray diffraction show that the capsid is composed of a specific number of identical subunits or capsomeres and the particular arrangement of the capsomeres is related to the shape of the virus and is a fundamental characteristic of the virus.

Viruses can multiply only in living cells and are obligatory intracellular parasites. When a virus and a cell come into contact they may interact in one of several ways.

1. The cell is insusceptible to the virus and the virus dies.
2. The virus penetrates the cell and ultimately causes the death of the cell (the lytic cycle). Four phases can be recognized in this cycle—adsorption, penetration, eclipse and release. During adsorption the virus adheres to specific sites on the surface of the cell and infection cannot occur if these are masked or changed. During penetration the virus passes into the host cell probably by pinocytosis, the lipid envelope if present being stripped off. Once within the host cell, the protein capsid of the virus is stripped off to release the viral nucleic acid into the cytoplasm. In the eclipse phase it is barely possible to detect the virus, but vital components are being synthesized by the host cell's own processes and assembled into virus particles. Most DNA viruses are assembled within the host cell nuclei, but the site of assembly of RNA viruses varies between the nucleus and the cytoplasm. In the release phase the assembled virus particles are extruded from the cell, the virus particles being covered with a lipid envelope from the host cell membrane in some viruses. Some viruses leak

steadily out of the cell as they are completed, while other viruses accumulate in the cell until they are released in a burst as the cell disintegrates.

A number of viral infections are characterized by the formation of acidophilic inclusions in either the nucleus or the cytoplasm, the exact nature of the inclusions still being doubtful. In some infections they consist of the virus itself, while in other infections they are products of the host cell formed under the influence of the virus. Nevertheless the inclusion bodies may be a useful diagnostic finding.

For the spread of infection to occur by the lytic cycle, virus must be released from infected cells into the extracellular environment to gain attachment to fresh cells. Some viruses, however (e.g. herpes simplex), can spread from infected to neighbouring cells by direct transfer, bypassing the extracellular environment. This mechanism of cell infection is usually associated with partial dissolution of the cell membranes and the formation of multinucleate giant cells.

3. The virus may penetrate the cell which then proliferates, and its progeny may develop the characteristics of malignant cells.

4. The virus may penetrate the cell and then disappear giving no immediate manifestations, only to reappear later as a result of externally applied stimuli. This phenomenon is called lysogeny and has only been demonstrated in bacteriophages (bacterial viruses). It has also been suggested that certain bacteria are able to produce bacteriophage in the complete absence of external phage particles, i.e. total viral synthesis by bacteria.

A similar mechanism is possibly of great importance in the pathogenesis of certain virus-induced tumours, and latent infection with the herpes simplex virus could have a similar mechanism.

5. Disease may result from viral infections due to immunological factors. Many theoretical relationships between viruses and immunological changes have been suggested, not all of which have been substantiated. These changes could be due either to the virus infecting cells of the immune system causing direct immunological derangements, or a normal immunological response reacting with virus-infected cells resulting in cell destruction, autoimmune responses, or the activation of biological mediators (*Bull. W.H.O.* 1972).

8:2:2 Diagnosis of viral infections

Three main methods are used in the diagnosis of viral infections, any of which may be used for most viruses, although one method is usually more suitable than the other two for the diagnosis of any particular infection in clinical practice.

8:2:2a ISOLATION AND IDENTIFICATION
OF THE VIRUS

As viruses are obligatory intracellular parasites they can be cultivated only in living cells, and experimental animals, fertilized eggs and tissue cultures are the three types of cell used in the laboratory. The majority of human viruses are most readily isolated using tissue cultures of mammalian cells. Experimental animals are necessary for isolating some viruses, principally the Coxsackie and arborvirus groups, and the chick embryo is the most sensitive method for isolating the influenza and pox viruses.

For the successful isolation of viruses the transport of specimens from the patient to the laboratory is important. The collection of specimens for virology does not differ in principle from the methods used in bacteriology, but unless taken to the laboratory within one hour of collection the specimens should be kept at 4°C or less. The specimens should be placed in a suitable screw-top container partly filled with a virus transport medium. Once the virus has been grown and isolated in the laboratory the identification of the virus may still be a problem. Some viruses produce characteristic macroscopical or microscopical changes in the cells in which they are cultured, but all viruses isolated in the laboratory should be identified by complement fixation or neutralization tests using specific antisera.

8:2:2b DEMONSTRATION OF VIRUS PARTICLES

Virus particles or characteristic histopathological changes may be found in affected tissues or material from the patient using either light, fluorescent or electron microscopy. For the diagnosis of viral infections by electron microscopy the lesions must be accessible and contain virus particles with a distinctive structure and in high concentration. Infections with the pox and herpes groups of viruses are the main ones to fufil these criteria (Flewett 1972a) and formalin-fixed material previously used for light microscopy may be used (Blank et al 1970). The diagnosis of some virus infections may be made by immunofluorescence, using tissue or material directly from the patient or following isolation of the virus in the laboratory. The indirect technique is usually more sensitive than the direct technique and many of the appropriate antisera are now commercially available (Gardner 1970).

8:2:2c DEMONSTRATION OF A SEROLOGICAL RESPONSE

For confirming the diagnosis of infection with a particular virus it is necessary to demonstrate a significant rise in antibody titre (at least fourfold) during the course of the disease. Two samples of serum are required, one taken as soon as possible and no later than 48 hours after the onset of the illness, and the second taken 2–3 weeks later. The diagnosis is therefore usually a retrospective one. The presence of antibodies may be demonstrated by neutralization tests, haemagglutination inhibition, immunofluorescence or complement fixation, the most appropriate method mainly depending on the virus under investigation.

The interpretation of the findings of the diagnostic methods may be difficult, as a virus which is isolated may only be a passenger or latent virus, or it may be associated with an unrecognized infection not directly related to the lesions under investigation. This particularly applies to possible tumour viruses. A rise in antibody titre has to be substantial for it to be significant in view of the experimental error involved in the investigations. Ideally for confirmation of the viral aetiology of a disease, the virus should be isolated and identified, and a significant rise in the antibody titre to that virus should be demonstrated during the course of the infection.

8:2:3 Antiviral agents

The value of antiviral agents in medicine has been questioned on the basis that, in many infections, virus growth may be near the maximum level before clinical symptoms develop. Some viruses, notably smallpox. but also herpes simplex, may continue to multiply for some time after symptoms are first noticed and so prompt antiviral treatment can be of value. Antiviral agents may be of more value in prophylaxis, preventing disease in close contacts of an infected person, than in treatment. Antiviral agents suitable for human infections are:

8:2:3a IMMUNOGLOBULIN

Passive prophylaxis using normal human immunoglobulin from convalescent or pooled sera has been successfully used in the prevention of some viral infections, e.g. measles and rubella, but is seldom of value against established infection when antibodies are already being actively produced.

The preparation and concentration of specific immunoglobulins in the future may be a considerable advantage (Miller 1970).

8:2:3b ANTIVIRAL CHEMOTHERAPY

Many substances are able to reduce cell metabolism and so reduce the amount of virus produced in virus infections. Unfortunately these effects are not specific for the virus itself and the host cells generally are affected so that the substances have little therapeutic value. Only three chemicals are at present of value in the prevention or treatment or viral infections.
1 Adamantanamine prevents the penetration of some viruses into the host cell, e.g. influenza and rubella, but its potential toxicity limits its value.
2 Iododeoxyuridine (IDU) is an analogue of thymidine which becomes incorporated into DNA, which then fails to function normally so that defective virus enzymes and capsid proteins are produced. It is only of value against DNA viruses, particularly herpes simplex virus. The incorporation of IDU into mammalian cells may possibly have a mutagenic effect and the use of such an agent in a self-limiting disease has been questioned by Hardwick et al (1969).
3 Isatin thiosemicarbazone affects the assembly or maturation of the virus particles in the lytic cycle and is of value in the prophylaxis of smallpox.

8:2:3c INTERFERON

This is a protein produced by a cell infected with a virus, which prevents the formation of virus specified proteins, i.e. the nucleic acid and the protein capsid. Interferons are species specific but have a broad spectrum of antiviral activity. They are poor antigens and of remarkably low toxicity, and after their discovery in 1957 it was hoped that they would be of great value in the treatment of viral infections. Their value, however, still remains to be determined, partly due to the great technical difficulties involved in the production of quantities of exogenous interferon sufficient for therapeutic use. A number of non-viral chemical and parasitic interferon inducers have been described, and it could well be that in the future exogenous interferon will be used for rapid protection followed by an inducer producing relatively much larger amounts of interferon after a delay of a few hours (Finter 1970).

8:2:4 Classification of viruses

There is no widely accepted classification of viruses and most systems of classification are based primarily on morphology, the type of nucleic acid present and the site of replication in the host cell. The following is a useful classification of human viruses with the groups arranged from the largest to the smallest viruses.

1. Pox group (DNA), e.g. smallpox virus, molluscum virus.
2. Myxovirus group (RNA), e.g. measles virus, mumps virus.
3. Herpes group (DNA), e.g. herpes simplex virus, varicella–zoster virus, EB virus, cytomegalic virus.
4. Adenovirus group (DNA)—causes respiratory infections.
5. Reovirus group (RNA)—causes respiratory and enteric infections.
6. Arborvirus group (RNA), e.g. yellow fever.
7. Papovavirus group (DNA), e.g. papilloma virus of man, polyoma virus.
8. Picornavirus group (RNA), e.g. Coxsackie viruses.
9. Virus-like particles, e.g. Australia antigen.

Viral diseases with oral manifestations will be discussed in this chapter, as well as viral diseases with no oral manifestations but which are particularly significant to anyone dealing with the oral cavity. Diseases with oral manifestations for which a viral aetiology has been suggested but not proven will also be mentioned.

8:2:5 Smallpox virus

Intraoral lesions are frequently seen in smallpox but are overshadowed by skin lesions.

8:2:6 Molluscum virus

This virus causes molluscum contagiosum, which clinically is characterized by a variable number of warty, dome-shaped nodules with umbilicated centres distributed over the body, particularly the face. Lesions on the lip and oral mucosa have been described (Clausen 1972) but are very rare.

8:2:7 Measles virus

The clinical features of measles infection are distinguished by a catarrhal phase lasting about 4 days before the characteristic rash appears. During this phase Koplik's spots can often be seen. These are tiny white spots with inflamed margins on the buccal and vestibular mucosa opposite the molar teeth, and they vary in number from a few to several hundreds. It has been suggested that Koplik's spots are Fordyce spots seen against an unusually erythematous buccal mucosa. Severe oral ulceration is often seen with measles in parts of Africa, malnutrition apparently being an important associated factor (Morley et al 1963).

8:2:8 Mumps virus

Involvement of the salivary glands occurs in almost all cases of mumps, usually the parotid glands but occasionally the submandibular or sublingual glands only are affected. The glands are swollen and painful and the openings of the ducts in the mouth may be inflamed and swollen. The virus can readily be isolated from the saliva.

8:2:9 Herpes simplex virus (HSV)

Primary infections with HSV are characterized by the acute onset of a systemic illness often with only slight local symptoms, the most frequent clinical presentation being acute herpetic gingivostomatitis. Following an incubation period of 4 or 5 days, the patient complains of malaise, irritability, headache, fever, and within a day or two the mouth becomes uncomfortable. Examination shows a usually widespread inflammation of the marginal and attached gingivae which are erythematous and oedematous. Numerous small vesicles develop anywhere on the oral mucosa and lips, but the vesicles soon ulcerate and become secondarily infected. The ulcers on the lips become crusted and if saliva dribbles from the mouth similar lesions may develop on the face. The cervical lymph glands are usually enlarged. Fresh crops of vesicles develop but the symptoms begin to subside about the sixth day of fever, and the oral lesions and lymphadenopathy take 10 to 14 days to resolve. In young children the infection may only be transient and the condition diagnosed as teething or tonsillitis (Knox 1968). In adults the infection is often dramatic with severe malaise and irritability.

Less frequent sites of primary infection are the eyes, upper respiratory tract, genitalia, central nervous system and skin. Primary implantation herpes of the hands is a particular problem to dental and medical personnel (Southam et al 1968), for if the virus is implanted into the skin in a non-immune person a severe local infection follows with vesicles, ulcers, local adenitis, and frequently a marked constitutional disturbance. Herpetic whitlow is a type of primary infection which affects one or several fingers, characteristically presenting with an extremely painful finger pulp and vesicles which initially contain clear fluid. Untreated the lesions take 3–4 weeks to heal (Stern *et al* 1959).

Serological studies indicate that about two out of every three primary herpetic infections are subclinical and pass unnoticed by the patient (Juel-Jensen & MacCallum 1972). Epidemiological studies indicate that the incidence of primary infections in the first two decades of life is related to socio-economic conditions. The apparent overall decrease in the incidence of primary herpetic infection in the United Kingdom over the last 20 years associated with an increasing incidence of primary infections in adults, is probably related to improved housing conditions with less overcrowding and increased awareness of hygiene (Smith *et al* 1967).

About one in three of those who have had a primary infection later develop recurrent infections which are characterized by marked local symptoms, unaccompanied by systemic illness. Herpes labialis is the most frequent type of recurrent infection, a cluster of vesicles which soon scab appearing on the lips a few hours after an itching or tingling feeling has been noticed in the site of the eruption. The lesions usually last for 2–3 days but sometimes persist for 2–3 weeks. The recurrences may be brought on by a number of different stimuli such as ultraviolet light, mechanical trauma or pyrexia, and the intervals between recurrences vary greatly. The lesions tend to recur in a similar site in any one individual.

Some writers consider that recurrent intraoral infections do not occur (McCarthy & Shklar 1964), but a number of proven cases have now been described (Griffin 1965; Southam 1969; Greenberg *et al* 1969). The typical features reported are single or small clusters of vesicles which rapidly break down into ulcers, occurring on the keratinized mucosa of the palate or gingiva and sometimes associated with herpes labialis. It may be impossible clinically to distinguish between such lesions and other, far more common types of recurrent oral ulceration. Less frequent sites of recurrent herpetic infection are the eyes, genitalia and the skin, where the lesions most frequently occur on the face. HSV has also been incriminated as the cause of facial palsy (McCormick 1972).

HSV infection occasionally occurs in the newborn. There is usually a definite close contact with open herpetic infection of some form, and the infant develops jaundice in the second week of life due to hepato-adrenal necrosis. There is a very high death rate and prevention is essential (MacCallum & Partridge 1968).

Disseminated HSV infection with a high mortality has been described in children between 2 months and 2 years of age. The cases described have all occurred in Africa and were related to malnutrition or coincided with some other infection, usually measles (Kipps et al 1967).

A diagnosis of herpetic infection can generally be made in the light of the clinical manifestations, but the diagnosis may be confirmed by a number of laboratory methods.

1 Isolation of the virus either in tissue culture or the chorio-allantoic membrane of the fertilized egg. HSV can be isolated from the mouths of 7% of healthy people (Buddingh et al 1953) and so there is a possibility of chance isolation.

2 Primary infections are associated with a rise in antibody titre, and the titre of neutralizing antibodies is more reliable than the titre of complement-fixing antibodies, as the latter may not rise in a mild primary infection (Dascomb et al 1955). A small rise in antibody titre may occur in the first or second recurrence after a primary infection. The initial antibody response is a marked increase in IgM followed after 21 days by a predominance of IgA and IgG (Tokumaru 1966).

3 Histological examination of an intact vesicle, though rarely possible, shows the vesicle to be intra-epithelial with characteristic giant and balloon cells at the lateral margins and base of the vesicle. Such an appearance is indistinguishable from chickenpox and zoster. Electron microscopy of either fresh or formalin-fixed material (Roy & Wolman 1969) and immunofluorescence (Gardner et al 1968) have both been used in the diagnosis of herpetic infections. Exfoliative cytological examination of the lesions may show characteristic changes (Southam et al 1968) due to either a giant cell strain of virus which produces large multinucleate giant cells or a proliferative strain of virus which produces balloon cells and occasional small giant cells.

The immunological response to the primary infection does not always prevent recurrent infections and the pathogenesis of the recurrent lesions has not been elucidated. A number of different mechanisms have been suggested, none of which has been proven.

1 The antigenic differences between strains of HSV isolated from consecutive recurrences of herpes labialis (Ashe & Scherp 1965) are consistent with exogenous reinfection by different strains. Such a mechanism has received little support, but Herrman (1967) and Juel-Jensen & MacCallum (1972) comment that such a mechanism is worth further investigation.

2 The most widely accepted hypothesis is that HSV remains in an inactive or latent state in the local tissues after the primary infection and

between the recurrences. The epithelial cells involved in the primary infection (Rustigan *et al* 1966) and the local nerves or nerve ganglia, are the likely sites for such a latent infection, but until the recent reports of the isolation of HSV from trigeminal ganglia (Bastian *et al* 1972; Baringer & Swoveland 1973; Rodda *et al* 1973) all attempts to unmask such a virus failed.

3   HSV can be isolated from saliva or tears in 7% of apparently healthy individuals (Buddingh *et al* 1953) and from respiratory secretions in a slightly higher percentage of patients with upper respiratory tract infections (Lingren *et al* 1968). Douglas & Couch (1970) isolated HSV from mixed saliva on at least one occasion in 8 out of 10 healthy individuals examined thrice weekly for 5 months, but the virus was never isolated from parotid saliva. Immunofluorescent studies show HSV in lacrymal gland duct cells in patients suffering from recurrent herpetic keratitis (Kaufman *et al* 1968) and the virus might similarly be present in salivary gland duct cells in some individuals. Rizzo & Ashe (1964) inoculated HSV into the oral mucosa of rabbits and noted an inward extension of such a primary infection into the minor salivary glands, but recurrent infections did not occur. Chronic virus multiplication in the upper respiratory tract and salivary glands (excluding the parotid) is therefore a possible source of HSV in recurrent infections, and the question then arises of why recurrent infections are so infrequent compared with the frequency with which virus is present in saliva.

4   Serum IgA levels in patients with recurrent herpes lesions are reported to be significantly less than in symptomless patients with HSV in their saliva (Greenberg & Brightman 1971). The protective role of IgA in mucocutaneous tissues may therefore be impaired in patients with recurrent infections.

5   Cell-mediated immunity is an important defence mechanism against viruses, and herpetic infections frequently occur in patients with myeloproliferative and lymphoproliferative disorders in which abnormalities of the immune response are frequent (Aston *et al* 1972). Wilton *et al* (1972) have investigated the cell-mediated and antibody responses to HSV in patients with primary and recurrent infections, and their findings suggest that susceptibility to recurrent infections is related to impairment of lymphocyte activity (reflected by impaired production of macrophage migration inhibition factor and lymphocyte cytotoxicity) and not to any impairment of lymphocyte sensitization or antibody production.

   The treatment of primary and recurrent intraoral and labial herpetic infections with IDU has been described by Jaffe & Lehner (1968). They found that the healing time of primary herpetic stomatitis was accelerated by 50% and the duration of symptoms and lesions in recurrent herpes labialis was considerably reduced. It was also suggested that prompt treatment of the primary infection might prevent recurrent infections. Hardwick et al (1969) have questioned the wisdom of employing a drug of potentially mutagenic activity in a self-limiting disease of children.

It is now agreed that there are two types of HSV with serological, biological and clinical differences. Type 1 virus is associated with infections of the skin and mucous membranes and type 2 virus is associated with infections of the genitalia. Sero-epidemiological studies have shown a relationship between carcinoma of the uterine cervix and HSV type 2 infection (Rawls et al 1970), but whether this is a causal relationship or a coincidental relationship due to a particular life style has still to be determined. Evidence also suggests a relationship between HSV type 1 infection and oral carcinoma. Squamous carcinoma of the lip has been described following herpes labialis (Wyburn-Mason 1957), but in view of the frequency of herpes labialis this is not very surprising. Tissue cultures infected with either HSV type 1 or 2 show chromosomal abnormalities similar to those which occur in human cancer (O'Neill & Miles 1969) and the virus may have a similar action to a cocarcinogen in experimental chemical carcinogenesis (Tanaka & Southam 1965). The virus may also participate in the malignant transformation of some oral leukoplakias (Lehner et al 1973).

8:2:10 Varicella-zoster virus

The viruses isolated from cases of chickenpox and cases of zoster are indistinguishable in the laboratory and the organism has been named varicella-zoster virus (*Lancet* 1971; Luby 1973). Primary infection with this virus is extremely common in childhood, presenting as chickenpox. Several crops of vesicles rapidly evolve on the trunk rather than on the arms and legs, and the rash is often transient but in adults may last for a week or more. Lesions may occur on the oral mucosa but are overshadowed by the skin lesions.

There is much evidence to support the view that the varicella-zoster behaves like HSV in that zoster is the manifestation of the recurrent infection following the primary infection of chickenpox, although unlike herpetic infections, second attacks of zoster are uncommon. As the patient has an immune reaction to the virus following the primary infection the lesions in zoster are localized, usually to the distribution of one or more sensory nerves. The characteristic unilateral vesicular eruption is frequently preceded by pain and paraesthesia for up to 2 weeks, and if the trigeminal nerve is involved the patient may complain of toothache (Nally & Ross 1971). Individual vesicles develop on an erythematous and oedematous base at staggered intervals. If the trigeminal nerve is involved the vesicles may be entirely intraoral. Involvement of motor nerves is rare, but isolated facial nerve palsy usually associated with vesicles in the distribution of the second division of the trigeminal nerve may occur. The most distressing feature of zoster is post-herpetic neuralgia caused by the dense fibrosis and the destruction of the sensory nerves and ganglia. Zoster increases in frequency and severity with advancing age and is quite often seen as a complication of lymphatic leukaemia, Hodgkin's disease and multiple myeloma, when the lesions may be generalized. The virus has been isolated from dorsal root ganglia during chickenpox (Cheatham *et al* 1956) and zoster (Esiri & Tomlinson 1972). It is generally accepted that the virus remains in a latent state in the sensory ganglia after chickenpox infection for the remainder of the life of the host, reactivation of the virus to cause zoster occurring when the host defences are depressed. However, the possibility of an entirely exogenous infection cannot be excluded (*Lancet* 1971).

If required, the laboratory diagnosis of chickenpox and zoster may be carried out by histological or exfoliative cytological examination of the vesicles, which have an appearance indistinguishable from that seen in HSV infections. The virus can be cultivated in tissue culture or serological identification of the virus from the lesions can be performed.

8:2:11 EB virus

This is a herpes-type virus named after its discoverers Epstein & Barr (1964), and was first discovered in electron micrographs of tissue cultures of lymphoblasts derived from Burkitt's lymphoma. It was later found, quite accidentally, that patients developed antibodies to this virus after an attack of infectious mononucleosis (Henle *et al* 1968), and EB virus can consistently be isolated from tissue cultures of peripheral lymphocytes from patients with this disease (*Brit. med. J.* 1971b). There is now little doubt that EB virus causes infectious monunucleosis.

Infectious mononucleosis (glandular fever) is usually an acute self-limiting disease seen in young adults (over 85% of cases occur between 15 and 30 years of age), characterized by malaise, excessive fatigue, fever and sore throat, and a significant lymphadenopathy develops in almost all patients. In about 25% of patients sharply circumscribed petechiae, symmetrically distributed at the juction of the soft and hard palate, develop between the 5th and 17th day of the illness (Caird & Holt 1958). Clinical features suggesting pericoronitis, acute ulcerative gingivitis or stomatitis may also be seen (Banks 1967). After an initial leukopenia, there is a leukocytosis with up to 40,000 cells per mm^3, the cells being predominantly mononuclear. Blood films may show large atypical lymphocytes. Serological diagnosis depends on the Paul–Bunnell reaction, which detects heterophile antibodies that agglutinate sheep red cells to a titre of more than 1 in 56. This test is positive in most cases of infectious mononucleosis at some stage of the disease and high titres may persist for many years. A positive reaction is found occasionally in normal people and in such conditions as serum sickness, leukaemia and reticulosis. In infectious mononucleosis the antibodies differ (Pullen 1973) in that they are removed after absorption with ox red cells but not with guinea-pig kidney suspension (Paul–Bunnell–Davidsohn test). Banatvala & Grylls (1969) found that patients who develop heterophile antibodies also have rising or high antibody titres to EB virus and these titres persist for a long period. It may be difficult therefore in an individual case to determine whether antibodies result from current or past infection.

Burkitt's lymphoma is a type of malignant lymphoma and it is the commonest form of malignant disease of children in Africa. Microscopically it has a characteristic appearance, composed of large, highly staining histiocytes scattered among sheets of round or polyhedral-shaped cells with large nuclei and scant cytoplasm. Although the tumour may involve almost any organ or tissue in the body, the orbit and jaws are the most frequent sites involved. Details of the changes in the jaws are given by Adatia (1970). Burkitt's lymphoma has a curious geographical distribution (Burkitt 1970) which suggests the participation of an insect vector and perhaps a viral aetiology. At least three viruses have been incriminated as possible aetiological agents (Stanley 1966), but EB virus is the one which has received the most support. Antibodies to this virus are invariably present in patients with Burkitt's lymphoma and the virus has been isolated in cultures of tumour tissue from many parts of the world. It now seems clear that some factor additional to the virus is involved, as infection with EB virus is very frequent. Burkitt (1969) suggests that EB virus usually induces either a subclinical infection or, less frequently, infectious mononucleosis. In environments where chronic lymphoreticular stimulation due to malaria or other endemic parasites occurs, infection with EB virus may lead to Burkitt's lymphoma.

8:2:12 Cytomegalovirus

Until fairly recently cytomegalic inclusion disease was recognized mainly as a histological diagnosis based on the necroscopy finding of giant cells with intranuclear and sometimes intracytoplasmic inclusions in the salivary glands and other organs of infants dying at, or shortly after, birth. It now seems that infection is a much more common event, as about 80% of healthy adults have antibodies to cytomegalovirus. Inapparent infection may be encountered on histological examination of salivary glands but the infection produces no oral symptoms except for a mild pharyngitis (Lamb 1971).

8:2:13 Papilloma virus of man

This virus causes infectious warts on the skin, which histologically show large vacuolated cells containing few or no kerato-hyalin granules in the upper-stratum malpighii and granular layers. The vacuolated cells have round, deeply basophilic nuclei, and electron microscopy shows that the nuclei are almost entirely replaced by virus particles (Almeida *et al* 1962). Such lesions are found only on the skin and lips. Squamous papillomas of the oral mucosa in man do not show the histological features of a virus infection and there is no evidence that they have a viral aetiology (Hertz 1972). Viruses, however, may cause oral papillomatosis in dogs (Cheville & Olson 1964) and rabbits (Rdzok *et al* 1966).

8:2:14 Polyoma virus

If polyoma virus is injected into suckling mice in the laboratory, an astonishing variety of tumours is produced, arising in many organs and tissues (Main 1972). The most frequent is salivary adenocarcinoma, but various odontogenic tumours, carcinomas and sarcomas are also produced (Lucas 1970). Wild mice are subject to natural infection with the polyoma virus, but the virus appears to reproduce so slowly that a type of harmless latent infection usually results and polyoma virus-induced tumours have not been described under natural conditions.

8:2:15 Coxsackie viruses

These viruses are divided into two groups, A and B, according to the histological lesions produced in mice, each group having many serotypes.

Two distinct infections with oral features are associated with Coxsackie A virus infection.

1 *Hand, foot and mouth disease.* The typical clinical features of this infection are numerous oral ulcers 2–8 mm in diameter, situated on the gingivae, tongue, buccal mucosa and palate, associated with vesicles and ulcers on the palms of the hands and the soles of the feet. Occasionally lesions occur on the backs of the fingers and toes, and other parts of the body, particularly the buttocks, may be affected in young children. The disease occurs predominantly in children below 9 years of age and within households, suggesting that spread usually takes place in conditions of close association. Influenza-like symptoms may be present for a day or two in adults before the characteristic lesions appear. The oral lesions may persist for up to 2 weeks, but the skin lesions are generally short lived and may not be seen in every case (Southam & Colley 1968).

2. *Herpangina.* The typical case of herpangina is seen during the summer and presents with the sudden onset of a mild illness with fever, anorexia, dysphagia and sore throat. Vesicles which rapidly break down into ulcers 1–2 mm in diameter are seen on the tonsils, palate and uvula. The symptoms persist for 2–3 days only (Parrot *et al* 1954).

The diagnosis of these infections can usually be made on clinical examination alone, particularly if the extremities are examined in suspected cases of hand, foot and mouth disease, as the lesions on the hands and feet may not be noticed by the patient. If confirmatory viral diagnosis is required specimens of faeces or material from the lesions should be injected into suckling mice and the subsequent development of a flaccid paralysis shows the presence of Group A Coxsackie virus. Final identification can be made in neutralization tests using the patient's own serum, but this may take several weeks and is rarely necessary. Duff (1968) suggested that specific subtypes of Coxsackie A virus were associated with epidemics or sporadic cases of hand, foot and mouth disease. Horstmann (1968), however, found that different types of picornavirus can give similar clinical features and that one virus can give different types of eruption in the same epidemic.

8:2:16 Australia antigen

This antigen was first detected in the blood of an Australian aborigine by Blumberg, Alter & Visnick (1965) and there is now good evidence that it is specifically associated with serum (Type B) hepatitis (Ferris 1972).

The morphology of the Australia antigen as seen in the electron microscope shares a number of features with known viral structure, and although the antigen is not the complete active virus responsible for the disease it provides a useful marker for the presence of the virus (Banatvala & Payne 1973). The antigen is now called the hepatitis-associated antigen (HB-Ag) and is found in the blood in 85% of patients at the end of the incubation period of serum hepatitis, which varies from 50 to 160 days, and at the height of the illness, which is usually within the first 12 days after the onset of the symptoms. The antigen normally disappears from the blood within 3 to 4 weeks, but in a few people it persists to give a chronic carrier state, particularly in individuals with some form of immunological deficiency. Disappearance of the antigen from the blood may be followed by the appearance in the blood of antibody to HB-Ag, and this antibody is found in about 1 in 3,000 people in the United Kingdom (Flewett 1972b). The severity of the disease varies from symptomless cases marked only by a transient antigenaemia, through anicteric cases with gastrointestinal symptoms to icteric attacks which may be fulminant (Sherlock 1973a).

The classical modes of infection by virus B are the transfusion of infected blood and the use of contaminated syringes and needles. Individuals particularly at risk are drug addicts and patients in renal units undergoing renal dialysis. Other modes of infection are now being recognized, and in a recent survey of acute Type B (serum) hepatitis it was found that sexual or domestic contact was the most likely source of infection in 40% of the cases (Heathcote & Sherlock 1973). The frequency with which HB-Ag can be detected in blood varies in different areas and in different communities. Examination of blood taken for transfusion shows HB-Ag in 0·16 to 1·8% of symptomless donors in Europe (Banke *et al* 1971) and this agrees with the less than 1% frequency of hepatitis following transfusion in the United Kingdom (Sherlock 1972), although it must be remembered that there is a ratio of 3-4 anicteric cases to one icteric case (Wallace 1970). Less frequent ways in which a person may be infected with virus B in blood include scratches, accidental needle pricks and cuts, especially as the injection of 0·0005 ml of contaminated whole blood is sufficient to transmit the infection (Sherlock 1963).

Dental treatment has been suspected of spreading serum hepatitis but evidence is largely circumstantial. Foley & Guthiem (1956) considered that over two-thirds of the cases of serum hepatitis which they had seen over a 2-year period were due to dental treatment, usually the extraction of teeth under local anaesthesia. Ross (1971) describes 4 patients out of a group of 53 cases of serum hepatitis, who admitted to no recent inoculations other than dental local anaesthesia and drilling of teeth, and Sherlock (1972) describes contaminated toothbrushes and dental instruments as sources of infection.

HB-Ag has been found in the saliva of 50% of mentally handicapped patients with high titres of HB-Ag in their serum (Ward et al 1972), the presence of the antigen not being dependent on the presence of occult blood. Whether the antigen is present in the saliva of patients with low HB-Ag titres is not known. As serum hepatitis has been transmitted orally by giving 0·5 ml of infected serum by mouth (Krugman et al 1967), saliva must be regarded as a potential source of infection.

No proven case of serum hepatitis resulting from dental treatment has been published, but the circumstantial evidence appears convincing. Transmission of infection during dental treatment can be prevented by using sterile instruments, and if disposable equipment is not available, autoclaving at 121°C for 15 minutes gives certain sterilization. Details of the effectiveness of various disinfectants are given by Cossart (1972).

In hospitals the accidental infection of medical, nursing or technical staff by injections or skin abrasions is not rare and a number of hospital outbreaks of serum hepatitis, usually associated with renal dialysis units, have been reported (Marmion & Tonkin 1972). The occupational risk of dentists becoming infected with serum hepatitis has been investigated by Jones et al (1972), who found that 175 dental hospital staff showed a similar evidence of infection with HB-Ag to medical and nursing personnel in hospital, which was slightly higher than that in the general population, although the number of individuals tested was small. Baunøe (1959) found that a history of hepatitis (both infectious and serum) in dentists in Denmark was as frequent as a similar history in physicians and lawyers.

Current evidence shows that patients in the late incubation period or acute phase of serum hepatitis and immunosuppressed HB-Ag carriers, typified by the infected dialysis or transplant patient, are a hazard. The precautions required in the dental care of such patients are described by Kirkpatrick & Morton (1971) and Donaldson (1972). Similar precautions should be carried out for patients who give a history of jaundice during the previous 3 months, but after this period the chances of patients with a past history of jaundice carrying infective virus in their blood is probably no higher than that of the general population (MacFarlane & Mason 1972b). The amount of HB-Ag in symptomless carriers is probably not related to the level of infective virus, and transfer of infection from such patients may be very low in the circumstances of ordinary dentist–patient contact. Serological subtypes of HB-Ag have been described, and although some studies show a relationship between virulence, carrier state and serology (Iwarson 1973), this now seems unlikely (Sherlock 1973b).

Procedures to reduce the risk of serum hepatitis in routine dental practice have not been evaluated, and at present the best advice is to ensure satisfactory sterilization of instruments and the avoidance of accidental injuries through the skin. The danger to patients of a dentist who is a chronic carrier of HB-Ag is not known, but present advice is that meticulous and frequent handwashing is essential and that gloves should be worn for tasks that present a particular risk (Chalmers & Alter 1971).

8:2:17 Diseases with a possible viral aetiology

Other diseases with oral manifestations for which a viral aetiology has been suggested but not as yet substantiated are:

1. *Focal epithelial hyperplasia.* This term was introduced by Archard et al (1965) to describe multiple, sessile smooth polyps on the oral mucosa of the lips and cheeks, which have an unusual racial distribution, being seen predominantly in Eskimos and American Indians (Clausen 1972). Histological examination of the lesions shows epithelial hyperplasia with a para- or non-keratinized surface. Many of the nuclei are vacuolated and occasional multinucleate giant cells are present. Electron microscopy shows intranuclear inclusion bodies, which Clausen (1969) interprets as evidence of a viral infection.

2. *Herpetiform ulceration.* Lehner & Sagebiel (1966) suggest a viral aetiology for this type of recurrent oral ulceration which is discussed in Chapter 9.

3. *Systemic lupus erythematosus.* Norton (1969) describes endothelial inclusions in active lesions of systemic lupus erythematosus which he interprets as either viral in nature of a reactive phenomenon of the cells at the site of active disease.

4. *Erythema multiforme.* This term means different things to different people (*Brit. Med. J.* 1972), but it is generally used to describe an inflammatory disease which may involve skin, genital, ocular and oral mucous membranes. As the name implies the lesions on the skin may be multiform and include macules, papules, vesicles and bullae. Vesicles and bullae may occur on the oral mucosa and they rapidly break down to form extensive and irregular ulcers. Extensive erosions covered with haemorrhagic crusts are typically seen on the lips, tongue and cheeks.

The disease is self-limiting over 2–6 weeks, but the lesions sometimes recur. Severe erythema multiforme starting abruptly with fever and extensive involvement of skin and mucous membrane is often referred to as Stevens–Johnson syndrome. The pathological process initially involves the superficial blood vessels with a cellular exudate of lymphocytes, histiocytes and erythrocytes which move up and into the epithelium with secondary degenerative changes in the epithelium (Ackerman et al 1971). Both subepithelial and intra-epithelial vesicles may develop in the oral mucosa (Cooke 1960; Wooten et al 1967), but intra-epithelial vesicles tend to predominate (Ackerman et al 1971). The aetiology is unknown but the disease can be regarded as a symptom complex following some type of immunological reaction to a number of different stimuli, which Shelley (1967) lists as drugs, contactants, internal malignancy, collagen diseases, vaccines, food, hormones and infections. Both bacteria and viruses have been implicated, herpes virus most frequently but also Coxsackie and measles viruses and mycoplasmas (Kennet 1968). The precipitating cause may not be found even after a detailed history, clinical examination, bacteriological and virological investigations. The treatment is mainly symptomatic, but systemic steroids may provide dramatic relief in severe cases and antibiotics may be given to prevent secondary bacterial infection.

8:3 References

ACKERMAN A.B., PENNEYS N.S. & CLARK W.H. (1971) Erythema multiforme exudativum: distinctive pathological process. *Brit. J. Derm.*, **84**, 554–566.

ADATIA A.K. (1970) Dental aspects. In BURKITT D.P. & WRIGHT D.H. *Burkitt's Lymphoma*, 34–42. E. & S. Livingstone, Edinburgh.

ALMEIDA JUNE D., HOWATSON A.F. & WILLIAMS M.G. (1962) Electron microscope study of human warts; sites of virus production and nature of the inclusion bodies. *J. invest. Derm.*, **38**, 337–345.

ARCHARD H.O., HECK J.W. & STANLEY H.R. (1965) Focal epithelial hyperplasia: an unusual oral mucosal lesion found in Indian children. *Oral Surg. Oral Med. & Oral Path.*, **20**, 201–212.

ASHE W.K. & SCHERP H.W. (1965) Antigenic variations in herpes simplex virus isolants from successive recurrences of herpes labialis. *J. Immunol.*, **94**, 385–394.

ASTON D.L., COHEN A. & SPINDLER MARGARET (1972) Herpesvirus hominis infection in patients with myeloproliferative and lymphoproliferative disorders. *Brit. med. J.*, **4**, 462–465.

BANATVALA J.E. & GRYLLS SALLY G. (1969) Serological studies in infectious mononucleosis. *Brit. med. J.*, **3**, 444–446.

BANATVALA J.E. & PAYNE C. (1973) Effects on plants of sera from patients with HB Ag-associated hepatitis. *Lancet*, **1**, 1359–1362.

BANKE O., DYBKJAER E., NORDENFELT E. & REINICKE V. (1971) Australia antigen and antibody in 10,000 Danish blood-donors. *Lancet*, **1**, 860–861 (letter).

BANKS P. (1967) Infectious mononucleosis. *Brit. J. oral Surg.*, **4**, 227–234.

BARINGER J.R. & SWOVELAND P. (1973) Recovery of herpes-simplex virus from human trigeminal ganglions. *New Engl. J. Med.*, **288**, 648–650.

BASTIAN F.O., RABSON A.S., LEE C.L. & TRALKA T.S. (1972) Herpes virus hominis isolation from human trigeminal ganglion. *Science*, **178**, 306–307.

BAUNØE J.H. (1959) Incidence of infectious hepatitis in Danish dentists. *Tandlaegebladet*, **63**, 407–417, in *Dental Abstracts*, 1960, **5**, 441.

BEELEY LINDA (1969) Teeth, Streptococcus viridans and subacute bacterial endocarditis. *Brit. dent. J.*, **127**, 424.

BENDER I.B., SELTZER S., TASHMAN S. & MELOFF G. (1963) Dental procedures in patients with rheumatic heart disease. *Oral Surg. Oral Med. & Oral Path.*, **16**, 466–473.

BLAKE G.C. (1968) The microbiology of acute ulcerative gingivitis with reference to the culture of oral trichomonads and spirochaetes. *Proc. R. Soc. Med.*, **61**, 131–136.

BLANK H., DAVIS C. & COLLINS CAROL (1970) Electron microscopy for the diagnosis of cutaneous viral infections. *Brit. J. Derm.*, **83**, 69–80.

BLUMBERG B.S., ALTER H.J. & VISNICH S. (1965) A 'new' antigen in leukemia sera. *J. Am. med. Ass.*, **191**, 541–546.

BRADLAW R.V. (1953) The dental stigmata of prenatal syphilis. *Oral Surg. Oral Med. & Oral Path.*, **6**, 147–158.

Brit. med. J. (1971a) Penicillin and the mouth flora. **2**, 63–4.

Brit. med. J. (1971b) Herpesvirus ubique. **4**, 574.

Brit. med. J. (1972) Erythema multiforme. **1**, 63–64.

BRITISH TUBERCULOSIS ASSOCIATION (1966) Tuberculosis among immigrants to England and Wales; a national survey in 1965. *Tubercle*, **47**, 145–156.

BROWN J.R. & LICHTENBERG F. VON (1970) Experimental actinomycosis in mice. *Arch. Path.*, **90**, 391–402.

BROWNE R.M. & O'RIORDAN B.C. (1966) A colony of Actinomyces-like organisms in a periapical granuloma. *Brit. dent. J.*, **120**, 603–606.

BUDDINGH G., SCHRUM D., LANIER J. & GUIDRY D. (1953) Studies of the natural history of herpes simplex infections. *Pediatrics*, **11**, 595–610.

Bull. Wld. Hlth. Org. 1972. Virus associated immunopathology. **47**, 257–264.

BURKITT D.P. (1969) Aetiology of Burkitt's lymphoma—an alternative hypothesis to a vectored virus. *J. nat. Cancer Inst.*, **42**, 19–28.

BURKITT D.P. (1970) Geographic aspects. In BURKITT D.P. & WRIGHT D.H. *Burkitt's Lymphoma*, 186–197. E. & S. Livingstone, Edinburgh.

CAIRD F.I. & HOLT P.R. (1958) The enanthem of glandular fever. *Brit. med. J.*, **1**, 85–87.

CALDWELL R.L., HURWITZ R.A. & GIROD D.A. (1971) Subacute bacterial endocarditis in children. *Am. J. Dis. Child.*, **122**, 312–315.

CAWSON R.A. (1960) Tuberculosis of the mouth and throat. *Brit. J. Dis. Chest*, **54**, 40–53.

CHALMERS T.C. & ALTER H.J. (1971) Management of the asymptomatic carrier of the hepatitis-associated (Australia) antigen. *New Engl. J. Med.*, **285**, 613–617.

CHEATHAM W.J., WELLER T.H., DOLAN T.F. & DOWER J.C. (1956) Varicella: report of 2 fatal cases with necroscopy, virus isolation and serologic studies. *Am. J. Path.*, **32**, 1015–1035.
CHEVILLE N.F. & OLSON C. (1964) Cytology of the canine oral papilloma. *Am. J. Path.*, **45**, 849–872.
CLAUSEN F.P. (1969) Histopathology of focal epithelial hyperplasia. *Tandlaegebladet*, **73**, 1013–1022.
CLAUSEN F.P. (1972) Rare oral disorders (molluscum contagiosum, localised keratoacanthoma, verrucae, condyloma acuminatum, and focal epithelial hyperplasia). *Oral Surg. Oral Med. & Oral Path.*, **34**, 604–618.
COBE H.M. (1954) Transitory bacteraemia. *Oral Surg. Oral Med. & Oral Path.*, **7**, 609–615.
COOKE B.E.D. (1960) The diagnosis of bullous lesions affecting the oral mucosa. *Brit. dent. J.*, **109**, 131–138.
COOKE B.E.D. (1970) Dental bacteriaemia. *Proc. R. Soc. Med.*, **63**, 263–267.
COSSART YVONNE E. (1972) Epidemiology of serum hepatitis. *Brit. med. Bull.*, **28**, 156–161.
CROXSON M.S., ALTMANN M.M. & O'BRIEN K.P. (1971) Dental status and recurrence of streptococcus viridans endocarditis. *Lancet*, **1**, 1205–1207.
CRUICKSHANK R. (1965) *Medical Microbiology*, 11th edition, 305. E. & S. Livingstone, Edinburgh.
DASCOMB H.E., ADAIR C.V. & ROGERS N.G. (1955). Serologic investigations of herpes simplex virus infections. *J. Lab. clin. Med.*, **46**, 1–11.
DONALDSON D. (1972) Homologous serum hepatitis and the dental treatment of renal dialysis and kidney transplant patients. *Brit. dent. J.*, **132**, 391–393.
DOUGLAS R.G. & COUCH R.B. (1970) A prospective study of chronic herpes simplex virus infection and recurrent herpes labialis in humans. *J. Immunol.*, **104**, 289–295.
DUFF M.F. (1968) Hand-foot-and-mouth syndrome in humans: Coxsackie A10 infections in New Zealand. *Brit. med. J.*, **2**, 661–664.
DURACK D.T. & PETERSDORF R.G. (1973) Chemotherapy of experimental streptococcal endocarditis. I. Comparison of commonly recommended prophylactic regimens. *J. clin. Invest.*, **52**, 592–598.
EMSLIE R.D. (1963) Cancrum oris. *Dental Practitioner*, **13**, 481–485.
ENWONWU C.O. (1972) Epidemiological and biochemical studies of necrotising ulcerative gingivitis and noma (cancrum oris) in Nigerian children. *Archs. of oral Biol.*, **17**, 1357–1371.
EPSTEIN M.A., ACHONG B.G. & BARR V.M. (1964) Virus particles in cultured lymphoblasts from Burkitt's lymphoma. *Lancet*, **1**, 702–703.
ESIRI M.M. & TOMLINSON A.H. (1972) Demonstration of virus in trigeminal nerve and ganglion by immunofluorescence and electron microscopy. *J. neurol. Sci.*, **15**, 35–48.
FERRIS A.A. (1972) Antigen in infectious hepatitis. *Brit. med. Bull.*, **28**, 131–133.
FINTER N.B. (1970) Interferons: therapeutic possibilities. In HEATH R.B. & WATERSON A.P. *Modern Trends in Virology*, Vol. 2, 262–283. Butterworths, London.
FLEMING H.A. (1970) Bacterial endocarditis. *Practitioner*, **204**, 238–245.

FLEWETT T.H. (1972a) Diagnosis of virus infections by electron microscopy. In CURRAN R.C. & HARNDEN D.G. *The Pathological Basis of Medicine*, 435–441. William Heinemann Medical Books Ltd, London.

FLEWETT T.H. (1972b) Cell and tissue reactions to viruses. In CURRAN R.C. & HARNDEN D.G. *The Pathological Basis of Medicine*, 414–434. William Heinemann Medical Books Ltd, London.

FOLEY F.E. & GUTHIEM R.N. (1956) Serum hepatitis following dental procedures: a presentation of 15 cases including 3 fatalities. *Ann. intern. Med.*, **45,** 369–380.

GARDNER P.S. (1970) Rapid diagnostic techniques in clinical virology. In HEATH R.B. & WATERSON A.P. *Modern Trends in Medical Virology*, Vol. 2, 15–50. Butterworths, London.

GARDNER P.S., MCQUILLAN JOYCE, BLACK M.M. & RICHARDSON J. (1968) Rapid diagnosis of herpesvirus hominis infections in superficial lesions by immunofluorescent antibody techniques. *Brit. med. J.*, **4,** 89–92.

GARROD L.P. & O'GRADY F. (1971) *Antibiotic and Chemotherapy*, 3rd edition, 347. E. & S. Livingstone, Edinburgh.

GARROD L.P. & WATERWORTH PAMELA K. (1962) Risks of dental extraction during penicillin treatment. *Brit. Heart J.*, **24,** 39–46.

GREENBERG M.S. & BRIGHTMAN V.J. (1971) Serum immunoglobulins in patients with recurrent intraoral herpes simplex infections. *J. dent. Res.*, **50,** 781.

GREENBERG M.S., BRIGHTMAN V.J. & SHIP I.I. (1969) Clinical and laboratory differentiation of recurrent intraoral herpes simplex virus infection following fever. *J. dent. Res.*, **48,** 385–391.

GRIFFIN J.W. (1965) Recurrent intraoral herpes simplex virus infection. *Oral Surg. Oral Med. & Oral Path.*, **19,** 209–213.

HAMPP E.G. & MERGENHAGEN S.E. (1961) Experimental infections with oral spirochaetes. *J. Infectious Dis.*, **109,** 43–61.

HAMPP E.G. & MERGENHAGEN S.E. (1963) Experimental intracutaneous fusobacterial and fusospirochaetal infections. *J. Infectious Dis.*, **112,** 84–99.

HANDELMAN S.L. & HAWES R.R. (1965) The effect of long-term systemic antibiotic administration on the numbers of salivary organisms. *Archs. oral Biol.*, **10,** 353–360.

HARDWICK J.L., LAJTHAL G., BESWICK T.S.L. & LONGSON M. (1969) Treatment of herpetic stomatitis with Idoxuridine. *Brit. dent. J.*, **126,** 247 (letter).

HAYWARD G.W. (1970) General review of acute and subacute bacterial endocarditis. In BEESON P.B. & RIDLEY M. *Bacterial Endocarditis*, 14–17. Royal College of Physicians, London.

HAYWARD G.W. (1973) Infective endocarditis: a changing disease. *Brit. med. J.*, **2,** 706–709, 764–766.

HEATHCOTE JENNY & SHERLOCK SHIRLEY (1973) Spread of acute type B hepatitis in London. *Lancet*, **1,** 1468–1470.

HENLE G., HENLE W. & DIEHL V. (1968) Relation of Burkitt's tumour-associated herpes-type virus to infectious mononucleosis. *Proc. nat. Acad. Sci.*, **59,** 94–101.

HERRMANN E.C. (1967) Experiences in laboratory diagnosis of herpes simplex, varicella-zoster, and vaccinia virus infections in routine medical practice. *Mayo Clinic Proc.*, **42,** 744–753.

HERTZ R.S. (1972) The occurrence of a verruca vulgaris on an intraoral skin graft. *Oral Surg. Oral Med. Oral Path.*, **34**, 934–942.
HEYLINGS R.T. (1967) Electron microscopy of acute ulcerative gingivitis (Vincent's type). *Brit. dent. J.*, **122**, 51–56.
HILSON G.R.F. (1970) Is chemoprophylaxis necessary? *Proc. R. Soc. Med.*, **63**, 267–271.
HOLM P. (1950) Studies on the aetiology of human actinomycosis; 'other microbes' of actinomycosis and their significance. *Acta path. microbiol. Scand.*, **27**, 736–751.
HOOK E.W. & KAYE D. (1962) Prophylaxis of bacterial endocarditis. *J. Chron. Dis.*, **15**, 635–646.
HORDER T.J. (1909) Infective endocarditis with an analysis of 150 cases and with special reference to the chronic form of the disease. *Quart. J. Med.*, **2**, 289–324.
HORSTMANN D.M. (1968) Viral exanthems and enanthems. *Pediatrics*, **41**, 867–870.
IWARSON S., MAGNIUS L., LINDHOLM S. & LUNDIN P. (1973) Subtypes of hepatitis B antigen in blood donors and post-transfusion hepatitis: clinical and epidemiological aspects. *Brit. med. J.*, **1**, 84–87.
JAFFE E.C. & LEHNER T. (1968) Treatment of herpetic stomatitis with Idoxuridine. *Brit. dent. J.*, **125**, 392–395.
JONES D.M., TOBIN J.O. & TURNER E.P. (1972) Australia antigen and antibodies to Epstein Barr virus, cytomegalovirus and rubella virus in dental personnel. *Brit. dent. J.*, **132**, 489–491.
JUEL-JENSEN B.E. & MACCALLUM F.O. (1972) *Herpes Simplex, Varicella and Zoster*. Heinemann, London.
KAUFMAN E.J., MASHIMO P.A., HAUSMANN, E., HANKS C.T. & ELLISON S.A. (1972) Fusobacterial infection: enhancement by cell free extracts of Bacteroides melaninogenicus possessing collagenolytic activity. *Archs. oral Biol.*, **17**, 577–580.
KAUFMAN H.E., BROWN D.C. & ELLISON E.D. (1968). Herpes virus in the lacrimal gland, conjunctiva and cornea of man—a chronic infection. *Am. J. Ophthalmol.*, **65**, 32–35.
KAY L.W. (1972) *Drugs in Dentistry*, 2nd edition, 88. John Wright & Sons Ltd, Bristol.
KENNETT S. (1968) Erythema multiforme affecting the oral cavity. *Oral Surg. Oral Med. & Oral Path.*, **25**, 366–373.
KING R.C. & CRAWFORD J.J. (1973) Study of bacteraemia following intraoral suture removal including use of prereduced anaerobically sterilised culture media. *J. dent. Res.*, Suppl. to Vol 52, abstract 249.
KIPPS A., BECKER W., WAINWRIGHT J. & MCKENZIE D. (1967). Fatal disseminated primary herpesvirus infection in children: epidemiology based on 93 nonneonatal cases. *S. Afr. med. J.*, **41**, 647–651.
KIRKPATRICK T.J. & MORTON J.B. (1971) Factors influencing the dental management of renal transplants and dialysis patients. *Brit. J. oral Surg.*, **9**, 57–64.
KNOX J.D.E. (1968) Trench mouth in children. *J. R. Coll. Gen. Pract.*, **16**, 23–30.
KRAUS F.W. (1958). The microbiology of the oral cavity and its systemic significance. *Dent. Clin. N. Am.*, July, 309–324.
KRUGMAN S., GILES JOAN P. & HAMMOND J. (1967) Infectious hepatitis. *J. Am. med. Ass.*, **200**, 365–373.

LAMB S.G. (1971) Cytomegalovirus infections. *Brit. J. Hosp. Med.*, **5,** 347–354.
Lancet (1971) Understanding zoster. **1,** 690.
LEHNER T. (1969) Immunoglobulin abnormalities in ulcerative gingivitis. *Brit. dent. J.*, **127,** 165–169.
LEHNER T. & CLARRY ELIZABETH D. (1966) Acute ulcerative gingivitis—an immunofluorescent investigation. *Brit. dent. J.*, **121,** 366–370.
LEHNER T. & SAGEBIEL R.W. (1966) Fine structural findings in recurrent oral ulceration. *Brit. dent. J.*, **121,** 454–456.
LEHNER T., WILTON J.M., SHILLITOE E. & IVANYI L. (1973) Cell mediated immunity and antibodies to herpesvirus hominis type 1 in oral leucoplakia and carcinoma. *Brit. J. Cancer*, **27,** 351–361.
LEINBACH R.C. (1965) Bacterial endocarditis prophylaxis: a comparison of current theory and practice. *J. dent. Med.*, **20,** 66–70.
LINDGREN K.M., DOUGLAS R.G. & COUCH R.B. (1968) Significance of herpesvirus hominis in respiratory secretions of man. *New Engl. J. Med.*, **278,** 517–523.
LISTGARTEN M.A. (1965) Electron microscope observations on the bacterial flora of acute necrotising ulcerative gingivitis. *J. Periodont.*, **36,** 328–339.
LÖE H. (1970) A review of the prevention and control of plaque. In MCHUGH W.D. *Dental Plaque*, 259–270. E. & S. Livingstone, Edinburgh.
LONG D.A. (1947) Effect of penicillin on bacterial flora of the mouth. *Brit. med. J.*, **2,** 819–821.
LUBY J.P. (1973) Varicella–zoster virus. *J. invest. Derm.*, **61,** 212–222.
LUCAS R.B. (1970) Odontogenic tumours in polyoma virus-infected mice. In *Fourth Proceedings of the International Academy of Oral Pathology*, 120–127. Gordon & Breach, New York.
MACCALLUM F.O. & PARTRIDGE J.W. (1968) Fetal–maternal relationships in herpes simplex. *Arch. Dis. Childh.*, **43,** 265–267.
MCCARTHY P.L. & SHKLAR G. (1964) *Diseases of the Oral Mucosa*, 80. McGraw-Hill, New York.
MCCORMICK D.P. (1972) Herpes simplex virus as cause of Bell's palsy. *Lancet*, **1,** 937–939.
MACDONALD J.B., SUTTON R.M., KNOLL M.L., MEDLENER E.M. & GRAINGER R.M. (1956) The pathogenic components of an experimental fusospirochaetal infection. *J. Infectious Dis.*, **98,** 15–20.
MACDONALD J.B., SOCRANSKY S. & GIBBONS R.J. (1963) Aspects of the pathogenesis of mixed anaerobic infections of mucous membranes. *J. dent. Res.*, **42,** 529–544.
MACFARLANE T.W. & MASON D.K. (1972a) Local environmental factors in the host resistance to the commensal microflora of the mouth. In MACPHEE T. *Host Resistance to Commensal Bacteria*, 64–75. Churchill Livingstone, Edinburgh and London.
MACFARLANE T.W. & MASON D.K. (1972b) The dentist and the prevention of serum hepatitis. *Brit. dent. J.*, **132,** 487–489.
MCGOWAN D.A. & TUOHY O. (1968) Dental treatment of patients with valvular heart disease. *Brit. dent. J.*, **124,** 519–520.

MAIN J.H.P. (1972) Developmental considerations: carcinogenesis and oncology. In SLAVKIN H.C. *Developmental Aspects of Oral Biology*, 385–405. Academic Press, New York and London.
MARMION B.P. & TONKIN R.W. (1972) Control of hepatitis in dialysis units. *Brit. med. Bull.*, **28**, 169–179.
MEYER I. & SHKLAR G. (1967) The oral manifestations of acquired syphilis. *Oral Surg. Oral Med. & Oral Path.*, **23**, 45–57.
MILLER D.L. (1970) The prophylactic and therapeutic uses of immunoglobulin in virus infections. In HEATH R.B. & WATERSON A.P. *Modern Trends in Medical Virology*, Vol. 2, 284–310. Butterworths, London.
MITCHELL R.G. (1966) Actinomycosis and the dental abscess. *Brit. dent. J.*, **120**, 423–429.
MORLEY D., WOODLAND MARGARET & MARTIN W.J. (1963). Measles in Nigerian children. *J. Hygiene, Camb.*, **61**, 115–134.
MURRAY M. & MOOSNICK F. (1941) Incidence of bacteraemia in patients with dental disease. *J. Lab. clin. Med.*, **26**, 801–802.
NALLY F.F. & ROSS I.H. (1971) Herpes zoster of the oral and facial structures. *Oral Surg. Oral Med. & Oral Path.*, **32**, 221–234.
NATHAN M.H., RADMAN W.P. & BARTON H.L. (1962) Osseous actinomycosis of the head and neck. *Am. J. Roentg.*, **87**, 1048–1053.
NORMAN J.E.DEB. (1970) Cervico-facial actinomycosis. *Oral Surg. Oral Med. & Oral Path.*, **29**, 735–745.
NORTON W.L. (1969) Endothelial inclusions in active lesions of systemic lupus erythematosus. *J. Lab. clin. Med.*, **74**, 369–379.
OKELL C.E. & ELLIOTT S.D. (1935) Bacteraemia and oral sepsis with special reference to the aetiology of subacute endocarditis. *Lancet*, **2**, 869–872.
O'NEIL R. (1963) Primary tuberculous ulceration of the gum in an adult. *Brit. dent. J.*, **115**, 330–332.
O'NEILL F.J. & MILES C.P. (1969) Chromosome changes induced by herpes simplex, types 1 and 2, in human cells. *Nature, Lond.*, **223**, 851–852.
PARROT R.H., WOLF S.I., NUDELMAN J., NAIDEN E., HUEBNER J., RICE E.C. & MCCULLOUGH N.B. (1954) Clinical and laboratory differentiation between herpangina and infectious (herpetic) gingivostomatitis. *Pediatrics*, **14**, 122–129.
PHILIPS I. (1972) Antibiotic sensitivity of oral non-haemolytic streptococci. In MACPHEE T. *Host Resistance to Commensal Bacteria*, 304–317. Churchill Livingstone, Edinburgh and London.
PINDBORG J.J., BHAT M. & PETERSEN B.R. (1967). Oral changes in South-Indian children with severe protein deficiency. *J. Periodont.*, **38**, 218–221.
PULLEN H. (1973) Infectious mononucleosis. *Brit. med. J.*, **1**, 350–352.
RAWLS W.E., GARDNER H.L. & KAUFMAN R.L. (1970) Antibodies to genital herpesvirus in patients with carcinoma of the cervix. *Am. J. Obst. Gyn.*, **107**, 710–716.
RDZOK E.J., SNIPKOWITZ N.L. & RICHTER W.R. (1966) Rabbit oral papillomatosis: ultrastructure of experimental infection. *Cancer Res.*, **26**, 160–165.
RIDLEY D.S. & JOPLING W.H. (1966) Classification of leprosy according to immunity. *Int. J. Leprosy*, **34**, 255–273.

RIDLEY M. (1970) Bacteriological diagnosis and control of antibiotic treatment in bacterial endocarditis. In BEESON P.B. & RIDLEY M. *Bacterial Endocarditis*, 49–65. Royal College of Physicians, London.
RIPPON J.W. (1972) Bacteria versus fungi. *New Engl. J. Med.*, **286**, 606 (letter).
RIZZO A.A. & ASHE W.K. (1964) Experimental herpetic ulcers in rabbit oral mucosa. *Archs. oral Biol.*, **9**, 713–724.
RODBARD S. (1963) Blood velocity and endocarditis. *Circulation*, **27**, 18–28.
RODDA S., JACK I. & WHITE D.O. (1973) Herpes-simplex virus from trigeminal ganglion. *Lancet*, **1**, 1395 (letter).
ROGOSA M., HAMPP E.G., NEVIN T.A., WAGNER H.N., DRISCOLL E.J. & BAER P.N. (1960) Blood sampling and cultural studies in the detection of postoperative bacteraemias. *J. Am. dent. Ass.*, **60**, 171–180.
ROSS CONSTANCE A.C. (1971) Viral hepatitis from dental procedures. *Brit. dent. J.*, **131**, 433 (letter).
ROSS P.W. (1972) The occurrence of potentially pathogenic bacteria in the mouth. In MACPHEE T. *Host Resistance to Commensal Bacteria*, 34–38. Churchill Livingstone, Edinburgh and London.
ROY S. & WOLMAN L. (1969) Electron microscopic observations on the virus particles in herpes simplex encephalitis. *J. clin. Path.*, **22**, 51–59.
RUSTIGAN R., SMULOW J.B., TYE M., GIBSON W.A. & SHINDELL E. (1966) Studies of latent infection of skin & oral mucosa in individuals with recurrent herpes simplex. *J. invest. Derm.*, **47**, 218–221.
SCHAFFER E.M. (1953) Biopsy studies of necrotising ulcerative gingivitis. *J. Periodont.*, **24**, 22–25.
SCHERP W. (1971) Dental caries: prospects for prevention. *Science*, **173**, 1199–1205.
SCHIOTT C.R., LÖE H., BORGLUM-JENSEN S., KILIAN M., DAVIES R.M. & GLAVIND K. (1970) The effect of chlorhexidine mouthrinses on the human oral flora. *J. periodont. Res.*, **5**, 84–89.
SCONYERS J.R., CRAWFORD J.J. & MORIARTY J.D. (1973) Relationship of bacteraemia to toothbrushing in patients with periodontitis. *J. Am. dent. Ass.*, **87**, 616–622.
SHEIHAM A. (1966) An epidemiological survey of acute ulcerative gingivitis in Nigerians. *Archs. oral Biol.*, **11**, 937–942.
SHELLEY W.B. (1967) Herpes simplex virus as a cause of erythema multiforme. *J. Am. med. Ass.*, **201**, 153–156.
SHERLOCK SHEILA (1963) *Diseases of the Liver and Biliary System*, 3rd edition, 264. Blackwell Scientific Publications, Oxford.
SHERLOCK SHEILA (1972) The course of long incubation (virus B) hepatitis. *Brit. med. Bull.*, **28**, 109–113.
SHERLOCK SHEILA (1973a) Acute virus hepatitis. *Practitioner*, **210**, 603–611.
SHERLOCK SHEILA (1973b) Chronic hepatitis B antigen disease. *J. R. Coll. of Physicians, Lond.*, **8**, 24–30.
SIMON D.S. & GOODWIN J.F. (1971) Should good teeth be extracted to prevent Streptococcus viridans endocarditis? *Lancet*, **1**, 1207–1209.
SMITH ISABEL, PEUTHERER J.F. & MACCALLUM F.O. (1967) Herpesvirus hominis antibody. *J. Hygiene, Camb.*, **65**, 395–408.
SMITT P.A.E.S. (1965) Some clinical and epidemiological aspects of Vincent's gingivitis. *Dent. Pract.*, **15**, 281–286.

SOMERS K., PATEL A.K., STEINER I., D'ARBELA P.G. & HUTT M.S.R. (1972) Infective endocarditis—an African experience. *Brit. Heart J.*, **34**, 1107–1112.
SOUTHAM J.C. (1969) Recurrent intra-oral herpes simplex infection. *Brit. dent. J.*, **127**, 276–279.
SOUTHAM J.C. & COLLEY I.T. (1968) Hand, foot and mouth disease. *Brit. dent. J.*, **125**, 298–301.
SOUTHAM J.C., CLARKE J. & COLLEY I.T. (1968) Viral diseases and the dental surgeon. *Dent. Pract.*, **19**, 45–49.
SOUTHAM J.C., COLLEY I.T. & CLARKE N.G. (1968) Oral herpetic infection in adults—clinical, histological and cytological features. *Brit. J. Derm.*, **80**, 248–256.
SOUTHAM J.C. & VENKATARAMAN B.K. (1973) Oral manifestations of leprosy. *Brit. J. oral Surg.*, **10**, 272–279.
SOWRAY J.H. (1967) Tuberculous facial sinuses. *Brit. dent. J.*, **123**, 291–294.
SPENCER W.H., THORNSBERRY C., MOODY M.D. & WENGER N.K. (1970). Rheumatic fever chemoproprophylaxis and penicillin-resistant gingival organisms. *Ann. intern. Med.*, **73**, 683–687.
SPRINGETT V.H. (1972) Tuberculosis—epidemiology in England and Wales. *Brit. med. J.*, **1**, 422–423.
STAMMERS A.F. (1946) Vincent's infection: Observations on the histopathology and their application to clinical practice. *Brit. dent. J.*, **81**, 4–15.
STANLEY N.F. (1966) The aetiology and pathogenesis of Burkitt's African lymphoma. *Lancet*, **1**, 961–962.
STEINER I., PATEL A.K., HUTT M.S.R. & SOMERS K. (1973) Pathology of infective endocarditis—a postmortem evaluation. *Brit. Heart J.*, **35**, 159–164.
STEPHEN K.W. & SPEIRS C.F. (1972) Oral environmental source of antibacterial drugs—the importance of gingival fluid. In MACPHEE T. *Host Resistance to Commensal Bacteria*, 76–83. Churchill Livingstone, Edinburgh and London.
STERN H., ELEK S.D., MILLARD M. & ANDERSON H.F. (1959) Herpetic whitlow—a form of cross-infection in hospitals. *Lancet*, **2**, 871–874.
TANAKA S. & SOUTHAM C.M. (1965) Joint action of herpes simplex virus and 3-methylcholanthrene in the production of papillomas in mice. *J. nat. Cancer Inst.*, **34**, 441–449.
TEMPEST M.N. (1966) Cancrum oris. *Brit. J. Surg.*, **53**, 949–969.
TOKUMARU T. (1966) A possible role of IgA-immunoglobulin in herpes simplex virus infection in man. *J. Immunol.*, **97**, 248–259.
TURK J.L. (1972) *Immunology in Clinical Medicine*, 2nd edition, 70. William Heinemann London.
WALLACE J. (1970) Viral hepatitis. *Scott. med. J.*, **15**, 311–314.
WARD R., WRIGHT A., BORCHERT P. & KLINE E. (1972) Hepatitis B antigen in saliva and mouth washings. *Lancet*, **2**, 726–727.
WERNER A.S., COBBS C.G., KAYE D. & HOOK E.W. (1967) Studies on the bacteremia of bacterial endocarditis. *J. Am. med. Ass.*, **202**, 199–203.
WILTON J.M.A., IVANYI L. & LEHNER T. (1971) Cell-mediated immunity and humoral antibodies in acute ulcerative gingivitis. *J. Periodont.*, **6**, 9–16.
WILTON J.M.A., IVANYI L. & LEHNER T. (1972) Cell mediated immunity in herpesvirus hominis infections. *Brit. med. J.*, **1**, 723–726.

WOOTEN J.W., KATZ H.I., HOFFMAN S. & LINK J.F. (1967) Development of oral lesions in erythema multiforme exudativum. *Oral Surg. Oral Med. Oral Path.*, **24,** 808-816.

WYBURN-MASON R. (1957) Malignant change following herpes simplex. *Brit. med. J.*, **2,** 615-616.

CHAPTER 9
ORAL ULCERATION: IMMUNOLOGICAL ASPECTS

A.E. DOLBY

9:0 Introduction

During recent years it has become apparent that certain diseases of the oral mucosa may have an immunological basis. Furthermore, immunological abnormalities in common with accompanying skin disease have been detected in some cases. Before considering these diseases it would be of value to examine the known mechanisms of immunological injury and the methods at present available for the demonstration of the involvement of these mechanisms in disease.

9:1 Mechanisms of Immunological Injury

Immunological reactions were at one time divided into the categories of humoral and cellular. The humoral reactions were those in which antibody was demonstrably involved, whereas the cellular reactions were those in which antibody did not appear to play a part and which appeared to be associated with the small lymphocyte. An attempt to classify the then existing knowledge of these humoral and cellular reactions was made by Gell & Coombs in 1963. Their classification into four main types of hypersensitivity reaction has considerably increased the understanding of the mechanisms of immunological injury.

9:1:1 Type I—the immediate hypersensitivity reaction

This is dependent upon antibodies of the IgE class which were originally termed reaginic antibodies. The IgE immunoglobulin is present in very low amounts in serum and has the unusual characteristic of being able to bind by its Fc, or crystallizable fragment (see Chapter 3) of the antibody molecule, to mast cells, basophils and epithelial cells. The $F(ab^1)_2$, or antibody portion, is thus available for interaction with the appropriate antigen. This interaction of antigen and antibody, when occurring on the surface of the mast cell, results in the exocytotic release of vasoactive amines such as histamine and 5-hydroxy tryptamine (but see Chapter 1). The classical example of such a reaction involving skin is the wheal and flare following a prick test with antigen. Since small antigenic molecules can pass through the oral mucosa (Tolo 1971), it would appear possible that reactions based on this IgE antibody mechanism could occur within the mouth. The fact that the incidence of such reactions is low when compared with skin or respiratory mucosa, has been difficult to explain. Of the suggested reasons one is the improved clearance afforded by saliva. Not only may this be mechanical, but immunoglobulin in saliva may react with such antigens. That the oral tissues are capable of responding in the same way as respiratory mucosa is seen in the oral manifestation of hereditary angioneurotic oedema. Although this disease is not immunologically activated it follows the same final pathway as the IgE-mediated immediate hypersensitivity reaction.

The disease is due to an autosomal dominant defect in the complement system (see below and Fig. 9.1) in which the patient lacks C1 esterase inhibitor (C1 INH). As a consequence, C1, the first component of complement, is more readily fixed in such patients leading to the release of 'C-Kinin' at the C2 stage of complement production. C-Kinin, a substance distinct from kallidin and bradykinin, produces symptoms similar to the type I immediate hypersensitivity reaction, and these symptoms may manifest themselves in the mouth.

Confirmation that the IgE-mediated type of hypersensitivity mechanism is responsible for the disease may be confirmed by the Prausnitz–Kustner test, a potentially hazardous procedure since it involves serum transfer. Serum from the patient is injected into a normal human recipient, followed after 18 hours by the injection at the same site of the suspected antigen. A wheal and erythema developing at the site implies a positive reaction.

It has been more difficult to achieve reliable *in vivo* methods of confirmation. Degranulation of rabbit basophils (Shelley 1963) and rat peritoneal mast cells (Schwartz *et al* 1966) by the patient's serum and suspected antigen have been employed, but it is possible that immunoglobulins other than IgE may contribute to this reaction. Antigen–antibody complexes formed when the patient's serum and antigen are allowed to diffuse towards each other through agar gel are usually not visible because of the very small

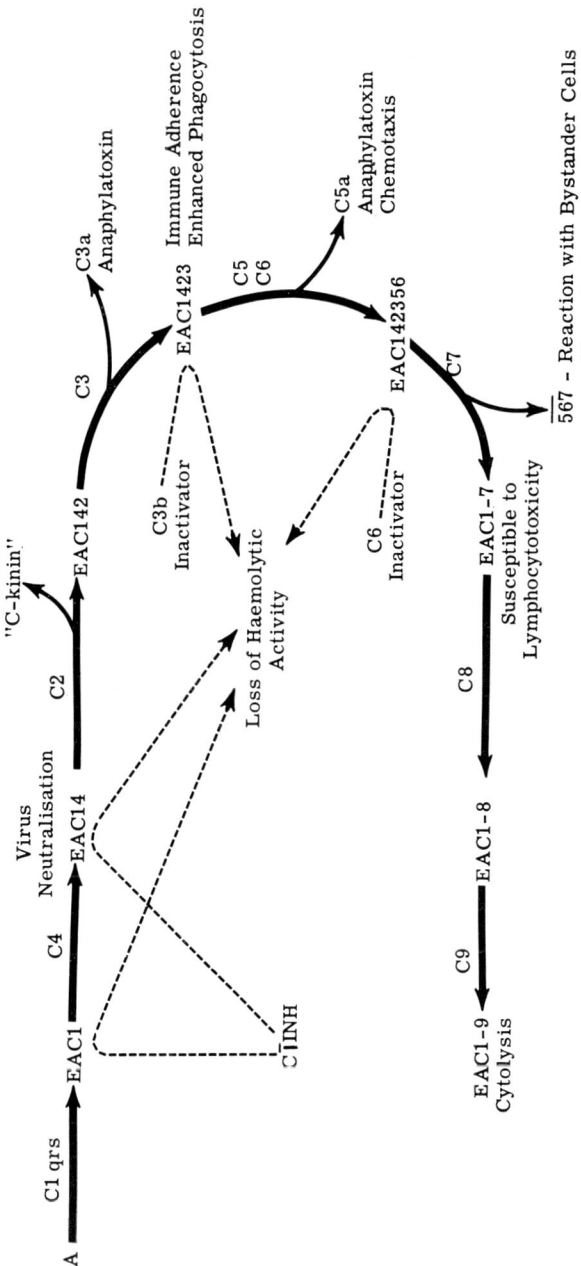

Fig. 9.1. The complement 'pathway'.

amounts involved. However, labelling of the antigen with radioisotope has enabled detection of these complexes (Ito et al 1969), so that measurement of the degree of hypersensitivity has become possible by an *in vitro* technique.

9:1:2 Type II reaction—the cytolytic or cytotoxic reaction

This reaction is complement dependent. Union of antibody, usually of the IgG type, and antigen occurs on, or in very close proximity to, the target cell and the complement system is activated through its normal cycle (Fig. 9.1).

The complement system consists of nine components which react sequentially, although the first three are in the unusual order of reaction C_1, C_4, C_2 (Fig. 9.1). The system is usually described in relation to erythrocytes (E), the combination of erythrocytes and antibody leading to activation of the first component of complement (EAC 1) from the precursor C q, r and s. Active C_1 splits C_4 and this reaction reveals a capacity in C_1 to bind C_2. The C_{42} enzyme or C_3 convertase cleaves C_3 into two fragments. The C_{423} enzyme on the complex splits C_5, the major part of which combines with C_6 to form the EAC 142356 intermediate. After reaction with C_7 the product becomes stable and reacts with C_8 and C_9 resulting in cell lysis or increased cell permeability. This simple description of what is a very complex pathway is further complicated by the fact that the terminal components may be activated by an alternate pathway commencing at the C_3 stage. This may be initiated for example by bacterial lipopolysaccharide interacting with serum, or by a site on the $F(ab)_2$ fraction of the antibody molecule (Ruddy et al 1972). The products of the complement reaction system shown in Fig. 9.1 are of considerable importance as will be seen below.

An example of the cytotoxic reaction is the purpura induced by the drug Sedormid; the drug binds to the platelets, the resulting drug platelet complexes serving as the antigen. The cell surface itself may represent the antigen so that, for example, in relation to oral mucosal cells, confirmation could be achieved by an *in vitro* examination of the phenomenon. Oral mucosal cells, incubated with the suspect serum, would undergo lysis. Complement is usually added in the form of fresh guinea-pig serum, a consistently good donor of complement. Assessment of cell death may be made in a variety of ways, ranging from the exclusion of dyes by still viable cells to the release of previously absorbed or adsorbed radioactive material into the incubation medium by dying cells. The type II reactions are rarely associated with the pathogenesis of skin disease and have so far not been implicated in oral mucosal disease.

9:1:3 Type III reaction, Arthus reaction—immune complex disease

In this reaction the combination of antigen with antibody leads to the formation of immune complexes which are ultimately harmful. The resulting immune complex disease is determined to a large extent by the site of formation or distribution of the complexes. Thus, in the Arthus

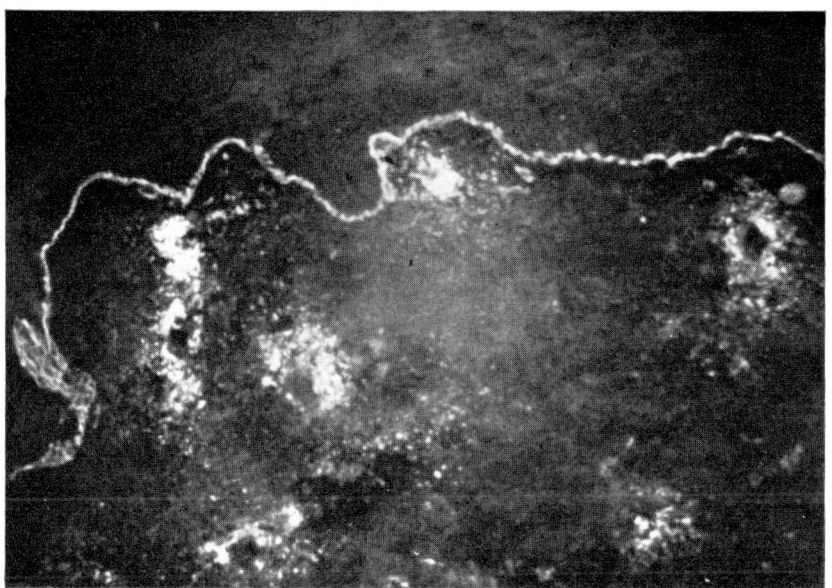

Fig. 9.2. Fluorescence photomicrograph. Oral mucosa of a rabbit with deposits of immune complexes around the arterioles and at the basement membrane zone. The animal had previously been injected intramuscularly with horse serum on several occasions and the submucosal injection was made 3 hours before this biopsy. $\times 140$. (By kind permission of Mr M. Addy, The Welsh National School of Medicine, Dental School, Cardiff.)

phenomenon, where antigen is present in the tissue and reacts with antibody within the vessel wall, a characteristic vasculonecrotic reaction ensues. Alternatively, complexes may form in the blood and continue to circulate, so that the sites at which they accumulate would give rise to varying clinical manifestations.

The vascular form of the type III reaction may be induced readily in rabbits. The animals are sensitized to an antigen, for example horse serum, and a submucosal or subcutaneous injection of this material produces a reaction in which acute vascular damage leads to necrosis of the overlying tissues (Fig. 9.2). The reaction of antigen with antibody within the vessel wall leads to activation of the complement system through its normal pathway (Fig. 9.1). Polymorphonuclear leukocytes are chemotactically attracted by the C_3, C_5 and C_{567} components of complement, to the site of deposition of the complexes, and appear to contribute to the vascular damage which results, possibly by the release of lysosomal hydrolases. An excess of antibody in the complexes increases the insolubility of the complex so that the titre of precipitating antibody in the animal's blood is of significance. Where insolubility is very high, the antibody–antigen complexes may persist for some time, resulting in granuloma formation.

The possibility that an epithelial lesion is due to this type of immune reaction may be suggested by the findings from a number of investigations. Thus the immune complexes that form within and around the vessel walls may be shown by fluorescent antibody techniques (Chapter 3). However, care must be taken to distinguish these deposits from the very considerable amount of antibody released in an inflammatory exudate, usually in high concentration around the vessels, even to the extent of complement components. The immunoglobulins present in such a case would still be soluble and it should be possible to remove them from the tissues by repeated washing. The histological appearance of such a reaction may also be suggestive of immune complex formation, since polymorphonuclear leukocytes would have been chemotactically attracted to the sites of maximum immune complex formation. Vascular damage would be prominent together with necrosis of overlying mucosa or skin but, again, these appearances are only suggestive of such a reaction. The two diseases which should be considered in relation to this type of reaction are pemphigus and bullous pemphigoid, since in both diseases there is circulating antibody that will combine with epithelial components.

Circulating immune complexes may deposit in skin or mucosa, and in systemic lupus erythematosus the occurrence of antinuclear antibody and nuclear material complexes which have combined and been deposited at the basement membrane zone are of value in diagnosis (Fig. 9.1) (Burnham *et al* 1963). In contrast to the complexes detectable at the basement membrane zone in bullous pemphigoid, one would not be able to detect by the same technique anti-basement membrane antibodies (see section 9.3) in the serum of the patient. Erythema multiforme may be another disease where the skin and mucosal lesions occur as a consequence of the deposition of immune complexes and in which the antigen could be bacterial, viral or drug induced (Amos 1973), but findings are at present only suggestive of this mechanism.

9:1:4 Type IV—cellular or delayed hypersensitivity reaction

Until some 20 years ago this was the least well understood of the hypersensitivity reactions. During the intervening period, the information that has been obtained, both in relation to the reaction and to the lymphocyte,

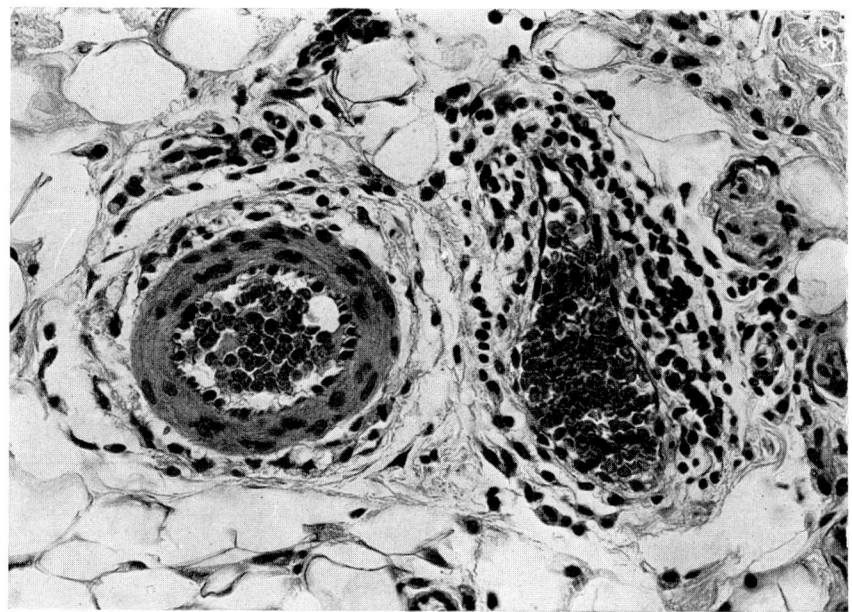

Fig. 9.3. Early Mikulicz's recurrent oral aphthous ulcer. Mononuclear cells surround two vessels at the base of the ulcer. ×280.

has led to a greater understanding of the phenomenon of delayed hypersensitivity. The combination of antigen in this reaction is usually with the T lymphocyte (Chapter 3) not with circulating antibody.

In the T cell system, combination with antigen leads to activation of the lymphocyte with not only the release of a range of soluble factors, but also the creation of an aggressive nature on the part of the lymphocyte itself. The soluble factors, or *lymphokines*, produced have a range of *in vitro* effects (Dumonde et al 1969). Thus the mitogenic factor results in mitogenesis in adjacent, uncommitted lymphocytes. The cytotoxic or cytopathic factor produces cell damage, including damage to adjacent uninvolved cells, and the macrophage migration inhibition factor prevents macrophages which have migrated to the area from leaving. An additional factor promotes an inflammatory response.

The histology of these reactions is fairly characteristic. At the earliest

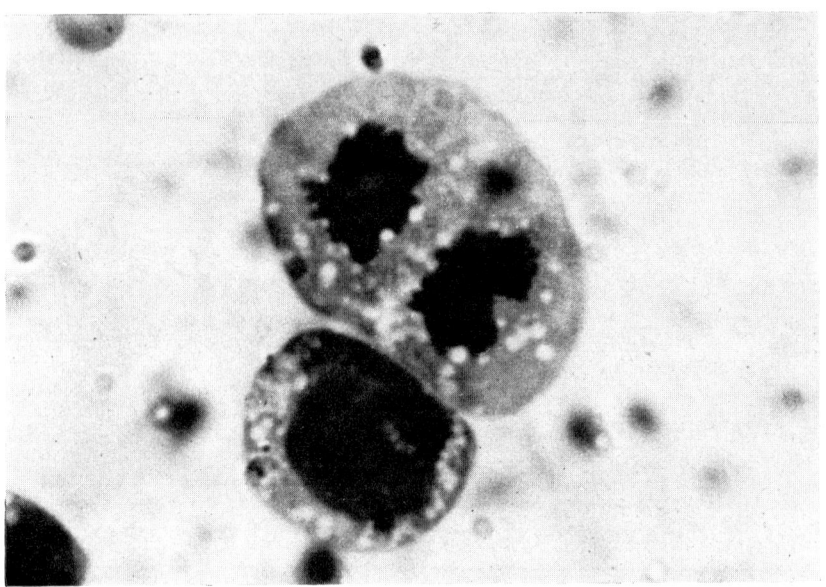

Fig. 9.4. 'Blast' transformation in peripheral blood lymphocytes cultured for 3 days with purified protein derivative. The cytoplasm is vesiculating and the uppermost 'blast' cell is about to undergo division. A portion of a non-responding lymphocyte can be seen in the top left-hand corner. ×353.

stage the inflammatory cell is the mononuclear cell, the polymorphonuclear leukocyte appearing at a later stage so that a mononuclear surround or 'cuff' to the blood vessels is a characteristic feature (Fig. 9.3). The blood vessels themselves may show end-arteriolar proliferation.

In vitro correlates of delayed hypersensitivity or cellular immunity

The recognition of the presence of an antigen-specific antibody-like receptor on the surface of a population of lymphocytes is made easier by the fact that lymphokines are produced, since these may be measured *in vitro*.

Measurement of lymphokine production

For measurement of the mitogenic factor, released lymphocytes may be separated from peripheral blood and incubated with the antigen in question. Prior to division the cells undergo a characteristic change known as 'blast transformation' (Fig. 9.4). The response to the antigen may be measured by assessing, after several days, the percentage of such 'blast transforming' lymphocytes on a slide preparation from the lymphocyte culture and comparing this with the percentage present in a control culture to which only saline had been added. More conveniently it may be estimated by measuring the uptake of radioactive DNA precursor, such as tritiated thymidine, since this occurs at a much higher level in responding lymphocytes. The two methods of measurement do not necessarily correlate.

Macrophage migration inhibition factor may be measured by making use of the knowledge that the factor is not species specific so that macrophages from an experimental animal may be employed. Thus guinea-pig peritoneal macrophages, induced in the peritoneal cavity by the prior injection into the cavity of sterile light paraffin oil, may be cultured in capillary tubes placed in small chambers. The culture medium consists of the supernatant from the lymphocyte cultures being tested (with and without antigen). If migration inhibition factor has been produced by the lymphocytes in the preceding cultures, the macrophages move only slightly, or not at all, from the end of the tube. In the control chamber migration will proceed unimpaired (Fig. 9.5).

The cytopathic or cytotoxic factor is antigen specific but produces differing cytopathic or cytotoxic effects depending upon the target cells employed. Assessment of cell death may be made as for antibody mediated cytolysis (vs) and assessment of altered cell metabolism may be made by estimating the degree of incorporation of radioactive protein precursors. Certain cell lines appear to be more susceptible than other (Williams & Granger 1968) and care has to be taken in interpreting such assays.

The inflammatory and cytotoxic or cytopathic effects of lymphokine are the effects which would appear most closely to simulate the disease process and are representative of immunological injury. Thus in those diseases where this type of hypersensitivity reaction is thought to be of importance it should be possible to show an enhanced response in terms of these *in vitro* correlates in persons suffering from the disease. Within the lesion interaction of specifically sensitized lymphocytes with the antigen

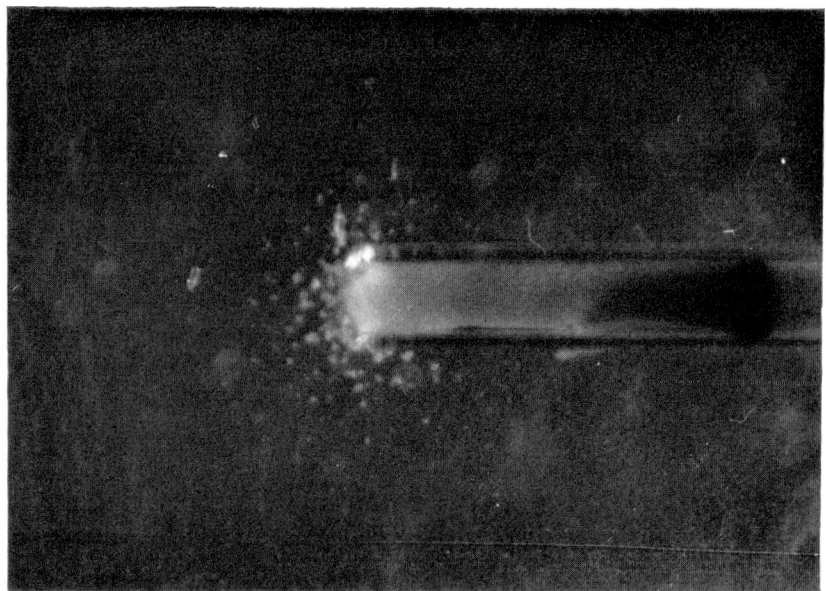

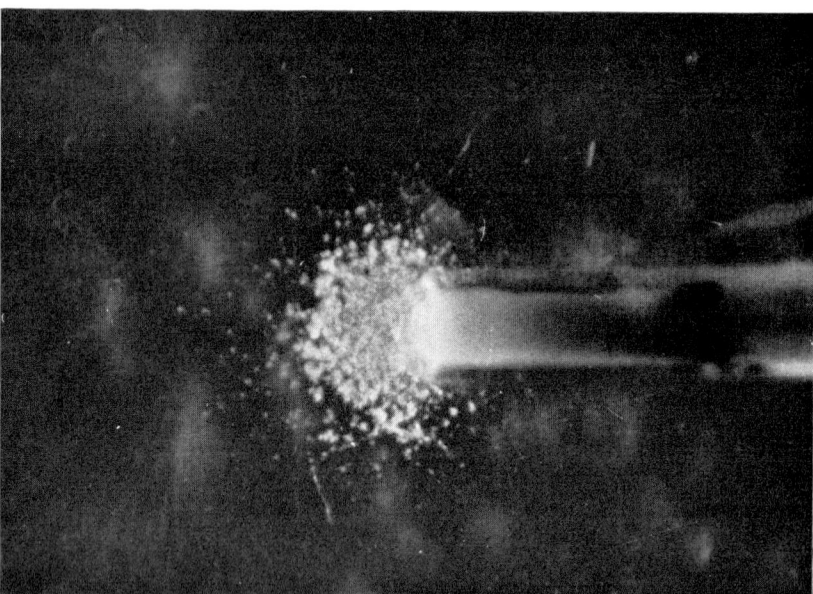

Fig. 9.5. Macrophage migration inhibition. Supernatants from lymphocyte cultures to one of which purified protein derivative has been added, were used in the chambers. In the chamber where the purified protein derivative has been added to the lymphocyte cultures migration is inhibited (upper picture). In the control chamber migration has occurred normally.

leads presumptively to the release of the soluble mediators and to the activation of the lymphocytes to an aggressive state. As a consequence, parenchymal cells, not necessarily involved in the reaction, may also be damaged, the so-called 'innocent bystander cells' of Waksman (1968).

Lymphocyte cytotoxicity

In addition to the lymphocyte cytotoxicity which occurs through the medium of the soluble mediator, other mechanisms leading to this phenomenon of target cell death have been detected:
1 In these two mechanisms contact between the lymphocyte and antigen-bearing target cell is essential for there to be a cytotoxic effect.
(*a*) The lymphocytes may become cytotoxic to target cells bearing histocompatibility antigens against which the T cells have been previously sensitized (Cerottini *et al* 1970).
(*b*) Where target cells have been coated by antibody cell-mediated lysis can occur through the medium of B cells from normal, unsensitized donors and in this, the intact Fc part of the anti 'anti target cell antibody' is essential, whereas complement is not (Larsson & Perlmann 1972).
2 Non-specific stimulation of lymphocytes by the plant mitogens, such as, for example, phytohaemagglutin or pokeweed mitogen, results in the production of, amongst other materials, a toxic soluble mediator which has been termed lymphotoxin (Granger & Kolb 1968).

Considerable corroborative evidence is required to demonstrate that an immune reaction is of significance in tissue injury in oral mucosal and skin disease. This is because the ultimate inflammatory response is remarkably similar in terms of the histopathological appearances and although these appearances may be suggestive of an immune reaction, it cannot be held as conclusive evidence. Certain oral mucosal and skin lesions have been shown to have an immunological component, the importance of which varies; these will be discussed under the various headings. In particular the gingival crevice area represents a site where an immune reaction is in progress continually and which may contribute to damage arising in that area.

9:1:5 Autoimmune disease; peripheral and central origin

During this discussion of the types of hypersensitivity reaction no reference has been made to the phenomenon of autoimmunity. It can be seen that an immune reaction with self components could take one of these four routes, and some examples will be quoted in the discussion of the diseases which follows. The concept of autoimmune disease presupposes a breakdown in the normal tolerance of the immune system for self antigens. This situation may arise in a number of ways. The self antigen may normally be sequestered from the lymphoreticular system so that autoantibody formation is not induced. Examples of such antigen which are quoted are lens tissue of the eye and thyroglobulin, whereas in fact the latter material appears in measurable amounts in the circulation. Again, antibody may 'cross-react' with a truly foreign antigen such as a bacterial or virus antigen and a previously non-antigenic self component. This is made possible by the fact that not all antigen combining sites are necessarily involved in an antigen–antibody reaction or lymphocyte–antigen reaction, and that the fit, although not perfect, may be sufficient to produce a response. This 'poor fit' situation was made use of many years ago in producing an immune responsiveness to smallpox by inoculation with the cowpox virus. Some immune complex diseases may also represent examples of autoimmune disease, for example in allergic glomerulonephritis where an antiglomerulo basement membrane antibody exists, autoantibody combines with glomerular basement membrane and local immune complexes are deposited. Viruses may contribute in another way since, from an intracellular site, they may induce the replication of foreign antigen intrinsically associated with the host cell surface, such antigens being termed neoantigens.

Autoimmune disease may arise as a consequence of the development of an abnormal clone of lymphocytes which do not recognize self antigen as self. In such a situation a variety of immunological abnormalities are often detectable, as is the case for example with systemic lupus erythematosus. This latter type of autoimmune disease has been termed central immunological fault autoimmunity, to distinguish it from the peripheral fault types described above (Turk 1969).

The recent finding that T and B cells may co-operate in their response to many antigens has raised another possible mechanism for the state of autoimmunity. B lymphocytes bearing antibody for autoantigens have been found in normal individuals (Bankhurst *et al* 1973) but in lower numbers than in diseased individuals. Control of the level of B lymphocytes which respond to autoantigens is thought to be dependent upon the T lymphocyte (Allison 1971). Thus the original concept of autoimmunity (Burnet & Fenner 1949) may be relevant only to T cells.

9:2 Recurrent Oral Ulceration

9:2:1 Mikulicz's recurrent oral aphthae (MROA)

Clinical features

Several surveys carried out during the last 15 years have resulted in a more definitive description of this disease (Sircus *et al* 1957; Farmer 1958; Cooke 1961). Small ulcers arise on the non-keratinized oral mucosa, in crops of from 1 to 6 and last for from 10 to 14 days. They occur at approximately 4-weekly intervals, with greater regularity in women than men, and are more common in women than men at a ratio of approximately 2 : 1. There is considerable pain, predominantly during the mid-part of the ulcer life. Occasionally the ulcers may be deeper or cover a larger area and then often heal with a scar. This difference in ulcer size has given rise to the distinction of minor and major oral aphthae (Truelove & Morris Owen 1958). The ulcers, although they may be produced by simple trauma, are clearly subject to other influences, for example, they occur predominantly in the luteal phase of the menstrual cycle in women (Dolby 1968). They appear also to undergo an increase in incidence at times of mental stress. A variety of aetiological agents has been proposed in the past, including bacterial and viral infection. In recent years a significant finding (Lehner 1964) has raised the possibility that an immune, or possibly autoimmune, reaction may be responsible for the disease.

9:2:2 Immunological findings in Mikulicz's recurrent oral aphthae

Patients suffering from this disease possess a raised titre of circulating antibody, predominantly of the IgM class, to a saline extract of foetal oral mucosa (Lehner 1964). Foetal, as opposed to non-foetal, oral mucosa was employed in the investigation in order to minimize the involvement of bacterial antigen contamination in the antibody assay. Slightly raised levels of this antibody are observed in other oral ulcerative diseases, but not to the same extent as in Mikulicz's recurrent oral aphthous ulceration. The antibodies have been detected by agglutination and immunodiffusion methods and are complement fixing. Thus the cytolytic or cytotoxic mechanism could be invoked to explain the tissue damage. The antibodies also exhibit some degree of specificity, there being no comparable reaction with saline extracts of viscera. There was some cross-reaction detectable with skin, suggesting a similarity of tissue antigens.

This finding was interpreted as evidence for an autoimmune basis for the disease, or as an indication of a cross-reaction occurring between antigens of an oral organism and of the oral mucosa itself. Both explanations could explain the tissue damage which ensues. Conversely, it is conceivable that the antibody arose because of the repeated exposure during the oral ulceration of a tissue antigen which had been previously sequestered from the immune system. The antibody would in such a case have arisen as a consequence of the disease rather than be a contributor to the aetiology.

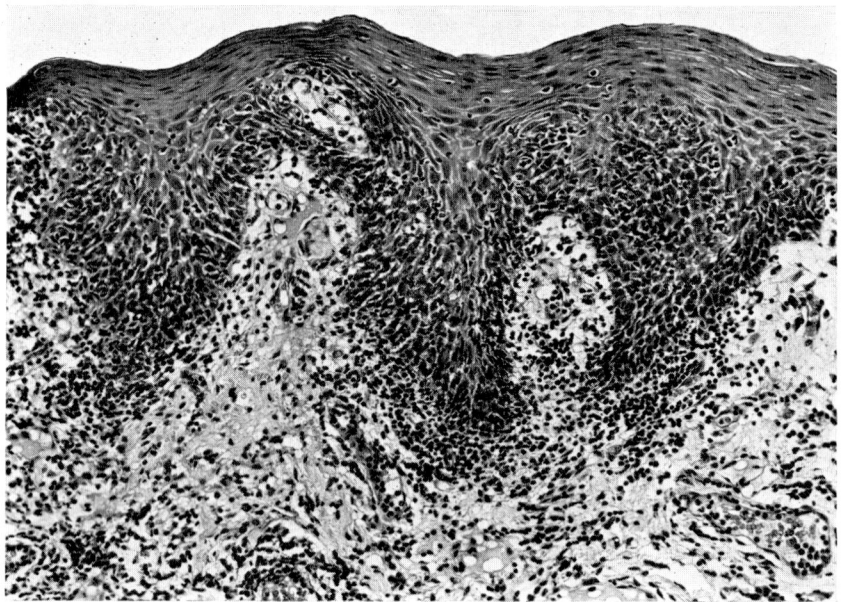

Fig. 9.6. The 'invasive destructive' event in Mikulicz's recurrent oral aphtous ulceration. Mononuclear cells are invading the basal layers of the epithelium and there is accompanying destruction of the basal layers of the epithelium. × 140.

Somewhat later (Lehner 1967) it was shown that these patients possess peripheral blood lymphocytes which were sensitized to the same antigen to a greater degree than control subjects. That is to say, they responded in culture by taking up more isotope-labelled DNA precursor when in the presence of foetal oral mucosa antigen than did the lymphocytes from control subjects. At about this time, a study of sequentially arranged biopsies of Mikulicz's oral aphthous ulcers (Graykowski et al 1966) demonstrated quite clearly that the epithelial damage was consistently associated with an infiltrate of lymphocytes, polymorphonuclear leukocytes not appearing until somewhat later (Fig. 9.6). Furthermore, mononuclear cuffing of blood vessels was a prominent feature in the early stages (Fig. 9.3). Thus there was considerable evidence to implicate a type IV hypersensitivity mechanism in the aetiology of the disease. That a cytotoxic component was operative was later shown when lymphocytes from patients suffering from Mikulicz's recurrent oral aphthous ulceration were incu-

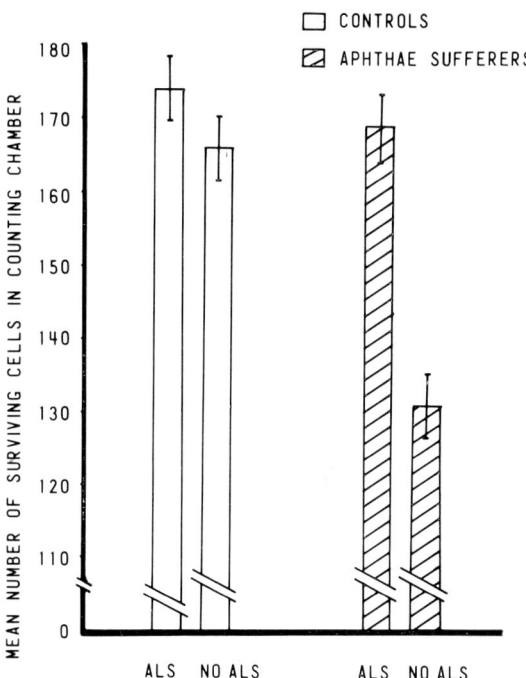

Fig. 9.7. Mikulicz's recurrent oral aphthous ulceration. Inhibition of the *in vitro* lymphocyte cytotoxicity for oral epithelial cells by prior incubation of the lymphocytes in anti-human lymphocyte serum raised in rabbits. (By kind permission of the editor of *Clinical and Experimental Immunology*.)

bated with oral epithelial cells *in vitro* (Dolby 1969). The survival of the oral epithelial cells was consistently worse with the lymphocytes from the Mikulicz's recurrent oral aphthous sufferers than with control subjects. This cytotoxic effect was probably of the direct type, not lymphokine mediated, since it was apparent within 24 hours and was probably of the T cell rather than B cell type, since the degree of target cell death was not increased by the addition of sera from the patients. However, for the antibody-dependent lymphocyte cytotoxicity mechanism, only very small quantities of antibody are required, inhibition occurring at higher concentrations. This mechanism may also be of importance. The cytotoxic effect could be abrogated by the addition of corticosteroids to the tissue culture or by the prior incubation of the lymphocytes in antilymphocyte serum prepared in rabbits (Fig. 9.7) (Dolby 1970). Experiments using serum alone, which had been previously determined as having a raised titre of antibody to foetal oral mucosa, showed that cytotoxicity could not be induced with the circulating antibody. The antigen responsible for initiating the lymphocytotoxic reaction presumably resides in, or on, the epithelial cell surface. Again, it may represent a cross-reaction between an antigen of oral mucosa and an antigen of an oral organism, in this instance mediated by a cellular immune mechanism. The production of the ulcers *in vivo* by mild trauma may therefore represent the release of antigen leading to the damage to cells observed *in vitro*. The pattern of the ulcer cycle is also suggestive of the cessation of an immune reaction following elimination of the antigen.

Thus the earlier investigations which sought an infective agent in the disease have been extended of late in a search for an organism to fill the role of the cross-reacting antigen. Patients suffering from Mikulicz's recurrent oral aphthous ulceration are hypersensitive in the cellular immune sense to adenovirus type I but not to herpes type I (Sallay *et al* 1971), so that this organism must be suspect. In another investigation patients suffering from the disease showed a reduced cellular immune response to *Streptococcus sanguis* (Francis & Oppenheim 1970), the organism which was not long before postulated as the causative organism (Barile & Graykowski 1963). Since these are the only three organisms which have yet been examined in relation to Mikulicz's recurrent oral aphthous ulceration and cellular hypersensitivity it is clearly too early to draw any conclusion as to the nature of a cross-reacting organism.

In the lymphocytotoxicity experiments described above, the antigen which initiated the reaction may have been revealed by the enzymatic treatment of the tissue preceding release of the cells from the mass of tissue. Not only may uncovering of the antigens have occurred but restructuring of the antigens is also theoretically possible, so that previously acceptable host antigens become foreign.

9:2:3 Herpetiform ulceration

Before describing this form of ulceration it should be emphasized that recurrent intraoral infection with herpes virus hominis type I does occur

(Chapter 8). The herpetiform variety of recurrent oral ulceration simulates the latter disease in so far as up to 100 ulcers may be present at one time; these later coalesce to give the appearance and characteristic discomfort pattern of Mikulicz's recurrent oral aphthous ulcers (Cooke 1961). The disease is much less common than Mikulicz's recurrent oral aphthous ulceration, and investigation has therefore been limited. The patients do not however possess a raised antibody titre to foetal oral mucosa (Lehner 1969), and on the basis of the immunological differences and the larger number of ulcers present at the outset, the disease must be distinguished from Mikulicz's recurrent oral aphthous ulceration. Electron microscopic studies of herpetiform ulceration have revealed intranuclear inclusion bodies suggestive of viral infection, but not of the herpes simplex type (Lehner & Sagebiel 1966). It was also observed that the cytoplasmic changes correlated with the delayed hypersensitivity reaction, suggesting that the same mechanism would appear to be operating in herpetiform ulceration as Mikulicz's recurrent oral aphthous ulceration, at least in terms of the tissue damage which occurs.

9:2:4 Behçet's syndrome

The existence of Behçet's syndrome as a separate entity has served to divide what some clinicians consider is a spectrum of disease (Touraine 1941). Thus Mikulicz's recurrent oral aphthous ulceration is sometimes accompanied by genital ulceration, which in women may have the same hormonally influenced pattern. Although not falling strictly into the triple symptom complex of Behçet they have none the less been termed by some clinicians 'partial cases' of Behçet's syndrome. Again it is often presumed that the oral ulceration is severe in nature and, although this is usually the case, ulcers of the minor Mikulicz's recurrent oral aphthous or herpetiform variety may occur (Lehner 1967). Unlike Mikulicz's recurrent oral aphthous ulceration, the disease occurs more commonly in men than in women (Dowling 1961), although there is a non-specific response of the skin to trauma as with that of oral mucosa to trauma in Mikulicz's recurrent oral aphthous ulceration. Thus the injection of, for example, normal saline in Behçet's syndrome will not infrequently result in an ulcer (Katzenellenbogen 1946). In the complete Behçet's syndrome there are widespread symptoms and signs in the form of iridocyclitis, neurological lesions and arthritis. Such extensions of the disease are similar to the extra gastrointestinal symptoms of ulcerative colitis, where circulating immune complexes have been detected (Doe et al 1973), and this mechanism may explain the unusual extraintegumental lesions of Behçet's syndrome.

Immunological abnormalities in Behçet's syndrome

Patients suffering from Behçet's syndrome also possess a variety of antibodies to tissue extracts, namely foetal oral mucosa, skin and colon (Oshima et al 1963). Unlike the antibody to foetal oral mucosa in recurrent aphthous ulceration, the titre of this antibody has been found to alter in parallel with the severity of the disease. A mononuclear surround to vessels is seen and the histopathological appearance is very similar to that of the experimental type IV invasive destructive lesions described by Waksman (1959). Thrombosis may occur, but a vasculonecrotic response may also be seen in delayed hypersensitivity reactions where the antigen level is high and where the tissue damage is still apparently due to lymphocyte activity. As with recurrent oral ulceration, an infective aetiology has been proposed for Behçet's syndrome in the past. Most recently a viral and mycoplasmal infection have been considered, but convincing evidence has not been produced. Thus the same mechanism may be operating in Behçet's syndrome as in Mikulicz's recurrent oral aphthous ulceration, namely an autoimmune response of the peripheral type with antigenic similarity between the various sites of involvement.

9:3 Pemphigus, Bullous Pemphigoid, Benign Mucous Membrane Pemphigoid

In contrast to the oral ulceration occurring in aphthous ulceration and Behçet's syndrome, the ulceration in these diseases is preceded by the formation of bullae. A fundamental histopathological distinction has existed for some time (Lever 1965), namely that the site of bulla formation differs in the two diseases. In pemphigus there is a loss of cohesion in the prickle cells with a separation of the overlying epithelium at that site. The space fills rapidly with fluid exudate and a flaccid bulla is produced. In bullous pemphigoid and benign mucous membrane pemphigoid there is a separation of the epidermis from the dermis and this space fills with exudate. The differing anatomical situations of the bullae usually enable histopathological differentiation of the two diseases, and cytological examination of the exudate from unerupted bullae will reveal acantholytic detached prickle cells or Tzanck cells only in pemphigus.

Mucosal surfaces are involved in both diseases, but skin rarely in benign mucous membrane pemphigoid. Oral lesions occur first in approximately one-quarter of pemphigus cases (Cooke 1960). Both diseases are sinister, pemphigus because it invariably led to death before the introduction of corticosteroid therapy, and benign mucous membrane pemphigoid because the symblepharon formation which occurs in the conjunctivae as a consequence of previous bulla formation may lead to blindness. These bullous diseases are often associated with another disease. For example pemphigus may occur in the presence of myasthenia gravis and the association of pemphigus with lupus erythematosus has led to the pemphigus erythematosus controversy, in which it is considered that lupus erythematosus with pemphigus is a different disease.

Immunological abnormalities in pemphigus

The immunological findings in pemphigus are so striking as to lead to an immediate suspicion that they are causally related to the disease. In pemphigus there is a raised titre of antibodies predominantly of the IgG class to the intercellular substance of the epithelium, while in bullous pemphigoid there is a raised titre of antibody to basement membrane material (Beutner *et al* 1964; Jordon *et al* 1967). IgM and IgA do not seem to be of such significance in these situations, although there are detectable levels of these antibodies also. The presence of these antigens was detected using the fluorescent antibody technique (see Chapter 3, Fig. 3.20).

In pemphigus the fluorescence is observed in the intercellular area of the epithelium, whilst in bullous pemphigoid it is present in the basement membrane area. Benign mucous membrane pemphigoid is, however, negative in this test with no fluorescence observed in either site. Confirmation of the intercellular nature of the antibody-binding site in pemphigus has been made by electron microscopic studies of this area after the application of labelled sera. Horseradish peroxidase coupled with anti-immunoglobulin gives electro-dense deposits which can be seen under the electron microscope (Wolff & Schreiner 1971). The antibodies demonstrated are apparently tissue specific; the intercellular material antibody will react only with the intercellular material of stratified squamous epithelium found in, for example, skin, oral mucosa or oesophagus (Beutner *et al* 1965), but will do so in a variety of species such as the human, monkey and guinea-pig. Muscle and gland are negative for the intercellular material antigen, whereas they are positive for the basement membrane antigen demonstrated by pemphigoid serum. This also is the case with skin, mucosa of lip, nose, cornea, showing that the basement membrane antigen is more widely distributed than that of the intercellular material antigen.

Pemphigus as a disease is endemic in certain parts of Brazil, where it is known as fogo selvagem, and the distribution is very suggestive of it being caused by an athropod-borne infectious organism (Beutner *et al* 1968). Antibody to intercellular material is found in this form of pemphigus and the possibility of the disease being due to cross-reaction between the antigen of the organism and the antigen of basement membrane material has been raised in much the same way, as this explanation has been put forward in relation to Mikulicz's recurrent oral aphthous ulceration.

The significance of the antibodies in the disease process has been a source of controversy for a long time. The test described above to demonstrate the antibodies is the indirect form of fluorescent antibody test. The direct form is not applicable to the lesion in pemphigus. In such a case a lesion from skin or mucosa from a patient would be treated with the serum in the hope that antibody binding would occur in the sites expected. However, it would not be unreasonable to presume that antibody binding had occurred *in vivo* previously, so filling the available binding sites for the antibody in the sera. However, *in vivo* binding of pemphigus antibodies can be demonstrated by injection into monkeys of pemphigus serum. That the immunoglobulin is acting as an antibody is supported *to some extent* by the fact that complement binding can also be detected by fluorescent antibody techniques at the same site as the binding of pemphigus serum takes place. The pemphigus antibody has a low affinity for the intercellular substance and the antibodies appear to be directed against different antigenic determinants of the intercellular substance.

The presence of these antibodies directed against different antigenic determinants is related also to the occurrence of such antibodies in patients who have received severe skin burns (Ablin *et al* 1969; Thivolet & Beyvin 1968), for it is presumed that the thermal trauma has revealed different antigenic determinants giving rise to the antibody. Although this would appear to refute the significance of pemphigus antibodies as a causative mechanism in pemphigus it should be remembered that such burn autoantibodies are transient, and pemphigus-like lesions may occur following severe burns (Chorzelski & Jablonska 1972).

Bullous pemphigoid and benign mucous membrane pemphigoid

Although these two diseases may be apparently difficult to distinguish from examination of the oral mucosa alone, it should be remembered that bullous pemphigoid is essentially a skin disease with occasional mucosal lesions, whereas benign mucous membrane pemphigoid is essentially a mucosal disease. Thus oral mucosal bullae arising as a consequence of separation at the dermo-epidermal junction should be considered benign mucous membrane pemphigoid in the absence of skin lesions. Confirmation of mucosal lesions in the genital region, nose or involving the cornea may be possible. The oral mucosal lesions of benign mucous membrane pemphigoid may simulate atrophic lichen planus in appearance with an erythematous zone surrounded by white striae. There is considerable scar formation leading to visual disturbances in the eye and to difficulty in the construction and retention of prostheses in the mouth.

Immunological abnormalities in bullous pemphigoid and benign mucous membrane pemphigoid

The major distinction between the two diseases is the presence of antibody to basement membrane material in bullous pemphigoid and the absence of such antibodies in benign mucous membrane pemphigoid. The existence of two similar diseases with such a fundamental difference in their immunopathology would suggest that they have completely different aetiological mechanisms. Again, as with pemphigus, tissue from different animal species may be used to detect the presence of these basement membrane antibodies, which are found to be positive in all stratified squamous epithelia and negative in other tissues such as muscle and gland.

Mechanism of action of the antibodies in pemphigus and bullous pemphigoid

Such a mechanism would be most like that of the type III reaction. Antibody binding to the antigens either of the intercellular material or the basement membrane would occur with activation of complement and subsequent attraction of polymorphonuclear leukocytes. The release of lysosomal material from these cells may explain the damage occurring in bullous pemphigoid, but since the acantholysis in pemphigus is not accompanied initially by the presence of these cells a different mechanism must be sought. Antibodies to components of epithelium have been produced in experimental animals, essentially by the injection of skin extracts treated so as to release antigen or to make the preparation antigenic. In such animals the application of dry ice to the skin afterwards results in the formation of acantholysis with bulla formation in the injected animals but not in uninjected animals (Grob & Inderbitzen 1967). The same material has been found to be capable of absorbing out the anti-intercellular material antibody from pemphigus serum in humans.

9:4 Periodontal Disease

There is now considerable experimental evidence to support a direct deleterious effect of dental plaque upon the gingival epithelial attachment. Thus, several investigations have shown that a variety of tissue culture cells function poorly, or not at all, in the presence of dental plaque extracts (Powell 1969; Levine *et al* 1971). However, periodontal disease is characterized also by an alteration in the attachment apparatus. This tissue possesses a high turnover rate and is therefore susceptible to damage by a process which interferes with the replacement mechanism. It is in this latter respect that the immunological aspects of periodontal disease may be of significance.

Chronic periodontal disease

Within the tissues investing the teeth involved by periodontal disease there is a marked immunological response. The inflammatory cell infiltrate contains many lymphocytes and plasma cells. The mechanisms by which tissue injury may arise within the gingiva depend partly upon the assumption that antigen can penetrate to the level of these cells. There is some indirect and direct evidence for this. Thus, small molecules have shown to be capable of penetrating the intact human gingival crevice (Cowley 1966; Fine *et al* 1969). In subhuman primates, detectable levels of circulating antibody have been produced with immunization via the gingival crevice route in which there had been no apparent break in continuity (Ranney & Zander 1970).

In a fundamental sense, it could be argued that the replacement of the supporting tissues of the tooth by tissue responding to this immunological challenge is not conducive to stability. However, there is a possibility that tissue damage may occur because of this immune response.

The *complement system* may be activated through the classical or alternate pathway. The predominant Ig produced in the gingiva (Chapter 3), IgG, is capable of complement activation when complexed with antigen. Cell damage and the production of the intermediate products which promote inflammatory changes in the surrounding tissue may then follow in the manner of a type III reaction. The alternate pathway may be activated by bacterial lipopolysaccharide from the gingival crevice with similar results. Bacterial endotoxin is capable of penetrating the intact gingival crevice of dogs (Schwartz et al 1972).

There is good evidence that the *type IV hypersensitivity reaction* may contribute to the destructive process. Thus patients suffering from periodontal disease possess an enhanced response to antigens of plaque (Ivanyi & Lehner 1970; Horton et al 1972b) as measured by the lymphocyte transformation test. Lymphocytes from these patients when stimulated by plaque antigen produce macrophage migration inhibition factor and lymphokine, which is cytotoxic for chicken red cells (Ivanyi et al 1972). The lymphokine produced has also been shown to be capable of inducing bone resorption in the tissue culture situation (Horton et al 1972a) and of being cytotoxic for mouse L-cells and human gingival fibroblasts (Horton et al 1973). An *in vitro* model of immunologically induced periodontal tissue destruction would appear to have been demonstrated by these investigations.

The third concept is perhaps the most disturbing in terms of control of the disease. In the area of tissue destruction antigenic changes in host tissue may occur so that a perpetuating mechanism is established. Thus in the experimental animal type IV hypersensitivity to the tissue surrounding a sterile cotton-wool granuloma can be induced by adjuvant augmentation (Powell & Baboolal 1973). 'Differentiation' antigens peculiar to a particular tissue (Boyse & Old 1969) may be sequestered from the immune system during development (Lachmann 1963) yet become uncovered by pathological processes. Certainly, enzymatic treatment of syngeneic cartilage can evoke a cellular immune response upon injection into the host animal (Langer et al 1972). In addition, it has been suggested that presentation of undeaminated host protein (deamination of protein is thought to be the basis of protein turnover) during an inflammatory response may invoke an autoimmune response to the material since it has not previously been encountered in that form (Westall 1973). Thus, the initiation of an immune response within the periodontal tissue may invoke a self-perpetuating immune reaction which also produces local tissue damage.

9:5 Lichen Planus

This disease may occur on the skin only, on the skin and mucous membrane or on the mucosa only. The aetiology of the disease is unknown although it is thought to be associated with stress or drug ingestion. The appearance of the lesion on the skin is the characteristic papule, which is purple with fine white striae—Wickham's striae. In the mouth the characteristic lesion is also the papule, although there may be atrophic changes—red glazed areas with a white surround. Occasionally the atrophic areas break down into shallow erosions.

With skin lesions there is intense itching but the lesions in the mouth give quite different symptoms. The atrophic or erosive areas are sensitive, producing pain with hot or spicy foods while the papules may actually go unnoticed, often only producing comment from a clinician who examines the mouth. The gingival margin may also be affected in oral lichen planus and in both skin and oral lichen planus bullae may occasionally form. The histological appearance of an oral papule is characteristic with acanthotic ridges, liquefaction degeneration of the basal layer and a dense band of mononuclear cells filling the upper third of the corium. In the atrophic form the epithelium is thin and perhaps absent. The liquefaction degeneration of the basal layers of the epithelium and the mononuclear infiltrate are still present.

Immunological abnormalities in lichen planus

The immunopathology of lichen planus has not been extensively investigated. The presence of an infiltrate predominantly composed of lymphocytes (Lehner 1971) and accompanying the basal cell liquefaction degeneration is suggestive of immunological damage via a cell-mediated immune reaction either primarily or secondarily through release of sequestered host antigens. There is a high rate of nuclear protein synthesis amongst cells of the mononuclear infiltrate which have been identified histochemically as lymphocytes (Lachapelle & de la Brassinne 1973), so that an *in vivo* 'blast transformation' response to antigen would appear possible. The rate of nuclear protein synthesis in the basal layers of the epithelium apparently reduces with increasing density of the mononuclear infiltrate (Walker & Dolby 1974), which may also be construed as evidence of an immunological event. Thus cell damage may be directly attributable to lymphocyte activity or the cell damage produced by another agency may have provoked an immune response to altered host antigens. The measurement of the *in vitro* cellular immune response to extracts of lichen planus skin lesions has so far produced inconclusive results (Sarkany & Gaylarde 1972) and we have not been able to demonstrate a humoral or lymphocyte (type 2 above) cytotoxicity mechanism (Dolby & Slade unpublished).

9:6 Antigens of Oral Mucosa and Skin

Tissue-specific antigens

Several 'tissue-related' antigens have been mentioned in the diseases described above. It should be remembered that an antigen is a substance which, in suitable circumstances, can stimulate a specific immune response and can react specifically with the antibody or cells associated with that response. Studies made upon the antigens of tissue have made wide use of the fact that an immune response can be induced by their injection into another animal. Thus Aoki *et al* (1969) were able to detect by immunoelectrophoresis 15 tissue-specific antigens of guinea-pig epidermis using rabbit antisera raised against a guinea-pig epidermal extract. Five of these antigens were specific to epidermis, not being found in other tissues, and so represent characteristic tissue components of guinea-pig epidermis.

The significance of the detection and characterization of tissue antigens lies in the fact that many investigations have shown that it has been possible to induce the production of *autoantibodies* to characteristic tissue components (Ablin *et al* 1969). Such autoantigens are known to exist in certain diseases and have been detected by an augmented immune response to antigen in patients suffering from the disease (Table 9.1). This has been the second major method of study of tissue antigens, the examination of patients' blood for antibodies to soluble extracts of tissue. More recently, this has been extended to the cellular immune response to tissue antigens. A method which has been widely employed, in addition to those *in vitro* methods described under type IV hypersensitivity, is that of leukocyte migration inhibition (Bendixen & Sjoberg 1969). The test is somewhat similar to the MMIF test save that human leukocytes only are employed. It is thought that lymphocyte/antigen interaction leads to the release of soluble mediators which inhibit migration in the other leukocytes present.

The antigenic purity of the tissue antigen preparation has usually been high in the animal investigations, whereas the tissue antigen preparations used in the examination of diseased states are, at least initially, fairly crude. Thus the foetal oral mucosa extract (Lehner 1964) may contain several antigenic components of varying importance. Characterization may be attempted by fractionation of the extract and tissue-specificity determination by assessment of the extent of cross-reactivity with other tissues (Lehner 1969; Dolby 1972). An example of good localization, but not characterization, is the detection of pemphigus 'antigen' by immuno-electron-microscopy (Wolff & Schreiner 1971). Tissue-specific antigens may be related to the pathogenesis of a disease because of their cross-reactivity with otherwise non-pathogenic organisms. The examination of

Table 9.1. Oral mucosal and skin antigens which may be related to disease

Antigen source	Disease	Method of demonstration
Foetal oral mucosa antigen	Behçet's syndrome	Haemagglutination (Oshima *et al* 1963) (Lehner 1969)
	Mikulicz's recurrent oral aphthous ulceration	Haemagglutination, complement fixation Gel diffusion (Lehner 1964) Lymphocyte transformation (Lehner 1967)
Extract of skin lesion	Behçet's syndrome	*In vivo* ulcer production (Jadassohn *et al* 1957)
Basement membrane antigen	Bullous pemphigoid	Fluorescent antibody test (Jordon *et al* 1967)
Intercellular material antigen	Pemphigus	Fluorescent antibody test (Beutner & Jordon 1964) Electron microscopy, ferritin labelled antibodies (Chorzelski *et al* 1968) Autoradiography, tritium labelled antibodies (Barnard *et al* 1970) Histochemical, peroxidase labelled Ig technique (Fukuyama *et al* 1969)

bacteria for such cross-reactivity constitutes another major area of investigation into tissue antigens which are apparently disease-related, for example in ulcerative colitis (Perlmann *et al* 1967) and Mikulicz's recurrent oral aphthous ulceration (Lehner 1972).

9:7 HLA Antigens and Oral Mucosal Disease

During recent years several investigations have been undertaken to examine the frequency distribution of HLA phenotypes in disease. In particular, patients with immunological disorders and diseases involving the lymphatic system have been examined.

It has been known for some time (McDevitt & Benacerraf 1969) that the immunological response of experimental animals to antigens is genetically controlled or influenced. Thus in mice the response to a synthetic polypeptide antigen is controlled by an autosomal dominant gene. This gene is also linked to the H-2 locus which determines the pattern of mouse histocompatibility antigens. Jerne's (1970) hypothesis (see also Chapter 3) would suggest that the degree of antibody diversity of an individual is restricted by the individual's histocompatibility pattern. Thus it would seem likely that the individual's pattern of histocompatibility antigens determines susceptibility to diseases in which there is a major immunological component, in particular to the diseases described in this chapter.

9:8 References

ABLIN R.J., MILGROM F., KANO K., RAPAPORT F.T. & BEUTER E.H. (1969) Pemphigus-like antibodies in patients with skin burns. *Vox. Sang.*, **16**, 73–75.

ALLISON A.C., DENMAN A.M. & BARNES R.D. (1971) Co-operating and controlling functions of thymus-derived lymphocytes in relation to autoimmunity. *Lancet*, **2**, 135–141.

AMOS H.E. (1973) Immunology of skin diseases. *Brit. J. Hosp. Med.*, **9**, No. 1, 43–48.

AOKI T., PARKER D. & TURK J.L. (1969) Analysis of soluble antigens in guinea pig epidermis. II Physico-chemical characterizations of tissue-specific antigens. *Immunol.*, **16**, 499–512.

BANKHURST A.D., TORRIGIANI G. & ALLISON A.C. (1973) Lymphocytes binding human thyroglobulin in healthy people and its relevance to tolerance for autoantigens. *Lancet*, **1**, 226–229.

BARILE M.F., GRAYKOWSKI E.A., DRISCOLL E.J. & RIGGS D.B. (1963) L form of bacteria isolated from recurrent aphthous stomatitis lesions. *Oral Surg. Oral Med. & Oral Path.*, **16**, No. 11, 1395–1402.

BARNARD E.A., OSTROWSKI K., CHORZELSKI T.P., MIKULSKI A., LONGNER A. & SAWICKI W. (1970) Autoradiographic detection of tritiated antibodies combined with antigens. In BEUTNER, CHORZELSKI & JORDON *Autosensitization in Pemphigus and Bullous Pemphigoid*, 54–55. Charles C. Thomas, Springfield, Illinois.

BENDIXEN G. & SJOBERG M. (1969) A leucocyte migration technique for in vitro detection of cellular (delayed type) hypersensitivity in man. *Dan. med. Bull.*, **16**, No. 1, 1–6.

BEUTNER E.H. & JORDAN R.E. (1964) Demonstration of skin antibodies in sera of pemphigus vulgaris patients by indirect immunofluorescent staining. *Proc. Soc. exp. Biol. Med.*, **117**, 505–510.

BEUTNER E.H., JORDON R. & CHORZELSKI T.P. (1968) The immunopathology of pemphigus and bullous pemphigoid. *J. invest. Derm.*, **51**, No. 2, 63–79.

BEUTNER E.H., LEVER W.F., WITEBSKY E., JORDON R. & CHERTOCK B. (1965) Autoantibodies in pemphigus vulgaris. Response to an intercellular substance of epidermis. *J. Am. med. Ass.*, **192**, 682–688.

BOYSE E.A. & OLD L.G. (1969) Some aspects of normal and abnormal cell surface genetics. *Ann. Rev. Genet.*, **3**, 269–290.

BURNETT F.M. & FENNER F. (1949) *The Production of Antibodies*, 2nd edition. Macmillan, London.

BURNHAM T.K., NEBLETT T.R. & FINE G. (1963) The application of the fluorescent antibody technique to the investigation of lupus erythematosus and various dermatoses. *J. invest. Derm.*, **41**, 451–456.

CEROTTINI J.C., NORDIN A.A. & BRUNNER K.T. (1970) In vitro cytotoxic activity of thymus cells sensitized to alloantigens. *Nature, Lond.*, **227**, 72–73.

CHORZELSKI T.P., BICZYSKO W., DABROWSKI J. & JARZABEK M. (1968) Ultrastructural localization of 'pemphigus' autoantibodies. *J. invest. Derm.*, **50**, 36–40.

CHORZELSKI T.P. & JABLONSKA S. (1972) Pemphigus as an autoimmune disease. *Brit. J. Derm.*, **87**, No. 1, 78 (correspondence).

COOKE B.E.D. (1960) The diagnosis of bullous lesions affecting the oral mucosa. *Brit. dent. J.*, **109**, No. 3, 83–96.

COOKE B.E.D. (1961) Recurrent Mikulicz's aphthae. *Dent. Pract.*, **12**, No. 4, 119–124.

COWLEY G.C. (1966) Gingival inflammation. Thesis, University of Edinburgh.

DOE W.F., BOOTH C.C. & BROWN D.L. (1973) Evidence for complement-binding immune complexes in adult coeliac disease, Crohn's disease and ulcerative colitis. *Lancet*, **1**, 402–403.

DOLBY A.E. (1968) Recurrent Mikulicz's oral aphthae. Their relation to the menstrual cycle. *Brit. dent. J.*, **124**, No. 8, 359–360.

DOLBY A.E. (1969) Recurrent aphthous ulceration. Effect of sera and peripheral blood lymphocytes upon oral epithelial tissue culture cells. *Immunol.*, **17**, No. 5, 709–714.

DOLBY A.E. (1970) Mikulicz's recurrent oral aphthae: The effect of antilymphocyte serum upon the in vitro cytotoxicity of lymphocytes from patients for oral epithelial cells. *Clin. exp. Immunol.*, **7**, No. 5, 681–686.

DOLBY A.E. (1972) The effect of lymphocytes from sufferers from recurrent aphthous ulceration upon colon cells in tissue culture. *Gut*, **13**, 387–389.

DOLBY A.E. & SLADE M. Failure to detect immune epithelial cytolysis in oral lichen planus. (In preparation.)

DOWLING G.B. (1961) Behçet's disease. *Proc. R. Soc. Med.*, **54**, 101–104.

DUMONDE D.C., WOLSTENCROFT R.A., PANAYI G.S., MATTHEW M., MORLEY J. & HOWSON W.T. (1969) Lymphokines: Non-antibody mediators of cellular immunity generated by lymphocyte activation. *Nature, Lond.*, **224**, 38–42.

FARMER E.D. (1958) Recurrent aphthous ulcers. *Dent. Pract.*, **8**, 177–184.

FINE D.H., PECHERSKY J.L. & MCKIBBEN D.H. (1969) The penetration of human gingival sulcular tissue by carbon particles. *Archs. oral Biol.*, **14**, 1117–1119.

FRANCIS T.C. & OPPENHEIM J.J. (1970) Impaired lymphocyte stimulation by some streptococcal antigens in patients with recurrent aphthous stomatitis and rheumatic heart disease. *Clin. exp. Immunol.*, **6**, 573–586.

FUKUYAMA K., DOUGLAS S.D., TUFFANELLI D.L. & EPSTEIN W.L. (1969) An immunohistochemical method for the localization of antibodies in cutaneous disease. *J. invest. Derm.*, **52**, 370–371.

GELL P.G.H. & COOMBS R.R.A. (1963) *Clinical Aspects of Immunology*, 317. Blackwell Scientific Publications, Oxford.

GRANGER G.A. & KOLB W.P. (1968) Lymphocyte in vitro cytotoxicity. Mechanisms of immune and non-immune small lymphocyte mediated target L cell destruction. *J. Immunol.*, **101**, No. 1, 111–119.

GRAYKOWSKI E.A., BARILE M.F., BOYD LEE W. & STANLEY H.R. (1966) Recurrent aphthous stomatitis. Clinical, therapeutic, histopathologic and hypersensitivity aspects. *J. Am. med. Ass.*, **196**, 637–644.

GROB P.J. & INDERBITZEN T.M. (1967) Pemphigus antigen and blood group substances A and B. *J. invest. Derm.*, **49**, 285–287.

HORTON J.E., LEIKEN S. & OPPENHEIM J.J. (1972b) Human lymphoproliferative reaction to saliva and dental plaque deposits; an in vitro correlation with periodontal disease. *J. Periodont.*, **43**, 522–527.

HORTON J.E., OPPENHEIM J.J. & MERGENHAGEN S.E. (1973) Elaboration of lymphotoxin by cultured human peripheral blood leucocytes stimulated with dental plaque deposits. *Clin. exp. Immunol.*, **13**, 383–393.

HORTON J.E., RAISZ L.G., SIMMONS H.A., OPPENHEIM J.J. & MERGENHAGEN S.E. (1972a) Bone resorbing activity in supernatant fluid from cultured human peripheral blood leukocytes. *Science*, **177**, 793–795.

ITO K., WICHER K. & ARBESMAN C.E. (1969) Insoluble immunoadsorbents containing anti-IgE; removal of reaginic activity and subsequent elution. *J. Immunol.*, **103**, 622–624.

IVANYI L. & LEHNER T. (1970) Stimulation of lymphocyte transformation by bacterial antigens in patients with periodontal disease. *Archs. oral Biol.*, **15**, 1089–1096.

IVANYI L., WILTON J.M.A. & LEHNER T. (1972) Cell mediated immunity in periodontal disease; cytotoxicity, migration inhibition and lymphocyte transformation studies. *Immunol.*, **22**, 141–145.

JADASSOHN W., FRANCESCHETTI A. & GOLAY M. (1953) A cutaneous reaction in a case of aphthous uveitis with recurring hypopyon (Behçet's syndrome). *Schweiz. med. Wochenschr.*, **38**, 1188.

JERNE N.K. (1970) The stomatic generation of immune recognition. *Eur. J. Immunol.*, **1**, 1–9.

JORDON R.E., BEUTNER E.H., WITEBSKY E., BLUMENTAL G., HALE W.L. & LEVER W.F. (1967) Basement zone antibodies in bullous pemphigoid. *J. Am. med. Ass.*, **200**, 751–756.

KATZENELLENBOGEN I. (1946) Recurrent aphthous ulceration of oral mucous membrane and genitals associated with recurrent hypopyon iritis (Behçet's syndrome). Report of three cases. *Brit. J. Derm. Syph.*, **58**, 161–172.

LACHAPELLE J.M. & DE LA BRASSINNE M. (1973) The proliferation of cells in the dermal infiltrate of lichen planus lesions. *Brit. J. Derm.*, **89**, 137–141.

LACHMAN P. (1963) Autoimmunity. In GELL & COOMBS, 567. Blackwell Scientific Publications, Oxford.

LANGER F., GROSS A.E. & GREAVES M.F. (1972) The autoimmunogenicity of articular cartilage. *Clin. exp. Immunol.*, **12**, 31–37.

LARSSON A. & PERLMANN P. (1972) Study of Fab and F(ab')$_2$ from rabbit IgG for capacity to induce lymphocyte-mediated target cell destruction. *Int. Arch. Allergy*, **43**, 80–88.

LEHNER T. (1964) Recurrent aphthous ulceration and autoimmunity. *Lancet*, **2**, 1154–1155.

LEHNER T. (1967) Behçet's syndrome and autoimmunity. *Brit. med. J.*, **1**, 465–467.

LEHNER T. (1969) Characterization of mucosal antibodies in recurrent aphthous ulceration and Behçet's syndrome. *Archs. oral Biol.*, **14**, 843–853.

LEHNER T. (1971) Quantitative assessment of lymphocytes and plasma cells in leukoplakia candidiasis and lichen planus. *J. dent. Res.*, **50**, No. 6, Part 2, 1661–1665.

LEHNER T. (1972) Immunological aspects of recurrent oral ulcers. *Oral Surg. Oral Med. & Oral Path.*, **33**, 80–85.

LEHNER T. & SAGEBIEL R.W. (1966) Fine structural findings in recurrent oral ulceration. *Brit. dent. J.*, **121**, 454–456.

LEVER W.F. (1965) In *Pemphigus and Pemphigoid*. Charles C. Thomas, Springfield, Illinois.

LEVINE M., ADAMS R.L.P. & COWLEY G.C. (1971) Effects of dental plaque extracts on HeLa cells in culture. *J. dent. Res.*, **50**, 672–673.

McDEVITT H.O. & BENACERRAF B. (1969) Genetic control of specific immune responses. *Advances in Immunol.*, **11**, 31–74.

OSHIMA Y., SHIMIZU T., YOKOHARI R., TOKIO M., KANO K., KAGAMI T. & NAGAYA N. (1963) Clinical studies on Behçet's syndrome. *Ann. Rheum. Dis.*, **22**, 36–45.

PERLMANN P., HAMMARSTROM S., LAGERCRANTZ R. & CAMPBELL D. (1967) Autoantibodies to colon in rats and human ulcerative colitis: cross reactivity with E. coli O 14 antigen. *Proc. Soc. exp. Biol. Med.*, **125**, 975–980.

POWELL R.N. (1969) The effect of bacterial plaque on gingival epithelium in vitro. *Dent. Pract.*, **20**, No. 4, 139–142.

POWELL R.N. & BABOOLAL R. (1973) The role of endogenous antigens in bone resorption. (Personal communication.)

RANNEY R.R. & ZANDER H.A. (1970) Allergic periodontal disease in sensitized squirrel monkeys. *J. Periodont.*, **41**, 12–21.

RUDDY S., GIGLI I. & AUSTEN K.F. (1972) The complement system of man. *New Engl. J. Med.*, **287**, No. 10, 489–495.

SALLAY K., DAN P., KULCSAR G. & NASZ I. (1971) Transformation of lymphocytes from patients with recurrent aphthae. *Revue d'Immunologie, Paris*, tome **35**, Nos. 1–2, 17–21.

SARKANY I. & GAYLARDE P.M. (1972) The pathogenesis of lichen planus. *Brit. J. Derm.*, **87**, No. 1, 817.

SCHWARTZ J. & VARDINON N. (1966) In vitro prevention of direct mast cell disruption by specific antibody. *Int. Arch. Allergy*, **30**, 67–74.

SCHWARTZ J., STINSON F.L. & PARKER R.B. (1972) The passage of tritiated bacterial endotoxin across intact gingivae crevicular epithelium. *J. Periodont.*, **43,** No. 5, 270–276.
SHELLEY W.B. (1963) Indirect basophil degranulation test for allergy to penicillin and other drugs. *J. Am. med. Ass.*, **184,** 171–178.
SIRCUS W., CHURCH R. & KELLEHER J. (1957) Recurrent aphthous ulceration of the mouth. A study of the natural history, aetiology and treatment. *Quart. J. Med.*, **26,** 235–249.
THIVOLET J. & BEYVIN A.J. (1968) Recherche par immunofluorescence d'auto anticorps seriques vis-a-vis des constituante de l'epiderme chez les brules. Personal communication. *Experientia*, **24,** 945.
TOLO K. (1971) A study of permeability of gingival pocket epithelium to albumin in guinea pigs and Norwegian pigs. *Archs. oral Biol.*, **16,** 881–888.
TOURAINE M.A. (1941) L'aphtose. *Bull. Soc. Franc. Derm. Syph.*, **48,** 61–104.
TRUELOVE S.C. & MORRIS-OWEN R.M. (1958) Treatment of aphthous ulceration of the mouth. *Brit. med. J.*, **1,** 603–607.
TURK J.L. (1969) In *Immunology of Clinical Medicine.* Heinemann Medical Books.
WAKSMAN B.H. (1959) Experimental allergic encephalomyelitis and the 'autoallergic' diseases. *Int. Arch. Allergy*, **14,** (Suppl.) 1–87.
WAKSMAN B.H. (1968) Discussion from Intersociety Symposium on in vitro correlates of delayed hypersensitivity. Presented at the 51st Meeting of the Federation of American Societies for Experimental Biology, Chicago, Ill. Apl. 1967. *Fed. Proc.*, **27,** 45, 1968.
WALKER D.M. & DOLBY A.E. (1974) The relationship between epithelial cell division and inflammatory cell infiltrate in oral lichen planus. *Brit. J. Derm.*, **91,** 549.
WESTALL F.C. (1973) An explanation for the determination of 'self' versus 'nonself' proteins. *J. theor. Biol.*, **38,** 139–141.
WILLIAMS T.W. & GRANGER G.A. (1968) Lymphocyte in vitro cytotoxicity: Lymphotoxins of several mammalian species. *Nature, Lond.*, **219,** 1076–1077.
WOLFF K. & SCHREINER E. (1971) Ultrastructural localization of pemphigus autoantibodies within the epidermis. *Nature, Lond.*, **229,** 59–61.

CHAPTER 10
DISTURBANCE OF SALIVARY GLAND SECRETION: SJÖGREN'S SYNDROME

D.M. CHISHOLM AND D.K. MASON

10:0 Introduction

Sjögren's syndrome, first described in 1933 (Sjögren 1933), consists of the triad of xerostomia, kerato-conjunctivitis sicca and, in half to two-thirds of patients, rheumatoid arthritis. Salivary gland and/or lacrimal gland enlargement may or may not be present. In some cases, rheumatoid arthritis may be replaced by another connective tissue disease such as polyarteritis nodosa, systemic lupus erythematosus, progressive systemic sclerosis, polymyositis or dermatomyositis. The presence of two of these three main components is generally sufficient for the diagnosis of the syndrome. The term 'sicca syndrome' is used when the connective tissue disorder is absent, i.e. xerostomia and kerato-conjunctivitis only are present.

The present chapter reviews recent investigations of the clinical manifestations, diagnostic techniques, histopathologic and laboratory findings, together with current approaches to treatment and management of Sjögren's syndrome. Particular attention is paid to the oral and salivary gland involvement.

10:1 General Features of Sjögren's Syndrome

Sjögren's syndrome is primarily a disorder which affects middle-aged females though, on occasion, males and younger individuals may be affected. The frequency with which Sjögren's syndrome is recognized depends largely upon the awareness of the examiner who first sees the patient (Shearn 1971).

Several studies suggest that Sjögren's syndrome is a common complication of rheumatoid arthritis alone (Holm 1949; Bloch & Bunim 1963; Shearn 1971). Our experience indicates that approximately 1% of patients

448 Chapter 10

with rheumatoid arthritis develop the salivary gland manifestations of the syndrome (Buchanan 1973). However, patients with the sicca syndrome accounted for 40% of all cases of Sjögren's syndrome recently reported by our group (Whaley et al 1973).

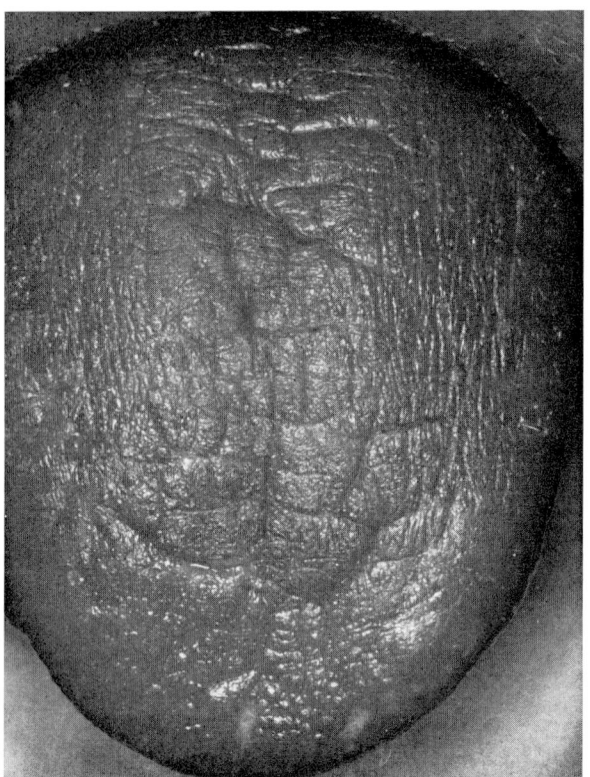

Fig. 10.1. Lingual changes in a 44-year-old patient with Sjögren's syndrome. Mucosal atrophy together with mild fissuring and lobulation is present.

With regard to the incidence of the syndrome, it is to be noted that among the connective tissue diseases, Sjögren's syndrome ranks second only to rheumatoid arthritis (Shearn 1971).

10:1:1 Clinical features

GENERAL MANIFESTATIONS

The symptoms, signs, laboratory findings and radiographic changes of patients with rheumatoid arthritis complicated by Sjögren's syndrome closely resemble those of classic rheumatoid arthritis. It is of interest that arthritic symptoms are the most frequent initial complaint of patients who develop full-blown Sjögren's syndrome (Bloch et al 1965; Shearn 1971). Kerato-conjunctivitis sicca manifests as a dryness, together with a gritty burning sensation of the eyes; redness, photophobia and discharge are other symptoms of note. Lacrimal gland enlargement is uncommon (Hughes & Whaley 1972). In view of the co-existence with various connective tissue diseases it is not surprising that recent investigations have

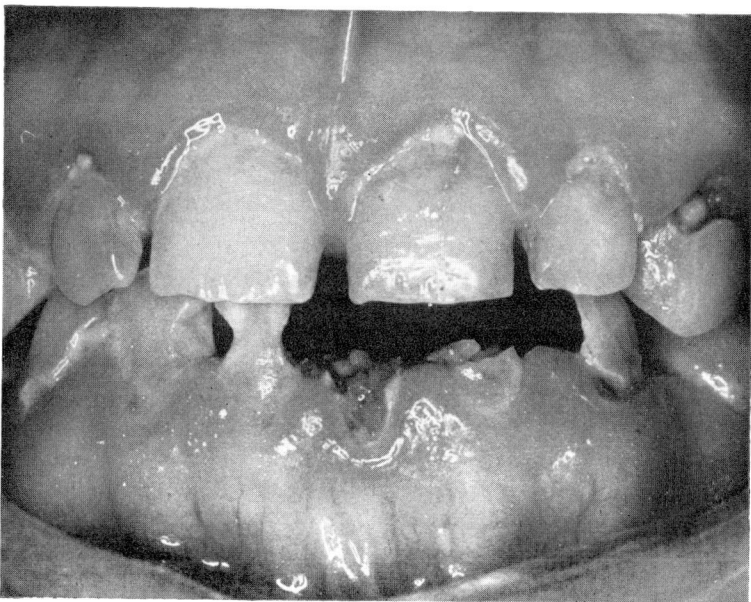

Fig. 10.2. Rapidly progressive dental caries in a 32-year-old female with Sjögren's syndrome.

revealed multisystem abnormalities in some patients with Sjögren's syndrome. In addition to dryness of the mouth and eyes, hypofunction of exocrine glands may lead to nasal, pharyngeal, vaginal and vulvar dryness. Dryness of the skin with pruritus and scaling, thrombocytopneic purpura and Raynaud's phenomenon are not infrequently seen. Various gastrointestinal, pulmonary, renal, neurological, cardiac and endocrine abnormalities in Sjögren's syndrome have been described and are well reviewed by Shearn (1971). Finally, the association between Sjögren's syndrome and malignant lymphoreticular disease is now well documented and will be discussed in more detail later in the chapter.

10:2 Oral Manifestations

(a) Xerostomia

Decreased salivation, difficulty in swallowing and mastication, increased fluid intake, abnormalities in taste sensation, oral mucosal soreness and ulceration are common symptoms. The oral mucous membranes appear dry, smooth and glazed, whilst lingual changes varying from slight

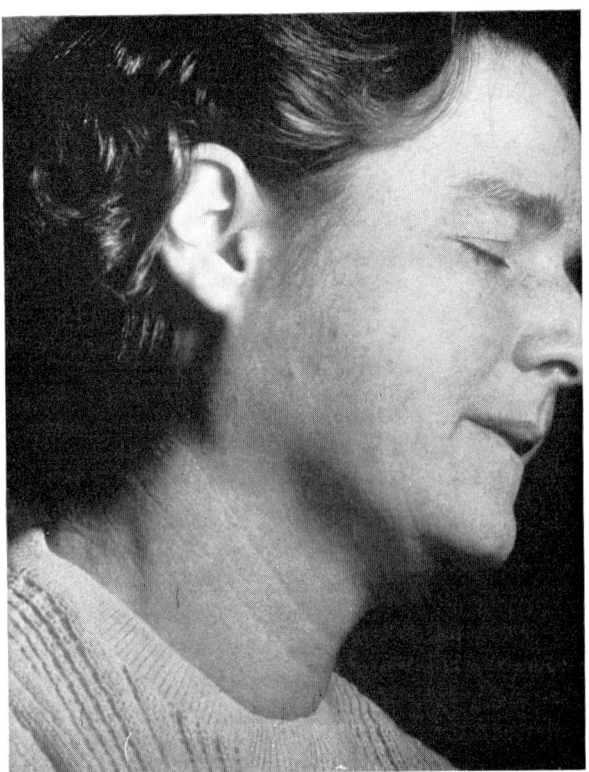

Fig. 10.3. Right parotid gland enlargement in a 46-year-old female with sicca syndrome.

reddening with mild fissuring to pronounced reddening with severe lobulation (Fig. 10.1) and deep fissuring are often present (Bertram 1967).

However, these mucosal signs are only suggestive of xerostomia due to Sjögren's syndrome, since they may present in a variety of disorders including pernicious anaemia, folic acid deficiency, sideropenic anaemia and malabsorption (Hjörting-Hansen & Bertram 1968).

Salivary Dysfunction

The histopathologic appearances of the oral epithelium in Sjögren's syndrome have recently been studied (Adams 1973). Although basal layer disruption, para-keratinization, lymphocytic infiltration and atrophy were features of note, they were inconsistent and could not be related to clinical features.

In patients with a natural dentition, a rapidly progressive dental caries may be observed (Fig. 10.2). Those patients with dentures have difficulty with retention. Recently, an association between Sjögren's syndrome and oral candidosis has been noted (MacFarlane & Mason 1973).

(b) Salivary gland enlargement

Bloch et al (1965) reported salivary gland enlargement to be present in half of 62 patients studied, but our experience over a 10-year period has been that although a history of salivary gland enlargement may be elicited from approximately 30% of patients, its presence is clinically apparent in only half that number. Most studies agree that salivary swelling in Sjögren's syndrome occurs bilaterally and that the parotid glands are more commonly affected (Fig. 10.3). It is of interest that Talal et al (1967) have reported that patients with Sjögren's syndrome who develop lymphoid neoplasia are more likely to show salivary gland enlargement.

10:3 Diagnostic Techniques

GENERAL

Rheumatoid arthritis and kerato-conjunctivitis sicca are diagnoses made by well-defined criteria. The American Rheumatism Association criteria (Ropes et al 1958) have been used in most recent studies. The diagnosis of kerato-conjunctivitis sicca is made by demonstrating diminished lacrimation by the use of the Schirmer tear test, and/or the finding of filamentary or punctate keratitis on slit lamp examination of the cornea after the instillation of rose bengal dye into the conjunctival sac (Williamson et al 1967).

ORAL

At the present time, there is no entirely satisfactory diagnostic test for the salivary gland component of Sjögren's syndrome. Xerostomia is a common clinical complaint with a multiplicity of causes and predisposing factors

(Bertram 1967; Mason & Glen 1967). In recent years, however, much attention has been directed towards the diagnostic value of salivary function tests such as flow rate estimation, labial salivary gland biopsy, hydrostatic sialography and pertechnetate scintiscanning (see Chapter 2), and these will now be considered:

(a) *Salivary flow rate estimation*

The factors which influence salivary flow rates, including methods of collecting saliva, have been reviewed (Bertram 1967). In addition to a diurnal variation (Hildes & Ferguson 1958) there is a wide range of flow

Table 10.1. Citric acid (5% solution) stimulated parotid flow rates (ml/min ± SEM) in 171 control subjects, 32 patients with sicca syndrome and 86 patients with Sjögren's syndrome.

		Age range (yrs): <20	21–40	41–60	61+
Controls	Male	1·49 ± 0·09	1·73 ± 0·09	1·69 ± 0·11	1·58 ± 0·16
	Female	1·99 ± 0·14	1·76 ± 0·09	1·36 ± 0·12	1·15 ± 0·08
Sicca syndrome	Male	—	—	—	0·43 ± 0·08
	Female	—	—	0·24 ± 0·08	0·27 ± 0·05
Sjögren's syndrome + rheumatoid arthritis	Male	—	—	0·93 ± 0·17	0·43 ± 0·05
	Female	—	0·56 ± 0·05	0·47 ± 0·07	0·41 ± 0·05

rate values in normal individuals which varies with age and sex (Chisholm 1970). It is important, therefore, that salivary flow rate values be interpreted against this background. In our clinic, parotid salivary flow rates are estimated using the method outlined by Mason *et al* (1967). A modified Carlson–Crittenden cup is placed over the parotid duct orifice, maintained in position by air suction applied through the outer chamber. During stimulation with 5% citric acid saliva is collected into graduated tubes. This method is a fairly reliable test of salivary gland function and 90% of patients with Sjögren's syndrome, observed over a 10-year period, had flow rate values (Table 10.1) below the normal range (Chisholm & Mason 1973). Reduced salivary flow rates in patients with Sjögren's syndrome have been reported by Bloch *et al* (1965) and Bertram (1967).

(b) Labial salivary gland biopsy

Although a biopsy of major salivary gland tissue would be of great value as a diagnostic aid, in view of the possible complication of salivary fistula

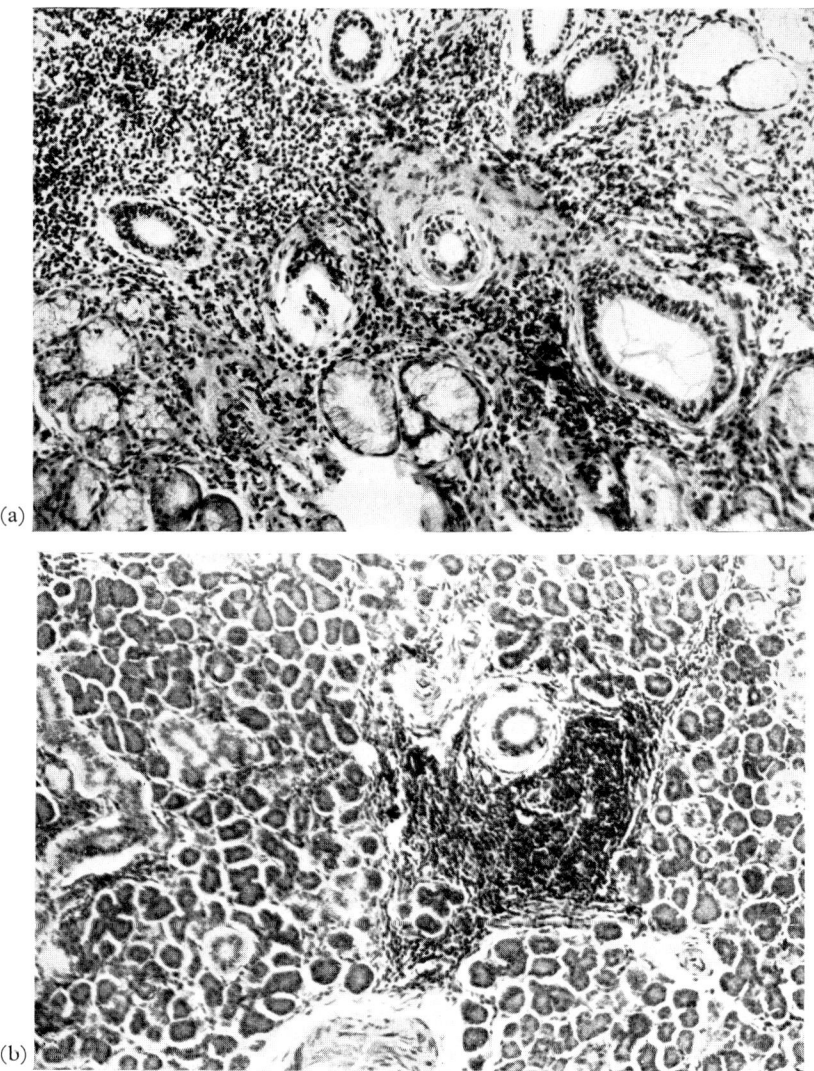

Fig. 10.4. Focal lymphocytic sialadenitis in Sjögren's syndrome:
(a) Labial gland.
(b) Submandibular gland ($\times 56$).

formation and damage to important neurovascular bundles, it cannot be recommended unless neoplasia is suspected. However, a biopsy of the intraoral minor salivary glands overcomes most of these problems. The presence of focal lymphocytic adenitis in the minor salivary glands, in a small number of cases of Sjögren's syndrome, has been reported (Cifarelli et al 1966; Calman & Reifman 1966; Mason 1966; Cahn 1967; Bertram 1967). Using the labial salivary glands, Chisholm & Mason (1968) studied the histopathologic features of groups of patients with various connective tissue disorders, including Sjögren's syndrome. In this and subsequent studies (Chisholm 1969; Chisholm et al 1971; Talal et al 1970; Berry et al

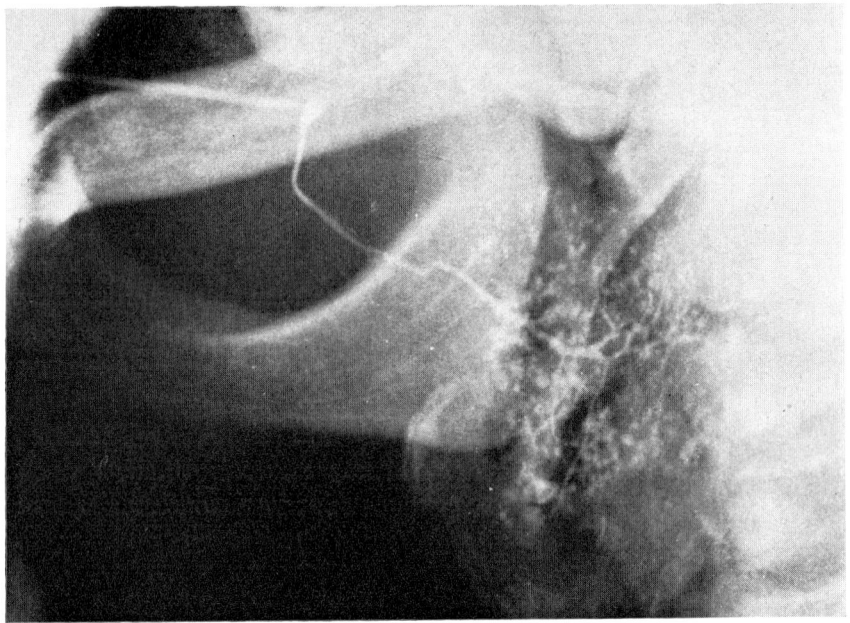

Fig. 10.5. Globular sialectasis of the parotid gland in a patient with Sjögren's syndrome.

1973), focal lymphocytic sialadenitis was demonstrated in approximately 70% of patients with Sjögren's syndrome (Fig. 10.4). The finding of focal lymphocytic adenitis in the labial salivary glands in approximately 20% of patients with rheumatoid arthritis alone is of interest, for this lesion may represent a subclinical form of Sjögren's syndrome in these patients (Chisholm & Mason 1968; Chisholm 1969). Conceptual support for the labial biopsy technique has been provided (Chisholm et al 1970) by a postmortem study in which focal lymphocytic sialadenitis could not be demonstrated in the labial glands. This study also showed that changes in the minor glands reflected those in their major counterparts.

(c) Hydrostatic sialography

Sialography is the radiographic demonstration of the salivary duct system following the introduction of a radio-opaque contrast medium through the duct orifice. The hydrostatic technique used in our clinic has been described by Park & Mason (1966) and allows a water-soluble contrast medium (Hypaque) to be introduced into the salivary duct system at a constant pressure. Interpretation of sialographic abnormalities is based on criteria laid down by Blatt et al (1956) and modified by Bloch et al (1965). Varying degrees of sialectasis (Fig. 10.5) are consistent findings in patients with Sjögren's syndrome (Bloch et al 1965; Mason 1966; Chisholm et al 1971; Blair 1973).

(d) Salivary scintiscanning

Salivary gland scanning appears promising as a method of assessing salivary gland function in man (Harden et al 1967; Veronesi et al 1967; Gates & Work 1967). ^{99m}Tc pertechnetate is an almost ideal scanning agent and, like iodide, is concentrated in the major salivary glands (Harden & Alexander 1967) and minor salivary glands (Chisholm et al 1971). Following recent work it appears, both qualitatively (Harden et al 1968; Abramson et al 1968; Grove & Di Chiro 1968) and quantitatively (Stephen et al 1971), that ^{99m}Tc pertechnetate uptake by the salivary glands is reduced in patients with Sjögren's syndrome. The recent study by Stephen et al (1971) showed that two-thirds of patients with Sjögren's syndrome had uptake values below the lowest value recorded in the control group. Furthermore, this investigation demonstrated that parotid gland involvement is more common than submandibular, that although the parotid glands may be involved without submandibular glands, the reverse does not hold, and finally that gland involvement is usually bilateral (Fig. 10.6). It is of interest that sequential salivary scintiscanning has been shown to parallel closely reduction in flow rates and sialographic abnormalities in the syndrome (Schall et al 1971).

Summary—clinical tests of salivary gland function

The relative value of these salivary gland function tests as diagnostic aids has been assessed by Chisholm & Mason (1973). They found reduced parotid flow rate to be the most sensitive index of salivary gland dysfunction in Sjögren's syndrome, followed by labial gland biopsy and

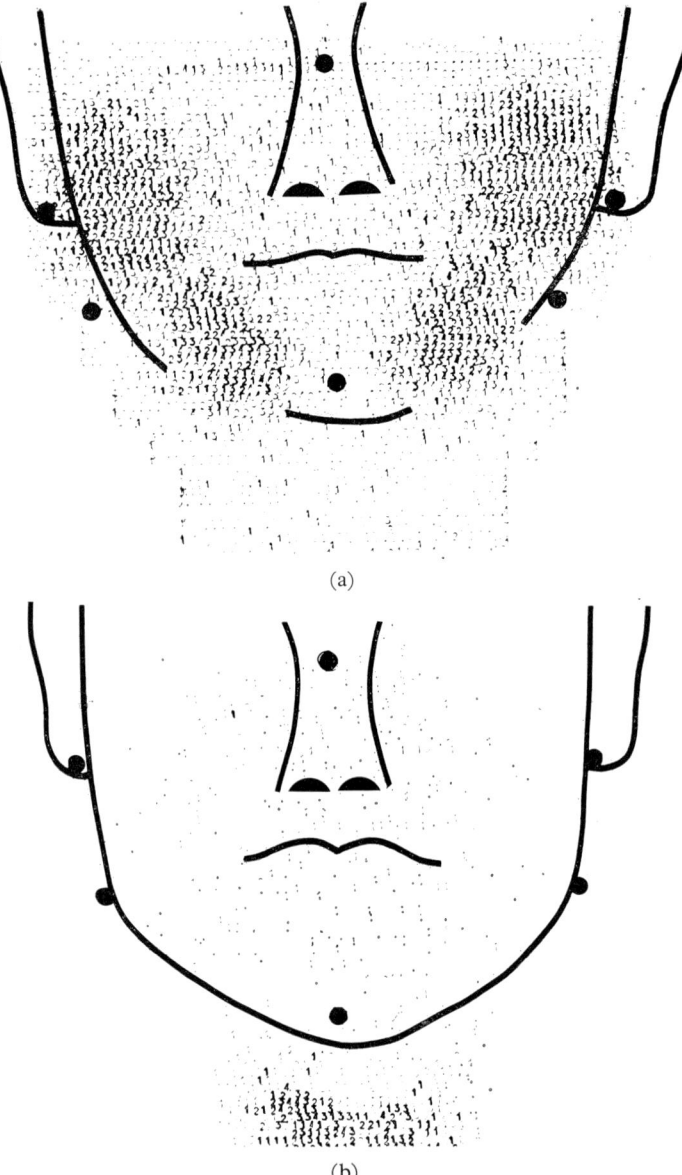

Fig. 10.6. Salivary gland scintiscanning using ^{99m}Tc pertechnetate.
(a) Normal uptake of isotope.
(b) No detectable uptake in a patient with Sjögren's syndrome.

sialography. Flow rate estimation, however, has the disadvantage of examining the secretions from one group of glands only. Since the parotid glands make the main contribution to whole saliva on stimulation, and are the most commonly involved clinically and as demonstrated by scintiscanning, we feel justified in recommending this technique as an initial screening test. Labial gland biopsy is a simple and safe technique and, in our experience, is well tolerated by patients. It is the only test which gives an indication of the nature of the disease process in the salivary glands. Sialography is time-consuming, since each gland has to be examined individually. The new method of quantitative scintiscanning with ^{99m}Tc pertechnetate is promising, but has not yet been fully evaluated as a test of salivary gland function in disease states. It has the advantage of examining both parotid and submandibular glands at the one time.

10:4 Laboratory Investigations

GENERAL

The remarkable prevalence of abnormal immunologic features represents a striking feature of Sjögren's syndrome. Indeed, the disease ranks second only to systemic lupus erythematosus in its abundance of serum autoantibodies, both organ specific and non-organ specific. Rheumatoid factor is present in 75–100% of patients with Sjögren's syndrome, even in the absence of rheumatoid arthritis (Bloch et al 1965). Antinuclear antibodies are found in approximately two-thirds of patients, speckled or nucleolar patterns being common (Beck 1961). Tests for lupus erythematosus cells are positive in roughly 10% of patients with Sjögren's syndrome (Bloch et al 1965). Autoantibodies to thyroglobulin and thyroid microsomes (Bloch & Bunim 1963), gastric parietal cell antibody (Buchanan et al 1966) and mitochondrial antibody (Whaley et al 1970) have been reported in Sjögren's syndrome. In vitro transformation of peripheral blood lymphocytes in response to phytohaemagglutinin and streptolysin O has been studied by Leventhal et al (1967). These studies showed significant reduction in response to these mitogenic agents in patients with Sjögren's syndrome, especially those cases complicated by rheumatoid arthritis or lymphoma, compared with controls. Leventhal et al (1967) have also shown that the skin of patients with Sjögren's syndrome has a reduced ability to become sensitized to the contact allergen 2,4-dinitrochlorobenzene (DNCB).

ORAL

An autoantibody to the cytoplasm of salivary duct cells has been demonstrated by indirect fluorescence (Bertram & Halberg 1964; Halberg et al 1965; MacSween et al 1967; Feltkamp & Van Rossum 1968). However, this antibody is considered to be a reflection of rheumatoid arthritis alone, rather than a manifestation of Sjögren's syndrome per se (Whaley et al 1969), and its pathogenic significance appears doubtful (Feltkamp & Van Rossum 1968). The inhibition of migration of cells by antigen is characteristic of hypersensitivities of the delayed type (see Chapter 9). Inhibition of macrophage migration in vitro by salivary gland extracts has been demonstrated in patients with Sjögren's syndrome (Søborg & Bertram 1968). Recently Berry et al (1972) using the leukocyte migration test showed reactivity to parotid gland extract antigen in 93% of patients with Sjögren's syndrome and that a good correlation existed between the degree of focal lymphocytic labial sialadenitis and reactivity in this test. From material obtained at labial salivary gland biopsy, Talal et al (1970) have demonstrated a greater synthesis of immunoglobulins, especially IgM and IgG, in Sjögren's syndrome compared with controls, whilst Anderson et al (1972) have demonstrated that the local synthesis of rheumatoid factor in labial salivary gland tissue is distinctive for Sjögren's syndrome.

The renewed interest in the role of infective agents including mycoplasmas in association with rheumatoid arthritis and other connective tissue disorders (Bartholomew 1965; Duthie et al 1967; Williams et al 1970) prompted our group to search for mycoplasmal infection in labial salivary gland tissue and parotid saliva in patients with Sjögren's syndrome. However, mycoplasma (M. orale type 1) was recovered from saliva in only one of 26 patients (Gordon et al 1971). Though disappointing, this study does not exclude the possibility of the occurrence of hitherto uncultivable agents or of 'latent' mycoplasmal infection in this and allied conditions. Recent mycologic studies from our laboratory have shown that an association exists between Sjögren's syndrome and oral candidosis (MacFarlane & Mason 1973). This finding is of special interest in view of the occurrence of chronic candidosis in patients with a wide variety of immune defects (Brit. med. J. 1972). Other factors which could explain this finding include lack of cleansing action or antibacterial factors in saliva, low pH of saliva, iron deficiency and the use of corticosteroid drugs. There is a paucity of information regarding the constituents of saliva from patients with Sjögren's syndrome. Recently Mandel & Baurmash (1973) reported significant elevations in sodium and chloride and reduction in phosphorus in saliva from patients with Sjögren's syndrome. In 1968, Fischer et al showed that the electrophoretic pattern of parotid saliva was specific for Sjögren's syndrome, anodal proteins migrating more rapidly with advancing severity of the disease. In Sjögren's syndrome, parotid salivary proteins have been separated by the more sensitive technique of isoelectric focusing in polyacrylamide gels (Chisholm et al 1973). This study demonstrated additional proteins, with low isoelectric points compared to control samples.

10:4:1 Histopathology and lymphoreticular neoplasia

GENERAL

The most characteristic histopathologic feature of affected tissue in Sjögren's syndrome is lymphocytic infiltration. Lymphoid infiltrates may be observed in the lacrimal glands, the mucus-secreting glands of the conjunctivae, the nasal cavity, pharynx, larynx, trachea and bronchi, leading to atrophy of these glands. The sweat glands may be similarly affected. Ultrastructural studies of renal biopsies have shown the presence of viral-like inclusion bodies within renal endothelial cells (Shearn et al 1970).

ORAL

The histopathologic features of the major salivary glands are well documented (Cardell & Gurling 1954; Bloch et al 1963; Ericson 1968) and include acinar atrophy, focal lymphocytic sialadenitis and ductal hyperplasia leading to the formation of 'epimyoepithelial' cell islands (Morgan & Castleman 1953). It is of interest that ultrastructural studies have failed to reveal the presence of myoepithelial cells in these cell islands (Boquist et al 1970; Kitamura et al 1970). The minor salivary glands show similar features to these described above for their major gland counterparts with the exception that epimyoepithelial cell islands do not appear to be a feature (Chisholm & Mason 1968; Eisenbud et al 1973; Talal et al 1971; Davies et al 1973). Histopathological features such as interstitial fibrosis, acinar atrophy and ductal changes in the labial glands have been semi-quantitated (Chisholm 1969; Davies et al 1973) and shown to be more severe in Sjögren's syndrome than in rheumatoid arthritis or other connective tissue disorders. It is of interest that virus-like particles, similar to murine C-type oncogenic virus, have been reported within endothelial cells and lymphocytes in the parotid gland (Albegger & Auböck 1972) and labial glands (Daniels *et al* 1973) in recent ultrastructural studies of biopsies from patients with Sjögren's syndrome.

Attempts to produce the salivary gland lesion of Sjögren's syndrome in experimental animals by immunization with salivary gland homogenates and Freund's adjuvant have met with limited success (Waterhouse 1963; Chan 1964). Perhaps the most exciting development in this field has been the discovery that a series of abnormalities resembling those of Sjögren's syndrome, occur spontaneously in NZB and NZBF mice. These abnormalities appear about the fourth month, hand in hand with other autoimmune phenomena and increase in severity with age, particularly in females. In these animals, salivary amylase is reduced and the salivary protein concentration is elevated. Recently, several reports of malignant lymphoma complicating Sjögren's syndrome have appeared (Bloch *et al* 1965; Hornbaker *et al* 1966; Mellors 1966; Talal *et al* 1967). Generally, such neoplastic change has an extra-salivary distribution, though recent reports have demonstrated that malignant transformation may originate within the salivary glands (Azzopardi & Evans 1971). The prolonged state of immunologic and lymphoid hyperactivity in patients with Sjögren's syndrome, especially those with the sicca syndrome, may be predisposing factors in the development of lymphoid neoplasia (Talal & Bunim 1964). Such patients are also more likely to show salivary gland enlargement (Talal *et al* 1967). Sjögren's syndrome, therefore, provides a link between disease affecting immunological responses and the development of neoplasia.

10:4:2 Pathogenetic considerations

Though the cause of Sjögren's syndrome remains unknown, it seems likely that a combination of genetic, immunologic, viral and/or environmental factors may play a role in the pathogenesis (Anderson & Talal 1971). There is strong evidence that Sjögren's syndrome should be considered an autoimmune disorder, since the criteria of such a disease as laid down by MacKay & Burnet (1963) are satisfied (Shearn 1971). The possibility that Sjögren's syndrome may have a hereditary component is based largely on observations of a familial incidence (Lisch 1937; Hamilton 1940; Coverdale 1955; Bloch *et al* 1965). A polygenic hereditary component, the expression of which depends upon certain environmental factors, as yet unknown, may exist in Sjögren's syndrome (Shearn 1971). Recently, the possible role of an infectious agent in the pathogenesis of Sjögren's syndrome and other connective tissue diseases and arthritides has received much attention (Shearn 1971). The implication of infectious agents in certain animal models of autoimmune disease, such as Aleutian mink disease, together with the concept of a slow virus disease, have accounted for this interest and are admirably reviewed by Shearn (1971).

10:5 Treatment and Management

A broad approach, directed both locally and systemically, is required in the treatment and management of the distressing symptoms of Sjögren's syndrome.

GENERAL

Approaches to treatment of rheumatoid arthritis or associated connective tissue disease are identical to those which would be employed if Sjögren's syndrome were absent. The measures aimed at reducing inflammation, pain, joint dysfunction and deformity have been reviewed (Shearn & Englemann 1968). The use of drugs such as salicylates, gold salts, corticosteroids and antimalarial drugs all have a place in the treatment of selected cases. The use of immunosuppressive drugs and antiviral agents such as amantadine have not been fully evaluated at the present time. The early recognition and treatment of kerato-conjunctivitis sicca with lubricating agents such as 1% methyl cellulose is essential if long-term complications such as corneal ulceration are to be avoided. The mucolytic agent acetylcysteine shows promise in the treatment of kerato-conjunctivitis sicca but requires further evaluation (Hughes & Whaley 1972).

ORAL

It is important that the oral mucous membranes be kept as moist as possible and, to this end, glycerine lozenges, methylcellulose (2% solution) as a lubricant and the salivary stimulant effect of boiled sweets may be of benefit to edentulous patients. A mouthwash containing citric acid (12·5 g), essence of lemon (20 ml) and glycerine (made up to 1 litre) has been used with success in our clinics. Patients should be encouraged to increase their fluid intake and the importance of meticulous oral and dental hygiene stressed. Local infections such as candidosis should be detected and treated with appropriate antifungal agents. Salivary gland swelling usually subsides, but painful recalcitrant swellings may be treated with analgesics and antibiotics. Irradiation is contra-indicated for persistent salivary swelling in view of the known association of Sjögren's syndrome and lymphoid neoplasia. The use of corticosteroids does not appear to improve the sicca symptoms (Bloch et al 1965). Drugs which may cause or increase xerostomia, such as some tranquillizers and hypotensive agents should be avoided or changed if possible. Parasympathominetic drugs are contra-indicated in some cases. Immunosuppressive drugs, such as cyclophosphamide, have been shown to cause an improvement of sicca symptoms in severe cases (Anderson et al 1971). However, this approach requires further study and cannot be recommended as a routine measure at the present time. In view of the known predisposition to drug allergy in Sjögren's syndrome (Bloch et al 1965) it is clear that the response to any drug administered should be carefully monitored.

10:6 References

ABRAMSON A.L., GOODMAN M. & KOLODNY H. (1968) Sjögren's syndrome. Additional diagnostic tools. Arch. Otolaryng., **88**, 91–94.

ADAMS D. (1973) Saliva, the mucus barrier and the health of the oral mucosa. Ph.D. Thesis, University of Wales.

ALBEGGER K.W. & AUBÖCK L. (1972) The evidence of 'virus-like' inclusions in myoepithelial sialadenitis of Sjögren's syndrome by electron microscopy. Arch. Klin. exp. Ohr., Nas. u. Kehek. Heilk., **203**, 153–165.

ANDERSON L.G. & TALAL N. (1971) The spectrum of benign to malignant lymphoproliferation in Sjögren's syndrome. Clin. exp. Immunol., **9**, 199–221.

ANDERSON L.G., CUMMINGS N.A., ASOFSKY R., HYLTON MARTHA B., TARPLEY T.M., TOMASI T.B., WOLF, R.O., SCHALL G.L. & TALAL N. (1972) Salivary gland immunoglobulin and rheumatoid factor synthesis in Sjögren's syndrome. Am. J. Med., **53**, 456–463.

AZZOPARDI J.G. & EVANS D.J. (1971) Malignant lymphoma of parotid associated with Mikulicz disease (benign lymphoepithelial lesion). J. clin. Path., **24**, 744–752.

BARTHOLOMEW L.E. (1965) Isolation and characterisation of mycoplasmas (PPLO) from patients with rheumatoid arthritis, systemic lupus erythematosus and Reiter's syndrome. Arth. Rheum., **8**, 376–388.

BECK J.S. (1961) Variations in the morphological patterns of 'auto-immune' nuclear fluorescence. Lancet, **1**, 1203–1204.

BERRY H., BACON P.A. & DAVIS J.D. (1972) Cell-mediated immunity in Sjögren's syndrome. Ann. rheum. Dis., **31**, 298–301.

BERTRAM U. (1967) Xerostomia. Clinical aspects, pathology and pathogenesis. Acta odont. Scand., **25**, Suppl. 49, 1–126.

BERTRAM U. & HALBERG P. (1964) A specific antibody against the epithelium of the salivary ducts in sera from patients with Sjögren's syndrome. Acta allerg. (Kbh.), **19**, 458–466.

BLAIR G.S. (1973) Oral and dental manifestations of adult rheumatoid arthritis. M.D.S. Thesis, University of Glasgow.
BLATT I.M., RUBIN P., FRENCH A.J., MAXWELL J.H. & HOLT J.F. (1965) Secretory sialography in diseases of the major salivary glands. *Ann. Otol.*, **65,** 293-304.
BLOCH K.J. & BUNIM J.J. (1963) Sjögren's syndrome and its relation to connective tissue diseases. *J. chron. Dis.*, **16,** 915-927.
BLOCH K.J., BUCHANAN W.W., WOHL M.J. & BUNIM J.J. (1965) Sjögren's syndrome. A clinical, pathological and serological study of sixty-two cases. *Med.*, **44,** 187-231.
BOQUIST L., KUMLIEN A. & ÖSTBERG Y. (1970) Ultrastructural findings in a case of benign lymphoepithelial lesion (Sjögren's syndrome). *Acta otolaryng.*, **70,** 216-226.
Brit. med. J. (1972) Editorial—Candida infection, **4,** 505-506.
BUCHANAN W.W., COX A.G., HARDEN R.McG., GLEN A.I.M., ANDERSON J.R. & GRAY K.G. (1966) Gastric studies in Sjögren's syndrome. *Gut*, **7,** 351-355.
BUCHANAN W.W. (1973) Personal communication.
CAHN L. (1967) A milder type (*forme fruste*) of Sjögren's syndrome. *Oral Surg.*, **23,** 25-28.
CALMAN H.I. & REIFMAN S. (1966) Sjögren's syndrome—report of a case. *Oral Surg.*, **21,** 158-160.
CARDELL B.S. & GURLING K.J. (1954) Observations on the pathology of Sjögren's syndrome. *J. Path. Bact.*, **68,** 137-146.
CHAN W.C. (1964) Experimental sialo-adenitis in guinea pigs. *J. Path. Bact.*, **88,** 592-595.
CHISHOLM D.M. (1969) Minor salivary gland pathology in Sjögren's syndrome and rheumatoid arthritis. In *Fourth Proceedings of the International Academy of Oral Pathology*, 44-56. Gordon & Breach, New York.
CHISHOLM D.M. (1970) The salivary glands and their secretions in connective tissue disease. Ph.D. Thesis, University of Glasgow.
CHISHOLM D.M., BEELEY J.A. & MASON D.K. (1973) Salivary proteins in Sjögren's syndrome: separation by isoelectric focusing in acrylamide gels. *Oral Surg.*, **35,** 620-630.
CHISHOLM D.M., BLAIR G.S., LOW P.S. & WHALEY K. (1971) Hydrostatic sialography as an index of salivary gland disease in Sjögren's syndrome. *Acta radiol.*, **11,** 577-585.
CHISHOLM D.M. & MASON D.K. (1968) Labial salivary gland biopsy in Sjögren's disease. *J. clin. Path.*, **21,** 656-660.
CHISHOLM D.M. & MASON D.K. (1973) *Brit. dent. J.*, **135,** 393-399.
CHISHOLM D.M., WATERHOUSE J.P. & MASON D.K. (1970) Lymphocytic sialadenitis in the major and minor glands: a correlation in postmortem subjects. *J. clin. Path.*, **23,** 690-694.
CIFARELLI P.S., BENNETT M.J. & ZAINO E.C. (1966) Sjögren's syndrome. *Arch intern. Med.*, **117,** 429-431.
COVERDALE H. (1948) Some unusual cases of Sjögren's syndrome. *Brit. J. Ophthal.* **32,** 669-673.
DANIELS T., SYLVESTER R., SILVERMAN S. & TALAL N. (1973) Virus-like structures occurring within labial salivary glands in Sjögren's syndrome. *I.A.D.R. Abstracts (North American Division)*, No. 428.

DAVIES J.D., BERRY H., BACON P.A., ISSA M.A. & SCHOFIELD J.J. (1973) Labial sialadenitis in Sjögren's syndrome and in rheumatoid arthritis. *J. Path.*, **109**, 307–314.

DUTHIE J.J.R., STEWART S., ALEXANDER W.R.M. & DAYHOFF R. (1967) Isolation of diphtheroid organisms from rheumatoid synovial membrane and fluid. *Lancet*, **1**, 142–143.

EISENBUD L., PLATT N., STERN M., D'ANGELO W. & SUMNER P. (1973) Palatal biopsy as a diagnostic aid in the study of connective tissue diseases. *Oral Surg.*, **35**, 642–648.

ERICSON S. (1968) The parotid gland in subjects with and without rheumatoid arthritis. *Acta radiol.*, Suppl. 275, 1–167.

FELTKAMP T.E. & VAN ROSSUM A.L. (1968) Antibodies to salivary duct cells and other autoantibodies in patients with Sjögren's syndrome and other idiopathic autoimmune diseases. *Clin. exp. Immun.*, **3**, 1–16.

FISCHER C.J., WYSHAK G.H. & WEISBERGER (1968) Sjögren's syndrome. Electrophoretic and immunological observations on serum and salivary proteins of man. *Archs. oral Biol.*, **13**, 257–270.

GATES G.A. & WORK W.P. (1967) Radioisotope scanning of the salivary glands. *Laryngoscope*, **77**, 861–875.

GORDON A.M., CHISHOLM D.M. & MASON D.K. (1971) Oral mycoplasmas in Sjögren's syndrome. *J. clin. Path.*, **24**, 810–815.

GROVE A.S. JR & DI CHIRO G. (1968) Salivary gland scanning with technetium ^{99m}pertechnetate. *Am. J. Roentgenol.*, **102**, 109–116.

HALBERG P., BERTRAM U., SÖBERG M. & NERUP J. (1965) Organ antibodies in disseminated lupus erythematosus. *Acta med. Scand.*, **178**, 291–295.

HAMILTON J.B. (1940) Keratitis sicca, including Sjögren's syndrome. *Trans. ophthal. Soc. Aust.*, **2**, 63–71.

HARDEN R.McG. & ALEXANDER W.D. (1967) The relation between the clearance of iodide and pertechnetate in human parotid saliva and salivary flow rate. *Clin. Sci.*, **33**, 425–431.

HARDEN R.McG., HILDITCH T.E., KENNEDY I., MASON D.K., PAPADOPOULOS S. & ALEXANDER W.D. (1967) Uptake and scanning of the salivary glands in man using pertechnetate ^{99m}Tc. *Clin. Sci.*, **32**, 49–55.

HARDEN R.McG., ALEXANDER W.D., SHIMMINS J. & RUSSELL R.J. (1968) Quantitative uptake measurements of ^{99m}Tc in salivary glands and stomach and concentration of ^{99m}Tc, ^{132}I and ^{82}Br in gastric juice and saliva. In FELLINGER K. & HOFER R. *Radioaktive Isotope in Klinik und Forschung*, **8**, 76–87.

HILDES J.A. & FERGUSON H. (1958) The concentration of electrolytes in normal human saliva. *Canad. J. Biochem.*, **33**, 217–223.

HJÖRTING-HANSEN E. & BERTRAM U. (1968) Oral aspects of pernicious anaemia. *Brit. dent. J.*, **125**, 266–270.

HOLM S. (1949) Keratoconjunctivitis sicca and the sicca syndrome. *Acta Ophthal.*, Suppl. **33**, 1–230.

HORNBAKER J.H., FOSTER E.A. & WILLIAMS G.S. (1966) Sjögren's syndrome and nodular reticulum cell sarcoma. *Arch. intern. Med.*, **118**, 449–452.

HUGHES G.R.V. & WHALEY K. (1972) Sjögren's syndrome. *Brit. med. J.*, **4**, 533–536.

KITAMURA T., KANDA T. & ISHIKAWA T. (1970) Parotid gland of Sjögren's syndrome. *Arch. Otolaryng.*, **91**, 64–70.

LEVENTHAL B.G., WALDORF D.S. & TALAL N. (1967) Impaired lymphocyte transformation and delayed hypersensitivity in Sjögren's syndrome. *J. clin. Invest.*, **46**, 1338-1345.
LISCH K. (1937) Über hereditäres Vorkomen des mit keratoconjunctivitis sicca verbundenen Sjögrenschen Symptomenkomplexes. *Arch. Augenheilk*, **110**, 357-369.
MACFARLANE T.W. & MASON D.K. (1973) The oral flora in Sjögren's syndrome. *I.A.D.R. Abstracts (British Division)*, No. 132.
MACKAY I.R. & BURNET F.M. (1963) *Autoimmune Diseases.* Charles C. Thomas, Springfield, Illinois.
MACSWEEN R.N.M., GOUDIE R.B., ANDERSON J.R., ARMSTRONG E.M., MURRAY M.A., MASON D.K., JASANI M.K., BOYLE J.A., BUCHANAN W.W. & WILLIAMSON J. (1967) Occurrence of antibody to salivary duct epithelium in Sjögren's disease, rheumatoid arthritis and other arthritides. A clinical and laboratory study. *Ann. Rheum. Dis.*, **26**, 402-411.
MANDEL I.D. & BAURMASH H. (1973) Biochemical profile in salivary gland disease. *I.A.D.R. Abstracts (North American Division)*, No. 672.
MASON D.K. (1966) Studies in salivary glands and their secretions in health and disease. M.D. Thesis, University of Glasgow.
MASON D.K. & GLEN A.I.M. (1967) The aetiology of xerostomia. *Dent. Mag. (Lond.)*, **84**, 235-238.
MASON D.K., HARDEN R.McG., BOYLE J.A., JASANI M.K., WILLIAMSON J. & BUCHANAN W.W. (1967) Salivary flow rates and iodide trapping capacity in patients with Sjögren's syndrome. *Ann. rheum. Dis.*, **26**, 311-315.
MELLORS R.C. (1966) Autoimmune disease in 4 NZBL/BL mice. *Blood*, **27**, 435-448.
MORGAN W.S. & CASTLEMAN B. (1953) A clinicopathologic study of Mikulicz's disease. *Am. J. Path.*, **29**, 471-489.
PARK W.M. & MASON D.K. (1966) Hydrostatic sialography. *Radiol.*, **86**, 116-122.
ROPES M.W., BENNETT G.A., COBB S., JACOX R. & JESSAR R.A. (1958) Diagnostic criteria for rheumatoid arthritis. *Bull. rheum. Dis.*, **9**, 175-184.
SCHALL G.L., ANDERSON L.G., WOLF R.O., HERDT JEAN R., TARPLEY T.M., CUMMINGS N.A., ZEIGER L.S. & TALAL T. (1971) Xerostomia in Sjögren's syndrome. *J. Am. med. Ass.*, **216**, 2109-2116.
SHEARN M.A. (1971) *Sjögren's Syndrome*, Vol. II in the series Major Problems in Internal Medicine. W.B. Saunders Co., Philadelphia.
SHEARN M.A. & ENGLEMAN E.P. (1968) *The Rheumatic Diseases.* Cyclopedia of Medicine, Surgery Specialties. F.A. Davis & Co., Philadelphia.
SHEARN M.A., TU W.H., STEPHENS B.G. & LEE J.C. (1970) Virus-like structures in Sjögren's syndrome. *Lancet*, **1**, 568-569.
SJÖGREN H. (1933) Zur Kenntnis der Keratoconjunctivitis sicca (Keratitis filiformis bei Hypofunktion der Träsendrüsen). *Acta Ophthal.*, Suppl. 2, **11**, 1-151.
SÖBORG M. & BERTRAM U. (1968) Cellular hypersensitivity in Sjögren's syndrome. *Acta med. Scand.*, **184**, 319-322.
STEPHEN K.W., CHISHOLM D.M., HARDEN R.McG., ROBERTSON J.W.K., WHALEY K. & STUART AGNES (1971) Diagnostic value of quantitative scintiscanning of the salivary glands in Sjögren's syndrome and rheumatoid arthritis. *Clin. Sci.*, **41**, 555-561.

TALAL N., ASOFSKY R. & LIGHTBODY P. (1970) Immunoglobulin synthesis by salivary gland lymphoid cells in Sjögren's syndrome. *J. clin. Invest.*, **49**, 49–54.
TALAL N. & BUNIM J.J. (1964) The development of malignant lymphoma in the course of Sjögren's syndrome. *Am. J. Med.*, **36**, 529–534.
TALAL N., SOKOLOFF L. & BARTH W.F. (1967) Extrasalivary lymphoid abnormalities in Sjögren's syndrome (reticulum cell sarcoma, 'Pseudolymphoma', macroglobulinemia). *Am. J. Med.*, **43**, 50–65.
VERONESI J., CASCINELLI N. & DAMASCELLI B. (1967) ^{131}I accumulation in a cystadenoma lymphomatosum of the parotid gland. *Brit. J. Radiol.*, **40**, 862–863.
WATERHOUSE J.P. (1963) Focal adenitis of salivary and lacrimal glands. M.D. Thesis, University of London.
WHALEY K., CHISHOLM D.M., GOUDIE R.B., DOWNIE W.W., DICK W.C., BOYLE J.A. & WILLIAMSON J. (1969) Salivary duct autoantibody in Sjögren's syndrome: Correlation with focal sialadenitis in the labial mucosa. *Clin. exp. Immunol.*, **4**, 273–282.
WHALEY K., GOUDIE R.B., WILLIAMSON J., NUKI G., DICK W.C. & BUCHANAN W.W. (1970) Liver disease in Sjögren's syndrome and rheumatoid arthritis. *Lancet*, **1**, 861–863.
WHALEY K., WILLIAMSON J., CHISHOLM D.M., WEBB J., MASON D.K. & BUCHANAN W.W. (1973) Sjögren's syndrome 1. Sicca components. *Quart. J. Med.*, **166**, 279–304.
WILLIAMS M.H., BROSTOFF J. & ROITT I.M. (1970) Possible role of *Mycoplasma fermentans* in pathogenesis of rheumatoid arthritis. *Lancet*, **2**, 277–280.
WILLIAMSON J., CANT J.S., MASON D.K., GREIG W.R. & BOYLE J.A. (1967) Sjögren's syndrome and thyroid disease. *Brit. J. Ophthal.*, **51**, 721–726.

CHAPTER 11
CANDIDAL INFECTION OF THE ORAL MUCOSA

D.M. WALKER

11:0 Taxonomy, Culture, Identification

Candida is a genus of yeast classified by Lodder (1970) in a fourth group of yeasts that do not reproduce sexually and form no ballisto spores. It exists in three principal forms: yeast cell or blastospore, pseudohypha and chlamydospore (Fig. 11.1). By definition candida reproduces asexually by budding of the round or oval yeast cell which elongates to form a pseudohypha. The first step for laboratory confirmation of a clinical diagnosis of candidal infection is to demonstrate the candidal pseudohyphae and spores with a Gram or PAS stain of smears or biopsy from the lesion. Secondly, material from a swab is cultured, aerobically at $37\,°C$ on Sabouraud's medium (Peptone maltose agar), candida being seen as a cream-coloured colony after 24 hours' incubation.

The following two cultural methods are adequate to identify candida subcultures as *Candida albicans* (Mackenzie 1966).
1 Cultured on a poorly nutrient medium such as corn meal agar it forms thick-walled spherical refractile chlamydospores.
2 Subcultured in human serum, *C. albicans* forms fine filaments ('germ tubes') (Taschdjian, Burchall & Kozinn 1960).

Sugar fermentation reactions can also be used to characterize *C. albicans* (Martin & Jones 1940). Of over 60 species of candida, *C. albicans* is most commonly implicated in human candidal infection (candidosis).

11:1 Candida as a Commensal Organism on Mucosa and Skin

As a saprophyte candida exists mainly in man and other host animals. In man it may occur as a commensal organism of the mouth most frequently, but also throat, large bowel and vagina. The prevalence of this candidal carrier state has varied according to the population studied and methodology for culture. The percentage of oral candidal carriers in subjects with clinically normal mouths has been carefully estimated as between 33 and 40% (Bartels & Blechman 1962) collecting stimulated saliva spat by the subject into a sterile universal container. This is a sensitive method (Lilienthal 1950). In the individual oral candida carrier with a

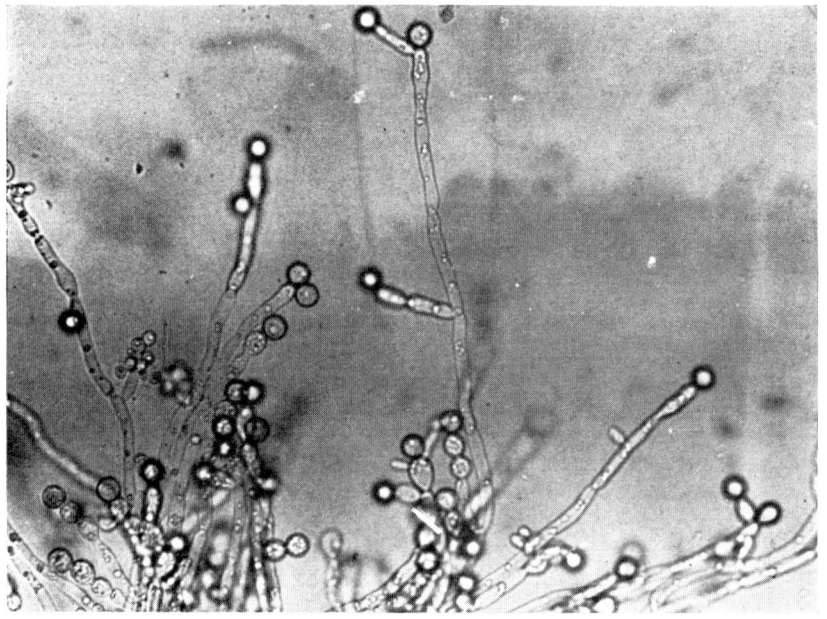

Fig. 11.1. *C. albicans* grown on corn meal agar, showing many spherical refractile chlamydospores, pseudohyphae and a few oval yeast cells. ×80.

clinically normal mouth, Williamson (1972a) estimated the number of candidal organisms in such salivary samples and noted a diurnal variation with an early morning peak in the dentate subject. Wearing dentures increased this candida count and reversed the diurnal curve. Conversely the mouths of non-carriers consistently failed to yield candida over the entire period of testing (Williamson 1972b). Adams (1974) found such oral candidal counts to be significantly greater than those from vaginal specimens of pregnant and non-pregnant women, and that the oral candidal counts became elevated in pregnancy. This influence of physiological factors on the density of the commensal population has been confirmed before for the vagina (Karnaky 1935; Jones & Martin 1938; Plass, Hesseltine & Borts 1931). These variations between oral candidal counts taken from different healthy subjects and fluctuation of the counts in any one individual limits their usefulness in diagnosis of oral candidal infection, that is there is an overlap between counts from carriers and those from individuals showing infection. A significant rise in the candidal count of any individual might on the other hand be an index of infection but is probably impracticable. Isolation of candida from the mouth in adults, even in pure culture, is not *per se* evidence of candidal infection (candidiasis syn. candidosis) and must be considered together with the clinical

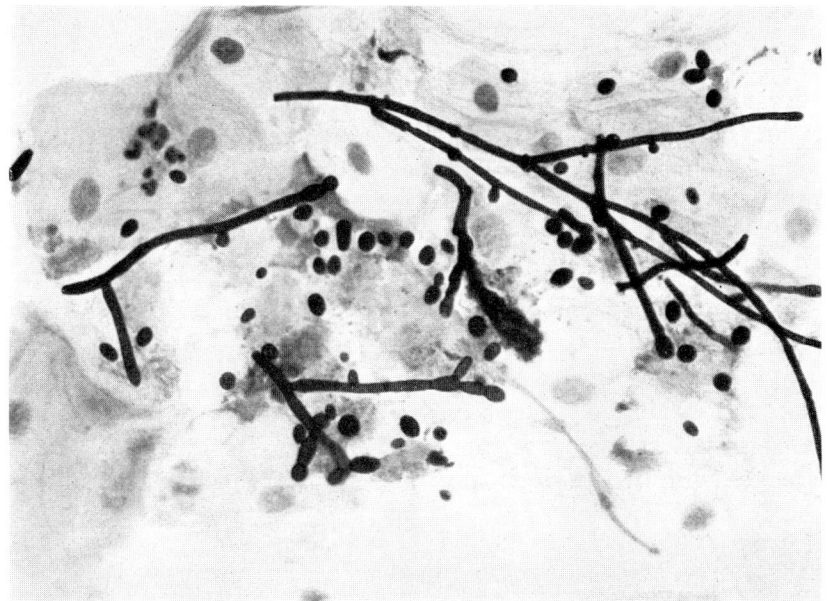

Fig. 11.2. Candidal hyphae and spores related to oral epithelial cells in smear from tongue of patient with thrush. Stained PAS. ×50.

findings. In the neonate, however, it is generally believed that a positive oral smear inevitably heralds clinical thrush (Taschdjian & Kozinn 1957; Kozinn *et al* 1958).

The morphology of the candidal organism obtained in material from a lesion, especially a smear, has been thought in the past to be valuable in distinguishing candidal infection from the carrier state, candidal hyphae indicating candidosis. Winner & Hurley (1964) weighed the evidence and found it inconclusive. In neonates Taschdjian *et al* (1957) showed that a change from predominantly yeast to predominantly hyphal forms indicated that oral thrush was imminent. In our experience in adults, hyphal forms are not found in significant numbers from healthy mouths. Conversely, in a case of oral candidosis verified by culture, where candidal forms are present in the oral smears, they always include hyphae (Fig. 11.2).

Presumably, since the carrier rate is so high in the general population, candida is constantly being transferred from person to person directly or indirectly. Although candidal contamination of the skin from mouth and other body cavities must constantly occur, it is not usually possible to culture candida from normal adult skin. Presumably the oral candidal population is kept within certain limits in any one carrier by a balance between proliferation in the mouth and loss in saliva and food by swallowing. The subsequent fate of these candidal organisms in the normal gastrointestinal tract has apparently not been studied. Whether such swallowed candidal organisms remain viable in their passage through the gut and contribute to the candidal large bowel population is not known. Occasionally candidal organisms of presumably oral origin assume importance in association with mycotic ulcers of the stomach (Ludlam & Henderson 1942) or direct invasion of the oesophagus in fatal thrush in infants. We do know how candida is acquired in oral thrush in the first few days of life due to Woodruff & Hesseltine's (1938) demonstration that a child's chance of contracting oral thrush was directly related to the presence of the fungus within the maternal vagina, the neonate presumably acquiring the organism during its passage through the birth canal. The nurse's fingers can also be a source of thrush in neonates (Ludlam & Henderson 1942).

11:2 Predisposing Factors

With the exception of neonates oral candidosis does not follow inoculation of the healthy subject with candidal organisms. The yeast is of such feeble invasiveness that host defence mechanisms prevent invasion and proliferation. Some prior local disturbance or systemic illness appears to be necessary before the commensal or acquired candidal organism can become pathogenic. The factors predisposing to subsequent candidosis have been listed by Winner & Hurley (1964) broadly as follows:

1 Physiological— infancy
— old age
— pregnancy
2 Drug-associated.

3 Endocrine.
4 Malabsorption.
5 Malnutrition.
6 Blood dyscrasias.
7 Post-operative states.
8 Malignant disease.

PHYSIOLOGICAL

Some of the factors predisposing to candidosis elsewhere in the body appear less important for the mouth. For example pregnancy predisposes to vaginal thrush (Plass, Hesseltine & Borts 1931; Hesseltine 1955) or the candidal carrier state (Mizuno 1961), and the post-menopausal state also predisposes to vaginal candidosis. More directly vaginal thrush occurred with greater frequency in pregnant women inoculated with cadida than non-pregnant women (Bland *et al* 1937). Susceptibility to oral thrush in pregnancy has not been satisfactorily proved, however. Presumably this is because the hormone-dependent changes in the vagina, such as increased glycogen content, the subsequent conversion of the glycogen to lactic acid and lowered pH, all favouring yeast growth (Gardner 1965; Cruickshank & Sharman 1934), do not occur in the oral mucosa. Similarly the reports of increased vaginal isolation of candida in women taking an oestrogen–progestogen contraceptive pill (Jackson & Spain 1968; Catterall 1971; Davis 1969) have not been confirmed for oral candidosis. In fact Rohatiner & Grimble (1970) concluded from their and other workers' findings that taking the contraceptive 'pill' did not predispose the subject to genital candidosis except where the oestrogen or progestogen content was high.

DRUG-ASSOCIATED

(*a*) *Antibiotics,* (*b*) *Steroids,* (*c*) *Immunosuppressive drugs*

The impression from the literature is that the incidence of thrush has probably declined since the last century, but it was not until 1940 that death due to candidosis was first recorded (Registrar General statistics). Since then the mortality has remained fairly constant, whereas that from bacterial disease and also for example actinomycosis has fallen steadily.

Improved diagnosis may be partly responsible for this continued trend of mortality, but the advent of broad spectrum antibiotics initially probably played a part. Many reports of a positive association between antibiotic therapy and candidosis are tendentious and lack appropriate controls. Seelig (1966a,b) reviewed the extensive literature concerning antibiotics in relation to candida infections and concluded that antibiotics caused proliferation of candida in the oral mucosa, stools and vagina.

Candidal superinfection is much higher in patients treated with tetracycline than penicillin or streptomycin (Weinstein, Goldfield & Chang 1954). Experimentally, rats treated with tetracycline and inoculated orally with *C. albicans* developed oral candidosis with hyphal infiltration of the oral epithelium, whereas the organisms tended to disappear in inoculated animals not given tetracycline (Russell & Jones 1973). The generally accepted explanation of oral candidosis associated with antibiotic therapy is that the normal oral bacterial flora checks candidal colonization (Young, Krasner & Yudkofsky 1956). When this resident flora is altered by antibiotic therapy the result is candidal overgrowth (see p. 475). Thus in germ-free rats, induced experimental oral candidosis persisted as long as tested (Russell *et al* 1974), whereas rats with a normal oral flora similarly inoculated, began to lose the candida.

Steroids

One's own clinical impression confirms early reports that patients on steroids, particularly in high systemic doses, do seem to be prone to oral candidosis (Lehner 1964a), and these candidal infections can contribute to death of some of these patients (Pillay *et al* 1968).

Topical steroids with a potentiated anti-inflammatory effect, such as beclomethasone diproprionate inhaled in powder form in asthma, definitely predisposed to oropharyngeal candidosis (Fig. 11.3) (Brompton Hospital—M.R.C. 1974). However, topical hydrocortisone is not followed by iatrogenic candidosis in our experience but this may be symptomless (Lehner & Ward 1970).

Local suppression of the immune or inflammatory changes may be the mechanism for this opportunist candidal proliferation; alternatively the steroid may cause toxic damage to the mucosa, but the atrophic changes following steroid application to skin have not been described in the oral mucosa.

The studies of Mankowski & Littleton (1954), Mankowski (1955), Henry & Fahlberg (1960) and Roth, Friedman & Syverton (1957) are

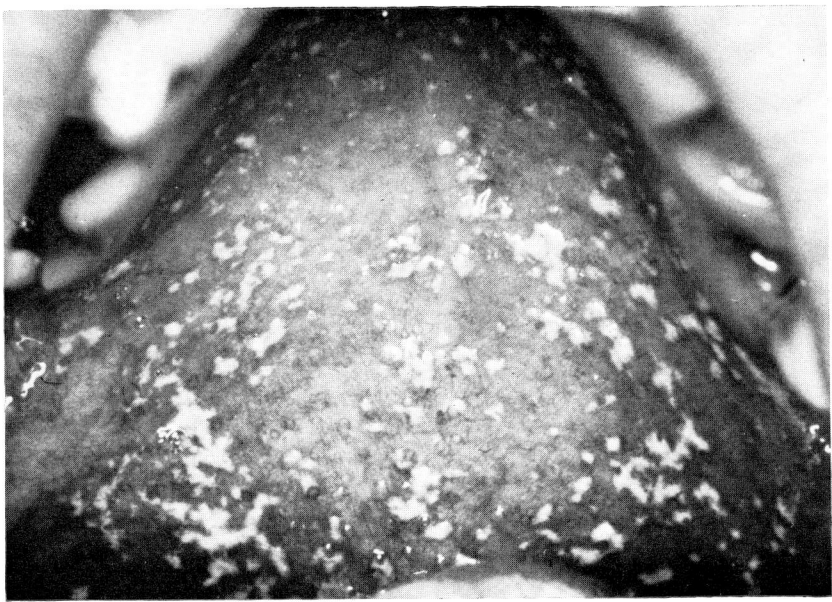

Fig. 11.3. Thrush in asthmatic 35-year-old woman, using beclomethasone inhaler.

broadly agreed that corticosteroids increased the pathogenicity of candida in mice in high systemic doses. The anti-inflammatory and immunosuppressive properties of steroids together with their tendency to raise the blood and tissue glucose concentrations make this steroid-induced enhancement of candidosis predictable.

Immunosuppressive therapy

Immunosuppressive drugs can cause a suppression of both cell-mediated and humoral immunity to candida (see below). Folb & Trounce (1970) found that patients on azathioprine and steroids or cyclophosphamide had a depressed *in vitro* lymphocyte transformation response to candida antigen as a marker of cell-mediated immunity. Humoral immunity was unimpaired. Carefully controlled studies on oral candidosis following immunosuppressive and antiproliferative drugs are lacking. The fact that the malignancy or autoimmune disease being treated may have an intrinsic immune defect adds complexity to the problem. The survival of such patients for long periods on immunosuppressive or antiproliferative agents has created a new population at risk from candidosis.

ENDOCRINE DISORDERS

Diabetics and patients suffering from hypoparathyroidism and hypoadrenocorticism are prone to candidal infections generally (Barlow & English 1973). Oral isolates of candida were obtained from 30% of diabetic children compared with 22% from healthy children (Basu *et al* 1961). However, in a more controlled study, Peters, Bahn & Barens 1966) could find no difference in oral candidal populations or oral candidosis in 600 patients including equal numbers of controlled and uncontrolled diabetics and normal subjects.

MALIGNANCY

Systemic candidosis is frequently seen in advanced malignant diseases (Hutter & Collins 1962), particularly lymphoreticular malignancy. It is difficult to evaluate malignant disease as a single factor in patients who may be debilitated and on different types of treatment.

BLOOD DYSCRASIAS

Patients with some of the blood dyscrasias do seem to be predisposed to systemic candidosis (Lannigan & Meynell 1959). The incidence of severe candidal infections increased to 40% of patients dying with acute leukaemia (all types) in a 10-year study, and was commoner than focal candidosis in patients on antimitotic, antibiotic or adrenocorticosteroid therapy. A low granulocyte or lymphocyte count was also associated with severe candidosis (Bobey 1966). Iron deficiency and candidosis is discussed below.

MALNUTRITION AND MALABSORPTION

The question of susceptibility to candidosis in malnutrition and malabsorption is not yet properly documented for oral infection. The low-serum vitamin A, pyridoxine and iron-deficiency states noted in a group of patients with chronic candidal infection of skin and mucosa by Wells *et al* (1972) are particularly interesting in this context, since it is possible that malabsorption either secondary to or as a causative factor in the candidosis may be occurring. High doses of vitamin A therapy were therefore tried in one such patient, and some improvement in the candidosis occurred before toxicity problems forced the vitamin A therapy to be terminated.

OTHER FACTORS. BLOOD GROUP

It is interesting that blood group O occurred almost universally in the 46 individuals with muco-cutaneous candidosis, including chronic oral candidosis alone, as classified by Wells *et al* (1972).

11:3 Non-specific Defence Mechanisms Controlling the Growth of Candida on Skin and Mucous Membranes

SALIVA

The mechanical flushing effect of saliva removes candidal organisms from the mouth and from the fitting surface of dentures and these organisms are then swallowed. This is one way in which the candidal organisms can be restricted and explains in part why candidal organisms are found in greater numbers on the fitting surface of an upper denture than that of the lower. The saliva also contains specific candidal antibodies, for example those detected by indirect immunofluorescence (Lehner 1965). Other antimicrobial properties of saliva have been dealt with elsewhere in this book (see Chapter 2). In clinical studies MacFarlane & Mason (1973) found 70% of patients with Sjogren's syndrome to have a history of oral candidosis. Adams (1973), in a small number of patients complaining of dry mouth, isolated candida more frequently from those actually found to have reduced salivary flow rates. However, experimental rats with hyoscine-induced xerostomia had no greater incidence of acute oral candidosis than the control group (Jones & Adams 1970). Qualitative differences such as the pH of the saliva may play a part; the candidal carrier rate of normal adults with saliva pH 5·0–6·5 was 90% compared with 56% of those with a pH of 6·5–7·0 (Young, Resca & Sullivan 1951).

Flora

It has been observed that *C. albicans* may enhance the growth of lactobacilli, an oral bacterial commensal (Young *et al* 1951), and that conversely lactobacilli, possibly by virtue of the lactic acid they produce, could inhibit the growth of *C. albicans* (Young *et al* 1956). *C. albicans* can liberate the complex vitamins needed by lactobacilli for its growth (Wilson & Goaz 1959, 1960). Antibiotic-induced disturbance of this symbiotic relationship can result in candidosis. This is confirmed by the experiments of Russell *et al* (1974) in which germ-free rats inoculated orally with candida, harboured the organism for as long as tested. In conventional rats similarly inoculated, the fungus could be recovered in only 50% of the animals at the conclusion.

BARRIER FUNCTION OF EPITHELIUM

We still do not clearly understand why candida is more frequently carried by or infects the oral mucosa rather than the skin. On the skin, local factors such as maceration, that is chronic damage to the skin by excess moisture, usually determine the presence and distribution of candidal infection in patients occurring commonly in the axillae, submammary folds and groins. Experimentally, an occlusive dressing is necessary before a candidal infection of the skin can be produced; merely damaging the skin is insufficient (Maibach & Kligman 1962). Normally dry intact skin with its thin fluid film derived from sweat, sebum and transudate and keratin layer is an efficient defensive barrier against candidosis; this film contains fatty acids with fungicidal properties. Candida is therefore not found on normal healthy adult skin. It is noteworthy that Maibach *et al* (1962) could not produce oral candidosis experimentally by inoculating buccal mucosa even after occluding it with Orabase. Presumably the oral mucosa is functionally adapted to a salivary or fluid environment so that experimental maceration could not be produced in this way.

Epithelial defects have not been detected in oral or muco-cutaneous candidosis (CMCC)—clinically the uninvolved mucosa or skin usually appears normal. It is noteworthy that Kirkpatrick, Rich & Bennett (1971) found 11 out of 12 patients with CMCC to have 'dysplastic' teeth; it would be interesting to know if hypoplasia of prenatally formed enamel or dentine occurs. This would confirm that this was a developmental (not acquired) ectodermal disorder which might be associated with a parallel ectodermal defect of skin or mucosae, predisposing to the candidosis.

FACTORS PROMOTING ORAL CANDIDOSIS
AND CANDIDAL CARRIER STATE

The oral mucosa is covered constantly by saliva in which candida can survive *in vitro* for appreciable periods. The fact that oral candidal infection usually first affects the non-keratinized mucosa in the dentate subject may indicate that the surface structure is also important. The importance of rates of shedding of epithelial squames and epithelial transit time needs to be determined.

Iron deficiency

Iron deficiency is thought to be an important predisposing factor in candidosis both confined to the mouth (Rose 1968) and in chronic mucocutaneous candidosis. In the latter group Higgs & Wells (1973) found that out of 31 patients 23 were iron deficient. Of this iron-deficient fraction, 8 had a frank iron-deficiency anaemia, but the remaining 15 had only latent iron deficiency diagnosed because of repeatedly low serum iron values, raised total iron binding capacities and reduced stainable iron in their bone marrow where examined. In the iron-deficient group a small controlled trial suggested improvement in their candidal infection with parenteral iron and antifungal therapy compared with those on antifungal therapy alone. The quality of the *oral epithelium* as a barrier to candidosis may be affected in iron deficiency. Jacobs (1960, 1961a,b) showed that the buccal epithelium in iron-deficient subjects is atrophic and deficient in iron-containing enzymes such as cytochrome oxidase. Secondly, this cytochrome-deficient oral epithelium may have for example impaired cell division and be less resistant to the normal wear and tear which in turn might predispose to candidosis. The epithelial cell kinetics of the iron-deficient mucosa now needs to be studied. A more ingenious explanation is offered by Higgs (1973), who said that the sulphydryl groups in the iron-deficient buccal epithelium are reduced (Jacobs (1961a) found them increased, however), and the resultant disturbance in the sulphydryl–disulphide equilibrium may in turn inhibit the enzyme controlling candidal yeast cell division which is known to act on disulphide groups. Enzymatic inhibition of yeast cell division without inhibition of metabolic intracellular activity leads to the elongated hyphal phase, that is the supposedly pathogenic form (Nickerson & Rij 1949; Nickerson & Falcone 1956). These investigations are primarily centred on the rare chronic muco-cutaneous candidosis. The possibility that the iron deficiency may be secondary to the candidosis has not been ruled out.

In the more common candidosis confined to the mouth the importance of iron deficiency as a predisposing factor has yet to be established. In a related study (Walker *et al* 1973) no differences in frequency of clinical candidosis or sizes of candidal populations were noted between iron-deficient subjects and appropriate controls, and no significant change occurred after iron therapy.

Lastly, iron-deficient subjects have a defect in cell-mediated immunity to candida antigen, both *in vivo* and *in vitro*, reversible with iron therapy (Joynson *et al* 1972) (Figs. 11.4, 11.5, 11.6).

In chronic candidal infections of the oral mucosa the infiltrating

478 Chapter 11

hyphae are limited to the superficial ageing layers of the oral epithelium (Figs. 11.7, 11.8), rarely, or never, reaching the prickle cell layer. This may indicate a functional or structural barrier to candidal invasion. Ultrastructural evidence that the hyphae grow intracellularly *through* oral

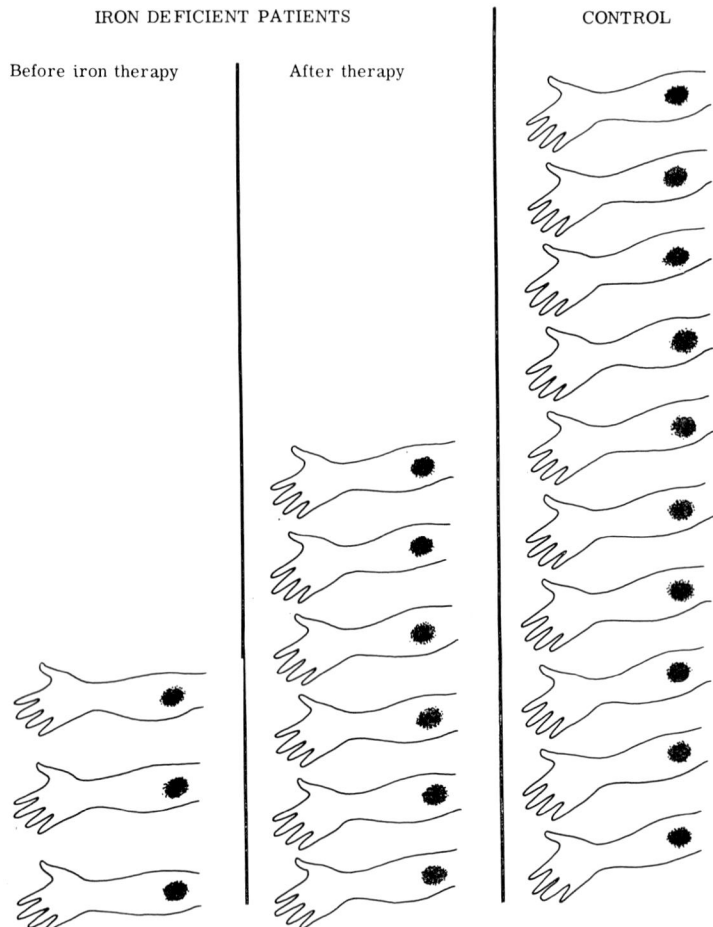

Fig. 11.4. Impaired *in vivo* immune response to candida antigen in iron deficiency. Positive skin reactions (indurated area >5 mm diameter) 48 hours after intradermal injection of 0·02 ml candida antigen.

epithelial cells in candidosis without respect to epithelial cell boundary (Montes & Wilborn 1968; Cawson & Rajasingham 1972) may indicate that the hyphae derive nutrients from the epithelial cell cytoplasm. Both the sulphydryl and disulphide local concentration may control candidal proliferation in the epithelium, by the mechanism referred to above.

CELLULAR DEFENCE

Polymorphs

Like bacteria, yeasts like *C. albicans* are phagocytosed by polymorphonuclear leucocytes and subsequently killed by intracellular digestion. Phagocytosis may be tested by the quantitative or qualitative nitro blue tetrazolium test (Baehner & Nathan 1967, 1968). The polymorph lysosomal

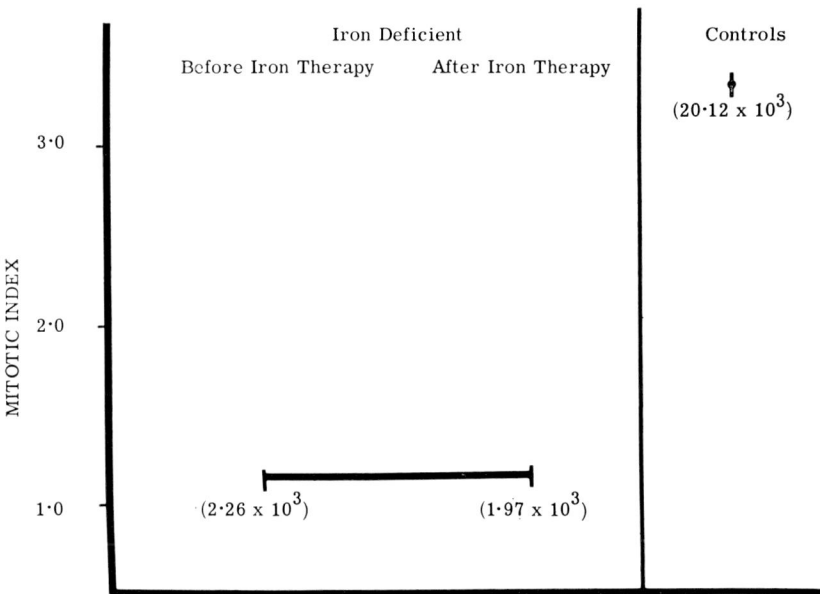

Fig. 11.5. Impaired cell-mediated immunity in iron deficiency. Lymphocyte transformation measured by tritiated thymidine uptake, in response to candida antigen in iron-deficient subjects, before and after (a limited amount of) iron therapy, compared with normal controls. Expressed as mean mitotic index (with counts per minute in brackets) ± SEM.

enzyme myeloperoxidase has also been held to be largely responsible for neutrophilic candidicidal activity and myeloperoxidase content to be an index of this function (Lehrer & Cline 1969a).

Lastly, serum factors have been demonstrated in some patients which prevent bactericidal activity of normal polymorphs. In oral candidosis, even when part of extensive muco-cutaneous candidosis, no abnormalities of these tests of polymorph function are generally demonstrated (Valdimarsson *et al* 1973). However, exceptionally, patients with disseminated candidosis have been shown to have leucocyte myeloperoxidase deficiency (Lehrer & Cline 1969b). The relationship of low granulocyte counts in acute leukaemia with severe candidosis has been dealt with above. The role of macrophages in candidicidal activity will be discussed in section 11.4.

INHIBITORY FACTORS IN SERUM

Using a method of Roth & Goldstein (1961) the serum of normal people has the property of inhibiting the growth of *C. albicans*. This is lacking in patients with Hodgkin's disease, acute leukaemia and multiple myeloma.

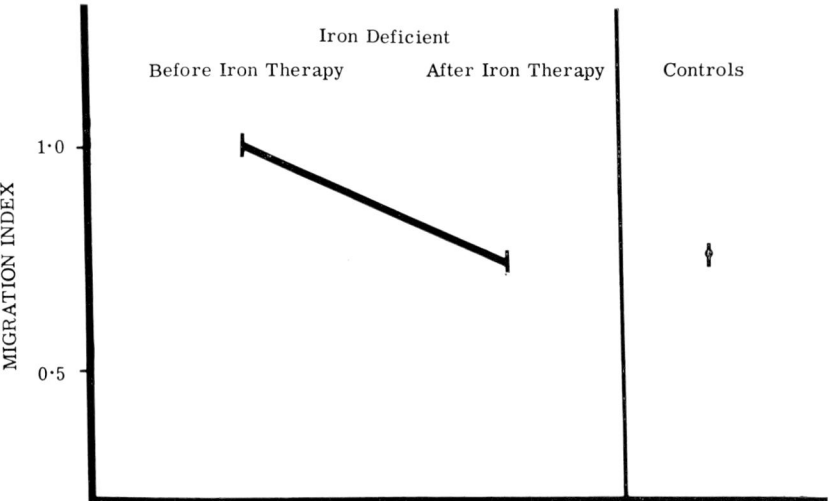

Fig. 11.6. Impaired cell-mediated immunity in iron deficiency (*in vitro*). Release of macrophage migration inhibitory factor from lymphocyte cultures in response to candida antigen from iron-deficient subjects, before and after (a limited amount of) iron therapy, compared with normal controls.

Expressed as percentage:

$$\frac{\text{area of guinea-pig macrophage migration with supernatants from lymphocyte cultures exposed to candida antigen}}{\text{area of guinea-pig macrophage migration with supernatants from lymphocytes with saline}}$$

This inhibitory factor was identified as transferrin by Caroline *et al* (1964).

Transferrin is a beta-globulin responsible for binding iron in plasma, is normally only one-third saturated and thus no free ionic iron is present in plasma. This unbound iron is a cultural requirement of *C. albicans* so that normal serum with its iron-avid transferrin inhibits its growth; addition of iron salts reverses this inhibitory effect. In acute leukaemia transferrin is fully saturated, the serum has no inhibitory effect *in vitro* and this could explain these patients' susceptibility to candidosis. However, patients with haemochromatosis have iron-saturated transferrin, yet do not seem prone to serious candidal infections.

Evidence for a different candidicidal factor was put forward by Louria

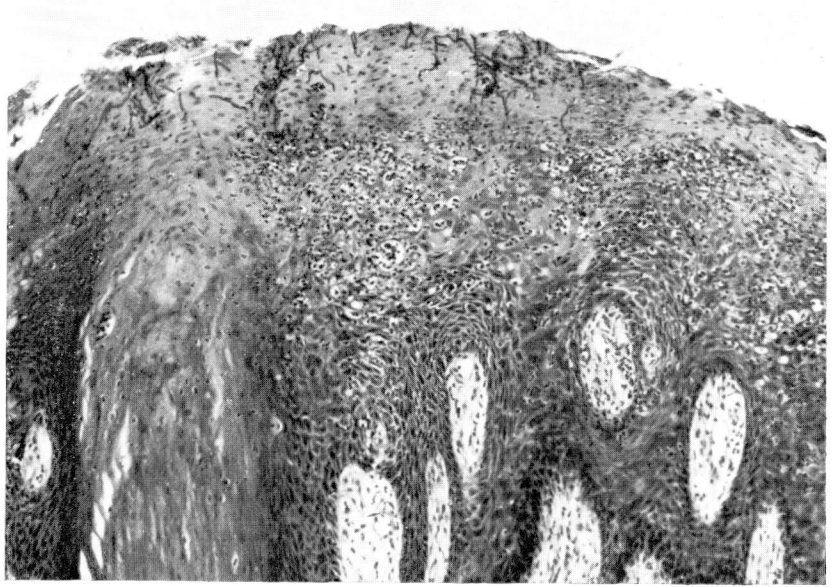

Fig. 11.7. Section of chronic hyperplastic candidosis involving tongue. Infiltrating candidal hyphae are orientated at right angles to surface and penetration is limited to superficial layers. Spaces containing polymorphs, i.e. deep to this zone. PAS ×50.

& Brayton (1964). When *C. albicans* was incubated in normal human serum, this factor reduced the number of colonies as estimated by the pour-plate technique by a factor of at least 10. Later Chilgren, Hong & Quie (1968) showed that the apparent reduction in number was due to clumping together of the organisms rather than killing them, and the factor was not an antibody. Serum from patients with chronic mucocutaneous candidosis contained a factor preventing this clumping of *C. albicans* by normal serum. This inhibitory factor was subsequently identified as candidal antibody.

POST-EXTRACTION CANDIDAL FUNGAEMIA AND DISSEMINATED CANDIDOSIS

Considering that the incidence of transient bacteraemia during dental treatment, especially extractions, can exceed 80% (Bender et al 1961), it is therefore surprising that it has not been possible to culture candida from any peripheral blood samples taken from 50 dental patients under-

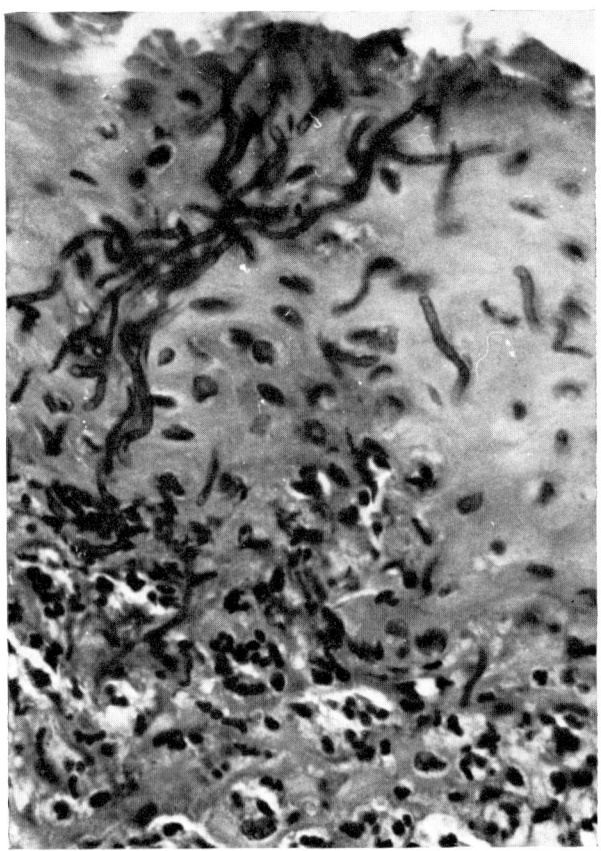

Fig. 11.8. Detail of same section as Fig. 11.7 to show candidal hyphae infiltrating superficial epithelium, deep to which are 'micro-abscesses' containing polymorphs. PAS ×100.

going treatment, mostly extractions (Lehner 1964b). Since then the increasing recognition of candidal endocarditis in patients after cardiac surgery, for example, indicates the necessity for repeating this study, taking care to neutralize the inhibitors such as transferrin or possibly using complement (and phagocyte) inhibitors such as sodium ethanol sulphonate. It is relevant that the polymorphs in normal whole blood are capable of ingesting 10^6 candidal organisms in 30 minutes *in vitro* (Louria *et al* 1964). It would be important to include patients with various types of oral candidosis in this study, that is with large oral candidal populations. Such information concerning the incidence of candidal fungaemia would be valuable in deciding whether or not to provide anticandidal prophylaxis (for example, minimal dose intravenous amphotericin B) as a prophylactic cover for dental extractions in patients at risk after cardiac surgery. From current knowledge this risk appears slight; venous catheters seem to be the main source of mycotic endocarditis post-operatively.

DISSEMINATED CANDIDOSIS

Disseminated candidosis, hitherto usually fatal, is a rare condition in which candidal colonization of almost every organ in the body can occur. This would suggest strongly that candidal fungaemia does occur, if rarely.

11:4 Immune Response to Candida

11:4:1 Humoral immunity

Agglutinating and precipitating antibodies present in human serum can be used to differentiate two antigenically distinct groups of *C. albicans*, A and B (Hasenclever, Mitchell & Loewe 1961). Candidal fluorescent antibody titres may be estimated in blood and saliva using an indirect technique (Lehner 1965, 1966b) (Fig. 11.9). Precipitating, agglutinating and fluorescent antibodies to candida and their immunoglobulin class IgG, IgM or IgA were determined in parallel from the same blood sample (Lehner *et al* 1972b). The precipitin activity resided in the IgG fraction and closely correlated with the IgG fluorescent antibody. The agglutinating and fluorescent antibody (Lehner 1970) belonged to the three major immunoglobulin classes IgG, IgM, IgA. In saliva the candidal antibody is IgA. In oral candidosis the candidal antibody titres of whole mixed saliva are elevated, immunoglobulin IgA predominating as it does in normal saliva.

ANTIGENIC STRUCTURE OF CANDIDA

Using the technique of immunoabsorption the same workers found that the agglutinating and fluorescent antibodies to candida are directed

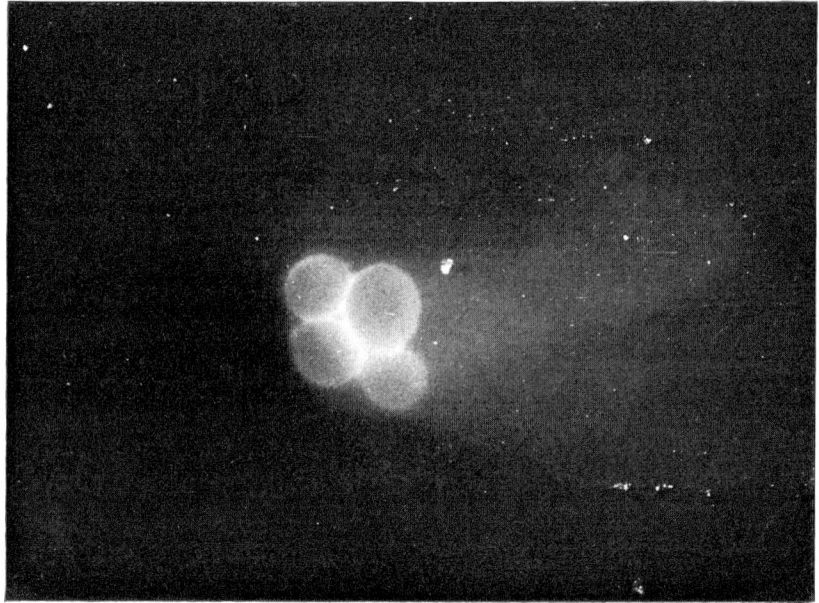

Fig. 11.9. Positive indirect immunofluorescent test for candidal antibody. To smear of *C. albicans*, serial dilutions of patient's serum added, and after washing, fluorescein-conjugated anti-human immunoglobulin added. Candidal antibody detected as continuous bright halo on yeast cell surface. ×320.

against the mannan (highly branched polysaccharide) determinant, which is probably a cell wall component. This was considered to be in line with Holborow & Loewi's (1967) finding that there is no evidence for delayed hypersensitivity developing towards polysaccharides.

Precipitating antibodies (precipitins) are directed to both mannan polysaccharide components and cytoplasmic protein antigens of candida (Stallybrass 1964).

THE DIAGNOSTIC USEFULNESS OF
CANDIDAL ANTIBODY ESTIMATIONS

Lehner (1965, 1966b) found higher fluorescent candidal antibody titres in saliva and serum from patients with oral candidosis than in carriers who in turn had higher titres from non-carriers. However, there is some overlap between these different groups at lower titres. In fact the confirmation of a clinical diagnosis of oral candidosis does not often present difficulties using a combination of culture for candida and epithelial smears.

In a chronic hyperplastic candidosis a PAS stain section of a biopsy will reveal candidal hyphae infiltrating the epithelium of the lesion.

However, deep-seated candidosis such as bronchopulmonary infections, mycotic endocarditis and disseminated candidosis generally represent vital diagnostic problems where conventional diagnostic methods seldom apply. Winner & Hurley (1964) concluded that the various types of antibodies used diagnostically were often confusing and contradictory. More recently precipitating antibodies (precipitins) to polysaccharide candida antigens were detected by Stallybrass (1964) only in disseminated candidosis but not in superficial candidosis. Taschdjian et al (1969) also found precipitins more reliable for diagnosing systemic candidosis than conventional methods. False positive precipitin tests do occur in cardiac surgery patients without mycotic endocarditis (Murray, Buckley & Turner, 1969). Lehner et al (1972b), however, found precipitins to whole candida extract in 6 of 10 patients with superficial candidosis only. The diagnostic value of serum precipitins to candidal protein antigen is not yet clear. Lehner et al (1972b) also described three cases where a raised fluorescent candidal antibody titre correctly identified a candidal endocarditis developing after cardiac surgery, whereas precipitating and agglutinating antibodies did not. By selecting a titre of 1/64 they suggested false positive rises in titre could be excluded.

In summary the practical value of estimating candidal antibodies for the clinical diagnosis of oral candidosis must be very limited at present. Furthermore the work to date on humoral immunity in oral candidosis usually makes unsupported assumptions with regard to candidal populations in the large bowel or vagina, for example. These extraoral sites may account for the scatter and overlap in antibody titres referred to previously.

PROTECTIVE OR DESTRUCTIVE ROLE OF
HUMORAL IMMUNITY IN ORAL CANDIDOSIS

The elevated titres of candidal antibodies in blood and saliva in chronic oral candidosis which may persist over many years suggest that no effective protection is given by these antibodies. Chilgren et al (1969) presented evidence of a salivary candidal IgA deficiency in two patients with mucocutaneous candidosis. Lehner et al (1972a) suggested similar salivary IgA deficiency in these patients, but this appeared to be relative in their study and not absolute. The penetration of salivary and serum IgA to candidal hyphae infiltrating the epithelium in chronic hyperplastic candidosis may be limited. In their intracellular position the organisms may be protected from the humoral–cellular defence mechanisms.

The impression is formed that humoral immunity is relatively unimportant in prevention or protection from oral candidosis and may merely reflect an increasing candidal antigenic stimulus. By contrast an intact cellular immunity seems important (q.v.). However these two components of the effector side of the immune response, cellular and humoral, can interact. For example, antigen–antibody complexes may be formed locally or systemically which can enhance lymphocyte transformation to candida antigen. Conversely antibodies may block immune receptors (Oppenheim 1969) The serum of one patient with muco-cutaneous candidosis inhibited lymphocyte transformation (Canales *et al* 1969).

11:4:2 Specific cellular immunity in candidosis

A state of delayed hypersensitivity mediated by specifically sensitized lymphocytes occurs in man in response to candida (Salvin 1963). Intradermal injection of a candidal extract has been used to measure this delayed hypersensitivity *in vivo* (e.g. Bencard antigen, Bencard, Brentford, Middlesex). Chilgren *et al* (1969) showed that a negative skin reaction can be rendered immediately positive in a subject by a transfusion of lymphocytes from a positive reactor, indicating the cell-mediated nature of the immune reaction.

Intradermal candidal skin tests have not been found satisfactory for diagnosis of occult candidosis; Lewis *et al* (1939) found 43% of patients with candidosis had negative skin tests whereas 46% of patients without the disease had a positive result. However, candida skin tests in our experience correlate quite satisfactorily with the *in vitro* measures of cell-mediated immunity to candida antigen. These *in vitro* markers of cell-mediated immunity include lymphocyte transformation as measured by 14 C- thymidine incorporation into DNA and lymphokine production, such as macrophage migration inhibitory factor. Cytotoxicity of specifically activated lymphocytes is another expression of cell-mediated immunity (CMI). Over 90% of the normal population can be shown to be sensitized to candida immunogen, a representative cytoplasmic antigen, by a combination of these *in vitro* and *in vivo* tests (Shannon *et al* 1966). Immune complexes of candida antigen–antibody are stated to enhance lymphocyte transformation more than the antigen alone by Lehner *et al* (1972a), without detailing their results.

DEFECTS OF CELLULAR IMMUNITY IN CANDIDOSIS

The realization of the importance of an intact cellular immunity in candidosis with fundamental implications for its treatment has been one of the exciting developments in this field in the past decade. A varying degree of impaired cell-mediated immunity has been described in patients with muco-cutaneous or chronic oral candidosis (Chilgren et al 1969). Groups of these patients have been investigated in more detail and certain common immune defects, predominantly cellular, have emerged. Excluding the patients with the rare immunodeficiency syndromes in which candidosis is often a minor feature, those patients with muco-cutaneous candidosis falling mainly into Group II of Wells et al (1972) will be considered. They show the following pattern of defect which can be ranked in severity type I (most severe) to type IV (no defect detectable) (Table 11.1) (Valdimarsson et al 1973).

Table 11.1. Tests of cell-mediated immunity in chronic muco-cutaneous candidosis with immune defects graded I (most severe) to IV (no defect detected) (+ = normal, − = absent). By courtesy Dr H. Valdimarsson and *Cellular Immunology*

	Lymphocyte transformation	Candida inhibitory factor present in serum	MIF	Skin testing for delayed hypersensitivity		
				Candida	PPD	DNCB
I	+	−	−	−	−	−
II	−	−	+	−	−	−
III	−	+	−	−	+	+
IV	+	−	+	+	+	+

Patients of *type I (greatest defect in CMI)* had no skin-delayed hypersensitivity to candida and other antigens. This cutaneous anergy correlated well with the impaired production of MIF by their lymphocytes in response to candida antigen (C_{ag}). However, these lymphocytes transformed normally in response to candida antigen.

Lesser CMI defects (types II, III) are found in less severely affected patients. In both types, lymphocyte transformation is impaired, but MIF production continued in type II. In type III this lymphocyte transformation (LTT) in autologous serum in response to candida antigen was inhibited by a specific inhibitory serum factor which did not inhibit LTT by PPD and/or DNCB. Cytotoxicity of the patient's lymphocytes was found to be normal.

It is most important to note that 10 out of 26 of the patients of Valdimarsson *et al* (1973) had no detectable immunological abnormality, although they had chronic candidosis. Valdimarsson arranged the immune defect into four types of progressive severity; Lehner *et al* (1972a) detected six grades. In fact these immune defects are likely to occupy a continuous spectrum and this could account for overlap between the clinico-genetic groups of muco-cutaneous candidosis defined by Wells *et al* (1972) (see below).

However, Lehner *et al* (1972a) were able to conclude that chronic oral candidosis, for example, has a more limited cellular defect (which they define) than candidosis affecting both mucosa and skin.

Primary or secondary nature of defects in cellular immunity

Whether the immune defects demonstrable in patients with chronic mucocutaneous or oral candidosis are primary and causative is actively under discussion. It is still possible in spite of the evidence cited above that the immunological hypo-responsiveness to candida antigen is a secondary acquired defect in at least some patients. This interpretation is favoured by case reports of Imperato *et al* (1968) and Paterson *et al* (1971), who described patients with muco-cutaneous candidosis with anergy to candida and other antigens. Following intravenous amphotericin B and in Imperato *et al*'s case parenteral iron also, marked clinical improvement occurred and with it a return towards normal delayed hypersensitivity *in vitro* and *in vivo*. The inference is that, exceptionally, a heavy load of candida antigen may depress the immune response. Immune defects detected in extensive candidosis should therefore be interpreted with caution, since they may be secondary and not play a primary role in the pathogenesis of candidosis.

Cellular–humoral interactions in candidosis

The ability of inhibitory factors in patients with muco-cutaneous candidosis to inhibit cell-mediated reactions *in vitro* suggests that interaction between cellular and humoral immunity does occur *in vitro* at least. The evidence that candidal antigen–antibody complexes can produce lymphocyte transformation more effectively than candidal antigen has already been referred to. The importance of cellular–humoral interactions *in vivo* has yet to be determined but is undoubtedly important.

MACROPHAGE FUNCTION IN CANDIDOSIS

Peritoneal macrophages from mice vaccinated with BCG have been shown to protect normal mice, if only temporarily, against virulent tubercle bacilli (Sever 1960). Macrophages from mice immunized with various extracts of candida could not retard the yeast's further growth once ingested by the macrophage. Macrophages from mice previously infected with candida could prevent intracellular growth of ingested candida and further dissemination of organism in the host. Serum factors did not affect this process (Winner 1972).

Macrophage function in man has been difficult to investigate up to now; its importance in candidosis is not yet evaluated. The fact that in muco-cutaneous candidosis MIF production can be lacking is important. It may mean that in chronic candidosis failure of MIF production results in macrophages failing to concentrate at a candidal invasion site. No amplification can then follow from lymphocyte–macrophage interaction which enhances the immune response (Unanue et al 1968). Alternatively the macrophages themselves may be abnormal, for example in defective antigen processing or poor release of their products. Investigation of macrophage function in candidosis is required.

IMMUNOLOGICAL REHABILITATION

Improvement or apparent complete cure in chronic muco-cutaneous candidosis has been recorded after transplantation of bone marrow (Buckley et al 1968) or thymus (Levy et al 1971), or transfusion of peripheral blood lymphocytes (Valdimarsson 1972a). All emphasize the importance of cellular immunity in muco-cutaneous candidosis and represent advances in the treatment of hitherto intractable skin and mucosal candidal infections. Graft-versus-host reactions are a hazard of such therapy unless donor and recipient are at least HLA compatible, i.e. are of matched histocompatibility antigens, and so there must be strong indications for such measures. Injections of transfer factor (Lawrence 1970), which is a cell-free extract of lymphocytes capable of restoration of defects of cellular immunity, has also been effective (Valdimarsson 1972b) in the treatment of muco-cutaneous candidosis. The effect of an injection lasts only a few months, however, and must be repeated. Its use carries no risk of graft-versus-host reaction.

11:5 Mechanisms of Pathogenesis

The mechanisms enabling candida to invade the tissues are not known. Some hierarchy in pathogenicity of the various species of candida can be established in man by experimental candidosis of the skin (Maibach *et al* 1962). In mice it has been assayed by estimating the lethal dose of organisms by intravenous injection. However, there is no *in vitro* test to identify whether a *C. albicans* organism from an oral swab is a pathogen in that patient or a commensal. Indeed although strains of *C. albicans* probably do vary in their ability to cause disease in man, little substantial proof exists that this is so. Instead studies in host–parasite relationship have concentrated on the variations in host factors which potentiate candidal infections (Beare *et al* 1972).

TOXICITY

Products of disintegrated candidal organisms do yield a potent (endo-) toxin capable of producing an acute pustular dermatitis under an occlusive dressing mimicking cutaneous candidosis. Maibach *et al* (1962) concluded that cutaneous candidosis must be classified as a primary irritant type contact dermatitis—no hypersensitive reactions needed to be invoked.

A comparatively long time ago, the pathogenicity of various strains of candida was studied to explain the puzzling way in which candida can behave as commensal or pathogen in a given host. In experimental candidosis in both animals (Hasenclever & Mitchell 1961) and man (Maibach *et al* 1962) the evidence is against significant variation in virulence between strains of *C. albicans*.

MORPHOLOGY AND PATHOGENICITY

The constant finding of the pseudohyphal form of candida in invasive candidosis (Gresham & Burns 1960; Kozinn & Taschdjian 1962) has prompted suggestions that the pseudohyphal form may be more pathogenic. Although hyphae may predominate in a tissue lesion of candidosis, yeasts are often also found in lesser numbers. These two forms and chlamydospores are all interconvertible. The evidence from *in vitro* experiments (Nickerson 1949, 1951; Nickerson & Chung 1954) is that whether candidal yeasts or hyphal form in any situation depends on the cultural conditions at that site. The predominance of the hyphal form in chronic hyperplastic candidosis lesions is probably just a product of the

Candidal Infection

intra-epithelial micro-environment (as referred to previously), rather than being evidence that this form is more pathogenic.

11:6 Classification of Oral Candidosis

In Tables 11.2–11.4, the valuable classification of Lehner (1966a) has been extended to incorporate more recent work by Higgs & Wells (1973, 1974). Muco-cutaneous candidosis is treated in some detail since the presenting complaint of almost every patient concerns his oral candidosis (Wells *et al* 1972). Associated skin or nail involvement may be relatively minor or asymptomatic.

11:7 Pathogenesis of Oral Mucosal Candidosis

The classification of oral candidosis, its clinical features and histopathology have been treated in standard texts and will not be enlarged upon here. Summarizing the concepts and evidence from previous sections, one may group the oral candidoses according to their pathogenesis as follows:
1   Defect in surface defence mechanisms:
(*a*) Carrier state.
(*b*) Acute pseudomembranous candidosis.
(*c*) Acute atrophic candidosis.
(*d*) Denture stomatitis.
2   Defect in immune mechanism, e.g. chronic hyperplastic candidosis.
(*a*) As part of muco-cutaneous candidosis.
(*b*) Confined to mouth.

11:7:1 Defect in surface defence mechanisms

The surface defence mechanisms against candidal infection of the oral mucosa are (i) surface film of saliva, (ii) oral microbial flora, (iii) oral epithelium, (iv) non-specific serum inhibitory factors, (v) non-specific phagocytosis—polymorphs are dealt with in section 11:4.
(*b*) & (*c*) Acute pseudomembranous and acute atrophic candidosis usually remain superficial infections confined to the mouth in persons with normal immunity to candida. Histologically the candidal hyphae and spores lie in an oedematous plaque on the surface of the oral epithelium,

Table 11.2. Classification of oral candidosis

GROUP I

Oral candidosis as part of muco-cutaneous candidosis occurring in patients with a profound immune deficiency syndrome. The patients usually die from other diseases and the muco-cutaneous candidosis remains superficial and not life-threatening

Syndrome	Inheritance	Distribution	Onset	Prognosis
Swiss type agammaglobulinaemia Hereditary thymic dysplasia Di George syndrome Chronic granulomatous disease of childhood	Congenital or genetically determined	Skin, oral mucosa, nails	Childhood	Usually die of associated disease in first few years of life

Table 11.3. Classification of oral candidosis

GROUP II

Chronic muco-cutaneous candidosis predominant feature but is not fatal, that is patients do not die from disseminated candidosis. Their candidosis remains superficial. In sub group 4 only the mouth is usually involved. All patients have chronic hyperplastic oral candidosis

Subgroup	Genetic group	Age onset	Type	Clinical features. Distribution of candidosis
1	Autosomal recessive	Early. Before 10 years of age	Familial chronic muco-cutaneous candidosis	Mouth, nails, skin. Other sites sometimes affected
2	Unknown	Early. Before 5 years of age	Diffuse chronic muco-cutaneous candidosis	Mouth, skin and nails extensively involved, often with granulomas. Eyes, pharynx and larynx. Susceptibility to other infection
3	Autosomal recessive	By second decade	Candida—endocrinopathy	Mouth, hypoparathyroidism, hypoadrenocorticism, hypothyroidism and diabetes mellitus
4	Probably not genetically determined	After age 30	Late onset	Chronic hyperplastic oral candidosis

Table 11.4. Classification of oral candidosis

GROUP III

This group includes common forms of oral candidosis, usually confined to the mouth. The candidosis is usually transient (1) and (2), easily treated and often a local or general predisposing factor is present

Subgroup			Age of onset	Genetic factors	Clinical features
1	Acute	Acute pseudomembranous candidosis (thrush)	Any age	None	Oral mucosa, but can rarely extend to oesophagus. Neonates and debilitated adults most commonly
2	Acute	Atrophic candidosis	Any age	None	Transient. Follows antibiotic therapy
3	Chronic	Chronic atrophic candidosis	Any age	None	'Denture sore mouth.' Occurs mostly exclusively on denture-bearing area of mucosa. Reversible on removing denture appliance

which is rapidly being shed. These infections, treated or untreated, tend to resolve in a matter of days in the normal person.
(*d*) *Chronic atrophic candidosis. Denture stomatitis.* See below.

11:7:2 Second stage. Defect in immune system—chronic hyperplastic candidosis (candidal leukoplakia)

(*a*) As part of muco-cutaneous candidosis.
(*b*) Confined to mouth—chronic oral candidosis.

If the immune system is defective the superficial candidosis resists therapy and becomes an established infiltrating persistent infection of the oral mucosa. The hyphae infiltrate the epithelium and are orientated at right angles to the surface but do not penetrate beyond the superficial glycogen-rich para-keratotic epithelial layer. There is an epithelial hyperplasia in response.

11:7:2a CHRONIC HYPERPLASTIC CANDIDOSIS AS PART OF MUCO-CUTANEOUS CANDIDOSIS

The distinguishing feature of this group is that they have chronic oral hyperplastic candidosis (syn.) candidal leukoplakia of early onset (Fig. 11.10), that is in the first 10 years of life. Histologically, they can be indistinguishable from candidal leukoplakia of late onset. Malignant change seems rare, but one such patient who developed oesophageal carcinoma at the relatively early age of 38 years has been reported (Kugelman *et al* 1963). In a few of these early onset muco-cutaneous candidosis patients successful immunological reconstitution of their immune defect has been achieved ridding them of their candidosis, as discussed in section 11:5. This would seem to argue forcibly that candida is directly causative in these types of candidal leukoplakias.

11:7:2b CHRONIC HYPERPLASTIC CANDIDOSIS— CONFINED TO MOUTH

These are all sporadic cases of late onset, i.e. over 35 years, commonly aged 50 or more (CHC). The main controversy over the causative role of candida in candida-infected white plaques or leukoplakias of the mouth concerns this group. As a clinical entity the group is ill defined, but this author excludes the 'denture stomatitis' included in this group by Higgs & Wells (1974) since (*a*) its onset can be at any age that a denture is first worn, (b) candidal colonization is predominantly of the fitting surface of the denture (Fig. 11.11) and not the mucosa (Davenport 1970). Nystatin

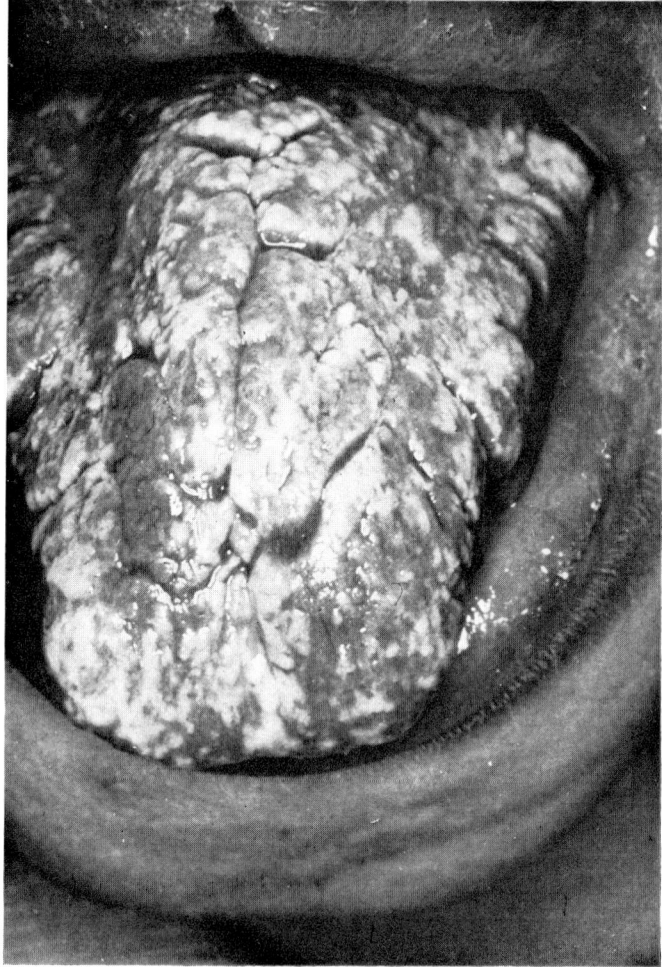

Fig. 11.10. Chronic muco-cutaneous candidosis. Chronic hyperplastic candidosis of tongue in boy in whom oral candidosis developed in the first few months of life. Eyes and nails also involved. Recurrent respiratory tract infections and bronchiectasis necessitating lobectomy of left lung.

therapy to eliminate the candidal organisms from the denture surface rather than the mucosa is successful (Budz-Jorgensen & Löe 1972; Douglas & Walker 1973). Denture-bearing mucosa exhibits an atrophic erythematous change and not a white patch due to epithelial hyperplasia. Dyskeratotic or malignant changes are never seen unlike candidal leukoplakia of late onset.

In a retrospective histological study of 138 leukoplakias Cawson (1966)

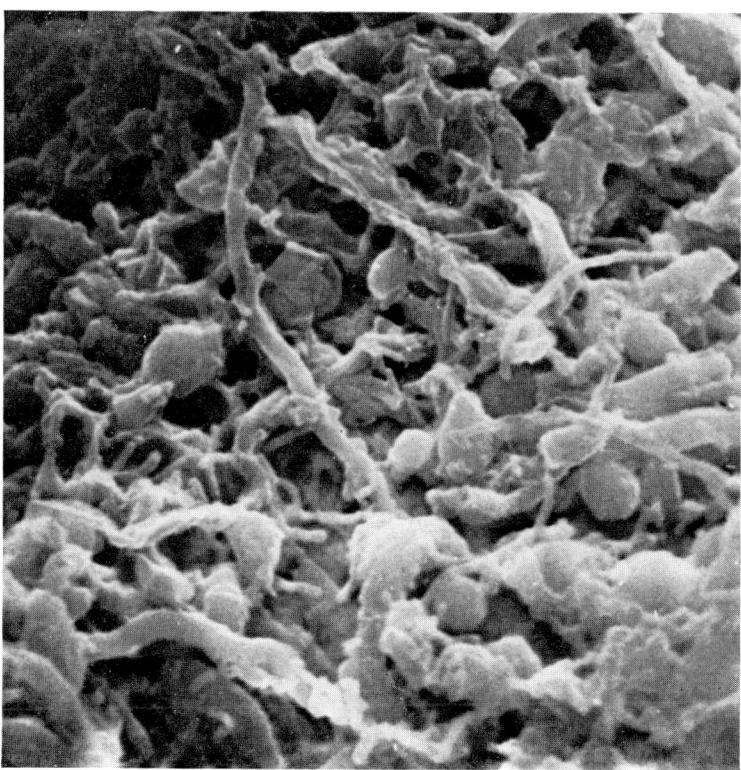

Fig. 11.11. Scanning electron photomicrograph of denture surface showing colonization of fitting surface. ×2500. (By courtesy of Dr W.H. Douglas and Mr R.T. Allison.)

diagnosed 15 as chronic hyperplastic candidosis and 6 of these had dyskeratosis. Of the 10 of these CHC which were followed up, 6 subsequently developed carcinoma compared with an overall incidence of malignant change in leukoplakias of about 2–4% in large series (Einhorn & Wersall 1967; Pindborg, Renstrup, Jolst & Roed-Petersen 1968). On the other hand McCarthy & Shklar (1964) held that in CHC candida was secondarily infecting a pre-existing pathological process such as leukoplakia. Certainly, in reviewing biopsy material from our department, candidal infiltration in oral carcinomas is very unusual.

The immune defect in chronic hyperplastic candidosis found by Lehner *et al* (1972) has been discussed above. To summarize, Oral Medicine clinics usually have been concerned with this group of patients presenting with chronic hyperplastic candidosis confined to the mouth. The role of candida is still undecided in this category of candidal leukoplakia, unlike the muco-cutaneous candidosis where candida appears to be causative. The production of this leukoplakia in man from a candidal culture is now the only unfulfilled Koch's postulate. Further work is necessary on the immunology of this CHC—late onset group—in a sufficiently large series with appropriate controls of other patients with non-candidal leukoplakias. It may well be that local defects in the epithelial barrier, for example secondary to iron deficiency, B complex or vitamin A deficiency, salivary factors, or macrophage function could be more important in determining the distribution of candidosis on skin and mucosa. Alternatively the fact that the candidal leukoplakias of late onset are the only group to have commonly malignant potential and never show any genetic basis, may indicate that they have entirely different pathogenesis. Research into the function and specificity of the cellular inflammatory infiltrate in the lamina propria of chronic hyperplastic candidosis in both early onset and late onset groups may help to separate the groups. The relative proportions of $T + B$ lymphocytes and macrophages in these lesions may soon be available if the rosetting techniques of Silveira *et al* (1972) and Edelson *et al* (1973) fulfil their promise. Immunoglobulin synthesis by the inflammatory infiltrate in chronic hyperplastic candidosis should now be studied to compare candidal leukoplakia, with and without epithelial atypia, with the oral lesions in the chronic muco-cutaneous candidosis by techniques described by Lai a Fat *et al* (1974). It is now possible to quantitate the number of immunoglobulin-bearing cells, their immunoglobulin class and semi-quantitatively estimate the amount of immunoglobulin synthesized in candidal lesions using these techniques. The specificity of this local immune response has not been established in the candidal lesions.

These investigations are not of purely scientific interest. Granted that candidal leukoplakias are premalignant lesions and that previous treatment has been ineffective, therapy to correct the immune defects of this group of patients will surely be tried following the favourable reports of treatment by restoration of immune competence in muco-cutaneous candidosis, which is by contrast not life threatening. The success or failure of such therapy would also shed light on the nature of candidal leukoplakia. Other methods, such as cryotherapy, with antifungal therapy are being evaluated.

11:8 References

ADAMS D. (1973) Saliva, the mucus barrier and the health of the oral mucosa. Ph.D. Thesis, University of Wales.
ADAMS D. (1974) Personal communication.
BAEHNER R.L. & NATHAN D.G. (1967) Leukocyte oxidase defective activity in chronic granulomatous disease. *Science*, **155**, 835-836.
BAEHNER R.L. & NATHAN D.G. (1968) Quantitative nitroblue tetrazolium test in chronic granulomatous disease. *New Engl. J. Med.*, **278**, 971-976.
BARLOW A.J.E. & ENGLISH M.P. (1973) In *Recent Advances in Dermatology*, No. 3, 33-68. Churchill Livingstone, Edinburgh and London.
BARTELS H.A. & BLECHMAN H. (1962) Survey of the yeast population in saliva and an evaluation of some procedures for identification of Candida albicans. *J. dent. Res.*, **41**, 1386.
BASU R., BASU N. & BANERJEE A.K. (1961) Incidence of Candida in the oral cavity. *Bull. Calcutta Sch. Trop. Med.*, **9**, 20.
BEARE J.M., GENTLES J.C. & MACKENZIE D.W.R. (1972) In ROOK A., WILKINSON D.S. & EBLING F.J.G. *Textbook of Dermatology*, 759. Blackwell, Oxford.
BENDER I.B., SELTZERS S., MELOFF G. & PREISMAN R.S. (1961) Conditions affecting sensitivity of techniques for detection of bacteraemia. *J. dent. Res.*, **40**, 951-959.
BLAND P.B., RAKOFF A.E. & PINCUS I.J. (1937) Experimental vaginal and cutaneous moniliasis: Clinical and laboratory study of certain monilias associated with vaginal, oral and cutaneous thrush. *Arch. Derm. Syph.* (Chic.), **36**, 760-780.
BODEY G.P. (1966) Fungal infections complicating acute leukaemia. *J. Chron. Dis.*, **15**, 667-687.
BRET J. & COUPE C.I. (1958) Vaginites et infection neo-natale. Etiologie des mycoses du nouveau-né. *Press med.*, **66**, 937-938.
BROMPTON HOSPITAL—MEDICAL RESEARCH COUNCIL COLLABORATIVE TRIAL (1974) Double blind trial comparing two dosage schedules of beclomethasone diprorionate aerosol in the treatment of chronic bronchial asthma. *Lancet*, **2**, 303-307.
BUCKLEY R.H., LUCAS Z.J., HATTLER B.G. JR, ZMIJEWSKI C.M. & AMOS D.B. (1968) Defective cellular immunity associated with chronic mucocutaneous moniliasis and recurrent staphylococcal botryomycosis: Immunological reconstitution by allogeneic bone marrow. *Clin. exp. Immunol.*, **3**, 153-169 Feb.
BUDTZ-JORGENSEN E., & LÖE H. (1972) Chlorhexidine as a denture disinfectant in the treatment of denture stomatitis. *Scand. J. dent. Res.*, **80**, 457-464.
CANALES L., MIDDLEMAS R.O. III, LOURO J.M. & SOUTH M.A. (1969) Immunological observations in chronic mucocutaneous candidiasis. *Lancet*, **2**, 567-571.
CAROLINE L., TASCHDJIAN C.L., KOZINN P.J. & SCHADE A.L. (1964) Reversal of serum fungistasis by addition of iron. *J. invest. Derm.*, **42**, (6), 415-419.
CATTERALL R.D. (1971) Influence of gestogenic contraceptive pills on vaginal candidosis. *Brit. J. Vener. Dis.*, **47**, 45-47.

CAWSON R.A. (1966) Chronic oral candidiasis and leukoplakia. *Oral Surg.*, **22**, 582–591.
CAWSON R.A. (1969) Leukoplakia and oral cancer. *Proc. R. Soc. Med.*, **62**, 610–615.
CAWSON R.A. & RAJASINGHAM K.C. (1972) Ultrastructural features of the invasive phase of Candida albicans. *Brit. J. Derm.*, **87**, 435–443.
CHILGREN R.A., HONG R. & QUIE P.G. (1968) Human serum interactions with Candida albicans. *J. Immunol.*, **101**, 128–132.
CHILGREN R.A., QUIE P.G., MEUWISSEN H., GOOD R.A. & HONG R. (1969) The cellular immune defect in chronic mucocutaneous candidiasis. *Lancet*, **1**, 1286–1288.
CRUICKSHANK R. & SHARMAN A. (1934) Biology of vagina in human subject; vaginal discharge of non-infective origin. *J. Obstet. gynec. Brit. Emp.*, **41**, 369–384.
DAVENPORT J.C. (1970) The oral distribution of Candida in denture stomatitis. *Brit. dent. J.*, **129**, 151–156.
DAVIS B.A. (1969) Vaginal moniliasis in private practice. *Obstet. & Gynec. (New York)*, **34**, 40–45.
DAVIS C.H. (1929) Trichomonas vaginalis; Donné, experimental and clinical observations. *Amer. J. Obstet. Gynec.*, **18**, 575–580.
DOUGLAS W.H. & WALKER D.M. (1973) Nystatin in denture liners—an alternative treatment of denture stomatitis. *Brit. dent. J.*, **135**, 55–59.
EDELSON R.L., SMITH R-W., FRANK M.M. & GREEN I. (1973) Identification of subpopulations of mononuclear cells in cutaneous infiltrates. I. Differentiation between B cells, T cells and histiocytes. *J. invest. Derm.*, **61**, 82–89.
EINHORN J. & WERSALL J. (1967) Incidence of oral carcinoma in patients with leukoplakia of the oral mucosa. *Cancer (Philad.)*, **20**, 2189–2193.
FOLB P.I. & TROUNCE J.R. (1970) Immunological aspects of Candida infection complicating steroid and immunosuppressive drug therapy. *Lancet*, **2**, 1112–1114.
GARDNER F.C. (1965) *Antibiot. News*, **21**, 1.
GRESHAM G.A. & BURNS M. (1960) Tissue invasion by Candida. In ROOK A. *Progress in the Biological Sciences in relation to Dermatology*, 174. Cambridge University Press, London.
HASENCLEVER H.F. & MITCHELL W.O. (1961) Antigenic studies of Candida. III. Comparative pathogenicity of Candida albicans Group A, Group B and Candida stellatoidea. *J. Bacteriol.*, **82**, 578–581.
HASENCLEVER H.F., MITCHELL W.O. & LOEWE J. (1961) Antigenic studies of Candida. II. Antigenic relationship of Candida albicans Group A and Group B to Candida stellatoidea and Candida tropicalis. *J. Bacteriol.*, **82**, 574–577.
HENRY B. & FAHLBERG W.J. (1960) The potentiating effect of hydrocortisone acetate and tetracycline on monilial infection in mice. *Antibiot. & Chemother. (Wash.)*, **10**, 114–120.
HESSELTINE H.C. (1955) Vulvitis, due to mycosis, atrophy and avitaminosis. *Am. Practit. & Digest Treat.*, **6**, 864–867.
HIGGS J.M. (1973) Chronic mucocutaneous candidiasis, iron deficiency and the effects of iron therapy. *Proc. R. Soc. Med.*, **66**, 802–804.
HIGGS J.M. & WELLS R.S. (1973) Chronic mucocutaneous candidiasis: new approaches to treatment. *Brit. J. Derm.*, **89**, 179–190.

HIGGS J.M. & WELLS R.S. (1974) Klassifizierung der chronischen muco-cutanen candidiasis mit Betrachtungen zum clinischen Bild und zur therapie. *Hautarzt*, **25,** 159-165.
HOLBOROW E.J. & LOEWI G. (1967) Delayed hypersensitivity and polysaccharide-containing antigens. *Brit. med. Bull.*, **23,** 72-75.
HUTTER R.V.P. & COLLINS H.S. (1962) The occurrence of opportunistic fungus infections in a cancer hospital. *Lab. Invest.*, **11,** 1035-1045.
IMPERATO P.J., BUCKLEY C.E. & CALLAWAY J.L. (1968) Candida granuloma: a clinical and immunological study. *Archs. Derm.*, **97,** 139-146.
JACKSON J.L. III & SPAIN W.T. (1968) Comparative study of combined and sequential antiovulatory therapy on vaginal monilialis. *Am. J. Obstet. Gynec.*, **101,** 1134-1135.
JACOBS A. (1960) The buccal mucosa in anaemia. *J. clin. Path.*, **13,** 463-468.
JACOBS A. (1961a) Carbohydrates and sulphur containing compounds in the anaemic buccal epithelium. *J. clin. Path.*, **14,** 610-614.
JACOBS A. (1961b) Iron containing enzymes in the buccal epithelium. *Lancet*, **2,** 1331-1333.
JONES C.P. & MARTIN D.S. (1938) Identification of yeast-like organisms isolated from vaginal tracts of pregnant and non-pregnant women. *Am. J. Obstet. Gynec.*, **35,** 98-106.
JONES J.H. & ADAMS D. (1970) Experimentally induced acute oral candidosis in the rat. *Brit. J. Derm.*, **83,** 670-673.
JOYNSON D.H.M., JACOBS A., WALKER D.M. & DOLBY A.E. (1972) Defect of cell-mediated immunity in patients with iron-deficiency anaemia. *Lancet*, **2,** 1058-1059.
KARNAKYK J. (1935) Trichomonas vaginalis and monilia albicans as causes of leukorrhoea. *South. M. J.*, **28,** 795-801.
KIRKPATRICK C.H., RICH R.R. & BENNETT J.E. (1971) Chronic mucocutaneous candidiasis: model building in cellular immunity. *Ann. intern. Med.*, **74,** 955-978.
KOZINN P.J., TASCHDJIAN C.L., WIENER H., DRAGUTSKY D. & MINSKY A. (1958) Neonatal candidiasis. *Pediat. Clin. N. Am.*, **5,** 803-815.
KOZINN P.J. & TASCHDJIAN C.L. (1962) Enteric candidiasis: diagnosis and clinical considerations. *Pediatrics*, **30,** 71-85.
KUGELMAN T.P., CRIPPS D.J. & HARRELL E.R. JR (1963) Candida granuloma with epidermophytosis. Report of a case and review of the literature. *Arch. Derm.*, **88,** 150-157.
LAI A FAT R.F.M., CORMANE R.H. & VAN FURTH R. (1974) An immunohisto-pathological study on the synthesis of immunoglobulins and complement in normal and pathological skin and adjacent mucous membranes. *Brit. J. Derm.*, **90,** 123-136.
LANNIGAN R. & MEYNELL M.J. (1959) Moniliasis in acute leukaemia. *J. clin. Path.*, **12,** 157-162.
LAWRENCE H.S. (1970) Transfer factor and cellular immune deficiency disease. *New Engl. J. Med.*, **283,** 411-419.
LEHNER T. (1964a) Oral thrush, or acute pseudomembranous candidiasis. *Oral Surg.*, **18,** 27-37.

LEHNER T. (1964b) Candidal fungaemia following extraction of teeth and its relationship to systemic candidiasis. *Brit. dent. J.*, **117,** 253–256.
LEHNER T. (1965) Immunofluorescent investigations of Candida albicans antibodies in human saliva. *Archs. oral Biol.*, **10,** 975–980.
LEHNER T. (1966a) Classification and clinico-pathological features of Candida infections in the mouth. In WINNER H.I. & HURLEY R. *Symposium on Candida Infections*, 119–137. Churchill-Livingstone, Edinburgh, 1966.
LEHNER T. (1966b) Immunofluorescent study of Candida albicans in candidiasis carriers and control. *J. Path. Bact.*, **91,** 97–104.
LEHNER T. (1967) Oral candidosis. *Dent. Pract.*, **17,** 209–216.
LEHNER T. (1970) Immunoglobulins in oral candidosis. *J. med. Microbiol.*, **3,** 475–481.
LEHNER T., BUCKLEY H.R. & MURRAY I.G. (1972b) The relationship between fluorescent agglutinating and precipitating antibodies to Candida albicans and their immunoglobulin classes. *J. clin. Path.*, **25,** 344–348.
LEHNER T. & WARD R.G. (1970) Iatrogenic oral candidosis. *Brit. J. Derm.*, **83,** 161–166.
LEHNER T., WILTON J.M. & IVANYI L. (1972a) Immunodeficiencies in chronic mucocutaneous candidosis. *Immunology*, **22,** 775–787.
LEHRER R.I. & CLINE M.J. (1969a) Interaction of Candida albicans with human leukocytes and serum. *J. Bacteriol.*, **98,** 996–1004.
LEHRER R.I. & CLINE M.J. (1969b) Leukocyte myeloperoxidase deficiency and disseminated candidiasis; the role of myeloperoxidase in resistance to Candida infection. *J. clin. Invest.*, **48,** 1478–1488.
LEVY R.L., HUANG S.W., BACH M.L., BACH F.H., HONG R., AMMANN A.J., BORTIN M. & KAY H.E.M. (1971) Thymic transplantation in a case of chronic mucocutaneous candidiasis. *Lancet*, **2,** 898–900.
LEWIS G.M., HOPPER M.E. & MONTGOMERY R.M. (1939) Infections of skin due to monilia albicans: I. Diagnostic value of intradermal testing with commercial extract of monilia albicans. *New York J. Med.*, **37,** 878.
LILIENTHAL B. (1950) Studies of flora of mouth, yeast like organism; some observations on their incidence in mouth. *Austral. J. exp. Biol. Med. Sci.*, **28,** 279–286.
LODDER J. (1970) *The yeasts. A taxonomic study*, 26. North Holland Publishing Co., Amsterdam and London.
LOURIA D.B. & BRAYTON R.G. (1964) A substance in blood lethal for Candida albicans. *Nature, Lond.*, **201,** 309.
LUDLAM G.B. & HENDERSON J.L. (1942) Neonatal thrush in a maternity hospital. *Lancet*, **1,** 64–70.
MCCARTHY P.L. & SHKLAR G. (1964) In *Diseases of the Oral Mucosa*. McGraw-Hill Book Co. Ltd, New York.
MACFARLANE T.W. & MASON D.K. (1973) The oral flora in Sjögren's syndrome (in the press).
MACKENZIE D.W.R. (1966) In WINNER H.I. & HURLEY R. *Symposium on Candida Infections*, 35. E. & S. Livingstone Ltd, Edinburgh and London.
MAIBACH H.K. & KLIGMAN A.M. (1962) The biology of experimental human cutaneous moniliasis (Candida albicans). *Arch. Derm. (Chic.)*, **85,** 233–257.

MANKOWSKI Z.T. (1955) The influence of hormonal conditions on experimental fungus infections. In *The Therapy of Fungus Diseases*, 90. Little, Brown & Co., Boston, Mass.

MANKOWSKI Z.T. & LITTLETON B.J. (1954) Action of cortisone and ACTH on experimental fungus infections. *Antibiot. & Chemother.*, **4**, 253–258.

MARTIN D.S. & JONES C.P. (1940) Further studies on the practical classification of the monilias. *J. Bact.*, **39**, 609–630.

MIZUNO S. (1961) *Studies on Candidiasis in Japan*, p. 19. Education Ministry of Japan.

MONTES L.F., CARTER R.E., MORELAND N. & CEBALLOS K. (1968) Generalised cutaneous candidiasis associated with diffuse myopathy and thymoma. *J. Am. Med. Ass.*, **204**, 351–354.

MONTES L.F. & WILBORN W.H. (1968) Ultrastructural features of host–parasite relationship in oral candidiasis. *J. Bact.*, **96**, 1349–1356.

MURRAY I.G., BUCKLEY H.R. & TURNER G.C. (1969) Serological evidence of Candida infection after open-heart surgery. *J. med. Microbiol.*, **2**, 463–469.

NICKERSON J.N. & RIJ N.J.W. (1949) The effect of sulfhydryl compounds, penicillin and cobalt on the cell division mechanism of yeasts. *Biochim. biophys. Acta*, **3**, 461–475.

NICKERSON W.J. (1949) Mechanism of cell division in pathogenic fungi. *Am. J. Bot.*, **36**, 812.

NICKERSON W.J. (1951) Physiological bases of morphogenesis in animal disease fungi. *Trans. N.Y. Acad. Sci.*, **13**, 140–145.

NICKERSON W.J. & CHUNG C.W. (1954) Genetic block in the cellular division. Mechanism of a morphological mutant of a yeast. *Am. J. Bot.*, **41**, 114–120.

NICKERSON W.J. & FALCONE G. (1956) Identification of protein disulfide reductase as a cellular division enzyme in yeasts. *Science*, **124**, 722–723.

OPPENHEIM J.J. (1969) Immunological relevance of antigen and antigen antibody complex induced lymphocyte transformation. *Ann. Allergy*, **27**, 305–315.

PATERSON P.Y., SEMO R., BLUMENSCHEIN G. & SWELSTAD J. (1971) Mucocutaneous candidiasis; anergy and a plasma inhibitor of cellular immunity: reversal after amphotericin B therapy. *Clin. exp. Immunol.*, **9**, 595–602.

PETERS R.B., BAHN A.N. & BARENS G. (1966) Candida albicans in the oral cavities of diabetics. *J. dent. Res.*, **45**, 771–777.

PILLAY V.K.G. et al (1968) Fungus infection in steroid-treated systemic lupus erythematosus. *J. Am. med. Ass.*, **205**, 261–265.

PINDBORG J.J. (1968) In *Atlas of Disease of the Oral Mucosa*. Munksgaard, Copenhagen.

PINDBORG J.J., RENSTRUP G., JOLST O. & ROED-PETERSEN B. (1968) Studies in oral leukoplakia: a preliminary report on the period prevalence of malignant transformation in leukoplakia based on a follow-up study of 248 patients. *J. Am. dent. Ass.*, **76**, 767–771.

PLASS E.D., HESSELTINE H.C. & BORTS I.H. (1931) Monilia vulvo-vaginitis. *Am. J. Obstet. Gynec.*, **21**, 320–334.

ROHATINER J.J. & GRIMBLE A. (1970) Genital candidiasis and oral contraceptives. *J. Obstet. Gynaec. Brit. Commonw.*, **77**, 1013–1015.

ROSE J.A. (1968) Aetiology of angular cheilosis: iron metabolism. *Brit. dent. J.*, **125**, 67–72.
ROTH F.J. JR, FRIEDMAN J. & SYVERTON J.T. (1957) Effects of roentgen radiation and cortisone on susceptibility of mice to Candida albicans. *J. Immunol.*, **78**, 122–127.
ROTH F.J. JR & GOLDSTEIN M.I. (1961) Inhibition of growth of pathogenic yeasts by human serum. *J. invest. Derm.*, **36**, 383–387.
RUSSELL C. & JONES J.H. (1973) Effects of oral inoculation of Candida albicans in tetracycline-treated rats. Colonisation of the mouths of germ-free and conventionalised rats with Candida albicans. *J. med. Microbiol.*, **6**, 275–280.
RUSSELL C., YOUNG C. & JONES J.H. (1974) Colonisation of the mouths of germ free and conventionalised rats with Candida albicans. *I.A.D.R. Abstract* (British Division), No. 73. Meeting Liverpool, April.
SALVIN S.B. (1963) Immunologic aspects of the mycoses. *Prog. Allergy.*, **7**, 213–331.
SEELIG M.S. (1966a) The role of antibiotics in the pathogenesis of Candida infections. *Am. J. Med.*, **40**, (6), 887–917.
SEELIG M.S. (1966b) Mechanisms by which antibiotics increase the incidence and severity of candidiasis and alter the immunological defences. *Bact. Rev.*, **30**, 442–459.
SEVER J.L. (1960) Passive transfer of resistance to tuberculosis through use of monocytes. *Proc. Soc. exp. Biol. Med.*, **103**, 326–329.
SHANNON D.C., JOHNSON G., ROSEN F.S. & AUSTEN K.F. (1966) Cellular reactivity to Candida albicans antigen. *New Engl. J. Med.*, **275**, 690–693.
SILVEIRA N.P., MENDES N.F. & TOLNAI M.E. (1972) Tissue localization of two populations of human lymphocytes distinguished by membrane receptors. *J. Immunol.*, **108**, 1456–1460.
STALLYBRASS F.C. (1964) Candida precipitins. *J. Path. Bact.*, **87**, 89–97.
TASCHDJIAN C.L. & KOZINN P.J. (1957) Laboratory and clinical studies on candidiasis in the new born infant. *J. Pediat.*, **50**, 426–433.
TASCHDJIAN C.L., BURCHALL J.J. & KOZINN P.J. (1960) Rapid identification of Candida albicans by filamentation on serum and serum substitutes. *Am. med. Ass. J. Dis. Child.*, **99**, 212–215.
TASCHDJIAN C.L., KOZINN P.J., FINK H., CRESTA M.B., CAROLINE L. & KANTROWITZ A.B. (1969) Postmortem studies of systemic candidiasis. I. Diagnostic validity of precipitin reaction and probable origin of sensitization to cytoplasmic candidal antigens. *Sabouraudia*, **7**, 110–117.
UNANUE E.R. & ASKONAS B.A. (1968) Persistence of immunogenicity of antigen after uptake by macrophages. *J. exp. Med.*, **127**, 915–926.
VALDIMARSSON H., MOSS P.D., HOLT P.J. & HOBBS J.R. (1972a) Treatment of chronic mucocutaneous candidiasis with leucocytes from HL-A compatible sibling. *Lancet*, **1**, 469–472.
VALDIMARSSON H., WOOD C.B., HOBBS J.R. et al (1972b) Immunological features in a case of chronic granulomatous candidiasis and its treatment with transfer factor. *Clin. exp. Immunol.*, **11**, 151–163.
VALDIMARSSON H., HIGGS J.M., WELLS R.S., YAMAMURA M., HOBBS J.R. & HOLT P.J.L. (1973) Immune abnormalities associated with chronic mucocutaneous candidiasis. *Cell. Immunol.*, **6**, 348–361.

WALKER D.M., DOLBY A.E., JOYNSON D.H.M. & JACOBS A. (1972) Candida and the immune defects in iron deficiency. *J. dent. Res.*, Suppl. to No. 5, **52**, 938–939.

WEINSTEIN L., GOLDFIELD M. & CHANG T.W. (1954) Infections occurring during chemotherapy; study of their frequency, type and predisposing factors. *New Engl. J. Med.*, **251**, 247–255.

WELLS R.S., HIGGS J.M., MACDONALD A., VALDIMARSSON H. & HOLT P.J.L. (1972) Familial chronic mucocutaneous candidiasis. *J. med. Genet.*, **9**, 302–310.

WILLIAMSON J.J. (1972a) Diurnal variation of Candida albicans counts in saliva. *Austr. dent. J.*, **17**, 54–60.

WILLIAMSON J.J. (1972b) A study of extent of variation in daily counts of Candida albicans in saliva. *Austr. dent. J.*, **17**, 1, 106–109.

WILSON T.E. & GOAZ P.W. (1959) The oral yeast–lacto bacillus relationship. *J. dent. Res.*, **38**, 1044–51.

WILSON T.E. & GOAZ P.W. (1960) The oral yeast–lacto bacillus relationship. III. Growth enhancement of lacto bacillus cagel by Candida albicans and saliva. *J. dent. Res.*, **39**, 365–371.

WINNER H.I. (1972) Studies on Candida. *Proc. R. Soc. Med.*, **65**, 433–436.

WINNER H.I. & HURLEY R. (1964) In *Candida Albicans*, 51. J. & A. Churchill Ltd, London.

WOODRUFF P.W. & HESSELTINE H.C. (1938) Relationship of oral thrush to vaginal mycosis and incidence of each. *Am. J. Obstet. Gynec.*, **36**, 467–471.

YOUNG G., KRASNER R.I., YUDKOFSKY P.L. (1956) Interactions of oral strains of Candida albicans and lactobacilli. *J. Bact.*, **72**, 525–529.

YOUNG G., RESCA H.G. & SULLIVAN M.T. (1951) The yeasts of the normal mouth and their relation to salivary acidity. *J. dent. Res.*, **30**, 426–430.

INDEX

Acanthosis nigricans 218
Acrodermatitis enteropathica 217
Actinomycosis, oral and facial lesions 377
Acute ulcerative gingivitis (acute necrotizing ulcerative gingivitis) 374
Addisons Disease, and oral mucosa 236
Adrenal cortex, and oral mucosa 236
Adreno-corticotrophic hormone, and oral mucosa 236
Age changes, skin, oral mucosa 88
  appendages and glands 92
  connective tissue 90
  epithelial turnover 90
  epithelium 88
Agranulocytosis, oral mucosa in 248
Amyloidosis, oral signs 223
Anaemia, oral mucosa in 247
Angular cheilitis
  in B_6 deficiency 260
  in folic acid deficiency 267
  in iron deficiency 272, 477
  in pellagra 258
  in riboflavin deficiency 254
Antibiotic stomatitis 373, 472
Antigens of oral mucosa and skin 439, Table 9:1
Aphthous ulceration
  Behçet's syndrome 431
  in B_{12} deficiency 265
  in folic acid deficiency 268
  herpetiform ulceration 430
  immunoglobulins in 178, 181, 427
  in iron deficiency 272
  Mikulicz's recurrent oral aphthae 427
  oestrogens and 245
  in relation to peptic ulceration 216
Appendages, oral mucosa and skin 5
Auto antigens 139, 198
  in periodontal disease 437
  in recurrent oral ulceration 427
Auto-immunity 425

Bacterial ecology of oral mucosa 371, 467
  effect of mutation 371
  infective transfer 372
Barrier function, of skin 2, 476
  of oral mucosa 2, 476
Basal cells 29, 88
Basal lamina 56
Basement membrane 56
  antibodies to in bullous pemphigoid 433
  functions 59
  origin 58
Behçet's syndrome 431
Benign mucous membrane pemphigoid 434
Blast cells 75
Blood coagulation, and saliva 126
Boeck's sarcoid (sarcoidosis)
  oral signs 222
Bullous pemphigoid
  immunofluorescence 181
  immunological aspects 435
Burkitt's lymphoma 398

Candidal leukoplakia 305, 340, 497
Candidosis, candida albicans as a commensal 467
  chronic hyperplastic 497
  classification 491, 492-494
  defence against 479
  disseminated 482
  immune response 483
  mucocutaneous, salivary immunoglobulins in 159
  pathogenesis 491
  predisposing factors 470
  and antibiotics 472
  and corticosteroids 472
  and immunosuppressive therapy 473
Candidosis, mucocutaneous, salivary immunoglobulins in 159

Carcinoma in situ 361
Cardiac disease, and oral bacteria 384, 482
Cell division 18
 age 25
 control 24
 diurnal rhythm 25
 endocrine status 26
 gingiva 23
 inflammation 27
 mitotic indices 22, Table 1:3
 phases 20
 progenitor compartment 19
 radioactive indices 22, Table 1:3
 rate 21
 stress 25
 sex 26
Cellular immunity 139, 421, 486, Fig. 3:2
Chalones 24
Chicken pox, oral mucosal lesions 392
Circulatory system, oral mucosa and skin 84
Clear cells 44, Table 1:4, 88
Collagen 77
 fibrilogenesis 78
 periodicity 78
 staining reactions 79
Complement 148
 in type II reaction 418
Connective tissue, oral mucosa and skin 64
Crohn's disease, and oral ulceration 217
Cystic fibrosis
 salivary immunoglobulins in 158
Cystinosis, oral signs 225
Cytotoxic factor
 (of lymphokine) 421
 in recurrent oral ulceration 429

Dermatomyositis, and neoplasia 218
 oral signs in 221
Dermis 11
Desmosome 31, Fig. 1:8
Desquamative gingivitis
 and hormones 245
 in lupoid hepatitis 219
Diabetes, and oral mucosa 240
 and candidosis 474

Elastic fibres 80
Eosinophilic granuloma, phase of, see histiocytosis, oral signs 228
Epithelial atypia 356
 computer analysis 359
 in diagnosis of premalignancy 357
 evaluation 359
 histological grading Fig. 7:1
Epithelium/connective tissue junction 55, 88
 epithelium interaction 60
Erythema multiforme
 and immune complex disease 420
 possible viral aetiology 404
Erythroplakia 342
Excretion, by skin 3
 by oral mucosa 4
Exfoliative cytology
 in diagnosis of premalignancy 362

Fluorescent antibody technique 164
 in candidosis 484
Focal epithelial hyperplasia 404
Fordyce spots 8, 115
 in measles 392
Fibroblasts 65, Fig. 1.18b

Giant cell arteritis
 oral signs and symptoms 222
Gingival sulcus
 immunoglobulins in fluid 159
 junctional epithelium 42
 permeability 42
Gingivitis
 experimental 189
 possible mechanisms in 198
Glossitis, in syphilis 382
 in folic acid deficiency 267
 in iron deficiency 272
 in pellagra 259
 in pernicious anaemia 264
 in riboflavin deficiency 257
 in vitamin B_6 deficiency 260
Glycogen 39, 88
Gonadotrophic hormones, and oral mucosa 235
Gonads, and oral mucosa 241
Granular layer 35, Fig. 1:11a
Granulocytes 76
Green's factor 121

Ground substance 82
　glycoproteins 83
　proteoglycans 83
　staining reactions 84
Growth hormone, and oral mucosa 235

Haemochromomatosis, oral signs 225
　and candidosis 481
Haemostasis 246
Hand, foot and mouth disease 401
Hand-Schüller-Christian disease
　oral signs 228
Hereditary angio-neurotic oedema 416
Herpangina 401
Herpes simplex infection
　and carcinoma of lip 303
　clinical features, diagnosis and treatment 393
　salivary immunoglobulins in recurrent 159
Herpes zoster infection and leukaemia 218
　oral lesions, diagnosis 397
Herpetiform ulceration 430
Histiocytes 67
Histiocytosis X, oral signs 228
Histocompatibility antigens and oral disease 440
Hemi-desmosomes 33, Fig. 1:16
Humoral immunity 139, 483, Fig. 3:2
Hurler's syndrome, oral signs 226
Hyperadrenocorticalism, and oral mucosa 238, 474
Hypersensitivity 138
　in acute ulcerative gingivitis 375
　in leprosy 380
　in syphilis 382
　in tuberculosis 378
　type I reaction 198, 415
　type II reaction 418
　type III reaction 419
　type IV reaction 421

IgA
　functions 193
　in gingiva 185
　in gingival crevice fluid 159
　in jaw cysts 161
　in major salivary glands 169
　in minor salivary glands 180
　in saliva 5, 152
　in sjögren's syndrome 158, 174, 181
　transfer Fig. 3:14
IgD
　in gingiva 190
IgE
　in gingiva 190
　in type I reaction 415
IgG
　in dental pulp 193
　functions 193
　in gingiva 185
　in gingival crevice fluid 159
　in jaw cysts 161
　in major salivary glands 168
　in pemphigus and pemphigoid 433, 435
　in saliva 152
　in Sjögren's syndrome 181
IgM
　functions 193
　in gingiva 185
　in gingival crevice fluid 159
　in jaw cysts 161
　in major salivary glands 169
　in Mikulicz's recurrent oral aphthae 427
　in saliva 154
　in Sjögren's syndrome 174
Immune complex disease
　and secondary syphilis 382
　and type III reaction 419
Immune response 137, Fig. 3:1
　to *Candida albicans* 479, 483
Immunodeficiency
　and candidosis 487, 495
　in recurrent herpes simplex infection 396
　in relation to gingivitis 191
Immunoglobulins 137
　classes and characteristics 144 Fig. 3:4
　detection 163
　in gingival crevice fluid 159
　in jaw cyst fluid 161
　in major salivary glands 168
　in minor salivary glands 180
　in oral mucosa 176

Immunoglobulins—*cont.*
  in palatine and pharyngeal tonsil 183
  quantitation 151
  in saliva 152
  in skin 176
  in sweat 181
Immunological injury 415
Infective endocarditis, and oral bacteria 384
Iron and oral mucosa
  deficiency 78, 272, 477
  oral cancer 327, 347

Junctional epithelium 42

Kelly-Paterson syndrome (Paterson-Brown Kelly syndrome) 327
Keratinization 11, 27, 89
  in epithelial atypia 357
  and folic acid 267
  in iron deficiency 274
  and vitamin A 254
Keratinized layer 38, 89
Keratinocytes 9
Keratohyaline granules 35, Fig. 1:11
Kopliks spots 392

Lactoferrin, in saliva 121
Lamina propria 11
Langerhans cells 45, Fig. 1:15, Table 1:4
Leprosy, oral involvement 381
Letterer-Siwe disease
  oral signs 228
Leukoplakia
  candidal 340, 497
  immunological aspects 353
  as premalignant lesion 337
  role in carcinoma 352
  simplex 338
  speckled 338
  stomatitis nicotina 341
  and syphilis 326
  verrucous 338
  and verrucous carcinoma 306
  and viral infection 354
Leucopaenia, oral mucosa in 248

Leukaemia, oral mucosa in 249
Lichen planus
  immunological aspects of oral 437
  oral cancer in 343
Lingual papillae
  in B_6 deficiency 260
  comparison with hair 8
  in folic acid deficiency 267
  in iron deficiency 272
  in pellagra 259
  in pernicious anaemia 264
  in riboflavin deficiency 257
Lipoid proteinosis (hyaloinosis cutis et mucosae)
  oral signs 226
Lymphocytes 72
  cytotoxicity 421
  in type IV reactions 421
Lymphokines 143, 421
Lysozyme, salivary 120, 150

Macrophage 67
  migration inhibition factor 423, 489, Fig. 9:5
Malabsorption, and oral ulceration 217
Mast cells 70, Fig. 1:20
Measles, oral mucosal lesions 392
Melanocyte 44
  in Addison's disease 236
  and B_{12} deficiency 264
  Table 1:4, Fig. 1:14
Melanocyte stimulating hormone and oral mucosa 238
Melanosome 54
Melkersson-Rosenthal syndrome 223
Membrane coating granule 33
Menopausal changes in oral mucosa 244, 471
Merkel cells 49, Table 1:4
Mikulicz's recurrent oral aphthae 427
Mitogenic factor
  of lymphokine 423
  in recurrent oral ulceration 428
Molluscum contagiosum, oral mucosal lesions 392
Muco-cutaneous junctions 13
Multiple mucosal neuroma syndrome 219
Mumps, oral mucosal lesions 393
Mycosis fungoides, oral signs 219

Nerves, oral mucosa and skin 86, 87

Oesophageal reflux 216
Oestrogens and oral mucosa 241
Oral mucosa, component tissues 5
  age changes 88, 244
  appendages 7
  circulatory system 84
  connective tissue 64
  effect of hormones 233, 471
  glycogen 39
  immunoglobulin of 176
  in iron deficiency 272
  lining 15, Fig. 1.5, Table 1.2
  masticatory 15, Fig. 1.5, Table 1.2
  metastases to 218
  nerves 86
  permeability 41, 123
  pigmentation 51, 238
  specialized 18
  stratification 9
Oral submucous fibrosis 346
Oxytalan fibres 82

Parathyroid glands, and oral mucosa 240, 474
Paterson-Brown Kelly syndrome (Kelly-Paterson syndrome) 327, 347
Pellagra, oral changes in 259
Pemphigus 432
  immunofluorescence 181
  peptic ulceration, in relation to aphthous ulceration 216
Pemphigoid, benign mucous membrane 434
  and malignant disease 218
  and uterine disease 218
Periodontitis
  possible mechanisms in 196, 436
Permeability, oral mucosa and skin 40, 122
Pernicious anaemia, oral mucosa in 264
Peutz-Jegher's syndrome 216
Phenylketonuria
  oral signs 227
Pigmentation, oral mucosa and skin 51
  in acanthosis nigricans 218

Pituitary gland, effect on oral mucosa 233
Plasma cells 76
  in dental pulp 193
  in gingiva 189
  in jaw cysts 193
  in salivary glands 175, 180
Plummer-Vinson syndrome (Paterson-Brown Kelly syndrome) 327, 347
Polyarteritis nodosa, classical and cutaneous, oral signs 221
Polycythaemia, oral mucosa in 248
Porphyria, oral signs 226
Pregnancy, changes in oral mucosa 244, 471
Premalignancy 336
  aetiology 352
  age significance 350
  diagnosis 356
  exfoliative cytology 362
  importance of site 348
  importance of size 351
  natural history 351
  premalignant lesions 337
  sex significance 350
Prickle cells 33 Fig. 1.9
Protein intake, and oral mucosa 252
Pyostomatitis vegetans 217

Reticulin fibres 79
Rheumatoid factor, in gingiva 190

Saliva
  antibacterial factors 120
  Australia antigen 403
  and blood coagulation 126
  and candidosis 128, 475
  composition 114
  factors affecting composition 116
  immunoglobulins 152
  mucosubstances 118
  reduced secretion 127
  in riboflavin deficiency 257
  secretion 114
  in Sjögren's syndrome 128, 450
  tests of function 129
  and vitamin C deficiency 271
Salivary glands 114
  in Sjögren's syndrome 450
Salivary mucins 118

Sarcoidosis (Boeck's sarcoid)
  oral signs 222
Scintiscanning, and salivation 129
Scleroderma (progressive systemic
  sclerosis), oral signs 220
Secretion, by skin 3
  by oral mucosa 4
Sensitivity, of skin 3
  of oral mucosa 3
Serum hepatitis and oral cavity
  402
Sialgrophy 129
Sjögren's syndrome
  diagnosis 451, 457
  general features 447
  IgA in labial glands 174
  and lymphoreticular neoplasia 459
  oral manifestations 450
  saliva 128
  salivary immunoglobulins 158, 174
  treatment 461
Skin component tissues 4, 11, Fig.
    1.1.
  age changes 88
  appendages 5
  circulatory system 84
  connective tissue 64
  glabrous and hairy 13, Table
    1.1.
  immunoglobulins of 178
  immunoglobulins of sweat 181
  nerves 86
  permeability 40, 122, 126
  pigmentation 51
  sebum 127
  stratification 9
  in temperature regulation 127
Small pox, oral mucosal lesions 392
Smoking, and oral mucosa 341, 321
Squamous cell carcinoma of lip 302
  aetiological factors 319
  incidence and mortality 306,
    Table 6:1, Figs. 6:1 – 6:6
  recording problems 318
  and smoking 321
Squamous cell carcinoma, of mouth
  aetiological factors 319
  alcohol 324
  buccal mucosa 305
  dental causes 328
  floor of mouth 304
  general clinical features 302

incidence and mortality 306,
  Table 6:1, Figs. 6:1 – 6:6
iron deficiency 327
leukoplakia in 337
occupation 314
palate 305
recording problems 318
sex incidence 309, Fig. 6:1
smoking 321
survival 314, Table 6:1
syphilis 326
tobacco chewing 323
tongue 303
verrucous 306
Squamous cell papilloma 344
Stomatitis nicotina 341
Stratification, oral mucosa and skin 9
Syphilis
  diagnosis 383
  oral cancer in 326, 345
  oral lesions in 381
Sytemic lupus erythematosus
  snd immune complexes 420
  aral signs 219
  ond viral disease 404

T + B cells 74, 139, 421
Thermal regulation, skin 3
  oral mucosa 3
Thiocyanate dependent factors
  in saliva 120
Thyroid gland, and oral mucosa 239
Tight junction 31, Fig. 1.8.
Tolerance, in immunity 141
Tongue
  in B_6 deficiency 260
  in folic acid deficiency 268
  in iron deficiency 274
  in pellagra 259
  in pernicious anaemia 264
  in riboflavin deficiency 257
  in syphilis 381
Tonofibrils 30
Tonofilaments 29
Tonsil, palatine + pharyngeal 183
Tuberculosis, oral mucosal lesions
  379

Ulcerative colitis, and oral ulceration
  217

Verrucous carcinoma of mouth 306
Verrucous leukoplakia of mouth 339
Viral disease
  aetiological mechanisms 387
  antiviral agents 390
  Australia antigen and serum hepatitis 401
  and Behçet's syndrome 432
  chicken pox 397
  classification 392
  cytomegalic inclusion disease 400
  diagnosis 388
  Epstein-Barr virus and Burkitt's lymphoma 398
  hand, foot and mouth disease 401
  herpangina 401
  and herpetiform ulceration 431
  herpes simplex 159, 303, 393
  infectious warts 400
  measles 392
  and Mikulicz's recurrent oral aphthae 430
  molluscum contagiosum 392
  mumps 393
  polyoma virus 400
  small pox 392
Vitamins and oral mucosa 254
  oral cancer and vitamin B deficiency 348
  vitamin C, and collagen 78

Warts, skin and oral mucosa 400
Wegener's granulomatosis, oral signs 221

Xanthomatosis
  oral signs 227